Third Edition

# *Clinical Skills Documentation Guide for*
# ATHLETIC TRAINING

**John M. Hauth, EdD, LAT, ATC**
Senior Director, Sports Medicine Relations
Center for Sports Medicine
Bethlehem, Pennsylvania

**Brian M. Gloyeske, MS, LAT, ATC**
St. Luke's University Health Network
Bethlehem, Pennsylvania

**Herbert K. Amato, DA, ATC**
Associate Vice Provost, University Programs
James Madison University
Harrisonburg, Virginia

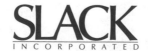
SLACK
INCORPORATED

www.Healio.com/books

ISBN: 978-1-61711-619-3

*Clinical Skills Documentation Guide for Athletic Training, Third Edition,* includes ancillary materials specifically available for faculty use. Please visit www.efacultylounge.com to obtain access.

The procedures and practices described in this publication should be implemented in a manner consistent with the professional standards set for the circumstances that apply in each specific situation. Every effort has been made to confirm the accuracy of the information presented and to correctly relate generally accepted practices. The authors, editors, and publisher cannot accept responsibility for errors or exclusions or for the outcome of the material presented herein. There is no expressed or implied warranty of this book or information imparted by it. Care has been taken to ensure that drug selection and dosages are in accordance with currently accepted/recommended practice. Off-label uses of drugs may be discussed. Due to continuing research, changes in government policy and regulations, and various effects of drug reactions and interactions, it is recommended that the reader carefully review all materials and literature provided for each drug, especially those that are new or not frequently used. Some drugs or devices in this publication have clearance for use in a restricted research setting by the Food and Drug and Administration or FDA. Each professional should determine the FDA status of any drug or device prior to use in their practice.

Any review or mention of specific companies or products is not intended as an endorsement by the author or publisher.

SLACK Incorporated uses a review process to evaluate submitted material. Prior to publication, educators or clinicians provide important feedback on the content that we publish. We welcome feedback on this work.

Published by:    SLACK Incorporated
                 6900 Grove Road
                 Thorofare, NJ 08086 USA
                 Telephone: 856-848-1000
                 Fax: 856-848-6091
                 www.Healio.com/books

Contact SLACK Incorporated for more information about other books in this field or about the availability of our books from distributors outside the United States.

Library of Congress Cataloging-in-Publication Data
Names: Amato, Herb, 1956- author. | Hauth, John M., author. | Gloyeske, Brian
  M., author.
Title: Clinical skills documentation guide for athletic training / John M.
  Hauth, Brian M. Gloyeske, Herbert K. Amato.
Description: Third edition. | Thorofare, NJ : Slack Incorporated, [2016] |
  Herb K. Amato's name appears first in the previous edition. | Includes
  bibliographical references.
Identifiers: LCCN 2016018679 (print) | LCCN 2016019196 (ebook) | ISBN
  9781617116193 (paperback) | ISBN 9781630913700 (Epub) | ISBN 9781630913717
  (Web)
Subjects: | MESH: Physical Education and Training | Sports Medicine--education
Classification: LCC RC1210 (print) | LCC RC1210 (ebook) | NLM QT 255 | DDC
  617.1/027--dc23
LC record available at https://lccn.loc.gov/2016018679

For permission to reprint material in another publication, contact SLACK Incorporated. Authorization to photocopy items for internal, personal, or academic use is granted by SLACK Incorporated provided that the appropriate fee is paid directly to Copyright Clearance Center. Prior to photocopying items, please contact the Copyright Clearance Center at 222 Rosewood Drive, Danvers, MA 01923 USA; phone: 978-750-8400; website: www.copyright.com; email: info@copyright.com

Printed in the United States of America.

Last digit is print number: 10 9 8 7 6 5 4 3 2 1

# *Dedication*

Twenty years from now you will be more disappointed by the things that you didn't do than by the ones you did do. So throw off the bowlines. Sail away from the safe harbor. Catch the trade winds in your sails. Explore. Dream. Discover.

—*Mark Twain*

To my parents, Ann and Marty Hauth, for providing me with every opportunity to explore, dream, and discover. And to all of my mentors from East Stroudsburg University and the University of Arizona, who inspired me to continually learn and serve this great profession. And to the many students, past and present, who keep me sharp and even more encouraged about the future than when I started 35 years ago. And finally, for Lynn, Amanda, Kendall, and Connor, who showed me what really matters.

—*John M. Hauth, EdD, LAT, ATC*

To my parents, Ken and Barb; I am reminded each day how grateful I am for your love, support, and encouragement. To my mentor and close friend John, who has shown me what passion, dedication, and hard work can achieve.

—*Brian M. Gloyeske, MS, LAT, ATC*

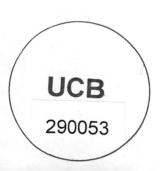

# Contents

---

*Clinical Skills Documentation Guide for Athletic Training, Third Edition,* includes ancillary materials specifically available for faculty use. Please visit www.efacultylounge.com to obtain access.

# *Acknowledgments*

We would like to extend our sincerest appreciation to Brien Cummings, Senior Acquisitions Editor, for his constant support and editorial and production assistance in the development of this manuscript. In addition, we are grateful to Dr. Herb Amato for providing us with the opportunity to work with him in revising and updating this Third Edition of *Clinical Skills Documentation Guide for Athletic Training*. Additionally, we would like to thank Dr. Keston Fulcher for sharing his expertise and significant contributions to the Program Assessment chapter.

The successful completion of this book could not have been accomplished without the hard work and determination of a number of individuals. We would like to especially thank Ashley N. Winkelspecht, MS, LAT, ATC, for her many contributions to this text. In addition, special thanks goes to Steven Malvasi, LAT, ATC; Melissa Frixione, LAT, ATC; and Kaitlyn Mohl, LAT, ATC, for their assistance in making this edition possible.

Lastly, we would like to extend our appreciation to Christy D. Hawkins, MS, ATC, and Steven L. Cole, MEd, ATC, CSCS, for the many contributions they made as coauthors on the first two editions.

# *About the Authors*

*John M. Hauth, EdD, LAT, ATC,* is the Senior Director of Sports Medicine Relationships at St. Luke's University Health Network in Bethlehem, Pennsylvania. Prior to his retirement from academe in January 2015, John held appointments as a tenured faculty member, program director, and associate dean at East Stroudsburg University of Pennsylvania. The University bestowed its highest faculty honor of Distinguished Professor in May 2010. He had been previously recognized for teaching excellence by the Pennsylvania Academy for the Profession of Teaching. He was inducted into the Pennsylvania Athletic Trainers Hall of Fame in 2009. He is an active member of the National Athletic Trainers' Association, having been presented the Association's Most Distinguished Athletic Trainer Award and Professional Development Excellence Award.

John has more than 30 years of experience as an athletic trainer, having worked in nearly every professional setting. He is licensed to practice as an athletic trainer by the PA State Board of Medicine and has been nationally certified (BOC) since 1983. He served as the Head Athletic Trainer for NCAA Division II Football and Division I Wrestling Teams from 1985 to 1997. John continues to work clinically as the Director of Athletic Training and Sports Medicine for the Lehigh Valley Steelhawks of the Professional Indoor Football League and at special events across the Lehigh Valley. In 2010, John served as a member of the Sports Medicine Staff for the XXI Central American and Caribbean Games in Mayaguez, Puerto Rico.

John resides in East Stroudsburg, Pennsylvania, with his wife, Lynn. They have three children: daughter Amanda and sons Kendall and Connor.

*Brian M. Gloyeske, MS, LAT, ATC,* is currently serving as an athletic trainer for St. Luke's University Health Network. He has practiced as a NATA BOC athletic trainer since 2010. Originally from Jackson Center, Ohio, Brian earned a Bachelor of Science in athletic training from the University of Toledo in 2010. He earned a Master of Science in athletic training from East Stroudsburg University of Pennsylvania in 2011, during which time he served as a graduate assistant athletic trainer at Warren Hills Regional High School, Washington, New Jersey.

Before joining St. Luke's full time in 2015, he spent 4 years as an instructor in a CAATE-accredited athletic training program at East Stroudsburg University of Pennsylvania. During his time at East Stroudsburg University, he worked clinically with collegiate dancers and the general population of the University and oversaw and provided athletic training services to the East Stroudsburg Youth Association Athletics. In addition, Brian served as the head athletic trainer for the Lehigh Valley Steelhawks of the Professional Indoor Football League. Currently, Brian serves as an assistant athletic trainer for Moravian College in Bethlehem, Pennsylvania, and coordinates the secondary school concussion education program for St. Luke's University Health Network.

*Herbert K. Amato, DA, ATC,* is currently an Associate Vice Provost at James Madison University (JMU) in Harrisonburg, Virginia. He was the Athletic Training Program Director at JMU from 1988 to 2006 and is still a tenured professor in the Department of Health Sciences. He has been actively involved in the education of athletic training students for 36 years at the university and high school levels. Dr. Amato has an extensive public speaking and consulting background and has published several articles in the areas of athletic training education and clinical practice. He was inducted into the Virginian Athletic Trainers' Hall of Fame in 2012. He is an active member of the National Athletic Trainers' Association, and has been presented the Association's 2003 Sayers "Bud" Miller Distinguished Educator Award.

Dr. Amato was the lead author for the first two editions of this book; however, he believes the now-lead authors are able to better portray the current needs of the profession. As co-founder of ACES, a preparatory workshop company that helps prepare students to take the BOC exam, Dr. Amato has stayed current in the field by developing assessment exams that mimic the blueprint of the national exam. In his current position, he is the chair of the Assessment Advisory Council and was the co-chair of the University-wide 10-year reaffirmation for The Southern Association of Colleges and Schools Commission on Colleges. This commission is the regional accreditor for JMU.

Dr. Amato is also active in service at the community, university, and national levels. He resides in Harrisonburg, Virginia, with his wife, Lori. They have three grown daughters, Casey, Lyndy, and Jessy.

## About the Contributing Author

*Keston H. Fulcher, PhD,* is an associate professor in the department of Graduate Psychology at James Madison University. Dr. Fulcher also is the Executive Director of the Center for Assessment and Research Studies. His research interests focus on integrating assessment with learning improvement, meta-assessment, and assessment and ethical reasoning.

# Introduction

The purpose of this book is to provide the athletic training educator, athletic training student, and athletic training preceptor with a reference that focuses on psychomotor competency, clinical skill, and ease of use. The Third Edition has been revised to include content that is reflective of contemporary athletic training practice and our commitment to developing a culture of evidence-based practice. In addition to changes in how the content is organized, the addition of a more global assessment (Clinical Integration Proficiencies) and the inclusion of skills from the Acute Care of Injuries and Illnesses and the Prevention and Health Promotion content areas represent the most significant updates to this text. These skills and global assessments represent, in part, the minimum requirements of an athletic training student's professional preparation. The purpose of the revisions is to cater to the three key elements in athletic training education: the student, preceptor, and educator.

Students can use this as a learning tool to take notes while being instructed in specific competencies. It can also be used as reference guide while practicing outside of class with the new, easy-to-follow, step-by-step instructions. As students learn these practical skills in the classroom or clinical environment, this book can be used as a guide to assist them as they work toward achieving entry-level competency. In addition, as the student reviews skills acquired throughout the clinical experience in preparation for cognitive skills, clinical decision making, and practical skills application integration of the BOC certification examination, he or she can use this book as a study guide and evaluation tool. Reference, supplies, and, wherever possible, statistical data are listed on each individual skill sheet. These skill sheets represent a comprehensive psychomotor checklist to determine skill competency.

The athletic training educator will also find this guide useful in ensuring clinical competence and learning over time. These faculty and clinical preceptor resources (Program Assessment chapter and Clinical Integration Proficiencies forms) can be easily accessed on SLACK Incorporated's website (www.efacultylounge.com). With clinical forms dedicated to specific competencies and the more global Clinical Integration Proficiencies, this guide will be of maximum benefit to program directors, clinical education coordinators, and course instructors. It is the authors' hope that the educators can best determine how to utilize the data gathered from these forms in a way that best fits their individual program. By employing the suggestions provided by Drs. Amato and Fulcher in the online chapter associated with this text, program directors can collect meaningful assessment data that can be used for program improvement and successful accreditation visits.

In many ways, it has been up to the athletic training preceptor to assess clinical competency with specific psychomotor skills. This task can seem daunting, and in many cases may take time away from being a focused health care provider. This guide has been specifically designed with this in mind. This edition includes global competency sheets designed to ensure that the student has real patient interactions and can be assessed on those patient interactions as a whole rather than individual skill competency (e.g., "student performance on the Lachman's test").

In addition, this book is formatted to record a student's progress in mastering psychomotor skills; therefore, it provides a history of that student's clinical strengths and weaknesses. With the help of the educator and preceptor, the student can create a plan and document his or her skill development over time.

# **I**

# **INTRODUCTION**

# 1

# CERTIFICATION OF ATHLETIC TRAINERS AND THE EVOLUTION OF PSYCHOMOTOR SKILL ASSESSMENT

In 1969, the National Athletic Trainers' Association (NATA) developed an examination to certify entry-level professionals. A function of any certification examination is to demonstrate to the public that an individual is qualified to perform specific duties without causing harm. The first certification examination included two sections: a written section and an oral/practical portion. The purpose of the written examination was to assess the candidate's basic knowledge of athletic training domains, and the goal of the oral/practical section of the examination was to test the clinical skills of the candidate.

Candidates were asked to complete skills in four categories (taping/wrapping, evaluation, rehabilitation, and emergency management) within a given time frame. Examples included asking the candidate to explain and demonstrate his or her ability to tape an ankle, evaluate a shoulder, construct a rehabilitation program for a medial collateral ligament sprain, and manage a patient suspected of heat illness. While the intent of the oral/practical section of the examination was to evaluate the clinical skills of a candidate, there was concern raised over the discrepancy between what was "explained" and what was "demonstrated."

Every 5 years, a *Role Delineation Study* (Job Analysis) is conducted as the initial step in updating the Board of Certification (BOC) examination. The first step in that process is for the BOC to appoint a committee of subject matter experts. Through their work, performance domains for the practice of athletic training are defined. These performance domains are further broken down into the tasks, knowledge areas, skills, and abilities expected of a professional in the field of athletic training.

The *Role Delineation Study, Third Edition*, published in 1995, led to changes in the design of the certification examination. The domain and task areas shifted from the previous study and resulted in a different configuration of the written examination. The oral/practical section of the examination was eliminated, giving rise to the practical examination wherein candidates were asked to demonstrate their ability to successfully perform specific psychomotor skills within a set time limit. Candidates were no longer expected to explain their actions during this section of the examination.

The BOC began to discuss options for transitioning the examination to a computer-based delivery method in 2002. By 2007, the BOC had transitioned to a fully integrated computer-based examination (CBE). On April 22, 2007, the final practical examinations were administered by the BOC to 1,229 candidates. After this date, the responsibility for ensuring psychomotor competency shifted to the individual athletic training programs accredited by the new specialized accreditor for athletic training—the Commission on

Hauth, J. M., Gloyeske, B. M., & Amato, H. K.
*Clinical Skills Documentation Guide for Athletic Training, Third Edition* (pp. 2-3).
© 2016 SLACK Incorporated.

Accreditation of Athletic Training Education (CAATE). It is critical that educational programs continue to stress the importance of psychomotor skill development through the use of regular practice and planned assessment activities. These skills reinforce essential knowledge critical for success of the BOC examination.

The current BOC examination is mapped to the *Role Delineation Study/Practice Analysis, Sixth Edition.* This edition and the associated BOC examination are valid from 2012-2017. This examination assesses the candidate's knowledge and skill in the following five domains:

1. Injury/Illness Prevention and Wellness Protection

2. Clinical Evaluation and Diagnosis

3. Immediate and Emergency Care

4. Treatment and Rehabilitation

5. Organizational and Professional Health and Well-Being

(Please note a *Role Delineation Study/Practice Analysis* will be coming out in March 2016 for review and will take effect April 2017.)

Successful performance on the certification examination for athletic trainers leads to BOC certification as an athletic trainer and the right to use the ATC credential.

While the current BOC examination does not require the satisfactory performance of psychomotor skills in a testing environment, athletic training programs must continue to emphasize the development and demonstration of these skills. The psychomotor skills are "physical activities associated with mental processes." Although the CBE evaluates athletic training students in areas pertaining to cognitive skills, clinical decision making, and practical skill application, it cannot assess the candidate's ability to physically perform skills on patients or simulated patients. Programs now bear the entire responsibility for demonstrating to the public that novice athletic trainers can perform essential athletic training skills without causing harm on completion of the accredited program.

It is critically important for examination candidates, program directors, clinical education coordinators, classroom faculty, and clinical preceptors to continually seek current guidelines of the format and requirements of the BOC examination. Readers should review the BOC website at www.bocatc.org for the latest information about certification eligibility and requirements. BOC certification is a prerequisite for licensure, certification, and/or registration in most states.

# 2

# HOW TO USE THIS BOOK

## Clinical Skill Assessments

Consistent with previous editions of the *Clinical Skills Documentation Guide for Athletic Training*, this new edition focuses primarily on skill assessment and the ability of students to demonstrate appropriate decision-making and clinical reasoning skills. The skill assessments are presented as specific outcomes, psychomotor skills, and integrated clinical proficiencies published in the Fifth Edition of NATA's *Athletic Training Education Competencies* (2011). Previous editions of this text were organized into general categories. The Third Edition is organized by the content area to which they have been assigned in the Competencies. This approach was adopted to assist program directors, clinical education coordinators, course instructors, students, and clinical preceptors to more easily organize and integrate its use in courses and clinical experiences.

The Third Edition has been revised to include content that is reflective of contemporary athletic training practice and our commitment to developing a culture of evidence-based practice. In addition to changes in how the content is organized, the addition of a more global assessment (Clinical Integration Proficiencies) and the inclusion of skills from the Acute Care of Injuries and Illnesses and the Prevention and Health Promotion content areas represent the most significant updates to this text. These skills and global assessments represent, in part, the minimum requirements of an athletic training student's professional preparation. The skills included in the Third Edition are used in the day-to-day duties of athletic training students as they progress toward mastery of the clinical skills and integrated clinical proficiencies.

To gain the most from *Clinical Skills Documentation Guide for Athletic Training, Third Edition*, athletic training students, course instructors, and clinical preceptors should review the following instructions on how to use the skill assessments (Figure 2-1). Each skill assessment is divided into four sections:

1. Introduction and instructions for specific clinical skills

2. Task form, score sheet, and evaluation box

3. Assessor comment section

4. Test environments—test information: statistics, references

The individual sections identified above will be further detailed and explained so that athletic training students, course instructors, and clinical preceptors can gain maximum benefits from this guide. In addition, program directors, clinical education coordinators, and program assessment officers can best determine how to utilize data from this guide in evaluating individual student ability, course and clinical education experiences, and overall program effectiveness.

Hauth, J. M., Gloyeske, B. M., & Amato, H. K.
*Clinical Skills Documentation Guide for Athletic Training, Third Edition* (pp. 4-7).
© 2016 SLACK Incorporated.

**Figure 2-1.** Sample Skill Assessment Sheet.

## Introduction and Instructions for Specific Clinical Skills

Figure 2-1 provides the reader with an example of a clinical skill assessment form. At the top of each skill assessment form, the reader can identify the section, region, and specific competency category. For example, in Figure 2-1A, the section is indicated in the title as the "Musculoskeletal System" and is followed by the region to which it has been assigned: "Region 6: Cervical Spine." The specific competency category, "Special Tests," is listed under the system and region classification.

The first section also includes the most basic information about the skill. For example, the NATA Education Competency designation by subject area ("CE") and skill ("21g") are listed at the top of the table. This is followed by the assigned BOC's Role Delineation Domain and Task numbers ("D2-0203"). The common name(s) of the clinical skill is included in the right side of the table at the top of the page ("Adson's Test"). Additional information in this section includes the supplies necessary or recommended for completing this task ("Supplies Needed: Table"). The final item in the first section is the instructions to be given to the student for each skill. These instructions include the name of the test or skill, what is intended to test for or rule out, and the time available for completing each task: "This problem allows you the opportunity to demonstrate an orthopedic test known as Adson's test to rule out thoracic outlet syndrome. You have 2 minutes to complete this task."

## The Score Sheet and Evaluation Box

The Score Sheet and Evaluation Box have been revised in the Third Edition to allow for the integration of the content areas and the knowledge and skills necessary to demonstrate mastery of the clinical skill. These components can be visualized in Figure 2-1B.

The top section of the task form and score sheet contains another listing of the name(s) for the clinical skill to be evaluated ("Adson's Test"). The right side for the score sheet and evaluation box includes three columns where the student and/or instructor can (1) identify where the skill is being tested ("Course or Site"), (2) identify who is assessing the skill ("Assessor"), and (3) identify the setting in which the skill is being assessed ("Environment"). The specific way in which the form is operationalized in programs will be decided on a local level. For instance, in column one, the skill could be assessed by a laboratory instructor of a specific course (430). Column two could show the assessment of the same skill in a clinical education course (489). Column three could outline how the skill was assessed in a capstone clinical experience by a preceptor.

The evaluation box includes the individual tasks required to execute the clinical skill. Blank circles, labeled Y or N (for yes or no), are provided next to each component of the clinical skill. A response of yes indicates that this component of the skill was completed correctly. A response of no indicates that the component of the skill listed was either performed incorrectly or not at all. The assessor should note that the evaluation of the individual elements is objective but also that they have not been weighted. Therefore, the final determination of pass or fail on any individual clinical skill should be viewed as somewhat subjective.

While a minimum threshold has been set for passing each skill, the authors stress that the level set for mastery is subjective and should be set by the clinical education coordinator and program director and shared with the clinical preceptors. This score is placed at the bottom of the Evaluation Box. For a student preparing for entry into the athletic training profession, the goal for mastery should be 100%. The student should strive to have as many yes circles checked as possible. In fact, these skill sheets have been organized to correspond with typical course/program structures and can be easily used for the instruction, practice, and testing of a skill. During instruction, students may use this score sheet, along with notes and other recommended references, to learn the skill.

Each of the skill sheets in this text were developed from several references. However, total agreement between these references does not occur in all cases, and for the purposes of this book, when disagreements occurred between the references, a decision was made based on the authors' knowledge and consultation with clinician-scholars. Course instructors and clinical preceptors are encouraged to use the discussion of such disagreements to enhance the learning experience for their students.

## The Assessor Comment Section

The Assessor Comment Section illustrated in Figure 2-1C provides the course instructor or clinical preceptor with a space to provide feedback and other important qualitative information to the student. Specific and measurable feedback can be shared with the student in an effort to help him or her better target his or her practice and skill review sessions. Instructors and clinical preceptors are encouraged to use this section because it can play a role in documenting improvement and attention to critical feedback.

## Test Environments/ Test Information (Statistics, References)

The bottom section of the clinical skill sheet includes information about the test environment (left side), as well as statistical information about the skill (if available) and the references used to review and construct the tasks included in the skill sheet (right side). This is illustrated in Figure 2-1D.

### TEST ENVIRONMENTS

The letters L, C, P, and A are used to indicate the environment in which the clinical skill assessment was completed. While the following information indicates the authors' definitions for using these environmental indicators, these indicators may be adjusted to fit the testing methods used in individual athletic training programs. This designation should be placed in the Evaluation Box in the space provided next to "Environment."

#### L: Laboratory/Classroom

The letter L indicates that the skill assessment occurred during a structured laboratory or classroom setting. These testing sessions may include formal laboratory tests, breakout sessions where testing occurs, or written examinations that include a practical test. This designation would most likely be used by a core or adjunct faculty member in a required athletic training program course.

### C: Clinical/Field Testing

The letter C indicates that the skill assessment occurred in the athletic training room, clinical setting, or on the athletic field or other venue where clinical experiences are completed. This assessment would have been completed by a clinical preceptor and is often based around the concept of the "teachable moment." Practice occurs during down time or structured clinical preceptor-student reviews in the clinical setting or during the observation of clinical skill when the student is performing it on a live (or simulated) patient.

### P: Practicum

The letter P indicates that the skill assessment occurred during scheduled testing at least one semester after the skill has been learned. This testing is included in practicum or proficiency courses, and there is often a clinical packet or online handbook/program associated with the completion of this clinical skill and the course. The practicum testing should not represent the first assessment of any given clinical skill.

### A: Assessment/Mock Exam

The letter A indicates that the skill assessment occurred during assessment testing. This type of testing evaluates the same clinical skill sets semester after semester or year to year. In isolation, this assessment provides the student with a picture of his or her strengths and weaknesses. Programmatically, this assessment provides the faculty, clinical education coordinator, and program director with data that can be used for assessment of program effectiveness and the need for curricular revision. Comparison between students in various cohorts can be completed to better understand variations in program outcomes. Please see the online chapter for additional information (www.efacultylounge.com).

## TEST INFORMATION

Valuable information about the clinical skill is included at the bottom of the sheet on the right hand side. To assist the student and clinical preceptor, the references and resources used to develop the skill sheet have been included. The reader is reminded that several resources were used in most cases and that there was disagreement in many cases. Students are encouraged to review the references to better understand the purpose of the skill, the structures under stress, the special considerations unique to the skill, and alternate or variations associated with the clinical skill/test.

Finally, the authors have added statistical information about the clinical skills/tests when available. In an effort to develop the student's commitment to evidence-based practice in athletic training, the authors encourage the students and clinical preceptors who use these sheets to investigate updates in this area and to use the clinical skills and therapeutic techniques based on the best research evidence whenever available.

# II

# PREVENTION AND HEALTH PROMOTION

# 3

# PREVENTION AND HEALTH PROMOTION

Hauth, J. M., Gloyeske, B. M., & Amato, H. K.
*Clinical Skills Documentation Guide for Athletic Training, Third Edition* (pp. 10-63).
© 2016 SLACK Incorporated.

## PREVENTION AND HEALTH PROMOTION
# KNOWLEDGE AND SKILLS

| *Prevention and Health Promotion* | | | | *Skill: Acquisition, Reinforcement, Proficiency* | | |
|---|---|---|---|---|---|---|
| **NATA EC 5th** | **BOC RD6** | **Equipment Maintenance** | **Page #** | | | |
| PHP-7 | D1-0104 | Cleaning of a Therapeutic Whirlpool | 13 | | | |
| PHP-7 | D3-0302 | Disposal of Contaminated Objects (Sharps, Saturated Gauze/Bandages) | 14 | | | |
| **EC 5th EC 5th** | **BOC RD6** | **Environmental Monitoring** | **Page #** | | | |
| PHP-13 | D1-0101, D1-0105 | Lightning Detection (Flash to Bang, 30/30 Rule, Lightning Detection Devices) | 15 | | | |
| PHP-13 | D1-0101, D1-0105 | Sling Psychrometer | 16 | | | |
| **NATA EC 5th** | **BOC RD6** | **Safe Weight Loss—Specific Gravity** | **Page #** | | | |
| PHP-14 | D1-0105 | Dipstick Urinalysis | 17 | | | |
| PHP-14 | D1-0105 | Refractometer (Specific Gravity) | 18 | | | |
| **NATA EC 5th** | **BOC RD6** | **General Medicine** | **Page #** | | | |
| PHP-15 | D3-0302 | Glucometer (Blood Glucose) | 19 | | | |
| PHP-17 | D3-0302 | Peak Flow Meter | 20 | | | |
| **NATA EC 5th** | **BOC RD6** | **Fitting Equipment** | **Page #** | | | |
| PHP-22 | D1-0103 | Fitting a Football Helmet | 21 | | | |
| PHP-22 | D1-0103 | Fitting Shoulder Pads | 22 | | | |
| PHP-22 | D1-0103 | Fitting a Mouthguard | 23 | | | |
| PHP-22 | D1-0103 | Fitting Running Shoes | 24 | | | |
| PHP-23 | D1-0103 | Fitting a Prophylactic Knee Brace | 25 | | | |
| PHP-23 | D1-0103 | Fitting a Prophylactic Ankle Brace | 26 | | | |
| **NATA EC 5th** | **BOC RD6** | **Taping and Wrapping** | **Page #** | | | |
| PHP-23 | D4-0403 | Taping to Prevent Hyperextension of the Elbow | 27 | | | |
| PHP-23 | D4-0403 | Taping – Shoulder Spica (Glenohumeral Joint) | 28 | | | |
| PHP-23 | D4-0403 | Shoulder Spica Elastic Wrap (Glenohumeral Joint) | 29 | | | |
| PHP-23 | D4-0403 | Wrist Taping Neutralization | 30 | | | |
| PHP-23 | D4-0403 | Thumb Spica Taping | 31 | | | |
| PHP-23 | D4-0403 | Collateral Interphalangeal Joint Taping | 32 | | | |
| PHP-23 | D4-0403 | Hip Spica Wrap (Hip Flexor) | 33 | | | |
| PHP-23 | D4-0403 | Hip Spica Wrap (Hip Adductor) | 34 | | | |
| PHP-23 | D4-0403 | Knee Compression Wrap | 35 | | | |
| PHP-23 | D4-0403 | Patellar Check Strap | 36 | | | |
| PHP-23 | D4-0403 | Closed Basketweave Ankle Taping | 37 | | | |
| PHP-23 | D4-0403 | Achilles Tendon Taping | 39 | | | |
| PHP-23 | D4-0403 | Longitudinal Arch Taping | 41 | | | |
| PHP-23 | D4-0403 | Great Toe Taping | 43 | | | |
| PHP-23 | D4-0403 | Taping Technique for Patellofemoral Stabilization | 45 | | | |
| PHP-23 | D4-0403 | Hardshell Doughnut Pad (Acromioclavicular Joint) | 46 | | | |

*(continued on the next page)*

## PREVENTION AND HEALTH PROMOTION
# KNOWLEDGE AND SKILLS

| NATA EC 5th | BOC RD6 | Fitness and Wellness | Page # | | | |
|---|---|---|---|---|---|---|
| PHP-28 | D1-0102 | Balance Test (Upper Extremity Proprioception) | 47 | | | |
| PHP-28 | D1-0102 | Endurance-Based Strength Test: % Fatigue (Middle Deltoid) | 48 | | | |
| PHP-28 | D1-0102 | Strength Test: % 1 x 10 Test (Shoulder Extensors) | 49 | | | |
| PHP-28 | D1-0102 | Strength Test: % 1 x 5 Test (Wrist Flexors) | 50 | | | |
| PHP-28 | D1-0102 | Strength Test: % Power Test (Triceps) | 51 | | | |
| PHP-28 | D1-0102 | Isokinetic Device Test (Shoulder) | 52 | | | |
| PHP-28 | D1-0102 | Functional Test (Upper Extremity) | 53 | | | |
| PHP-28 | D1-0102 | Balance Test (Lower Extremity Proprioception) | 54 | | | |
| PHP-28 | D1-0102 | Endurance-Based Strength Test: % Fatigue (Tibialis Anterior) | 55 | | | |
| PHP-28 | D1-0102 | Strength Test: % 1 x 10 Test (Hamstring) | 56 | | | |
| PHP-28 | D1-0102 | Strength Test: % 1 x 5 Test (Ankle Plantar Flexors) | 57 | | | |
| PHP-28 | D1-0102 | Strength Test: % Power Test (Knee Extensors) | 58 | | | |
| PHP-28 | D1-0102 | Isokinetic Device Test (Knee) | 59 | | | |
| PHP-28 | D1-0102 | Functional Test (Lower Extremity) | 60 | | | |
| NATA EC 5th | BOC RD6 | Weight Management and Body Composition | Page # | | | |
| PHP-44 | D1-0105 | Body Composition (Skinfold Caliper) | 62 | | | |
| PHP-44 | D1-0105 | Body Composition (Bioimpedance) | 63 | | | |

**PREVENTION AND HEALTH PROMOTION**
# EQUIPMENT MAINTENANCE

| NATA EC 5th | BOC RD6 | SKILL |
|---|---|---|
| PHP-7 | D1-0104 | Cleaning of a Therapeutic Whirlpool |

**Supplies Needed:** Whirlpool, appropriate protection equipment, cleaner, brush, water source

*This problem allows you the opportunity to demonstrate the appropriate* **cleaning of a therapeutic whirlpool.** *You have 5 minutes to complete this task.*

| Cleaning of a Therapeutic Whirlpool | Course or Site<br>Assessor<br>Environment | | | | | |
|---|---|---|---|---|---|---|
| | | Test 1 | | Test 2 | | Test 3 |
| **Equipment maintenance** | | Y | N | Y | N | Y | N |
| Uses appropriate personal protective attire | | ○ | ○ | ○ | ○ | ○ | ○ |
| Drains the whirlpool | | ○ | ○ | ○ | ○ | ○ | ○ |
| Refills the tub with hot water (120 degrees) | | ○ | ○ | ○ | ○ | ○ | ○ |
| Adds a cleaning agent (antibacterial/chlorine bleach) | | ○ | ○ | ○ | ○ | ○ | ○ |
| Turns on the turbine for 1 minute (water level must be sufficient not to cause damage) | | ○ | ○ | ○ | ○ | ○ | ○ |
| Drains the whirlpool | | ○ | ○ | ○ | ○ | ○ | ○ |
| Cleans the interior of the whirlpool (with a brush and appropriate cleaner) | | ○ | ○ | ○ | ○ | ○ | ○ |
| Rinses the interior of the whirlpool | | ○ | ○ | ○ | ○ | ○ | ○ |
| Cleans the exterior of the whirlpool (uses appropriate cleaner) | | ○ | ○ | ○ | ○ | ○ | ○ |
| **Total** | | __/9 | | __/9 | | __/9 | |
| **Must achieve >7 to pass this examination** | | Ⓟ | Ⓕ | Ⓟ | Ⓕ | Ⓟ | Ⓕ |

| Assessor:<br>Date: | Test 1 Comments: |
|---|---|
| Assessor:<br>Date: | Test 2 Comments: |
| Assessor:<br>Date: | Test 3 Comments: |

**TEST ENVIRONMENTS**
**L:** Laboratory/Classroom
**C:** Clinical/Field Testing
**P:** Practicum
**A:** Assessment/Mock Exam

**TEST INFORMATION**
**Test Statistics:** N/A
**Reference(s):** Starkey (2013)

PREVENTION AND HEALTH PROMOTION
# EQUIPMENT MAINTENANCE

| NATA EC 5th | BOC RD6 | SKILL |
|---|---|---|
| PHP-7 | D3-0302 | Disposal of Contaminated Objects (Sharps, Saturated Gauze/Bandages) |

**Supplies Needed:** Hazardous waste container, personal protective equipment

*This problem allows you the opportunity to demonstrate the appropriate* **disposal of contaminated objects**. *You have 3 minutes to complete this task.*

| Disposal of Contaminated Objects (Sharps, Saturated Gauze/Bandages) | Course or Site Assessor Environment ___ ___ ___ | | Test 1 | | Test 2 | | Test 3 | |
|---|---|---|---|---|---|---|---|---|
| **Tester's knowledge of procedures and regulations** | | | **Y** | **N** | **Y** | **N** | **Y** | **N** |
| Sharps are objects that can penetrate a worker's skin (needles, scalpels, broken glass) and, if contaminated, can infect worker with a blood-borne pathogen | | | ○ | ○ | ○ | ○ | ○ | ○ |
| Uses safer medical devices, safer procedures, and PPE (needles with built-in protection, uses the "scoop" technique to recap needles, uses tongs, uses gloves, uses facemask, uses goggles/glasses) | | | ○ | ○ | ○ | ○ | ○ | ○ |
| Prompt disposal of sharps into sharps container | | | ○ | ○ | ○ | ○ | ○ | ○ |
| Container must be in an assessable location where sharps are used, must be puncture-resistant, leak-proof, appropriately labeled/color-coded red, and must be closeable | | | ○ | ○ | ○ | ○ | ○ | ○ |
| Containers must be replaced routinely and not overfilled | | | ○ | ○ | ○ | ○ | ○ | ○ |
| When being replaced, must make sure container is closed, and it may need to be placed in a second container if being shipped | | | ○ | ○ | ○ | ○ | ○ | ○ |
| Contact OSHA for any emergencies or advice (800)-321-OSHA (6742) | | | ○ | ○ | ○ | ○ | ○ | ○ |
| | Total | | ___/7 | | ___/7 | | ___/7 | |
| | **Must achieve >5 to pass this examination** | | Ⓟ | Ⓕ | Ⓟ | Ⓕ | Ⓟ | Ⓕ |
| **Assessor:** **Date:** | **Test 1 Comments:** | | | | | | | |
| **Assessor:** **Date:** | **Test 2 Comments:** | | | | | | | |
| **Assessor:** **Date:** | **Test 3 Comments:** | | | | | | | |

**TEST ENVIRONMENTS**
**L:** Laboratory/Classroom
**C:** Clinical/Field Testing
**P:** Practicum
**A:** Assessment/Mock Exam

**TEST INFORMATION**
**Test Statistics:** N/A
**Reference(s):** OSHA Fact Sheet

# ENVIRONMENTAL MONITORING

| NATA EC 5th | BOC RD6 | SKILL |
|---|---|---|
| PHP-13 | D1-0101, D1-0105 | Lightning Detection (Flash to Bang, 30/30 Rule, Lightning Detection Devices) |

**Supplies Needed:** Lightning detection device, weather service application

*This problem allows you the opportunity to demonstrate the ability to appropriately use* **lightning detection.** *You have 3 minutes to complete this task.*

| Lightning Detection (Flash to Bang, 30/30 Rule, Lightning Detection Devices) | Course or Site Assessor Environment | | Test 1 | | Test 2 | | Test 3 | |
|---|---|---|---|---|---|---|---|---|
| **Guidelines of lightning safety** | | **Y** | **N** | **Y** | **N** | **Y** | **N** | |
| Establish a chain of command | | ○ | ○ | ○ | ○ | ○ | ○ | |
| Name a designated weather watcher | | ○ | ○ | ○ | ○ | ○ | ○ | |
| Have a means of subscribing to a weather-monitoring system (lightning detection device, weather service application) | | ○ | ○ | ○ | ○ | ○ | ○ | |
| Designate a safe shelter for each outdoor venue (building with four solid walls, electrical, plumbing) | | ○ | ○ | ○ | ○ | ○ | ○ | |
| Use the flash-to-bang count to determine when to go to safety (begin counting after seeing a lightning flash, stop when thunder is heard, and divide this count by 5 to determine the distance; e.g., 30 seconds = 6 miles away) | | ○ | ○ | ○ | ○ | ○ | ○ | |
| Once activity has been suspended, wait at least 30 minutes after the last lightning flash to resume activity | | ○ | ○ | ○ | ○ | ○ | ○ | |
| Avoid being at, or being near, the highest point in an open field | | ○ | ○ | ○ | ○ | ○ | ○ | |
| Know the lightning safety position (crouching on the ground, weight on balls of feet, feet together, head low, ears covered) | | ○ | ○ | ○ | ○ | ○ | ○ | |
| **Total** | | _____ /8 | | _____ /8 | | _____ /8 | | |
| **Must achieve >6 to pass this examination** | | Ⓟ | Ⓕ | Ⓟ | Ⓕ | Ⓟ | Ⓕ | |

| Assessor: Date: | Test 1 Comments: |
|---|---|
| Assessor: Date: | Test 2 Comments: |
| Assessor: Date: | Test 3 Comments: |

**TEST ENVIRONMENTS**
**L:** Laboratory/Classroom
**C:** Clinical/Field Testing
**P:** Practicum
**A:** Assessment/Mock Exam

**TEST INFORMATION**
**Test Statistics:** N/A
**Reference(s):** Gorse et al. (2010)

**PREVENTION AND HEALTH PROMOTION**
# ENVIRONMENTAL MONITORING

| NATA EC 5th | BOC RD6 | SKILL |
|---|---|---|
| PHP-13 | D1-0101, D1-0105 | Sling Psychrometer |

**Supplies Needed:** Sling psychrometer, water source, pencil/pen

*This problem allows you the opportunity to demonstrate the ability to appropriately use a **sling psychrometer**. You have 3 minutes to complete this task.*

| Sling Psychrometer | Course or Site<br>Assessor<br>Environment | | Test 1 | | Test 2 | | Test 3 | |
|---|---|---|---|---|---|---|---|---|
| | | | **Y** | **N** | **Y** | **N** | **Y** | **N** |
| **Tester places measuring device in appropriate position** | | | **Y** | **N** | **Y** | **N** | **Y** | **N** |
| Moistens wet bulb for 1 minute | | | ○ | ○ | ○ | ○ | ○ | ○ |
| Slides instrument into measuring position | | | ○ | ○ | ○ | ○ | ○ | ○ |
| **Tester follows correct procedures for using measuring device** | | | **Y** | **N** | **Y** | **N** | **Y** | **N** |
| Stands in the center of the practice area, out of shade | | | ○ | ○ | ○ | ○ | ○ | ○ |
| Twirls sling psychrometer for about 2 minutes | | | ○ | ○ | ○ | ○ | ○ | ○ |
| Slides instrument into proper position to read | | | ○ | ○ | ○ | ○ | ○ | ○ |
| **Tester uses measurement according to accepted guidelines** | | | **Y** | **N** | **Y** | **N** | **Y** | **N** |
| Records measurements correctly | | | ○ | ○ | ○ | ○ | ○ | ○ |
| | | **Total** | ___/6 | | ___/6 | | ___/6 | |
| | **Must achieve >4 to pass this examination** | | Ⓟ | Ⓕ | Ⓟ | Ⓕ | Ⓟ | Ⓕ |

| Assessor:<br>Date: | Test 1 Comments: |
|---|---|
| Assessor:<br>Date: | Test 2 Comments: |
| Assessor:<br>Date: | Test 3 Comments: |

**TEST ENVIRONMENTS**
**L:** Laboratory/Classroom
**C:** Clinical/Field Testing
**P:** Practicum
**A:** Assessment/Mock Exam

**TEST INFORMATION**
**Test Statistics:** N/A
**Reference(s):** Manufacturer's recommendations

**PREVENTION AND HEALTH PROMOTION**
## SAFE WEIGHT LOSS—SPECIFIC GRAVITY

| NATA EC 5th | BOC RD6 | SKILL |
|---|---|---|
| PHP-14 | D1-0105 | Dipstick Urinalysis |

**Supplies Needed:** Clean specimen cup, dipstick, manufacturer's recommendations for time and interpretation

*This problem allows you the opportunity to demonstrate the ability to appropriately perform a* **dipstick urinalysis***. You have 3 minutes to complete this task.*

| Dipstick Urinalysis | Course or Site Assessor Environment _____ _____ _____ | | Test 1 | | Test 2 | | Test 3 | |
|---|---|---|---|---|---|---|---|---|
| **Tester prepares patient** | | | **Y** | **N** | **Y** | **N** | **Y** | **N** |
| Gives instructions to the patient | | | ○ | ○ | ○ | ○ | ○ | ○ |
| **Tester performs test according to accepted guidelines** | | | **Y** | **N** | **Y** | **N** | **Y** | **N** |
| Instructs the patient to discard the initial flow of urine into a toilet bowl | | | ○ | ○ | ○ | ○ | ○ | ○ |
| Delivers a "clean catch" specimen (mid-stream) into a specimen cup | | | ○ | ○ | ○ | ○ | ○ | ○ |
| Collects about 2 ounces of urine | | | ○ | ○ | ○ | ○ | ○ | ○ |
| Immerses dipstick into the specimen cup for the recommended time (see manufacturer's recommendations) | | | ○ | ○ | ○ | ○ | ○ | ○ |
| Records the results (matches the proper colors of the dipstick to the values provided by the manufacturer) | | | ○ | ○ | ○ | ○ | ○ | ○ |
| | | Total | ___/6 | | ___/6 | | ___/6 | |
| | Must achieve >4 to pass this examination | | Ⓟ | Ⓕ | Ⓟ | Ⓕ | Ⓟ | Ⓕ |
| **Assessor:** **Date:** | **Test 1 Comments:** | | | | | | | |
| **Assessor:** **Date:** | **Test 2 Comments:** | | | | | | | |
| **Assessor:** **Date:** | **Test 3 Comments:** | | | | | | | |

**TEST ENVIRONMENTS**
**L:** Laboratory/Classroom
**C:** Clinical/Field Testing
**P:** Practicum
**A:** Assessment/Mock Exam

**TEST INFORMATION**
**Test Statistics:** N/A
**Reference(s):** Starkey & Brown (2015)

## PREVENTION AND HEALTH PROMOTION
# SAFE WEIGHT LOSS—SPECIFIC GRAVITY

| NATA EC 5th | BOC RD6 | SKILL |
|---|---|---|
| PHP-14 | D1-0105 | Refractometer (Specific Gravity) |

**Supplies Needed:** Refractometer, urine specimen, distilled water, cleaning cloth/tissue, gloves

*This problem allows you the opportunity to demonstrate the ability to appropriately use a* **refractometer** *to find* **specific gravity***. You have 3 minutes to complete this task.*

| Refractometer (Specific Gravity) | Course or Site Assessor Environment | | Test 1 | | Test 2 | | Test 3 | |
|---|---|---|---|---|---|---|---|---|
| **Tester/patient preparation** | | | Y | N | Y | N | Y | N |
| Instructs the patient to collect a urine sample | | | ○ | ○ | ○ | ○ | ○ | ○ |
| Calibrates the refractometer by placing distilled water on the glass as the sample and adjusting the scale to read 1.000 (should be done after every 10 samples or so) | | | ○ | ○ | ○ | ○ | ○ | ○ |
| **Tester performs test according to accepted guidelines** | | | Y | N | Y | N | Y | N |
| Opens the flap at the end of the refractometer | | | ○ | ○ | ○ | ○ | ○ | ○ |
| Cleans with distilled water and cloth | | | ○ | ○ | ○ | ○ | ○ | ○ |
| Places a drop of urine on the glass plate and closes the flap | | | ○ | ○ | ○ | ○ | ○ | ○ |
| Holds the refractometer up toward an area of natural light and looks through the eye piece | | | ○ | ○ | ○ | ○ | ○ | ○ |
| Reads the specific gravity level off the scale (a part of the contrast line crosses the scale) | | | ○ | ○ | ○ | ○ | ○ | ○ |
| Specific gravity ranges from 1.000 (equivalent to water) and 1.035 (very dehydrated), but usually a value of 1.020 or greater is considered dehydrated | | | ○ | ○ | ○ | ○ | ○ | ○ |
| Total | | | __/8 | | __/8 | | __/8 | |
| Must achieve >6 to pass this examination | | | Ⓟ | Ⓕ | Ⓟ | Ⓕ | Ⓟ | Ⓕ |

| Assessor: Date: | Test 1 Comments: |
|---|---|
| Assessor: Date: | Test 2 Comments: |
| Assessor: Date: | Test 3 Comments: |

**TEST ENVIRONMENTS**
**L:** Laboratory/Classroom
**C:** Clinical/Field Testing
**P:** Practicum
**A:** Assessment/Mock Exam

**TEST INFORMATION**
**Test Statistics:** N/A
**Reference(s):** Armstrong & Pandolf (1988)
Casa et al. (2000)

PREVENTION AND HEALTH PROMOTION
# GENERAL MEDICINE

| NATA EC 5th | BOC RD6 | SKILL |
|:---:|:---:|:---:|
| PHP-15 | D3-0302 | Glucometer (Blood Glucose) |

**Supplies Needed:** Glucometer, glucose testing strip, adhesive bandage, alcohol prep pad, gauze, lancet and/or lancing device

*This problem allows you the opportunity to demonstrate the ability to appropriately use a* **glucometer** *to find* **blood glucose***. You have 3 minutes to complete this task.*

| Glucometer (Blood Glucose) | Course or Site<br>Assessor<br>Environment | Test 1 | | Test 2 | | Test 3 | |
|:---|:---:|:---:|:---:|:---:|:---:|:---:|:---:|
| **Tester/patient preparation** | | **Y** | **N** | **Y** | **N** | **Y** | **N** |
| The tester washes hands | | ○ | ○ | ○ | ○ | ○ | ○ |
| The tester uses surgical gloves | | ○ | ○ | ○ | ○ | ○ | ○ |
| The tester preps the patient by cleaning the area with an alcohol wipe | | ○ | ○ | ○ | ○ | ○ | ○ |
| **Tester performs test according to accepted guidelines** | | **Y** | **N** | **Y** | **N** | **Y** | **N** |
| Performs a fingerstick using a lancet (wipes away the first drop of blood) | | ○ | ○ | ○ | ○ | ○ | ○ |
| Collects blood using a test strip | | ○ | ○ | ○ | ○ | ○ | ○ |
| Inserts test strip into a glucose meter | | ○ | ○ | ○ | ○ | ○ | ○ |
| **Tester/patient post instructions** | | **Y** | **N** | **Y** | **N** | **Y** | **N** |
| Wipes off the involved areas (patient/room) | | ○ | ○ | ○ | ○ | ○ | ○ |
| Ensures adequate hemostasis at the fingerstick site | | ○ | ○ | ○ | ○ | ○ | ○ |
| Properly disposes of surgical gloves, lancet, gauze, and capillary tube | | ○ | ○ | ○ | ○ | ○ | ○ |
| Cleans glucometer as needed and washes hands | | ○ | ○ | ○ | ○ | ○ | ○ |
| Records results | | ○ | ○ | ○ | ○ | ○ | ○ |
| | Total | ___/11 | | ___/11 | | ___/11 | |
| | Must achieve >8 to pass this examination | Ⓟ | Ⓕ | Ⓟ | Ⓕ | Ⓟ | Ⓕ |

| Assessor:<br>Date: | Test 1 Comments: |
|:---|:---|
| Assessor:<br>Date: | Test 2 Comments: |
| Assessor:<br>Date: | Test 3 Comments: |

**TEST ENVIRONMENTS**
**L:** Laboratory/Classroom
**C:** Clinical/Field Testing
**P:** Practicum
**A:** Assessment/Mock Exam

**TEST INFORMATION**
**Test Statistics:** N/A
**Reference(s):** Manufacturer's guidelines

# PREVENTION AND HEALTH PROMOTION
## GENERAL MEDICINE

| NATA EC 5th | BOC RD6 | SKILL |
|---|---|---|
| PHP-17 | D3-0302 | Peak Flow Meter |

**Supplies Needed:** Peak flow meter, mouthpiece

*This problem allows you the opportunity to demonstrate the ability to appropriately use a **peak flow meter**. You have 3 minutes to complete this task.*

| Peak Flow Meter | Course or Site / Assessor / Environment | | Test 1 | | Test 2 | | Test 3 | |
|---|---|---|---|---|---|---|---|---|
| | | | | | | | | |
| **Tester places patient in appropriate position** | | | Y | N | Y | N | Y | N |
| Standing | | | ○ | ○ | ○ | ○ | ○ | ○ |
| **Tester placed in proper position** | | | Y | N | Y | N | Y | N |
| Stands in front of the patient | | | ○ | ○ | ○ | ○ | ○ | ○ |
| **Tester performs test according to accepted guidelines** | | | Y | N | Y | N | Y | N |
| Resets the indicator of the peak flow meter by shaking or swinging the meter until the colored indicator is resting within the diamond shape near the mouthpiece | | | ○ | ○ | ○ | ○ | ○ | ○ |
| Instructs the patient to take as deep a breath as possible | | | ○ | ○ | ○ | ○ | ○ | ○ |
| Instructs the patient to put the mouthpiece in his/her mouth (sealing lips around it) | | | ○ | ○ | ○ | ○ | ○ | ○ |
| The patient should blow out as hard and as fast as possible | | | ○ | ○ | ○ | ○ | ○ | ○ |
| Read the peak expiratory flow as the number indicated by the new position of the colored indicator | | | ○ | ○ | ○ | ○ | ○ | ○ |
| **Total** | | | ___/7 | | ___/7 | | ___/7 | |
| **Must achieve >5 to pass this examination** | | | Ⓟ | Ⓕ | Ⓟ | Ⓕ | Ⓟ | Ⓕ |

| Assessor: Date: | Test 1 Comments: |
|---|---|
| Assessor: Date: | Test 2 Comments: |
| Assessor: Date: | Test 3 Comments: |

**TEST ENVIRONMENTS**
**L:** Laboratory/Classroom
**C:** Clinical/Field Testing
**P:** Practicum
**A:** Assessment/Mock Exam

**TEST INFORMATION**
**Test Statistics:** N/A
**Reference(s):** Gorse et al. (2010)

**PREVENTION AND HEALTH PROMOTION**
# FITTING EQUIPMENT

| NATA EC 5th | BOC RD6 | SKILL |
|---|---|---|
| PHP-22 | D1-0103 | Fitting a Football Helmet |

**Supplies Needed:** Football helmet

*This problem allows you the opportunity to demonstrate the ability to properly* **fit a football helmet**. *You have 5 minutes to complete this task.*

| Fitting a Football Helmet | Course or Site Assessor Environment | | Test 1 | | Test 2 | | Test 3 | |
|---|---|---|---|---|---|---|---|---|
| **Tester/patient preparation** | | **Y** | **N** | **Y** | **N** | **Y** | **N** | |
| Wets the patient's hair | | ○ | ○ | ○ | ○ | ○ | ○ | |
| **Tester properly fits helmet** | | **Y** | **N** | **Y** | **N** | **Y** | **N** | |
| Helmet should fit snugly around all parts of the patient's head (front, sides, crown), with no gaps between the cheek pads and face | | ○ | ○ | ○ | ○ | ○ | ○ | |
| Helmet should cover the base of the skull | | ○ | ○ | ○ | ○ | ○ | ○ | |
| Helmet should not come down over the eyes (should be 3/4 inch above the patient's eyebrows) | | ○ | ○ | ○ | ○ | ○ | ○ | |
| The ear holes should match | | ○ | ○ | ○ | ○ | ○ | ○ | |
| The facemask should be three finger-widths from the nose | | ○ | ○ | ○ | ○ | ○ | ○ | |
| Helmet should not shift when manual pressure is applied | | ○ | ○ | ○ | ○ | ○ | ○ | |
| Helmet should not recoil when axially loaded | | ○ | ○ | ○ | ○ | ○ | ○ | |
| The chin strap should be an equal distance from the center of the helmet | | ○ | ○ | ○ | ○ | ○ | ○ | |
| **Total** | | ___/9 | | ___/9 | | ___/9 | | |
| **Must achieve >7 to pass this examination** | | Ⓟ | Ⓕ | Ⓟ | Ⓕ | Ⓟ | Ⓕ | |

| Assessor:<br>Date: | Test 1 Comments: |
|---|---|
| Assessor:<br>Date: | Test 2 Comments: |
| Assessor:<br>Date: | Test 3 Comments: |

**TEST ENVIRONMENTS**
**L:** Laboratory/Classroom
**C:** Clinical/Field Testing
**P:** Practicum
**A:** Assessment/Mock Exam

**TEST INFORMATION**
**Test Statistics:** N/A
**Reference(s):** Prentice (2014)

PREVENTION AND HEALTH PROMOTION
# FITTING EQUIPMENT

| NATA EC 5th | BOC RD6 | SKILL |
|---|---|---|
| PHP-22 | D1-0103 | Fitting Shoulder Pads |

**Supplies Needed:** Football shoulder pads

*This problem allows you the opportunity to demonstrate the ability to properly* **fit shoulder pads***.*
*You have 5 minutes to complete this task.*

| Fitting Shoulder Pads | Course or Site Assessor Environment | | Test 1 | | Test 2 | | Test 3 | |
|---|---|---|---|---|---|---|---|---|
| **Tester/patient preparation** | | | Y | N | Y | N | Y | N |
| The width of the shoulder is measured to determine the proper size of pad | | | O | O | O | O | O | O |
| The inside shoulder pad should cover the tip of the shoulder in a direct line with the lateral aspect of the shoulder | | | O | O | O | O | O | O |
| The epaulets and cups should cover the deltoid muscle and allow movements required by the patient's position | | | O | O | O | O | O | O |
| The neck opening must allow the patient to raise the arms overhead without sliding | | | O | O | O | O | O | O |
| If a split-clavicle shoulder pad is used, the channel for the top of the shoulder must be in the proper position | | | O | O | O | O | O | O |
| Straps underneath the arm must hold the pads firmly in place but not be too constricting | | | O | O | O | O | O | O |
| After fitting, make sure the pads do not shift when the patient puts on the jersey | | | O | O | O | O | O | O |
| **Total** | | | ___/7 | | ___/7 | | ___/7 | |
| **Must achieve >5 to pass this examination** | | | P | F | P | F | P | F |
| Assessor: Date: | Test 1 Comments: | | | | | | | |
| Assessor: Date: | Test 2 Comments: | | | | | | | |
| Assessor: Date: | Test 3 Comments: | | | | | | | |

**TEST ENVIRONMENTS**
**L:** Laboratory/Classroom
**C:** Clinical/Field Testing
**P:** Practicum
**A:** Assessment/Mock Exam

**TEST INFORMATION**
**Test Statistics:** N/A
**Reference(s):** Prentice (2014)

**PREVENTION AND HEALTH PROMOTION**
# FITTING EQUIPMENT

| NATA EC 5th | BOC RD6 | SKILL |
|---|---|---|
| PHP-22 | D1-0103 | Fitting a Mouthguard |

**Supplies Needed:** Mouthguard, water source

*This problem allows you the opportunity to demonstrate the ability to properly* **fit a mouthguard.**
*You have 3 minutes to complete this task.*

| Fitting a Mouthguard | Course or Site Assessor Environment | | | | | | |
|---|---|---|---|---|---|---|---|
| | | Test 1 | | Test 2 | | Test 3 | |
| **Tester applies protective device** | | Y | N | Y | N | Y | N |
| Places mouthguard in hot water (about 170 degrees) until pliable (about 3 seconds) | | ○ | ○ | ○ | ○ | ○ | ○ |
| Removes mouthguard and shakes off excess water | | ○ | ○ | ○ | ○ | ○ | ○ |
| Asks the patient to bite down on back of mouthguard | | ○ | ○ | ○ | ○ | ○ | ○ |
| Asks the patient to apply suction to remove excess air | | ○ | ○ | ○ | ○ | ○ | ○ |
| Asks the patient to remove mouthguard once molded (about 1 minute) | | ○ | ○ | ○ | ○ | ○ | ○ |
| Asks the patient to run mouthguard under cold water for a few seconds | | ○ | ○ | ○ | ○ | ○ | ○ |
| | Total | ___/6 | | ___/6 | | ___/6 | |
| **Must achieve >4 to pass this examination** | | Ⓟ | Ⓕ | Ⓟ | Ⓕ | Ⓟ | Ⓕ |
| **Assessor:** **Date:** | **Test 1 Comments:** | | | | | | |
| **Assessor:** **Date:** | **Test 2 Comments:** | | | | | | |
| **Assessor:** **Date:** | **Test 3 Comments:** | | | | | | |

**TEST ENVIRONMENTS**
**L:** Laboratory/Classroom
**C:** Clinical/Field Testing
**P:** Practicum
**A:** Assessment/Mock Exam

**TEST INFORMATION**
**Test Statistics:** N/A
**Reference(s):** Prentice (2014)

## PREVENTION AND HEALTH PROMOTION
# FITTING EQUIPMENT

| NATA EC 5th | BOC RD6 | SKILL |
|---|---|---|
| PHP-22 | D1-0103 | Fitting Running Shoes |

**Supplies Needed:** Tape measure, shoes

*This problem allows you the opportunity to demonstrate the ability to properly* **fit running shoes**.
*You have 5 minutes to complete this task.*

| Fitting Running Shoes | Course or Site<br>Assessor<br>Environment | Test 1 | | Test 2 | | Test 3 | |
|---|---|---|---|---|---|---|---|
| **Tester/patient preparation** | | **Y** | **N** | **Y** | **N** | **Y** | **N** |
| Measures both feet (left may differ from right) | | O | O | O | O | O | O |
| Simulates the conditions in which the patient will be using them (socks, certain movements such as jumping or cutting) | | O | O | O | O | O | O |
| **Tester makes sure shoes fit properly** | | **Y** | **N** | **Y** | **N** | **Y** | **N** |
| Have a strong heel counter that fits well around foot | | O | O | O | O | O | O |
| Good flexibility in the forefoot where toes bend | | O | O | O | O | O | O |
| Midsole that is moderately soft but does not flatten out | | O | O | O | O | O | O |
| **Special considerations** | | **Y** | **N** | **Y** | **N** | **Y** | **N** |
| High heel for individuals with a tight Achilles tendon | | O | O | O | O | O | O |
| Considers the patient's arch (high arch, flat footed) | | O | O | O | O | O | O |
| Considers the "style" of the shoe that the patient needs (e.g., running, jumping) | | O | O | O | O | O | O |
| Evaluates for orthotics and inserts, if needed | | O | O | O | O | O | O |
| Makes sure the patient is wearing shoe properly and lacing it properly | | O | O | O | O | O | O |
| **Total** | | ____/10 | | ____/10 | | ____/10 | |
| **Must achieve >7 to pass this examination** | | (P) | (F) | (P) | (F) | (P) | (F) |

| Assessor:<br>Date: | Test 1 Comments: |
|---|---|
| Assessor:<br>Date: | Test 2 Comments: |
| Assessor:<br>Date: | Test 3 Comments: |

**TEST ENVIRONMENTS**
**L:** Laboratory/Classroom
**C:** Clinical/Field Testing
**P:** Practicum
**A:** Assessment/Mock Exam

**TEST INFORMATION**
**Test Statistics:** N/A
**Reference(s):** Prentice (2014)

## PREVENTION AND HEALTH PROMOTION
# FITTING EQUIPMENT

| NATA EC 5th | BOC RD6 | SKILL |
|---|---|---|
| PHP-23 | D1-0103 | Fitting a Prophylactic Knee Brace |

**Supplies Needed:** Prophylactic knee brace

*This problem allows you the opportunity to demonstrate the ability to properly* **fit a prophylactic knee brace***. You have 5 minutes to complete this task.*

| Fitting a Prophylactic Knee Brace | Course or Site / Assessor / Environment | | Test 1 | | Test 2 | | Test 3 | |
|---|---|---|---|---|---|---|---|---|
| | | **Y** | **N** | **Y** | **N** | **Y** | **N** | |
| **Tester places patient and limb in appropriate position** | | Y | N | Y | N | Y | N |
| Standing with knee flexed at 15 to 30 degrees | | ○ | ○ | ○ | ○ | ○ | ○ |
| **Tester applies protective device to injured area** | | Y | N | Y | N | Y | N |
| Selects appropriate-sized prophylactic brace | | ○ | ○ | ○ | ○ | ○ | ○ |
| Applies sleeve over knee joint | | ○ | ○ | ○ | ○ | ○ | ○ |
| **Tester evaluates protective device after application** | | Y | N | Y | N | Y | N |
| Has the patient actively flex the knee joint | | ○ | ○ | ○ | ○ | ○ | ○ |
| Ensures snug fit above and below the knee joint | | ○ | ○ | ○ | ○ | ○ | ○ |
| Ensures alignment of brace elements with joint line | | ○ | ○ | ○ | ○ | ○ | ○ |
| Confirms comfort and functionality of brace | | ○ | ○ | ○ | ○ | ○ | ○ |
| Total | | __/7 | | __/7 | | __/7 | |
| Must achieve >5 to pass this examination | | Ⓟ | Ⓕ | Ⓟ | Ⓕ | Ⓟ | Ⓕ |

| Assessor: Date: | Test 1 Comments: |
|---|---|
| Assessor: Date: | Test 2 Comments: |
| Assessor: Date: | Test 3 Comments: |

**TEST ENVIRONMENTS**
**L:** Laboratory/Classroom
**C:** Clinical/Field Testing
**P:** Practicum
**A:** Assessment/Mock Exam

**TEST INFORMATION**
**Test Statistics:** N/A
**Reference(s):** Prentice (2014)

## PREVENTION AND HEALTH PROMOTION
# FITTING EQUIPMENT

| NATA EC 5th | BOC RD6 | SKILL |
|---|---|---|
| PHP-23 | D1-0103 | Fitting a Prophylactic Ankle Brace |

**Supplies Needed:** Prophylactic ankle brace, chair

*This problem allows you the opportunity to demonstrate the ability to properly* **fit a prophylactic ankle brace**. *You have 5 minutes to complete this task.*

| Fitting a Prophylactic Ankle Brace | Course or Site Assessor Environment | | Test 1 | | Test 2 | | Test 3 | |
|---|---|---|---|---|---|---|---|---|
| | | | Y | N | Y | N | Y | N |
| **Tester places patient and limb in appropriate position** | | | Y | N | Y | N | Y | N |
| Seated or supine | | | O | O | O | O | O | O |
| Ankle in neutral position | | | O | O | O | O | O | O |
| **Tester applies protective device to injured area** | | | Y | N | Y | N | Y | N |
| Selects appropriate-sized prophylactic brace | | | O | O | O | O | O | O |
| Applies sleeve over ankle joint | | | O | O | O | O | O | O |
| Laces brace and tightens to comfort of the patient | | | O | O | O | O | O | O |
| **Tester evaluates protective device after application** | | | Y | N | Y | N | Y | N |
| Ensures snug fit above and below the ankle joint | | | O | O | O | O | O | O |
| Confirms comfort and functionality of brace | | | O | O | O | O | O | O |
| Has the patient actively dorsiflex and plantar flex the ankle joint | | | O | O | O | O | O | O |
| Has the patient actively invert and evert the ankle joint | | | O | O | O | O | O | O |
| Confirms that inversion is limited by brace | | | O | O | O | O | O | O |
| Performs assessment bilaterally (if needed) | | | O | O | O | O | O | O |
| **Total** | | | /11 | | /11 | | /11 | |
| **Must achieve >8 to pass this examination** | | | P | F | P | F | P | F |
| Assessor: Date: | Test 1 Comments: | | | | | | | |
| Assessor: Date: | Test 2 Comments: | | | | | | | |
| Assessor: Date: | Test 3 Comments: | | | | | | | |

**TEST ENVIRONMENTS**
**L:** Laboratory/Classroom
**C:** Clinical/Field Testing
**P:** Practicum
**A:** Assessment/Mock Exam

**TEST INFORMATION**
**Test Statistics:** N/A
**Reference(s):** Prentice (2014)

## PREVENTION AND HEALTH PROMOTION
# TAPING AND WRAPPING

| NATA EC 5th | BOC RD6 | SKILL |
|---|---|---|
| PHP-23 | D4-0403 | Taping to Prevent Hyperextension of the Elbow |

**Supplies Needed:** Pre-wrap, heel and lace pads, 2- or 3-inch elastic tape, adherent spray, skin lubricant, taping scissors

*This problem allows you the opportunity to demonstrate the ability to properly* **tape to prevent hyperextension of the elbow**. *You have 4 minutes to complete this task.*

| Taping to Prevent Hyperextension of the Elbow | Course or Site Assessor Environment | | Test 1 | | Test 2 | | Test 3 |
|---|---|---|---|---|---|---|---|
| **Proper position of patient** | | Y | N | Y | N | Y | N |
| Seated or standing | | O | O | O | O | O | O |
| Extends elbow to the point of pain (backs off approximately 10 to 20 degrees) | | O | O | O | O | O | O |
| Contracts biceps and forearm | | O | O | O | O | O | O |
| **Taping technique** | | Y | N | Y | N | Y | N |
| Applies tape adhesive/applies pre-wrap (optional) | | O | O | O | O | O | O |
| Applies anchor(s) to skin, mid-to-upper humerus | | O | O | O | O | O | O |
| Applies anchor(s) to skin, mid-to-lower forearm | | O | O | O | O | O | O |
| Applies (five strips) longitudinal fan to anterior surface of the elbow | | O | O | O | O | O | O |
| Reinforces the center of fan | | O | O | O | O | O | O |
| Secures fan at proximal and distal | | O | O | O | O | O | O |
| Applies closures to secure holes and loose ends | | O | O | O | O | O | O |
| Closes with stretch tape or elastic compression wrap | | O | O | O | O | O | O |
| **Support and neatness** | | Y | N | Y | N | Y | N |
| Prevents elbow from moving into full extension | | O | O | O | O | O | O |
| Maintains good circulation to the hand | | O | O | O | O | O | O |
| No holes and/or loose ends | | O | O | O | O | O | O |
| **Total** | | ____/14 | | ____/14 | | ____/14 | |
| **Must achieve >10 to pass this examination** | | Ⓟ | Ⓕ | Ⓟ | Ⓕ | Ⓟ | Ⓕ |

| Assessor:<br>Date: | Test 1 Comments: |
|---|---|
| Assessor:<br>Date: | Test 2 Comments: |
| Assessor:<br>Date: | Test 3 Comments: |

**TEST ENVIRONMENTS**
**L:** Laboratory/Classroom
**C:** Clinical/Field Testing
**P:** Practicum
**A:** Assessment/Mock Exam

**TEST INFORMATION**
**Test Statistics:** N/A
**Reference(s):** Beam (2012)

## PREVENTION AND HEALTH PROMOTION
# TAPING AND WRAPPING

| NATA EC 5th | BOC RD6 | SKILL |
|---|---|---|
| PHP-23 | D4-0403 | Taping – Shoulder Spica (Glenohumeral Joint) |

**Supplies Needed:** Elastic tape, 1.5-inch white tape, gauze/Band-Aids, pre-wrap

*This problem allows you the opportunity to demonstrate the ability to properly perform a* **shoulder spica taping** *of the* **glenohumeral joint** *to help prevent* **external rotation**. *You have 3 minutes to complete this task.*

| Taping – Shoulder Spica (Glenohumeral Joint) | Course or Site _____ _____ _____ Assessor _____ _____ _____ Environment _____ _____ _____ | | | | | |
|---|---|---|---|---|---|---|
| | | Test 1 | | Test 2 | | Test 3 |
| **Proper position of patient** | | Y | N | Y | N | Y | N |
| Standing | | ○ | ○ | ○ | ○ | ○ | ○ |
| Shoulder abducted with the hand resting on ASIS | | ○ | ○ | ○ | ○ | ○ | ○ |
| Contracts biceps | | ○ | ○ | ○ | ○ | ○ | ○ |
| For a male patient, cover both nipples with either gauze or Band-Aids; for a female patient, tape over a sports bra | | ○ | ○ | ○ | ○ | ○ | ○ |
| **Wrapping technique** | | Y | N | Y | N | Y | N |
| Taping begins at the distal portion of the affected upper arm and moves anteriorly, encircling the affected arm | | ○ | ○ | ○ | ○ | ○ | ○ |
| Continues the tape across the anterior portion of the chest, under the opposite arm, and across the back | | ○ | ○ | ○ | ○ | ○ | ○ |
| Repeats the above procedure a second time, ending by encircling the affected upper arm | | ○ | ○ | ○ | ○ | ○ | ○ |
| Places a check rein between the upper arm and the torso (optional) | | ○ | ○ | ○ | ○ | ○ | ○ |
| **Support and neatness** | | Y | N | Y | N | Y | N |
| Prevents abduction and external rotation of the shoulder | | ○ | ○ | ○ | ○ | ○ | ○ |
| Maintains good circulation to the hands and fingers | | ○ | ○ | ○ | ○ | ○ | ○ |
| No holes and/or loose ends | | ○ | ○ | ○ | ○ | ○ | ○ |
| Total | | ___/11 | | ___/11 | | ___/11 | |
| Must achieve >8 to pass this examination | | Ⓟ | Ⓕ | Ⓟ | Ⓕ | Ⓟ | Ⓕ |

| Assessor: Date: | Test 1 Comments: |
|---|---|
| Assessor: Date: | Test 2 Comments: |
| Assessor: Date: | Test 3 Comments: |

**TEST ENVIRONMENTS**
**L:** Laboratory/Classroom
**C:** Clinical/Field Testing
**P:** Practicum
**A:** Assessment/Mock Exam

**TEST INFORMATION**
**Test Statistics:** N/A
**Reference(s):** Beam (2012)

## PREVENTION AND HEALTH PROMOTION
# TAPING AND WRAPPING

| NATA EC 5th | BOC RD6 | SKILL |
| --- | --- | --- |
| PHP-23 | D4-0403 | Shoulder Spica Elastic Wrap (Glenohumeral Joint) |

**Supplies Needed:** Elastic wrap (6- or 4-inch double), 1.5-inch white tape

*This problem allows you the opportunity to demonstrate the ability to properly perform a* **shoulder spica elastic wrap** *in order to help support the* **glenohumeral joint**. *You have 3 minutes to complete this task.*

| Shoulder Spica Elastic Wrap (Glenohumeral Joint) | Course or Site Assessor Environment | | Test 1 | | Test 2 | | Test 3 | |
| --- | --- | --- | --- | --- | --- | --- | --- | --- |
| **Proper position of patient** | | **Y** | **N** | **Y** | **N** | **Y** | **N** | |
| Standing | | O | O | O | O | O | O | |
| Shoulder abducted with hand resting on low back (elbow flexed) | | O | O | O | O | O | O | |
| Contracts biceps | | O | O | O | O | O | O | |
| Instructs the patient to breathe deeply (expand the chest) | | O | O | O | O | O | O | |
| **Wrapping technique** | | **Y** | **N** | **Y** | **N** | **Y** | **N** | |
| Using 6-inch elastic (double) wrap, begins at the distal aspect of the biceps muscles and encircles the arm, pulling the wrap from posterior to anterior | | O | O | O | O | O | O | |
| Continues the wrap across the chest, beneath the opposite arm, around the back, and encircles the upper arm | | O | O | O | O | O | O | |
| Repeats the above steps until the wrap runs out | | O | O | O | O | O | O | |
| Secures the wrap with elastic tape and adhesive tape | | O | O | O | O | O | O | |
| **Support and neatness** | | **Y** | **N** | **Y** | **N** | **Y** | **N** | |
| Provides support to the GH joint | | O | O | O | O | O | O | |
| Maintains good circulation to the hand and fingers | | O | O | O | O | O | O | |
| No gaps and/or loose ends | | O | O | O | O | O | O | |
| **Total** | | ___ /11 | | ___ /11 | | ___ /11 | | |
| **Must achieve >8 to pass this examination** | | Ⓟ | Ⓕ | Ⓟ | Ⓕ | Ⓟ | Ⓕ | |

| Assessor: Date: | Test 1 Comments: |
| --- | --- |
| Assessor: Date: | Test 2 Comments: |
| Assessor: Date: | Test 3 Comments: |

**TEST ENVIRONMENTS**
**L:** Laboratory/Classroom
**C:** Clinical/Field Testing
**P:** Practicum
**A:** Assessment/Mock Exam

**TEST INFORMATION**
**Test Statistics:** N/A
**Reference(s):** Beam (2012)

PREVENTION AND HEALTH PROMOTION
# TAPING AND WRAPPING

| NATA EC 5th | BOC RD6 | SKILL |
|---|---|---|
| PHP-23 | D4-0403 | Wrist Taping Neutralization |

**Supplies Needed:** 1.5-inch white tape, pre-wrap

*This problem allows you the opportunity to demonstrate the ability to properly perform* **wrist taping neutralization** *to prevent* **flexion/extension of the wrist**. *You have 3 minutes to complete this task.*

| Wrist Taping Neutralization | Course or Site ___ ___ ___ <br> Assessor ___ ___ ___ <br> Environment ___ ___ ___ | | | | | |
|---|---|---|---|---|---|---|
| | | Test 1 | | Test 2 | | Test 3 |
| **Proper position of patient** | | Y | N | Y | N | Y | N |
| Seated or standing | | O | O | O | O | O | O |
| Wrist position into neutral (0 degrees) | | O | O | O | O | O | O |
| **Taping technique** | | Y | N | Y | N | Y | N |
| Applies 2-inch anchor around the distal forearm | | O | O | O | O | O | O |
| Applies a smaller anchor around the hand (second to fifth metacarpal heads) | | O | O | O | O | O | O |
| Constructs a fan of tape ("X"-shaped), extending from proximal to distal anchors (fan placed on dorsal side to prevent hyperflexion and on palmar side to prevent hyperextension) | | O | O | O | O | O | O |
| Applies a second set of anchors (holding the fan down) | | O | O | O | O | O | O |
| Applies tape in a figure-8 pattern, encircling the wrist | | O | O | O | O | O | O |
| Closes with a spiral taping from proximal anchor to distal anchor | | O | O | O | O | O | O |
| **Support and neatness** | | Y | N | Y | N | Y | N |
| Prevents hyperextension and flexion of the wrist (good support) | | O | O | O | O | O | O |
| Maintains good circulation to the hand and fingers | | O | O | O | O | O | O |
| No gaps and/or loose ends | | O | O | O | O | O | O |
| Total | | ___/11 | | ___/11 | | ___/11 | |
| Must achieve >8 to pass this examination | | P | F | P | F | P | F |

| Assessor:<br>Date: | Test 1 Comments: |
|---|---|
| Assessor:<br>Date: | Test 2 Comments: |
| Assessor:<br>Date: | Test 3 Comments: |

**TEST ENVIRONMENTS**
**L:** Laboratory/Classroom
**C:** Clinical/Field Testing
**P:** Practicum
**A:** Assessment/Mock Exam

**TEST INFORMATION**
**Test Statistics:** N/A
**Reference(s):** Beam (2012)

PREVENTION AND HEALTH PROMOTION
# TAPING AND WRAPPING

| NATA EC 5th | BOC RD6 | SKILL |
|---|---|---|
| PHP-23 | D4-0403 | Thumb Spica Taping |

**Supplies Needed:** 1-inch white tape or elastic tape, 1.5-inch white tape, pre-wrap (optional)

*This problem allows you the opportunity to demonstrate the ability to properly perform a* **thumb spica taping** *in order to support the* **first metacarpophalangeal joint** *of the hand. You have 3 minutes to complete this task.*

| Thumb Spica Taping | Course or Site Assessor Environment | Test 1 | | Test 2 | | Test 3 | |
|---|---|---|---|---|---|---|---|
| | | Y | N | Y | N | Y | N |
| **Proper position of patient** | | Y | N | Y | N | Y | N |
| Standing or seated | | ○ | ○ | ○ | ○ | ○ | ○ |
| Hand pronated and slightly extended | | ○ | ○ | ○ | ○ | ○ | ○ |
| Thumb slightly flexed/fingers abducted | | ○ | ○ | ○ | ○ | ○ | ○ |
| **Taping technique** | | Y | N | Y | N | Y | N |
| Applies an anchor around the distal forearm just above the ulnar condyle | | ○ | ○ | ○ | ○ | ○ | ○ |
| Applies a figure-8 around the thumb, starting at the ulnar condyle, across the dorsal aspect of the hand, around the limb, across the palmar aspect of the hand, and back to the ulnar condyle | | ○ | ○ | ○ | ○ | ○ | ○ |
| Repeats the above step one to two more times | | ○ | ○ | ○ | ○ | ○ | ○ |
| Secures tape with an anchor around the wrist with 1.5-inch white tape | | ○ | ○ | ○ | ○ | ○ | ○ |
| **Support and neatness** | | Y | N | Y | N | Y | N |
| Provides support and stability to the MP joint | | ○ | ○ | ○ | ○ | ○ | ○ |
| Maintains good circulation to the hand and thumb (check capillary refill) | | ○ | ○ | ○ | ○ | ○ | ○ |
| No holes and/or loose ends | | ○ | ○ | ○ | ○ | ○ | ○ |
| Total | | /10 | | /10 | | /10 | |
| Must achieve >7 to pass this examination | | Ⓟ | Ⓕ | Ⓟ | Ⓕ | Ⓟ | Ⓕ |

| Assessor: Date: | Test 1 Comments: |
|---|---|
| Assessor: Date: | Test 2 Comments: |
| Assessor: Date: | Test 3 Comments: |

**TEST ENVIRONMENTS**
**L:** Laboratory/Classroom
**C:** Clinical/Field Testing
**P:** Practicum
**A:** Assessment/Mock Exam

**TEST INFORMATION**
**Test Statistics:** N/A
**Reference(s):** Beam (2012)

# TAPING AND WRAPPING

| NATA EC 5th | BOC RD6 | SKILL |
|---|---|---|
| PHP-23 | D4-0403 | Collateral Interphalangeal Joint Taping |

**Supplies Needed:** 1-inch white tape

*This problem allows you the opportunity to demonstrate the ability to properly perform a* **collateral interphalangeal joint taping**. *You have 3 minutes to complete this task.*

| Collateral Interphalangeal Joint Taping | Course or Site Assessor Environment | | Test 1 | | Test 2 | | Test 3 | |
|---|---|---|---|---|---|---|---|---|
| **Proper position of patient** | | | **Y** | **N** | **Y** | **N** | **Y** | **N** |
| Standing or seated | | | O | O | O | O | O | O |
| Finger slightly flexed (PIP joint) | | | O | O | O | O | O | O |
| Fingers abducted (spread apart) | | | O | O | O | O | O | O |
| **Taping technique** | | | **Y** | **N** | **Y** | **N** | **Y** | **N** |
| Applies anchor strips proximal and distal to the PIP joint | | | O | O | O | O | O | O |
| Applies a strip of tape, beginning on the anterior proximal anchor, crossing the medial joint line, under the finger, and ending on the posterior distal anchor | | | O | O | O | O | O | O |
| Applies a strip of tape from the anterior distal anchor, across the medial joint line, under the finger, and ending on the posterior proximal anchor | | | O | O | O | O | O | O |
| Repeats the above two steps, crossing the lateral joint line | | | O | O | O | O | O | O |
| Secures the tape with a second set of proximal and distal anchors | | | O | O | O | O | O | O |
| **Support and neatness** | | | **Y** | **N** | **Y** | **N** | **Y** | **N** |
| Prevents valgus and varus stress on the PIP joint | | | O | O | O | O | O | O |
| Maintains good circulation to the finger (check capillary refill) | | | O | O | O | O | O | O |
| Proper tape positioning with no loose ends | | | O | O | O | O | O | O |
| **Total** | | | ___/11 | | ___/11 | | ___/11 | |
| **Must achieve >8 to pass this examination** | | | Ⓟ | Ⓕ | Ⓟ | Ⓕ | Ⓟ | Ⓕ |

| Assessor: Date: | Test 1 Comments: |
|---|---|
| Assessor: Date: | Test 2 Comments: |
| Assessor: Date: | Test 3 Comments: |

**TEST ENVIRONMENTS**
**L:** Laboratory/Classroom
**C:** Clinical/Field Testing
**P:** Practicum
**A:** Assessment/Mock Exam

**TEST INFORMATION**
**Test Statistics:** N/A
**Reference(s):** Beam (2012)

PREVENTION AND HEALTH PROMOTION
# TAPING AND WRAPPING

| NATA EC 5th | BOC RD6 | SKILL |
|---|---|---|
| PHP-23 | D4-0403 | Hip Spica Wrap (Hip Flexor) |

**Supplies Needed:** 6-inch double elastic wrap, elastic tape, 1.5-inch white tape

*This problem allows you the opportunity to demonstrate the ability to properly perform a* **hip spica wrap** *for an injury to the* **hip flexor***. You have 3 minutes to complete this task.*

| Hip Spica Wrap (Hip Flexor) | Course or Site / Assessor / Environment | | | | | |
|---|---|---|---|---|---|---|
| | | Test 1 | | Test 2 | | Test 3 |
| **Proper position of patient** | | Y | N | Y | N | Y | N |
| Standing | | ○ | ○ | ○ | ○ | ○ | ○ |
| Hip in slight flexion (heel may be propped up on small block) | | ○ | ○ | ○ | ○ | ○ | ○ |
| Foot/lower leg in neutral position (quadriceps contracted) | | ○ | ○ | ○ | ○ | ○ | ○ |
| **Wrapping technique** | | Y | N | Y | N | Y | N |
| Beginning at the proximal end of the thigh, wraps a 6-inch elastic wrap down to the distal lateral aspect of the quadriceps (pulls down and out) | | ○ | ○ | ○ | ○ | ○ | ○ |
| Spirals back up the thigh (pulls up and out), overlapping each layer by half the wrap's width | | ○ | ○ | ○ | ○ | ○ | ○ |
| At the proximal end of the thigh, continues the wrap around the waist, across the back, around the torso, and back to the proximal hip | | ○ | ○ | ○ | ○ | ○ | ○ |
| Repeats the above steps until the wrap is gone (start and finish on the thigh) | | ○ | ○ | ○ | ○ | ○ | ○ |
| Secures the wrap with elastic and white tape around the thigh | | ○ | ○ | ○ | ○ | ○ | ○ |
| **Support and neatness** | | Y | N | Y | N | Y | N |
| Provides support and stability | | ○ | ○ | ○ | ○ | ○ | ○ |
| Good circulation to the lower leg and foot | | ○ | ○ | ○ | ○ | ○ | ○ |
| No gaps and/or loose ends | | ○ | ○ | ○ | ○ | ○ | ○ |
| Total | | ___/11 | | ___/11 | | ___/11 | |
| Must achieve >8 to pass this examination | | Ⓟ | Ⓕ | Ⓟ | Ⓕ | Ⓟ | Ⓕ |

| Assessor: Date: | Test 1 Comments: |
|---|---|
| Assessor: Date: | Test 2 Comments: |
| Assessor: Date: | Test 3 Comments: |

**TEST ENVIRONMENTS**
**L:** Laboratory/Classroom
**C:** Clinical/Field Testing
**P:** Practicum
**A:** Assessment/Mock Exam

**TEST INFORMATION**
**Test Statistics:** N/A
**Reference(s):** Beam (2012)

**PREVENTION AND HEALTH PROMOTION**
# TAPING AND WRAPPING

| NATA EC 5th | BOC RD6 | SKILL |
|---|---|---|
| PHP-23 | D4-0403 | Hip Spica Wrap (Hip Adductor) |

**Supplies Needed:** Elastic wrap (6- or 4-inch double), elastic tape, 1.5-inch white tape

*This problem allows you the opportunity to demonstrate the ability to properly perform a* **hip spica wrap (hip adductor)** *for an injury to the groin area. You have 3 minutes to complete this task.*

| Hip Spica Wrap (Hip Adductor) | Course or Site Assessor Environment | | Test 1 | | Test 2 | | Test 3 | |
|---|---|---|---|---|---|---|---|---|
| **Proper position of patient** | | **Y** | **N** | **Y** | **N** | **Y** | **N** | |
| Standing | | ○ | ○ | ○ | ○ | ○ | ○ | |
| Hip in slight flexion (heel may be propped up on small block) | | ○ | ○ | ○ | ○ | ○ | ○ | |
| Foot/lower leg in slight internal rotation (quadriceps contracted) | | ○ | ○ | ○ | ○ | ○ | ○ | |
| **Wrapping technique** | | **Y** | **N** | **Y** | **N** | **Y** | **N** | |
| Beginning at the proximal end of the thigh, wraps 6-inch elastic wrap down to the medial aspect of the quadriceps (pulls down and in) | | ○ | ○ | ○ | ○ | ○ | ○ | |
| Spirals back up the thigh (pulls up and in), overlapping each layer by half the wrap's width | | ○ | ○ | ○ | ○ | ○ | ○ | |
| At the proximal end of the thigh, continues the wrap around the waist, pulling across the abdomen, around the torso, and back to the proximal hip | | ○ | ○ | ○ | ○ | ○ | ○ | |
| Repeats the above steps until the wrap is gone (start and finish on the thigh) | | ○ | ○ | ○ | ○ | ○ | ○ | |
| Secures the wrap with elastic and white tape around the thigh | | ○ | ○ | ○ | ○ | ○ | ○ | |
| **Support and neatness** | | **Y** | **N** | **Y** | **N** | **Y** | **N** | |
| Provides support and stability | | ○ | ○ | ○ | ○ | ○ | ○ | |
| Good circulation to the lower leg and foot | | ○ | ○ | ○ | ○ | ○ | ○ | |
| No gaps and/or loose ends | | ○ | ○ | ○ | ○ | ○ | ○ | |
| **Total** | | ____/11 | | ____/11 | | ____/11 | | |
| **Must achieve >8 to pass this examination** | | Ⓟ | Ⓕ | Ⓟ | Ⓕ | Ⓟ | Ⓕ | |

| Assessor: Date: | Test 1 Comments: |
|---|---|
| Assessor: Date: | Test 2 Comments: |
| Assessor: Date: | Test 3 Comments: |

**TEST ENVIRONMENTS**
**L:** Laboratory/Classroom
**C:** Clinical/Field Testing
**P:** Practicum
**A:** Assessment/Mock Exam

**TEST INFORMATION**
**Test Statistics:** N/A
**Reference(s):**   Beam (2012)

PREVENTION AND HEALTH PROMOTION
# TAPING AND WRAPPING

| NATA EC 5th | BOC RD6 | SKILL |
|---|---|---|
| PHP-23 | D4-0403 | Knee Compression Wrap |

**Supplies Needed:** Table, 6-inch elastic wrap (single), white adhesive tape, ice bag with ice

*This problem allows you the opportunity to demonstrate the ability to properly perform a* **knee compression wrap** *to secure an ice bag over the medial pole of the patella. You have 3 minutes to complete this task.*

| Knee Compression Wrap | Course or Site / Assessor / Environment | Test 1 | | Test 2 | | Test 3 | |
|---|---|---|---|---|---|---|---|
| **Proper position of patient** | | Y | N | Y | N | Y | N |
| Supine | | ○ | ○ | ○ | ○ | ○ | ○ |
| Knee slightly flexed | | ○ | ○ | ○ | ○ | ○ | ○ |
| Places ice bag in appropriate area | | ○ | ○ | ○ | ○ | ○ | ○ |
| **Wrapping technique** | | Y | N | Y | N | Y | N |
| Begins wrapping the leg with a 6-inch elastic wrap (single), beginning about 6 inches below the knee | | ○ | ○ | ○ | ○ | ○ | ○ |
| Spirals up the leg, overlapping each layer by half the wrap's width, covering the ice bag | | ○ | ○ | ○ | ○ | ○ | ○ |
| Wrap should end above the knee at about mid-quadriceps | | ○ | ○ | ○ | ○ | ○ | ○ |
| Secures the wrap with white adhesive tape | | ○ | ○ | ○ | ○ | ○ | ○ |
| **Support and neatness** | | Y | N | Y | N | Y | N |
| Provides compression to the knee (holds ice bag in place) | | ○ | ○ | ○ | ○ | ○ | ○ |
| Maintains good circulation to the foot | | ○ | ○ | ○ | ○ | ○ | ○ |
| No gaps and/or loose ends | | ○ | ○ | ○ | ○ | ○ | ○ |
| Total | | ___/10 | | ___/10 | | ___/10 | |
| Must achieve >7 to pass this examination | | Ⓟ | Ⓕ | Ⓟ | Ⓕ | Ⓟ | Ⓕ |

| Assessor: Date: | Test 1 Comments: |
|---|---|
| Assessor: Date: | Test 2 Comments: |
| Assessor: Date: | Test 3 Comments: |

**TEST ENVIRONMENTS**
**L:** Laboratory/Classroom
**C:** Clinical/Field Testing
**P:** Practicum
**A:** Assessment/Mock Exam

**TEST INFORMATION**
**Test Statistics:** N/A
**Reference(s):** Beam (2012)

## PREVENTION AND HEALTH PROMOTION
# TAPING AND WRAPPING

| NATA EC 5th | BOC RD6 | SKILL |
|---|---|---|
| PHP-23 | D4-0403 | Patellar Check Strap |

**Supplies Needed:** 2-inch heavyweight elastic tape, 0.5-inch white tape

*This problem allows you the opportunity to demonstrate the ability to properly perform a* **patellar check strap** *to help reduce symptoms of* **patellar tendinitis***. You have 3 minutes to complete this task.*

| Patellar Check Strap | Course or Site<br>Assessor<br>Environment | | | | | | |
|---|---|---|---|---|---|---|---|
| | | Test 1 | | Test 2 | | Test 3 | |
| **Proper position of patient** | | **Y** | **N** | **Y** | **N** | **Y** | **N** |
| Standing | | ○ | ○ | ○ | ○ | ○ | ○ |
| Knee slightly flexed (lower leg muscles relaxed) | | ○ | ○ | ○ | ○ | ○ | ○ |
| **Taping technique** | | **Y** | **N** | **Y** | **N** | **Y** | **N** |
| Cuts about 25 to 30 inches of the 2-inch elastic tape and folds it lengthwise, adhering both sides together | | ○ | ○ | ○ | ○ | ○ | ○ |
| Anchors a strip of tape between the inferior pole of patella and tibial tuberosity, applying direct pressure on patellar tendon | | ○ | ○ | ○ | ○ | ○ | ○ |
| Applies tape in a circling motion from lateral to medial across tendon (moderate tension) | | ○ | ○ | ○ | ○ | ○ | ○ |
| Repeats above step until tape is gone | | ○ | ○ | ○ | ○ | ○ | ○ |
| Anchors 0.5-inch white tape to secure tape and circles around 2 to 4 times | | ○ | ○ | ○ | ○ | ○ | ○ |
| **Support and neatness** | | **Y** | **N** | **Y** | **N** | **Y** | **N** |
| Reduces stress on the patellar tendon | | ○ | ○ | ○ | ○ | ○ | ○ |
| Good circulation to the lower leg, no numbness or tingling | | ○ | ○ | ○ | ○ | ○ | ○ |
| Clean looking | | ○ | ○ | ○ | ○ | ○ | ○ |
| | Total | ___/10 | | ___/10 | | ___/10 | |
| | Must achieve >7 to pass this examination | Ⓟ | Ⓕ | Ⓟ | Ⓕ | Ⓟ | Ⓕ |

| Assessor:<br>Date: | Test 1 Comments: |
|---|---|
| Assessor:<br>Date: | Test 2 Comments: |
| Assessor:<br>Date: | Test 3 Comments: |

**TEST ENVIRONMENTS**
**L:** Laboratory/Classroom
**C:** Clinical/Field Testing
**P:** Practicum
**A:** Assessment/Mock Exam

**TEST INFORMATION**
**Test Statistics:** N/A
**Reference(s):**   Beam (2012)

PREVENTION AND HEALTH PROMOTION
# TAPING AND WRAPPING

| NATA EC 5th | BOC RD6 | SKILL |
|---|---|---|
| PHP-23 | D4-0403 | Closed Basketweave Ankle Taping |

**Supplies Needed:** Table, 1.5-inch white tape, pre-wrap (optional), adhesive spray, heel/lace pads

*This problem allows you the opportunity to demonstrate the ability to properly perform a* **closed basketweave ankle taping** *to help prevent* **excessive inversion of the ankle**. *You have 3 minutes to complete this task.*

| Closed Basketweave Ankle Taping | Course or Site<br>Assessor<br>Environment<br>Test 1 | | Test 2 | | Test 3 | |
|---|---|---|---|---|---|---|
| **Proper position of patient** | **Y** | **N** | **Y** | **N** | **Y** | **N** |
| Seated with leg supported in full extension, lower leg hanging off the table (just enough for tape) | O | O | O | O | O | O |
| Ankle/foot dorsiflexed to 0 degrees (maintain throughout) | O | O | O | O | O | O |
| **Taping technique** | **Y** | **N** | **Y** | **N** | **Y** | **N** |
| Sprays ankle with adhesive spray (optional) | O | O | O | O | O | O |
| Places heel/lace pads on anterior/posterior ankle joint line | O | O | O | O | O | O |
| Secures pads with pre-wrap and covers the taping area (base of gastrocnemius to base of fifth metatarsal) | O | O | O | O | O | O |
| Places two anchors around the lower leg at the base of the gastrocnemius | O | O | O | O | O | O |
| Places another anchor around the instep (proximal to base of fifth metatarsal) | O | O | O | O | O | O |
| Applies a stirrup (medial to lateral) | O | O | O | O | O | O |
| Places a horseshoe around the foot just below the malleoli | O | O | O | O | O | O |
| Repeats the above two steps two additional times (each time overlapping by half the width of the tape) | O | O | O | O | O | O |
| Applies two figure-8's, starting at the dorsal aspect of the ankle | O | O | O | O | O | O |
| Applies two heel locks to each side of the ankle | O | O | O | O | O | O |
| Closes tapping with horseshoes, overlapping by half, from distal to proximal | O | O | O | O | O | O |
| Places final anchor around the instep, proximal to base of fifth metatarsal | O | O | O | O | O | O |
| **Support and neatness** | **Y** | **N** | **Y** | **N** | **Y** | **N** |
| Limits excessive inversion | O | O | O | O | O | O |
| Maintains good circulation to the foot and toes | O | O | O | O | O | O |
| No holes, loose ends, or wrinkles | O | O | O | O | O | O |
| **Total** | ____/17 | | ____/17 | | ____/17 | |

*(continued on the next page)*

| Must achieve >12 to pass this examination | Ⓟ | Ⓕ | Ⓟ | Ⓕ | Ⓟ | Ⓕ |
|---|---|---|---|---|---|---|
| **Assessor:** <br> **Date:** | **Test 1 Comments:** | | | | | |
| **Assessor:** <br> **Date:** | **Test 2 Comments:** | | | | | |
| **Assessor:** <br> **Date:** | **Test 3 Comments:** | | | | | |

## TEST ENVIRONMENTS
**L:** Laboratory/Classroom
**C:** Clinical/Field Testing
**P:** Practicum
**A:** Assessment/Mock Exam

## TEST INFORMATION
**Test Statistics:** N/A
**Reference(s):** Beam (2012)

# TAPING AND WRAPPING

| NATA EC 5th | BOC RD6 | SKILL |
|---|---|---|
| PHP-23 | D4-0403 | Achilles Tendon Taping |

**Supplies Needed:** Table, 3-inch heavyweight elastic tape, 2-inch elastic tape, 1.5-inch white tape

*This problem allows you the opportunity to demonstrate the ability to properly perform an* **Achilles tendon taping** *to help prevent* **ankle dorsiflexion***. You have 3 minutes to complete this task.*

| Achilles Tendon Taping | Course or Site Assessor Environment | Test 1 | | Test 2 | | Test 3 | |
|---|---|---|---|---|---|---|---|
| **Proper position of patient** | | Y | N | Y | N | Y | N |
| Prone with lower leg off the table | | ○ | ○ | ○ | ○ | ○ | ○ |
| Finds the painful range of motion by dorsiflexing ankle | | ○ | ○ | ○ | ○ | ○ | ○ |
| Places involved foot in a pain-free range and maintains this position | | ○ | ○ | ○ | ○ | ○ | ○ |
| **Taping technique** | | Y | N | Y | N | Y | N |
| Applies two anchors around the distal lower leg (base of gastrocnemius) with 1.5-inch white tape | | ○ | ○ | ○ | ○ | ○ | ○ |
| Applies one anchor around the ball of the foot with 2-inch elastic tape | | ○ | ○ | ○ | ○ | ○ | ○ |
| Anchors a strip of 3-inch heavyweight elastic tape to the distal surface of the anchor around the foot, pull up toward calcaneus | | ○ | ○ | ○ | ○ | ○ | ○ |
| Continues to pull up with moderate tension and ends on the anchors around the lower leg | | ○ | ○ | ○ | ○ | ○ | ○ |
| Anchors another strip to the dorsal surface of the anchor around the foot, pulling up toward the calcaneus, and cuts the tape about 3 to 4 inches below the anchors on the lower leg | | ○ | ○ | ○ | ○ | ○ | ○ |
| Cuts this strip in half down the middle and wraps each end around the lower leg in a spiral pattern (moderate tension), finishing on the distal lower leg | | ○ | ○ | ○ | ○ | ○ | ○ |
| Applies two to four more of these same strips | | ○ | ○ | ○ | ○ | ○ | ○ |
| Secures the strips with 1.5-inch white tape or elastic tape | | ○ | ○ | ○ | ○ | ○ | ○ |
| **Support and neatness** | | Y | N | Y | N | Y | N |
| Limits excessive dorsiflexion | | ○ | ○ | ○ | ○ | ○ | ○ |
| Good circulation to foot | | ○ | ○ | ○ | ○ | ○ | ○ |
| No holes and/or loose ends | | ○ | ○ | ○ | ○ | ○ | ○ |
| | Total | ___/14 | | ___/14 | | ___/14 | |

*(continued on the next page)*

| Must achieve >10 to pass this examination | Ⓟ | Ⓕ | Ⓟ | Ⓕ | Ⓟ | Ⓕ |
|---|---|---|---|---|---|---|
| **Assessor:** <br> **Date:** | **Test 1 Comments:** | | | | | |
| **Assessor:** <br> **Date:** | **Test 2 Comments:** | | | | | |
| **Assessor:** <br> **Date:** | **Test 3 Comments:** | | | | | |

**TEST ENVIRONMENTS**
**L:** Laboratory/Classroom
**C:** Clinical/Field Testing
**P:** Practicum
**A:** Assessment/Mock Exam

**TEST INFORMATION**
**Test Statistics:** N/A
**Reference(s):**   Beam (2012)

## PREVENTION AND HEALTH PROMOTION
# TAPING AND WRAPPING

| NATA EC 5th | BOC RD6 | SKILL |
|---|---|---|
| PHP-23 | D4-0403 | Longitudinal Arch Taping |

**Supplies Needed:** Table, 1-inch white tape

*This problem allows you the opportunity to demonstrate the ability to properly perform a* **longitudinal arch taping***. You have 3 minutes to complete this task.*

| Longitudinal Arch Taping | Course or Site Assessor Environment _____ _____ | | Test 1 | | Test 2 | | Test 3 |
|---|---|---|---|---|---|---|---|
| **Proper position of patient** | | **Y** | **N** | **Y** | **N** | **Y** | **N** |
| Seated (leg supported in full extension) | | O | O | O | O | O | O |
| Ankle/foot slightly plantar flexed | | O | O | O | O | O | O |
| **Taping technique** | | **Y** | **N** | **Y** | **N** | **Y** | **N** |
| Places an anchor at the head of the metatarsals | | O | O | O | O | O | O |
| Begins at the first metatarsal head and attaches a strip of tape, bringing it along the medial foot (anterior to posterior), around the heel and diagonally along the plantar side of the foot, and back to the first metatarsal head | | O | O | O | O | O | O |
| Repeats above step | | O | O | O | O | O | O |
| Makes a teardrop beginning on the plantar side of the third metatarsal head, back around the heel, and returning to the starting point | | O | O | O | O | O | O |
| Repeats above step | | O | O | O | O | O | O |
| Places the tape on the plantar side of the fifth metatarsal head and draws the tape diagonally across the foot to the medial side of the heel, around heel, and back to the lateral head of the fifth metatarsal | | O | O | O | O | O | O |
| Repeats the above step | | O | O | O | O | O | O |
| Places strips of tape along the plantar surface of the foot, pulling the tape from lateral to medial, beginning distally and moving proximally (each strip should overlap by half) | | O | O | O | O | O | O |
| Places tape around the heads of the metatarsals to secure | | O | O | O | O | O | O |
| **Support and neatness** | | **Y** | **N** | **Y** | **N** | **Y** | **N** |
| Provides support to the longitudinal arch | | O | O | O | O | O | O |
| Maintains good circulation throughout the foot | | O | O | O | O | O | O |
| No holes and/or loose ends | | O | O | O | O | O | O |
| Total | | ____/14 | | ____/14 | | ____/14 | |

*(continued on the next page)*

| Must achieve >10 to pass this examination | Ⓟ | Ⓕ | Ⓟ | Ⓕ | Ⓟ | Ⓕ |
|---|---|---|---|---|---|---|
| **Assessor:** <br> **Date:** | **Test 1 Comments:** | | | | | |
| **Assessor:** <br> **Date:** | **Test 2 Comments:** | | | | | |
| **Assessor:** <br> **Date:** | **Test 3 Comments:** | | | | | |

**TEST ENVIRONMENTS**
**L:**  Laboratory/Classroom
**C:**  Clinical/Field Testing
**P:**  Practicum
**A:**  Assessment/Mock Exam

**TEST INFORMATION**
**Test Statistics:** N/A
**Reference(s):**  Beam (2012)

## PREVENTION AND HEALTH PROMOTION
# TAPING AND WRAPPING

| NATA EC 5th | BOC RD6 | SKILL |
|---|---|---|
| PHP-23 | D4-0403 | Great Toe Taping |

**Supplies Needed:** Table, 1-inch white tape, elastic tape

*This problem allows you the opportunity to demonstrate the ability to properly perform a* **great toe taping***. You have 3 minutes to complete this task.*

| Great Toe Taping | Course or Site Assessor Environment | | Test 1 | | Test 2 | | Test 3 |
|---|---|---|---|---|---|---|---|
| **Proper position of patient** | | **Y** | **N** | **Y** | **N** | **Y** | **N** |
| Seated (leg supported in full extension) | | O | O | O | O | O | O |
| First metatarsal placed in a neutral position | | O | O | O | O | O | O |
| **Taping technique** | | **Y** | **N** | **Y** | **N** | **Y** | **N** |
| Places 2-inch elastic anchor around mid-foot (lateral to medial) and 1-inch white tape anchor around the distal great toe | | O | O | O | O | O | O |
| A fan of four to six strips of white tape should be placed on the dorsal side of the foot, beginning on the distal anchor and attaching on the proximal anchor | | O | O | O | O | O | O |
| A fan of four to six strips of white tape should be placed on the plantar side of the foot, beginning on the distal anchor and attaching on the proximal anchor | | O | O | O | O | O | O |
| Using a continuous strip of elastic tape, make a figure-8 around the great toe and mid-foot, aiding the abduction of the first metatarsal joint | | O | O | O | O | O | O |
| Secure the figure-8 with white tape | | O | O | O | O | O | O |
| **Support and neatness** | | **Y** | **N** | **Y** | **N** | **Y** | **N** |
| Limits excessive motion of the first MP joint (flexion/extension) | | O | O | O | O | O | O |
| Maintains good circulation of the great toe (check capillary refill) | | O | O | O | O | O | O |
| No holes and/or loose ends | | O | O | O | O | O | O |
| Total | | ___/10 | | ___/10 | | ___/10 | |

*(continued on the next page)*

| Must achieve >7 to pass this examination | P | F | P | F | P | F |
|---|---|---|---|---|---|---|
| **Assessor:**<br>**Date:** | **Test 1 Comments:** | | | | | |
| **Assessor:**<br>**Date:** | **Test 2 Comments:** | | | | | |
| **Assessor:**<br>**Date:** | **Test 3 Comments:** | | | | | |

**TEST ENVIRONMENTS**
**L:** Laboratory/Classroom
**C:** Clinical/Field Testing
**P:** Practicum
**A:** Assessment/Mock Exam

**TEST INFORMATION**
**Test Statistics:** N/A
**Reference(s):** Beam (2012)

# TAPING AND WRAPPING

| NATA EC 5th | BOC RD6 | SKILL |
|---|---|---|
| PHP-23 | D4-0403 | Taping Technique for Patellofemoral Stabilization |

**Supplies Needed:** Table, Leukotape, cover roll tape

*This problem allows you the opportunity to demonstrate the ability to properly perform a* **taping technique for patellofemoral stabilization**. *You have 3 minutes to complete this task.*

| Taping Technique for Patellofemoral Stabilization | Course or Site<br>Assessor<br>Environment | | | | | | |
|---|---|---|---|---|---|---|---|
| | | Test 1 | | Test 2 | | Test 3 | |
| **Proper position of patient** | | **Y** | **N** | **Y** | **N** | **Y** | **N** |
| Supine or seated | | O | O | O | O | O | O |
| Knee fully extended | | O | O | O | O | O | O |
| **Taping technique** | | **Y** | **N** | **Y** | **N** | **Y** | **N** |
| Assesses the patella for tilt and rotation | | O | O | O | O | O | O |
| Applies cover roll tape to protect the affected area | | O | O | O | O | O | O |
| Corrects tilt of the patella by applying Leukotape from the lateral border of the patella and pulling medially to the medial femoral condyle (or opposite if needed) | | O | O | O | O | O | O |
| Corrects external rotation of the patella by applying Leukotape from the inferior pole of the patella and pulling upward at a 45-degree angle (or opposite if needed) | | O | O | O | O | O | O |
| **Support and neatness** | | **Y** | **N** | **Y** | **N** | **Y** | **N** |
| Provides proper support to patellofemoral joint | | O | O | O | O | O | O |
| No holes and/or loose ends | | O | O | O | O | O | O |
| Assesses the patient for pain while performing functional activities | | O | O | O | O | O | O |
| **Total** | | ___/9 | | ___/9 | | ___/9 | |
| **Must achieve >7 to pass this examination** | | Ⓟ | Ⓕ | Ⓟ | Ⓕ | Ⓟ | Ⓕ |

| Assessor:<br>Date: | Test 1 Comments: |
|---|---|
| Assessor:<br>Date: | Test 2 Comments: |
| Assessor:<br>Date: | Test 3 Comments: |

**TEST ENVIRONMENTS**
L: Laboratory/Classroom
C: Clinical/Field Testing
P: Practicum
A: Assessment/Mock Exam

**TEST INFORMATION**
**Test Statistics:** N/A
**Reference(s):** Beam (2012)

PREVENTION AND HEALTH PROMOTION
# TAPING AND WRAPPING

| NATA EC 5th | BOC RD6 | SKILL |
|---|---|---|
| PHP-23 | D4-0403 | Hardshell Doughnut Pad (Acromioclavicular Joint) |

**Supplies Needed:** Thermomoldable material, heating sources, foam/felt, elastic tape, white tape, scissors

*This problem allows you the opportunity to demonstrate the ability to properly create a* **hardshell doughnut pad (acromioclavicular joint)**. *You have 4 minutes to complete this task.*

| Hardshell Doughnut Pad (Acromioclavicular Joint) | Course or Site Assessor Environment | | Test 1 | | Test 2 | | Test 3 | |
|---|---|---|---|---|---|---|---|---|
| **Proper position of patient** | | | **Y** | **N** | **Y** | **N** | **Y** | **N** |
| Cuts foam to create doughnut pad, appropriate size for the patient | | | ○ | ○ | ○ | ○ | ○ | ○ |
| Cuts hole in pad to fit the patient's AC joint | | | ○ | ○ | ○ | ○ | ○ | ○ |
| Cuts thermomoldable material to same size as doughnut pad | | | ○ | ○ | ○ | ○ | ○ | ○ |
| Heats thermomoldable material until pliable | | | ○ | ○ | ○ | ○ | ○ | ○ |
| Molds a convex dome in thermomoldable material | | | ○ | ○ | ○ | ○ | ○ | ○ |
| Secures thermomoldable material to doughnut pad with elastic tape | | | ○ | ○ | ○ | ○ | ○ | ○ |
| **Tester applies protective device to injured area** | | | **Y** | **N** | **Y** | **N** | **Y** | **N** |
| Secures finished pad over the AC joint (if needed) | | | ○ | ○ | ○ | ○ | ○ | ○ |
| | | Total | ___/7 | | ___/7 | | ___/7 | |
| | Must achieve >5 to pass this examination | | Ⓟ | Ⓕ | Ⓟ | Ⓕ | Ⓟ | Ⓕ |
| Assessor: Date: | Test 1 Comments: | | | | | | | |
| Assessor: Date: | Test 2 Comments: | | | | | | | |
| Assessor: Date: | Test 3 Comments: | | | | | | | |

**TEST ENVIRONMENTS**
L:  Laboratory/Classroom
C:  Clinical/Field Testing
P:  Practicum
A:  Assessment/Mock Exam

**TEST INFORMATION**
**Test Statistics:** N/A
**Reference(s):**   Beam (2012)

## PREVENTION AND HEALTH PROMOTION
# FITNESS AND WELLNESS

| NATA EC 5th | BOC RD6 | SKILL |
|---|---|---|
| PHP-28 | D1-0102 | Balance Test (Upper Extremity Proprioception) |

**Supplies Needed:** Fully inflated ball (basketball), stopwatch

*This problem allows you the opportunity to demonstrate the ability to properly perform a* **balance test** *for* **upper extremity proprioception***. You have 5 minutes to complete this task.*

| Balance Test (Upper Extremity Proprioception) | Course or Site Assessor Environment | | Test 1 | | Test 2 | | Test 3 | |
|---|---|---|---|---|---|---|---|---|
| **Proper position of patient** | | | **Y** | **N** | **Y** | **N** | **Y** | **N** |
| Prone (push-up position) | | | ○ | ○ | ○ | ○ | ○ | ○ |
| **Tester performs test according to accepted guidelines** | | | **Y** | **N** | **Y** | **N** | **Y** | **N** |
| Places the basketball under the patient's uninvolved limb | | | ○ | ○ | ○ | ○ | ○ | ○ |
| Moves the opposite limb away from the floor | | | ○ | ○ | ○ | ○ | ○ | ○ |
| Instructs the patient to balance on the uninvolved limb (as long as possible or for a maximum of 1 minute) | | | ○ | ○ | ○ | ○ | ○ | ○ |
| Repeats the above three steps with the involved limb | | | ○ | ○ | ○ | ○ | ○ | ○ |
| Compares time in a balanced position (determines deficit) | | | ○ | ○ | ○ | ○ | ○ | ○ |
| Total | | | _____/6 | | _____/6 | | _____/6 | |
| Must achieve >5 to pass this examination | | | Ⓟ | Ⓕ | Ⓟ | Ⓕ | Ⓟ | Ⓕ |

| Assessor: Date: | Test 1 Comments: |
|---|---|
| Assessor: Date: | Test 2 Comments: |
| Assessor: Date: | Test 3 Comments: |

**TEST ENVIRONMENTS**
**L:** Laboratory/Classroom
**C:** Clinical/Field Testing
**P:** Practicum
**A:** Assessment/Mock Exam

**TEST INFORMATION**
**Test Statistics:** N/A
**Reference(s):** Prentice (2014)

**PREVENTION AND HEALTH PROMOTION**
# FITNESS AND WELLNESS

| NATA EC 5th | BOC RD6 | SKILL |
|:---:|:---:|:---:|
| PHP-28 | D1-0102 | Endurance-Based Strength Test: % Fatigue (Middle Deltoid) |

**Supplies Needed:** 10-pound dumbbell, stopwatch

*This problem allows you the opportunity to demonstrate the ability to properly perform an* **endurance-based strength test: % fatigue (middle deltoid)**. *You have 5 minutes to complete this task.*

| Endurance-Based Strength Test: % Fatigue (Middle Deltoid) | Course or Site Assessor Environment | | | | | |
|---|---|---|---|---|---|---|
| | | Test 1 | | Test 2 | | Test 3 |
| **Proper position of patient** | | **Y** | **N** | **Y** | **N** | **Y** | **N** |
| Standing or seated | | O | O | O | O | O | O |
| Arms hanging to the side | | O | O | O | O | O | O |
| **Tester performs test according to accepted guidelines** | | **Y** | **N** | **Y** | **N** | **Y** | **N** |
| Instructs the patient to hold a 10-pound dumbbell with the uninvolved limb | | O | O | O | O | O | O |
| Instructs the patient to fully abduct the shoulder (slow, controlled pace) | | O | O | O | O | O | O |
| Continues until the patient cannot complete the next repetition or for 1 minute continuously (count the number of repetitions completed) | | O | O | O | O | O | O |
| Completes the above three steps with the uninvolved limb | | O | O | O | O | O | O |
| Compares the number of repetitions completed (determines deficit) | | O | O | O | O | O | O |
| **Total** | | ___/7 | | ___/7 | | ___/7 |
| **Must achieve >5 to pass this examination** | | Ⓟ | Ⓕ | Ⓟ | Ⓕ | Ⓟ | Ⓕ |

| Assessor: Date: | Test 1 Comments: |
|---|---|
| Assessor: Date: | Test 2 Comments: |
| Assessor: Date: | Test 3 Comments: |

**TEST ENVIRONMENTS**
**L:** Laboratory/Classroom
**C:** Clinical/Field Testing
**P:** Practicum
**A:** Assessment/Mock Exam

**TEST INFORMATION**
**Test Statistics:** N/A
**Reference(s):** Baechle & Earle (2008)

| NATA EC 5th | BOC RD6 | SKILL |
|---|---|---|
| PHP-28 | D1-0102 | Strength Test: % 1 x 10 Test (Shoulder Extensors) |

**Supplies Needed:** Lateral pulldown machine (ideally)

*This problem allows you the opportunity to demonstrate the ability to properly perform a* **strength test: % 1 x 10 test (shoulder extensors)***. You have 5 minutes to complete this task.*

| Strength Test: % 1 x 10 Test (Shoulder Extensors) | Course or Site Assessor Environment | | Test 1 | | Test 2 | | Test 3 | |
|---|---|---|---|---|---|---|---|---|
| **Proper position of patient** | | | Y | N | Y | N | Y | N |
| Seated or kneeling | | | O | O | O | O | O | O |
| **Tester performs test according to accepted guidelines** | | | Y | N | Y | N | Y | N |
| Instructs the patient to grip the wall pulley/lateral pulldown machine with the uninvolved limb | | | O | O | O | O | O | O |
| Instructs the patient to fully adduct the shoulder and flex the elbow (slow, controlled pace) | | | O | O | O | O | O | O |
| Continues until the patient cannot complete the 11th repetition (choose a weight that the patient can only complete 10 repetitions) | | | O | O | O | O | O | O |
| Repeats the above three steps with the involved limb (same weight) | | | O | O | O | O | O | O |
| Compares the number of repetitions completed (determines deficit) | | | O | O | O | O | O | O |
| Total | | | __/6 | | __/6 | | __/6 | |
| Must achieve >5 to pass this examination | | | P | F | P | F | P | F |
| Assessor: Date: | Test 1 Comments: | | | | | | | |
| Assessor: Date: | Test 2 Comments: | | | | | | | |
| Assessor: Date: | Test 3 Comments: | | | | | | | |

**TEST ENVIRONMENTS**
**L:** Laboratory/Classroom
**C:** Clinical/Field Testing
**P:** Practicum
**A:** Assessment/Mock Exam

**TEST INFORMATION**
**Test Statistics:** N/A
**Reference(s):** Baechle & Earle (2008)

**PREVENTION AND HEALTH PROMOTION**
# FITNESS AND WELLNESS

| NATA EC 5th | BOC RD6 | SKILL |
|---|---|---|
| PHP-28 | D1-0102 | Strength Test: % 1 x 5 Test (Wrist Flexors) |

**Supplies Needed:** Table, dumbbell

*This problem allows you the opportunity to demonstrate the ability to properly perform a* **strength test: % 1 x 5 test (wrist flexors)**. *You have 5 minutes to complete this task.*

| Strength Test: % 1 x 5 Test (Wrist Flexors) | Course or Site Assessor Environment | | Test 1 | | Test 2 | | Test 3 | |
|---|---|---|---|---|---|---|---|---|
| **Proper position of patient** | | | **Y** | **N** | **Y** | **N** | **Y** | **N** |
| Seated | | | ○ | ○ | ○ | ○ | ○ | ○ |
| Wrist supported hanging off the edge of the table | | | ○ | ○ | ○ | ○ | ○ | ○ |
| Forearm supinated to 90 degrees | | | ○ | ○ | ○ | ○ | ○ | ○ |
| **Tester performs test according to accepted guidelines** | | | **Y** | **N** | **Y** | **N** | **Y** | **N** |
| Instructs the patient to hold the dumbbell with the uninvolved limb | | | ○ | ○ | ○ | ○ | ○ | ○ |
| Instructs the patient to fully flex the wrist (slow, controlled pace) | | | ○ | ○ | ○ | ○ | ○ | ○ |
| Continues until the patient cannot complete the sixth repetition (choose a weight that the patient can only do five repetitions) | | | ○ | ○ | ○ | ○ | ○ | ○ |
| Repeats the above three steps with the involved limb (same weight) | | | ○ | ○ | ○ | ○ | ○ | ○ |
| Compares the number of repetitions completed (determines deficit) | | | ○ | ○ | ○ | ○ | ○ | ○ |
| Total | | | ___ /8 | | ___ /8 | | ___ /8 | |
| **Must achieve >6 to pass this examination** | | | Ⓟ | Ⓕ | Ⓟ | Ⓕ | Ⓟ | Ⓕ |

| Assessor: Date: | Test 1 Comments: |
|---|---|
| Assessor: Date: | Test 2 Comments: |
| Assessor: Date: | Test 3 Comments: |

**TEST ENVIRONMENTS**
**L:** Laboratory/Classroom
**C:** Clinical/Field Testing
**P:** Practicum
**A:** Assessment/Mock Exam

**TEST INFORMATION**
**Test Statistics:** N/A
**Reference(s):** Baechle & Earle (2008)

# FITNESS AND WELLNESS

| NATA EC 5th | BOC RD6 | SKILL |
|---|---|---|
| PHP-28 | D1-0102 | Strength Test: % Power Test (Triceps) |

**Supplies Needed:** Table, 10-pound dumbbell, stopwatch

*This problem allows you the opportunity to demonstrate the ability to properly perform a* **strength test: % power test (triceps)***. You have 5 minutes to complete this task.*

| Strength Test: % Power Test (Triceps) | Course or Site Assessor Environment | | Test 1 | | Test 2 | | Test 3 |
|---|---|---|---|---|---|---|---|
| **Proper position of patient** | | **Y** | **N** | **Y** | **N** | **Y** | **N** |
| Supine or seated | | ○ | ○ | ○ | ○ | ○ | ○ |
| **Tester performs test according to accepted guidelines** | | **Y** | **N** | **Y** | **N** | **Y** | **N** |
| Instructs the patient to hold the 10-pound dumbbell with the uninvolved limb | | ○ | ○ | ○ | ○ | ○ | ○ |
| Instructs the patient to fully extend the elbow (as quickly as possible) | | ○ | ○ | ○ | ○ | ○ | ○ |
| Continues contractions as quickly as possible for 20 seconds (time can vary) | | ○ | ○ | ○ | ○ | ○ | ○ |
| Repeats the above three steps with the involved limb (same weight) | | ○ | ○ | ○ | ○ | ○ | ○ |
| Compares the number of repetitions completed (determines deficit) | | ○ | ○ | ○ | ○ | ○ | ○ |
| Total | | ___/6 | | ___/6 | | ___/6 | |
| Must achieve >5 to pass this examination | | Ⓟ | Ⓕ | Ⓟ | Ⓕ | Ⓟ | Ⓕ |
| Assessor: Date: | Test 1 Comments: | | | | | | |
| Assessor: Date: | Test 2 Comments: | | | | | | |
| Assessor: Date: | Test 3 Comments: | | | | | | |

**TEST ENVIRONMENTS**
**L:** Laboratory/Classroom
**C:** Clinical/Field Testing
**P:** Practicum
**A:** Assessment/Mock Exam

**TEST INFORMATION**
**Test Statistics:** N/A
**Reference(s):** Baechle & Earle (2008)

PREVENTION AND HEALTH PROMOTION
# FITNESS AND WELLNESS

| NATA EC 5th | BOC RD6 | SKILL |
|---|---|---|
| PHP-28 | D1-0102 | Isokinetic Device Test (Shoulder) |

**Supplies Needed:** Isokinetic device

*This problem allows you the opportunity to demonstrate the ability to properly perform an* **isokinetic device test**. *This specific scenario requires you to set up the* **shoulder** *for* **abduction/adduction** *at* **90, 180, and 270 degrees per second**. *You have 5 minutes to complete this task.*

| Isokinetic Device Test (Shoulder) | Course or Site Assessor Environment | | Test 1 | | Test 2 | | Test 3 | |
|---|---|---|---|---|---|---|---|---|
| | | | Y | N | Y | N | Y | N |
| **Proper position of patient** | | | Y | N | Y | N | Y | N |
| Seated | | | O | O | O | O | O | O |
| **Tester performs proper set up for the isokinetic device** | | | Y | N | Y | N | Y | N |
| Makes sure all components of the isokinetic device are in proper working order | | | O | O | O | O | O | O |
| Proper attachments are connected and secured to isokinetic device | | | O | O | O | O | O | O |
| Shoulder joint is in line with the axis of isokinetic dynamometer | | | O | O | O | O | O | O |
| Lever arm is adjusted to match the length of the involved limb | | | O | O | O | O | O | O |
| All straps are properly placed and secured (if appropriate) | | | O | O | O | O | O | O |
| **Tester performs test according to accepted guidelines** | | | Y | N | Y | N | Y | N |
| Proper warm-up is provided | | | O | O | O | O | O | O |
| Proper instructions are given | | | O | O | O | O | O | O |
|    Moves limb through full range of motion | | | O | O | O | O | O | O |
|    Generates maximal contraction for each repetition | | | O | O | O | O | O | O |
|    Moves limb as hard and as fast as possible | | | O | O | O | O | O | O |
| Velocities are preset at 90, 180, and 270 degrees per second prior to the start of each set | | | O | O | O | O | O | O |
| Number of repetitions are given and explained to the patient | | | O | O | O | O | O | O |
| Isokinetic test is administered and recorded/printed | | | O | O | O | O | O | O |
| Total | | | ___/14 | | ___/14 | | ___/14 | |
| Must achieve >10 to pass this examination | | | P | F | P | F | P | F |

| Assessor: Date: | Test 1 Comments: |
|---|---|
| Assessor: Date: | Test 2 Comments: |
| Assessor: Date: | Test 3 Comments: |

**TEST ENVIRONMENTS**
**L:** Laboratory/Classroom
**C:** Clinical/Field Testing
**P:** Practicum
**A:** Assessment/Mock Exam

**TEST INFORMATION**
**Test Statistics:** N/A
**Reference(s):** Prentice (2014)

PREVENTION AND HEALTH PROMOTION
# FITNESS AND WELLNESS

| NATA EC 5th | BOC RD6 | SKILL |
|---|---|---|
| PHP-28 | D1-0102 | Functional Test (Upper Extremity) |

**Supplies Needed:** Tennis ball, baseball, glove

*This problem allows you the opportunity to demonstrate the ability to properly perform a* **functional test** *for the* **upper extremity.** *You have 5 minutes to complete this task.*

| Functional Test (Upper Extremity) | Course or Site / Assessor / Environment | Test 1 | | Test 2 | | Test 3 | |
|---|---|---|---|---|---|---|---|
| **Proper position of patient** | | Y | N | Y | N | Y | N |
| Standing | | ○ | ○ | ○ | ○ | ○ | ○ |
| **Tester performs test according to accepted guidelines** | | Y | N | Y | N | Y | N |
| Instructs the patient to go through the motions of throwing and letting go of the tennis ball | | ○ | ○ | ○ | ○ | ○ | ○ |
| Instructs the patient to throw the ball so it hits a wall about 15 feet away | | ○ | ○ | ○ | ○ | ○ | ○ |
| Progression: Hits the wall and rolls back to the patient | | ○ | ○ | ○ | ○ | ○ | ○ |
| Progression: Hits the wall, bounces once, then back to the patient | | ○ | ○ | ○ | ○ | ○ | ○ |
| Progression: Hits the wall and comes back to the patient in the air | | ○ | ○ | ○ | ○ | ○ | ○ |
| Instructs the patient to throw the ball to a partner 20 feet away | | ○ | ○ | ○ | ○ | ○ | ○ |
| Progression: 1 to 60 throws | | ○ | ○ | ○ | ○ | ○ | ○ |
| Progression: Increases velocity of the throws | | ○ | ○ | ○ | ○ | ○ | ○ |
| Progression: Uses a glove to catch the ball | | ○ | ○ | ○ | ○ | ○ | ○ |
| Instructs the patient to throw the ball to a partner 30 feet away | | ○ | ○ | ○ | ○ | ○ | ○ |
| Progression: 1 to 60 throws | | ○ | ○ | ○ | ○ | ○ | ○ |
| **Total** | | /12 | | /12 | | /12 | |
| **Must achieve >9 to pass this examination** | | Ⓟ | Ⓕ | Ⓟ | Ⓕ | Ⓟ | Ⓕ |

| Assessor: Date: | Test 1 Comments: |
|---|---|
| Assessor: Date: | Test 2 Comments: |
| Assessor: Date: | Test 3 Comments: |

**TEST ENVIRONMENTS**
**L:** Laboratory/Classroom
**C:** Clinical/Field Testing
**P:** Practicum
**A:** Assessment/Mock Exam

**TEST INFORMATION**
**Test Statistics:** N/A
**Reference(s):** Prentice (2014)

## PREVENTION AND HEALTH PROMOTION
# FITNESS AND WELLNESS

| NATA EC 5th | BOC RD6 | SKILL |
|:---:|:---:|:---:|
| PHP-28 | D1-0102 | Balance Test (Lower Extremity Proprioception) |

**Supplies Needed:** Deflated soccer ball, stopwatch

*This problem allows you the opportunity to demonstrate the ability to properly perform a* **balance test** *for* **lower extremity proprioception**. *You have 5 minutes to complete this task.*

| Balance Test (Lower Extremity Proprioception) | Course or Site Assessor Environment | | Test 1 | | Test 2 | | Test 3 | |
|---|---|---|:---:|:---:|:---:|:---:|:---:|:---:|
| | | | Y | N | Y | N | Y | N |
| **Proper position of patient** | | | Y | N | Y | N | Y | N |
| Standing | | | ○ | ○ | ○ | ○ | ○ | ○ |
| **Tester performs test according to accepted guidelines** | | | Y | N | Y | N | Y | N |
| Places a deflated soccer ball under the patient's uninvolved limb | | | ○ | ○ | ○ | ○ | ○ | ○ |
| Removes the opposite limb away from the floor | | | ○ | ○ | ○ | ○ | ○ | ○ |
| Instructs the patient to balance on the uninvolved limb (as long as possible or for a maximum of 1 minute) | | | ○ | ○ | ○ | ○ | ○ | ○ |
| Repeats the above three steps with the involved limb | | | ○ | ○ | ○ | ○ | ○ | ○ |
| Compares time in a balanced position (determines deficit) | | | ○ | ○ | ○ | ○ | ○ | ○ |
| Total | | | ___/6 | | ___/6 | | ___/6 | |
| Must achieve >5 to pass this examination | | | Ⓟ | Ⓕ | Ⓟ | Ⓕ | Ⓟ | Ⓕ |
| **Assessor:** **Date:** | Test 1 Comments: | | | | | | | |
| **Assessor:** **Date:** | Test 2 Comments: | | | | | | | |
| **Assessor:** **Date:** | Test 3 Comments: | | | | | | | |

**TEST ENVIRONMENTS**
**L:** Laboratory/Classroom
**C:** Clinical/Field Testing
**P:** Practicum
**A:** Assessment/Mock Exam

**TEST INFORMATION**
**Test Statistics:** N/A
**Reference(s):** Prentice (2014)

PREVENTION AND HEALTH PROMOTION
# FITNESS AND WELLNESS

| NATA EC 5th | BOC RD6 | SKILL |
|---|---|---|
| PHP-28 | D1-0102 | Endurance-Based Strength Test: % Fatigue (Tibialis Anterior) |

**Supplies Needed:** Table, cuff weight, stopwatch

*This problem allows you the opportunity to demonstrate the ability to properly perform an* **endurance-based strength test: % fatigue (tibialis anterior)**. *You have 5 minutes to complete this task.*

| Endurance-Based Strength Test: % Fatigue (Tibialis Anterior) | Course or Site Assessor Environment ——— ——— ——— | | | | | |
|---|---|---|---|---|---|---|
| | | Test 1 | | Test 2 | | Test 3 |
| **Proper position of patient** | | Y | N | Y | N | Y | N |
| Seated (leg off table) | | O | O | O | O | O | O |
| Knee flexed to 90 degrees | | O | O | O | O | O | O |
| **Tester performs test according to accepted guidelines** | | Y | N | Y | N | Y | N |
| Fastens the 10-pound cuff weight around the foot of the uninvolved limb | | O | O | O | O | O | O |
| Instructs the patient to fully dorsiflex the ankle (slow, controlled pace) | | O | O | O | O | O | O |
| Continues until the patient cannot complete the next repetition or for 1 minute continuously (count the repetitions completed) | | O | O | O | O | O | O |
| Repeats the above three steps with the involved limb | | O | O | O | O | O | O |
| Compares the number of repetitions completed (determines deficit) | | O | O | O | O | O | O |
| **Total** | | ___/7 | | ___/7 | | ___/7 |
| **Must achieve >5 to pass this examination** | | (P) | (F) | (P) | (F) | (P) | (F) |

| Assessor: Date: | Test 1 Comments: |
|---|---|
| Assessor: Date: | Test 2 Comments: |
| Assessor: Date: | Test 3 Comments: |

**TEST ENVIRONMENTS**
**L:** Laboratory/Classroom
**C:** Clinical/Field Testing
**P:** Practicum
**A:** Assessment/Mock Exam

**TEST INFORMATION**
**Test Statistics:** N/A
**Reference(s):** Baechle & Earle (2008)

PREVENTION AND HEALTH PROMOTION
# FITNESS AND WELLNESS

| NATA EC 5th | BOC RD6 | SKILL |
|---|---|---|
| PHP-28 | D1-0102 | Strength Test: % 1 x 10 Test (Hamstring) |

**Supplies Needed:** Weight machine hamstring curl

*This problem allows you the opportunity to demonstrate the ability to properly perform a* **strength test: % 1 x 10 test (hamstring)**. *You have 5 minutes to complete this task.*

| Strength Test: % 1 x 10 Test (Hamstring) | Course or Site / Assessor / Environment | | | | | | |
|---|---|---|---|---|---|---|---|
| | | Test 1 | | Test 2 | | Test 3 | |
| **Proper position of patient** | | **Y** | **N** | **Y** | **N** | **Y** | **N** |
| Prone | | ○ | ○ | ○ | ○ | ○ | ○ |
| **Tester performs test according to accepted guidelines** | | **Y** | **N** | **Y** | **N** | **Y** | **N** |
| Selects the appropriate weight needed for the uninvolved limb | | ○ | ○ | ○ | ○ | ○ | ○ |
| Instructs the patient to fully flex the knee (slow, controlled pace) | | ○ | ○ | ○ | ○ | ○ | ○ |
| Continues until the patient cannot complete the 11th repetition (choose a weight that the patient can only do 10 repetitions) | | ○ | ○ | ○ | ○ | ○ | ○ |
| Repeats the above steps with the involved limb (same weight) | | ○ | ○ | ○ | ○ | ○ | ○ |
| Compares the number of repetitions completed (determines deficit) | | ○ | ○ | ○ | ○ | ○ | ○ |
| **Total** | | ___/6 | | ___/6 | | ___/6 | |
| **Must achieve >5 to pass this examination** | | Ⓟ | Ⓕ | Ⓟ | Ⓕ | Ⓟ | Ⓕ |
| **Assessor:** **Date:** | **Test 1 Comments:** | | | | | | |
| **Assessor:** **Date:** | **Test 2 Comments:** | | | | | | |
| **Assessor:** **Date:** | **Test 3 Comments:** | | | | | | |

**TEST ENVIRONMENTS**
**L:** Laboratory/Classroom
**C:** Clinical/Field Testing
**P:** Practicum
**A:** Assessment/Mock Exam

**TEST INFORMATION**
**Test Statistics:** N/A
**Reference(s):** Baechle & Earle (2008)

PREVENTION AND HEALTH PROMOTION
# FITNESS AND WELLNESS

| NATA EC 5th | BOC RD6 | SKILL |
|---|---|---|
| PHP-28 | D1-0102 | Strength Test: % 1 x 5 Test (Ankle Plantar Flexors) |

**Supplies Needed:** Leg press machine (ideally)

*This problem allows you the opportunity to demonstrate the ability to properly perform a* **strength test: % 1 x 5 test (ankle plantar flexors)**. *You have 5 minutes to complete this task.*

| Strength Test: % 1 x 5 Test (Ankle Plantar Flexors) | Course or Site Assessor Environment | | | | | |
|---|---|---|---|---|---|---|
| | | Test 1 | | Test 2 | | Test 3 |
| **Proper position of patient** | | **Y** | **N** | **Y** | **N** | **Y** | **N** |
| Seated | | ○ | ○ | ○ | ○ | ○ | ○ |
| Knee extended to 0 degrees | | ○ | ○ | ○ | ○ | ○ | ○ |
| **Tester performs test according to accepted guidelines** | | **Y** | **N** | **Y** | **N** | **Y** | **N** |
| Selects the appropriate weight needed for the uninvolved limb | | ○ | ○ | ○ | ○ | ○ | ○ |
| Instructs the patient to fully plantar flex the ankle (slow, controlled pace) | | ○ | ○ | ○ | ○ | ○ | ○ |
| Continues until the patient cannot complete the sixth repetition (choose a weight that the patient can only complete five repetitions) | | ○ | ○ | ○ | ○ | ○ | ○ |
| Repeats the above steps with the involved limb (same weight) | | ○ | ○ | ○ | ○ | ○ | ○ |
| Compares the number of repetitions completed (determines deficit) | | ○ | ○ | ○ | ○ | ○ | ○ |
| **Total** | | ___/7 | | ___/7 | | ___/7 |
| **Must achieve >5 to pass this examination** | | Ⓟ | Ⓕ | Ⓟ | Ⓕ | Ⓟ | Ⓕ |
| **Assessor:** **Date:** | **Test 1 Comments:** | | | | | |
| **Assessor:** **Date:** | **Test 2 Comments:** | | | | | |
| **Assessor:** **Date:** | **Test 3 Comments:** | | | | | |

**TEST ENVIRONMENTS**
**L:** Laboratory/Classroom
**C:** Clinical/Field Testing
**P:** Practicum
**A:** Assessment/Mock Exam

**TEST INFORMATION**
**Test Statistics:** N/A
**Reference(s):** Baechle & Earle (2008)

PREVENTION AND HEALTH PROMOTION
# FITNESS AND WELLNESS

| NATA EC 5th | BOC RD6 | SKILL |
|---|---|---|
| PHP-28 | D1-0102 | Strength Test: % Power Test (Knee Extensors) |

**Supplies Needed:** Table, cuff weight, stopwatch

*This problem allows you the opportunity to demonstrate the ability to properly perform a* **strength test: % power test (knee extensors)**. *You have 5 minutes to complete this task.*

| Strength Test: % Power Test (Knee Extensors) | Course or Site Assessor Environment | Test 1 | | Test 2 | | Test 3 | |
|---|---|---|---|---|---|---|---|
| **Proper position of patient** | | Y | N | Y | N | Y | N |
| Seated (knee flexed) | | ○ | ○ | ○ | ○ | ○ | ○ |
| **Tester performs test according to accepted guidelines** | | Y | N | Y | N | Y | N |
| Fastens the 10-pound cuff weight to the distal tibia/fibula of the uninvolved limb | | ○ | ○ | ○ | ○ | ○ | ○ |
| Instructs the patient to fully extend the knee as quickly as possible | | ○ | ○ | ○ | ○ | ○ | ○ |
| Continues contractions as quickly as possible for 20 seconds (time may vary) | | ○ | ○ | ○ | ○ | ○ | ○ |
| Repeats the above three steps for the involved limb (same weight and time) | | ○ | ○ | ○ | ○ | ○ | ○ |
| Compares the number of repetitions completed (determines deficit) | | ○ | ○ | ○ | ○ | ○ | ○ |
| **Total** | | ___/6 | | ___/6 | | ___/6 | |
| **Must achieve >5 to pass this examination** | | Ⓟ | Ⓕ | Ⓟ | Ⓕ | Ⓟ | Ⓕ |
| **Assessor: Date:** | **Test 1 Comments:** | | | | | | |
| **Assessor: Date:** | **Test 2 Comments:** | | | | | | |
| **Assessor: Date:** | **Test 3 Comments:** | | | | | | |

**TEST ENVIRONMENTS**
**L:** Laboratory/Classroom
**C:** Clinical/Field Testing
**P:** Practicum
**A:** Assessment/Mock Exam

**TEST INFORMATION**
**Test Statistics:** N/A
**Reference(s):** Baechle & Earle (2008)

**PREVENTION AND HEALTH PROMOTION**
# FITNESS AND WELLNESS

| NATA EC 5th | BOC RD6 | SKILL |
|---|---|---|
| PHP-28 | D1-0102 | Isokinetic Device Test (Knee) |

**Supplies Needed:** Isokinetic device

*This problem allows you the opportunity to demonstrate the ability to properly perform an* **isokinetic device test** *for the* **knee** *for* **flexion/extension** *at* **60, 120, and 210 degrees per second**. *You have 5 minutes to complete this task.*

| Isokinetic Device Test (Knee) | Course or Site Assessor Environment | | Test 1 | | Test 2 | | Test 3 | |
|---|---|---|---|---|---|---|---|---|
| | | | Y | N | Y | N | Y | N |
| **Proper position of patient** | | | Y | N | Y | N | Y | N |
| Seated | | | ○ | ○ | ○ | ○ | ○ | ○ |
| **Tester performs proper set up for the isokinetic device** | | | Y | N | Y | N | Y | N |
| Makes sure all components of the isokinetic device are in proper working order | | | ○ | ○ | ○ | ○ | ○ | ○ |
| Makes sure proper attachments are connected and secured | | | ○ | ○ | ○ | ○ | ○ | ○ |
| Knee joint is in line with the axis of the isokinetic dynamometer | | | ○ | ○ | ○ | ○ | ○ | ○ |
| Lever arm is adjusted to match the length of the involved limb | | | ○ | ○ | ○ | ○ | ○ | ○ |
| All straps are properly placed and secured (if appropriate) | | | ○ | ○ | ○ | ○ | ○ | ○ |
| **Tester performs test according to accepted guidelines** | | | Y | N | Y | N | Y | N |
| Proper warm-up is provided | | | ○ | ○ | ○ | ○ | ○ | ○ |
| Proper instructions are given | | | ○ | ○ | ○ | ○ | ○ | ○ |
| Moves limb through full range of motion | | | ○ | ○ | ○ | ○ | ○ | ○ |
| Generates maximal contraction for each repetition | | | ○ | ○ | ○ | ○ | ○ | ○ |
| Moves limb as hard and as fast as possible | | | ○ | ○ | ○ | ○ | ○ | ○ |
| Velocities are set to appropriate degrees per second prior to the start of each set | | | ○ | ○ | ○ | ○ | ○ | ○ |
| Number of repetitions are given and explained to the patient | | | ○ | ○ | ○ | ○ | ○ | ○ |
| Isokinetic test is administered and recorded/printed | | | ○ | ○ | ○ | ○ | ○ | ○ |
| | | **Total** | ___/14 | | ___/14 | | ___/14 | |
| | **Must achieve >10 to pass this examination** | | Ⓟ | Ⓕ | Ⓟ | Ⓕ | Ⓟ | Ⓕ |
| **Assessor:** **Date:** | **Test 1 Comments:** | | | | | | | |
| **Assessor:** **Date:** | **Test 2 Comments:** | | | | | | | |
| **Assessor:** **Date:** | **Test 3 Comments:** | | | | | | | |

**TEST ENVIRONMENTS**
**L:** Laboratory/Classroom
**C:** Clinical/Field Testing
**P:** Practicum
**A:** Assessment/Mock Exam

**TEST INFORMATION**
**Test Statistics:** N/A
**Reference(s):** Prentice (2014)

| NATA EC 5th | BOC RD6 | SKILL |
|:---:|:---:|:---:|
| PHP-28 | D1-0102 | Functional Test (Lower Extremity) |

**Supplies Needed:** Cones, whistle, sport equipment

*This problem allows you the opportunity to demonstrate the ability to properly perform a* **functional test** *for the* **lower extremity***. You have 5 minutes to complete this task.*

| Functional Test (Lower Extremity) | Course or Site Assessor Environment | Test 1 | | Test 2 | | Test 3 | |
|---|---|:---:|:---:|:---:|:---:|:---:|:---:|
| **Proper position of patient** | | **Y** | **N** | **Y** | **N** | **Y** | **N** |
| Standing | | O | O | O | O | O | O |
| **Tester performs test according to accepted guidelines** | | **Y** | **N** | **Y** | **N** | **Y** | **N** |
| Instructs the patient to warm up | | O | O | O | O | O | O |
| Cutting activities progress from easy to difficult | | O | O | O | O | O | O |
| Progression consists of speed | | O | O | O | O | O | O |
|    Progression: Half speed | | O | O | O | O | O | O |
|    Progression: Three-quarter speed | | O | O | O | O | O | O |
|    Progression: Full speed | | O | O | O | O | O | O |
| Progression consists of direction | | O | O | O | O | O | O |
|    Progression: Activities to the left | | O | O | O | O | O | O |
|    Progression: Activities to the right | | O | O | O | O | O | O |
| Progression consists of angles/degrees | | O | O | O | O | O | O |
|    Progression: Running forward cutting at a 15-degree angle | | O | O | O | O | O | O |
|    Progression: Running forward cutting at a 45-degree angle | | O | O | O | O | O | O |
|    Progression: Running forward cutting at a 90-degree angle | | O | O | O | O | O | O |
| Progression consists of commands | | O | O | O | O | O | O |
|    Progression: Instructs the patient to cut left or right at the cone | | O | O | O | O | O | O |
|    Progression: Instructs the patient to cut left or right on the whistle | | O | O | O | O | O | O |
| Progression consists of sport-specific activities | | O | O | O | O | O | O |
|    Progression: Catching, dribbling, etc. | | O | O | O | O | O | O |
| **Total** | | ____/19 | | ____/19 | | ____/19 | |

*(continued on the next page)*

| Must achieve >14 to pass this examination | Ⓟ | Ⓕ | Ⓟ | Ⓕ | Ⓟ | Ⓕ |
|---|---|---|---|---|---|---|
| **Assessor:** <br> **Date:** | **Test 1 Comments:** | | | | | |
| **Assessor:** <br> **Date:** | **Test 2 Comments:** | | | | | |
| **Assessor:** <br> **Date:** | **Test 3 Comments:** | | | | | |

## TEST ENVIRONMENTS
**L:** Laboratory/Classroom
**C:** Clinical/Field Testing
**P:** Practicum
**A:** Assessment/Mock Exam

## TEST INFORMATION
**Test Statistics:** N/A
**Reference(s):** Prentice (2014)

**PREVENTION AND HEALTH PROMOTION**
# WEIGHT MANAGEMENT AND BODY COMPOSITION

| NATA EC 5th | BOC RD6 | SKILL |
|---|---|---|
| PHP-44 | D1-0105 | Body Composition (Skinfold Caliper) |

**Supplies Needed:** Caliper, pencil/paper

*This problem allows you the opportunity to demonstrate the ability to properly perform* **body composition** *using a* **skinfold caliper***. You have 3 minutes to complete this task.*

| Body Composition (Skinfold Caliper) | Course or Site<br>Assessor<br>Environment _____ | | | | | |
|---|---|---|---|---|---|---|
| | Test 1 | | Test 2 | | Test 3 | |
| **Proper position of patient** | **Y** | **N** | **Y** | **N** | **Y** | **N** |
| Standing | O | O | O | O | O | O |
| Disrobes to shorts (male) or shorts and a sports bra (female) | O | O | O | O | O | O |
| **Tester placed in proper position** | **Y** | **N** | **Y** | **N** | **Y** | **N** |
| Triceps: Vertical pinch at midline of posterior upper arm | O | O | O | O | O | O |
| Subscapular: Oblique pinch below inferior angle of scapula | O | O | O | O | O | O |
| Suprailiac: Oblique pinch just above the iliac crest | O | O | O | O | O | O |
| Abdominal: Vertical pinch 1 inch to the right of umbilicus | O | O | O | O | O | O |
| Quadriceps: Vertical pinch at mid-thigh | O | O | O | O | O | O |
| **Tester performs test according to accepted guidelines** | **Y** | **N** | **Y** | **N** | **Y** | **N** |
| All measurements should be taken on the right side of the body | O | O | O | O | O | O |
| Grasps area with thumb and forefinger | O | O | O | O | O | O |
| Pulls skin and fat away from underlying muscle tissue | O | O | O | O | O | O |
| Pinches area with caliper | O | O | O | O | O | O |
| Reads caliper dial within 2 seconds of pinching area | O | O | O | O | O | O |
| Repeats measurement two to three times for each area | O | O | O | O | O | O |
| Takes average of the two to three measurements and records results | O | O | O | O | O | O |
| **Total** | ___/14 | | ___/14 | | ___/14 | |
| **Must achieve >10 to pass this examination** | Ⓟ | Ⓕ | Ⓟ | Ⓕ | Ⓟ | Ⓕ |

| Assessor:<br>Date: | Test 1 Comments: |
|---|---|
| Assessor:<br>Date: | Test 2 Comments: |
| Assessor:<br>Date: | Test 3 Comments: |

**TEST ENVIRONMENTS**
**L:** Laboratory/Classroom
**C:** Clinical/Field Testing
**P:** Practicum
**A:** Assessment/Mock Exam

**TEST INFORMATION**
**Test Statistics:** N/A
**Reference(s):** Manufacturer's
recommendations

PREVENTION AND HEALTH PROMOTION
# WEIGHT MANAGEMENT AND BODY COMPOSITION

| NATA EC 5th | BOC RD6 | SKILL |
|---|---|---|
| PHP-44 | D1-0105 | Body Composition (Bioimpedance) |

**Supplies Needed:** Body fat/hydration monitor

*This problem allows you the opportunity to demonstrate the ability to properly perform* **body composition** *using* **bioimpedance***. You have 5 minutes to complete this task.*

| Body Composition (Bioimpedance) | Course or Site Assessor Environment | | Test 1 | | Test 2 | | Test 3 |
|---|---|---|---|---|---|---|---|
| **Proper set up of equipment** | | Y | N | Y | N | Y | N |
| Presses the on/set button to wake up the unit | | ○ | ○ | ○ | ○ | ○ | ○ |
| Presses the on/set button to cycle through the settings | | ○ | ○ | ○ | ○ | ○ | ○ |
| Puts in the patient's gender, height, weight, and age | | ○ | ○ | ○ | ○ | ○ | ○ |
| Presses the start button | | ○ | ○ | ○ | ○ | ○ | ○ |
| **Tester sets proper patient position** | | Y | N | Y | N | Y | N |
| Instructs the patient to grip each handle/conductive pads in each hand | | ○ | ○ | ○ | ○ | ○ | ○ |
| Instructs the patient to hold the device in front of him/her with arms perpendicular to his/her body (make sure hands are clean and dry) | | ○ | ○ | ○ | ○ | ○ | ○ |
| Within a few seconds, the unit will automatically measure fat and hydration percentages | | ○ | ○ | ○ | ○ | ○ | ○ |
| The tester properly interprets the patient's results as either too lean, lean, normal, high body fat, or very high body fat (see chart in manual for exact percentages) | | ○ | ○ | ○ | ○ | ○ | ○ |
| **Total** | | \_\_\_\_/8 | | \_\_\_\_/8 | | \_\_\_\_/8 | |
| **Must achieve >6 to pass this examination** | | ⓟ | Ⓕ | ⓟ | Ⓕ | ⓟ | Ⓕ |
| **Assessor:** **Date:** | Test 1 Comments: | | | | | | |
| **Assessor:** **Date:** | Test 2 Comments: | | | | | | |
| **Assessor:** **Date:** | Test 3 Comments: | | | | | | |

**TEST ENVIRONMENTS**
**L:** Laboratory/Classroom
**C:** Clinical/Field Testing
**P:** Practicum
**A:** Assessment/Mock Exam

**TEST INFORMATION**
**Test Statistics:** N/A
**Reference(s):** Manufacturer's recommendations

# III

# CLINICAL EXAMINATION AND DIAGNOSIS

# 4

# MUSCULOSKELETAL SYSTEM— REGION 1: FOOT AND TOES

Hauth, J. M., Gloyeske, B. M., & Amato, H. K.
*Clinical Skills Documentation Guide for Athletic Training, Third Edition* (pp. 66-91).
© 2016 SLACK Incorporated.

## MUSCULOSKELETAL SYSTEM—REGION 1: FOOT AND TOES
# KNOWLEDGE AND SKILLS

| *Musculoskeletal System—Region 1: Foot and Toes* | | | | *Skill: Acquisition, Reinforcement, Proficiency* | | |
|---|---|---|---|---|---|---|
| **NATA EC 5th** | **BOC RD6** | **Palpation** | **Page #** | | | |
| CE-21b, CE-20c | D2-0202 | Palpation: Foot and Toes – 01 | 68 | | | |
| CE-21b, CE-20c | D2-0202 | Palpation: Foot and Toes – 02 | 69 | | | |
| CE-21b, CE-20c | D2-0202 | Palpation: Foot and Toes – 03 | 70 | | | |
| **NATA EC 5th** | **BOC RD6** | **Manual Muscle Testing** | **Page #** | | | |
| CE-21c | D2-0203 | MMT: Abductor Hallucis | 71 | | | |
| CE-21c | D2-0203 | MMT: Adductor Hallucis | 72 | | | |
| CE-21c | D2-0203 | MMT: Extensor Digitorum Longus/Brevis | 73 | | | |
| CE-21c | D2-0203 | MMT: Extensor Hallucis Longus/Brevis | 74 | | | |
| CE-21c | D2-0203 | MMT: Flexor Digitorum Brevis | 75 | | | |
| CE-21c | D2-0203 | MMT: Flexor Digitorum Longus | 76 | | | |
| CE-21c | D2-0203 | MMT: Flexor Hallucis Brevis | 77 | | | |
| CE-21c | D2-0203 | MMT: Flexor Hallucis Longus | 78 | | | |
| **NATA EC 5th** | **BOC RD6** | **Osteokinematic Joint Motion** | **Page #** | | | |
| CE-21d | D2-0203 | Goniometric Assessment: Metatarsophalangeal Joint Great Toe (Flexion/Extension) | 79 | | | |
| CE-21d | D2-0203 | Goniometric Assessment: Tarsal Inversion | 80 | | | |
| CE-21d | D2-0203 | Goniometric Assessment: Tarsal Eversion | 81 | | | |
| **NATA EC 5th** | **BOC RD6** | **Capsular and Ligamentous Stress Testing** | **Page #** | | | |
| CE-21e | D2-0203 | Valgus Stress Test for the Metatarsophalangeal and Interphalangeal Joints | 82 | | | |
| CE-21e | D2-0203 | Varus Stress Test for the Metatarsophalangeal and Interphalangeal Joints | 83 | | | |
| **NATA EC 5th** | **BOC RD6** | **Joint Play (Arthrokinematics)** | **Page #** | | | |
| CE-21f | D2-0203 | Intermetatarsal Glide Assessment | 84 | | | |
| CE-21f | D2-0203 | Midtarsal Joint Play | 85 | | | |
| CE-21f | D2-0203 | Tarsometatarsal Joint Play | 86 | | | |
| **NATA EC 5th** | **BOC RD6** | **Special Tests** | **Page #** | | | |
| CE-21g, CE-20e | D2-0203 | Dorsiflexion-Eversion Test | 87 | | | |
| CE-21g, CE-20e | D2-0203 | Long Bone Compression Test | 88 | | | |
| CE-21g, CE-20e | D2-0203 | Mulder Sign for Intermetatarsal Neuroma | 89 | | | |
| CE-21g, CE-20e | D2-0203 | Navicular Drop Test | 90 | | | |
| CE-21g, CE-20e | D2-0203 | Test for Supple Pes Planus (Windlass Test) | 91 | | | |

## MUSCULOSKELETAL SYSTEM—REGION 1: FOOT AND TOES
# PALPATION

| NATA EC 5th | BOC RD6 | SKILL |
|---|---|---|
| CE-21b, CE-20c | D2-0202 | Palpation: Foot and Toes – 01 |

**Supplies Needed:** Table

*This problem allows you the opportunity to demonstrate your ability to* **palpate** *the* **foot and toes**. *You have 2 minutes to complete this task.*

| Palpation: Foot and Toes – 01 | Course or Site Assessor Environment _____ _____ _____ | | | | | |
|---|---|---|---|---|---|---|
| | | Test 1 | | Test 2 | | Test 3 | |
| | | Y | N | Y | N | Y | N |
| First MTP joint | | ◯ | ◯ | ◯ | ◯ | ◯ | ◯ |
| Navicular tuberosity | | ◯ | ◯ | ◯ | ◯ | ◯ | ◯ |
| Flexor hallucis longus tendon | | ◯ | ◯ | ◯ | ◯ | ◯ | ◯ |
| Posterior tibial pulse | | ◯ | ◯ | ◯ | ◯ | ◯ | ◯ |
| First cuneiform | | ◯ | ◯ | ◯ | ◯ | ◯ | ◯ |
| Dome of the talus | | ◯ | ◯ | ◯ | ◯ | ◯ | ◯ |
| Sesamoid bones of the great toe | | ◯ | ◯ | ◯ | ◯ | ◯ | ◯ |
| Total | | ___/7 | | ___/7 | | ___/7 | |
| Must achieve >4 to pass this examination | | Ⓟ | Ⓕ | Ⓟ | Ⓕ | Ⓟ | Ⓕ |

| Assessor: Date: | Test 1 Comments: |
|---|---|
| Assessor: Date: | Test 2 Comments: |
| Assessor: Date: | Test 3 Comments: |

**TEST ENVIRONMENTS**
**L:** Laboratory/Classroom
**C:** Clinical/Field Testing
**P:** Practicum
**A:** Assessment/Mock Exam

**TEST INFORMATION**
**Test Statistics:** N/A
**Reference(s):** Starkey & Brown (2015)

## MUSCULOSKELETAL SYSTEM—REGION 1: FOOT AND TOES
# PALPATION

| NATA EC 5th | BOC RD6 | SKILL |
|---|---|---|
| CE-21b, CE-20c | D2-0202 | Palpation: Foot and Toes – 02 |

**Supplies Needed:** Table

*This problem allows you the opportunity to demonstrate your ability to* **palpate** *the* **foot and toes**.
*You have 2 minutes to complete this task.*

| Palpation: Foot and Toes – 02 | Course or Site Assessor Environment | Test 1 | | Test 2 | | Test 3 | |
|---|---|---|---|---|---|---|---|
| | | Y | N | Y | N | Y | N |
| First metatarsal | | ○ | ○ | ○ | ○ | ○ | ○ |
| Talar head | | ○ | ○ | ○ | ○ | ○ | ○ |
| Sustentaculum tali | | ○ | ○ | ○ | ○ | ○ | ○ |
| Fifth metatarsal | | ○ | ○ | ○ | ○ | ○ | ○ |
| Second cuneiform | | ○ | ○ | ○ | ○ | ○ | ○ |
| Extensor digitorum longus | | ○ | ○ | ○ | ○ | ○ | ○ |
| Dorsalis pedis pulse | | ○ | ○ | ○ | ○ | ○ | ○ |
| | Total | __/7 | | __/7 | | __/7 | |
| | Must achieve >4 to pass this examination | Ⓟ | Ⓕ | Ⓟ | Ⓕ | Ⓟ | Ⓕ |
| **Assessor:** **Date:** | **Test 1 Comments:** | | | | | | |
| **Assessor:** **Date:** | **Test 2 Comments:** | | | | | | |
| **Assessor:** **Date:** | **Test 3 Comments:** | | | | | | |

**TEST ENVIRONMENTS**
**L:** Laboratory/Classroom
**C:** Clinical/Field Testing
**P:** Practicum
**A:** Assessment/Mock Exam

**TEST INFORMATION**
**Test Statistics:** N/A
**Reference(s):** Starkey & Brown (2015)

## MUSCULOSKELETAL SYSTEM—REGION 1: FOOT AND TOES
# PALPATION

| NATA EC 5th | BOC RD6 | SKILL |
|---|---|---|
| CE-21b, CE-20c | D2-0202 | Palpation: Foot and Toes – 03 |

**Supplies Needed:** Table

*This problem allows you the opportunity to demonstrate your ability to* **palpate** *the* **foot and toes**.
*You have 2 minutes to complete this task.*

| Palpation: Foot and Toes – 03 | Course or Site<br>Assessor<br>Environment | | | | | |
|---|---|---|---|---|---|---|
| | | Test 1 | | Test 2 | | Test 3 |
| | | Y | N | Y | N | Y | N |
| Calcaneonavicular ligament | | ○ | ○ | ○ | ○ | ○ | ○ |
| Medial talar tubercle | | ○ | ○ | ○ | ○ | ○ | ○ |
| Cuboid | | ○ | ○ | ○ | ○ | ○ | ○ |
| Peroneal tubercle | | ○ | ○ | ○ | ○ | ○ | ○ |
| Third cuneiform | | ○ | ○ | ○ | ○ | ○ | ○ |
| Styloid process of the fifth metatarsal | | ○ | ○ | ○ | ○ | ○ | ○ |
| Medial calcaneal tubercle | | ○ | ○ | ○ | ○ | ○ | ○ |
| **Total** | | __/7 | | __/7 | | __/7 | |
| **Must achieve >4 to pass this examination** | | Ⓟ | Ⓕ | Ⓟ | Ⓕ | Ⓟ | Ⓕ |
| Assessor:<br>Date: | Test 1 Comments: | | | | | | |
| Assessor:<br>Date: | Test 2 Comments: | | | | | | |
| Assessor:<br>Date: | Test 3 Comments: | | | | | | |

**TEST ENVIRONMENTS**
**L:** Laboratory/Classroom
**C:** Clinical/Field Testing
**P:** Practicum
**A:** Assessment/Mock Exam

**TEST INFORMATION**
**Test Statistics:** N/A
**Reference(s):** Starkey & Brown (2015)

## MUSCULOSKELETAL SYSTEM—REGION 1: FOOT AND TOES
# MANUAL MUSCLE TESTING

| NATA EC 5th | BOC RD6 | SKILL |
|---|---|---|
| CE-21c | D2-0203 | MMT: Abductor Hallucis |

**Supplies Needed:** Table

*This problem allows you the opportunity to demonstrate a* **manual muscle test** *for the* **abductor hallucis.** *You have 2 minutes to complete this task.*

| MMT: Abductor Hallucis | Course or Site Assessor Environment | | | | | |
|---|---|---|---|---|---|---|
| | | Test 1 | | Test 2 | | Test 3 |
| | | Y | N | Y | N | Y | N |
| **Tester places patient and limb in appropriate position** | | Y | N | Y | N | Y | N |
| Supine or seated – foot and ankle should be off the table | | O | O | O | O | O | O |
| **Tester placed in proper position** | | Y | N | Y | N | Y | N |
| Stabilizes the foot by grasping the heel firmly | | O | O | O | O | O | O |
| **Tester performs test according to accepted guidelines** | | Y | N | Y | N | Y | N |
| Instructs the patient to actively pull the forefoot in adduction | | O | O | O | O | O | O |
| Applies resistance to the medial aspect of the first proximal phalanx (direction of abduction) | | O | O | O | O | O | O |
| Holds resistance for 5 seconds | | O | O | O | O | O | O |
| Performs assessment bilaterally | | O | O | O | O | O | O |
| **Identifies implications** | | Y | N | Y | N | Y | N |
| Correctly grades the MMT | | O | O | O | O | O | O |
| Total | | __/7 | | __/7 | | __/7 | |
| Must achieve >4 to pass this examination | | Ⓟ | Ⓕ | Ⓟ | Ⓕ | Ⓟ | Ⓕ |

| Assessor: Date: | Test 1 Comments: |
|---|---|
| Assessor: Date: | Test 2 Comments: |
| Assessor: Date: | Test 3 Comments: |

**TEST ENVIRONMENTS**
**L:** Laboratory/Classroom
**C:** Clinical/Field Testing
**P:** Practicum
**A:** Assessment/Mock Exam

**TEST INFORMATION**
**Test Statistics:** N/A
**Reference(s):** Kendall et al. (2005)

## MUSCULOSKELETAL SYSTEM—REGION 1: FOOT AND TOES
# MANUAL MUSCLE TESTING

| NATA EC 5th | BOC RD6 | SKILL |
|:---:|:---:|:---:|
| CE-21c | D2-0203 | MMT: Adductor Hallucis |

**Supplies Needed:** Table

*This problem allows you the opportunity to demonstrate a* **manual muscle test** *for the* **adductor hallucis.**
*You have 2 minutes to complete this task.*

| MMT: Adductor Hallucis | Course or Site<br>Assessor<br>Environment<br>Test 1 | | Test 2 | | Test 3 | |
|---|:---:|:---:|:---:|:---:|:---:|:---:|
| **Tester places patient and limb in appropriate position** | **Y** | **N** | **Y** | **N** | **Y** | **N** |
| Supine or seated – foot and ankle should be off the table, great toe placed in slight extension | ○ | ○ | ○ | ○ | ○ | ○ |
| **Tester placed in proper position** | **Y** | **N** | **Y** | **N** | **Y** | **N** |
| Stabilizes the foot by grasping the heel firmly | ○ | ○ | ○ | ○ | ○ | ○ |
| **Tester performs test according to accepted guidelines** | **Y** | **N** | **Y** | **N** | **Y** | **N** |
| Instructs the patient to actively pull the forefoot in abduction and toe into flexion | ○ | ○ | ○ | ○ | ○ | ○ |
| Applies resistance to the lateral aspect of the first proximal phalanx (direction of adduction and extension) | ○ | ○ | ○ | ○ | ○ | ○ |
| Holds resistance for 5 seconds | ○ | ○ | ○ | ○ | ○ | ○ |
| Performs assessment bilaterally | ○ | ○ | ○ | ○ | ○ | ○ |
| **Identifies implications** | **Y** | **N** | **Y** | **N** | **Y** | **N** |
| Correctly grades the MMT | ○ | ○ | ○ | ○ | ○ | ○ |
| **Total** | ___/7 | | ___/7 | | ___/7 | |
| **Must achieve >4 to pass this examination** | Ⓟ | Ⓕ | Ⓟ | Ⓕ | Ⓟ | Ⓕ |

| Assessor:<br>Date: | Test 1 Comments: |
|---|---|
| Assessor:<br>Date: | Test 2 Comments: |
| Assessor:<br>Date: | Test 3 Comments: |

**TEST ENVIRONMENTS**
**L:** Laboratory/Classroom
**C:** Clinical/Field Testing
**P:** Practicum
**A:** Assessment/Mock Exam

**TEST INFORMATION**
**Test Statistics:** N/A
**Reference(s):** Kendall et al. (2005)

## MUSCULOSKELETAL SYSTEM—REGION 1: FOOT AND TOES
# MANUAL MUSCLE TESTING

| NATA EC 5th | BOC RD6 | SKILL |
|---|---|---|
| CE-21c | D2-0203 | MMT: Extensor Digitorum Longus/Brevis |

**Supplies Needed:** Table

*This problem allows you the opportunity to demonstrate a* **manual muscle test** *for the* **extensor digitorum longus/brevis muscles**. *You have 2 minutes to complete this task.*

| MMT: Extensor Digitorum Longus/Brevis | Course or Site Assessor Environment | | Test 1 | | Test 2 | | Test 3 | |
|---|---|---|---|---|---|---|---|---|
| | | | Y | N | Y | N | Y | N |
| **Tester places patient and limb in appropriate position** | | | Y | N | Y | N | Y | N |
| Supine or seated – foot and ankle should be off the table | | | O | O | O | O | O | O |
| **Tester placed in proper position** | | | Y | N | Y | N | Y | N |
| Examiner stabilizes the foot in slight plantar flexion and eversion | | | O | O | O | O | O | O |
| **Tester performs test according to accepted guidelines** | | | Y | N | Y | N | Y | N |
| Instructs the patient to actively extend all joints – second to fifth | | | O | O | O | O | O | O |
| Applies resistance to the dorsal surface of the toes (direction of flexion) | | | O | O | O | O | O | O |
| Holds resistance for 5 seconds | | | O | O | O | O | O | O |
| Performs assessment bilaterally | | | O | O | O | O | O | O |
| **Identifies implications** | | | Y | N | Y | N | Y | N |
| Correctly grades the MMT | | | O | O | O | O | O | O |
| | Total | | ___/7 | | ___/7 | | ___/7 | |
| | Must achieve >4 to pass this examination | | Ⓟ | Ⓕ | Ⓟ | Ⓕ | Ⓟ | Ⓕ |
| **Assessor:** **Date:** | Test 1 Comments: | | | | | | | |
| **Assessor:** **Date:** | Test 2 Comments: | | | | | | | |
| **Assessor:** **Date:** | Test 3 Comments: | | | | | | | |

**TEST ENVIRONMENTS**
**L:** Laboratory/Classroom
**C:** Clinical/Field Testing
**P:** Practicum
**A:** Assessment/Mock Exam

**TEST INFORMATION**
**Test Statistics:** N/A
**Reference(s):** Kendall et al. (2005)

## MUSCULOSKELETAL SYSTEM—REGION 1: FOOT AND TOES
# MANUAL MUSCLE TESTING

| NATA EC 5th | BOC RD6 | SKILL |
|---|---|---|
| CE-21c | D2-0203 | MMT: Extensor Hallucis Longus/Brevis |

**Supplies Needed:** Table

*This problem allows you the opportunity to demonstrate a* **manual muscle test** *for the* **extensor hallucis longus/brevis muscles**. *You have 2 minutes to complete this task.*

| MMT: Extensor Hallucis Longus/Brevis | Course or Site Assessor Environment | | Test 1 | | Test 2 | | Test 3 | |
|---|---|---|---|---|---|---|---|---|
| **Tester places patient and limb in appropriate position** | | | Y | N | Y | N | Y | N |
| Supine or seated – foot and ankle should be off the table | | | ○ | ○ | ○ | ○ | ○ | ○ |
| **Tester placed in proper position** | | | Y | N | Y | N | Y | N |
| Stabilizes the foot in slight plantar flexion | | | ○ | ○ | ○ | ○ | ○ | ○ |
| **Tester performs test according to accepted guidelines** | | | Y | N | Y | N | Y | N |
| Instructs the patient to actively extend the first phalanx | | | ○ | ○ | ○ | ○ | ○ | ○ |
| Applies resistance to the dorsal surface of the great toe (direction of flexion) | | | ○ | ○ | ○ | ○ | ○ | ○ |
| Holds resistance for 5 seconds | | | ○ | ○ | ○ | ○ | ○ | ○ |
| Performs assessment bilaterally | | | ○ | ○ | ○ | ○ | ○ | ○ |
| **Identifies implications** | | | Y | N | Y | N | Y | N |
| Correctly grades the MMT | | | ○ | ○ | ○ | ○ | ○ | ○ |
| Total | | | ___/7 | | ___/7 | | ___/7 | |
| Must achieve >4 to pass this examination | | | Ⓟ | Ⓕ | Ⓟ | Ⓕ | Ⓟ | Ⓕ |

| Assessor: Date: | Test 1 Comments: |
|---|---|
| Assessor: Date: | Test 2 Comments: |
| Assessor: Date: | Test 3 Comments: |

**TEST ENVIRONMENTS**
**L:** Laboratory/Classroom
**C:** Clinical/Field Testing
**P:** Practicum
**A:** Assessment/Mock Exam

**TEST INFORMATION**
**Test Statistics:** N/A
**Reference(s):** Kendall et al. (2005)

## MUSCULOSKELETAL SYSTEM—REGION 1: FOOT AND TOES
# MANUAL MUSCLE TESTING

| NATA EC 5th | BOC RD6 | SKILL |
|---|---|---|
| CE-21c | D2-0203 | MMT: Flexor Digitorum Brevis |

**Supplies Needed:** Table

*This problem allows you the opportunity to demonstrate a* **manual muscle test** *for the* **flexor digitorum brevis muscle.** *You have 2 minutes to complete this task.*

| MMT: Flexor Digitorum Brevis | Course or Site Assessor Environment | | Test 1 | | Test 2 | | Test 3 | |
|---|---|---|---|---|---|---|---|---|
| **Tester places patient and limb in appropriate position** | | **Y** | **N** | **Y** | **N** | **Y** | **N** | |
| Supine or seated – foot and ankle should be off the table | | O | O | O | O | O | O | |
| **Tester placed in proper position** | | **Y** | **N** | **Y** | **N** | **Y** | **N** | |
| Stabilizes the proximal phalanges and maintains a neutral foot position | | O | O | O | O | O | O | |
| **Tester performs test according to accepted guidelines** | | **Y** | **N** | **Y** | **N** | **Y** | **N** | |
| Instructs the patient to actively flex the PIP joints of the second to fifth digits | | O | O | O | O | O | O | |
| Applies resistance to the plantar surface of the middle phalanx of the four toes (direction of extension) | | O | O | O | O | O | O | |
| Holds resistance for 5 seconds | | O | O | O | O | O | O | |
| Performs assessment bilaterally | | O | O | O | O | O | O | |
| **Identifies implications** | | **Y** | **N** | **Y** | **N** | **Y** | **N** | |
| Correctly grades the MMT | | O | O | O | O | O | O | |
| **Total** | | ___/7 | | ___/7 | | ___/7 | | |
| **Must achieve >4 to pass this examination** | | Ⓟ | Ⓕ | Ⓟ | Ⓕ | Ⓟ | Ⓕ | |

| Assessor: Date: | Test 1 Comments: |
|---|---|
| Assessor: Date: | Test 2 Comments: |
| Assessor: Date: | Test 3 Comments: |

**TEST ENVIRONMENTS**
**L:** Laboratory/Classroom
**C:** Clinical/Field Testing
**P:** Practicum
**A:** Assessment/Mock Exam

**TEST INFORMATION**
**Test Statistics:** N/A
**Reference(s):** Kendall et al. (2005)

MUSCULOSKELETAL SYSTEM—REGION 1: FOOT AND TOES
# MANUAL MUSCLE TESTING

| NATA EC 5th | BOC RD6 | SKILL |
|---|---|---|
| CE-21c | D2-0203 | MMT: Flexor Digitorum Longus |

**Supplies Needed:** Table

*This problem allows you the opportunity to demonstrate a* **manual muscle test** *for the* **flexor digitorum longus muscle**. *You have 2 minutes to complete this task.*

| MMT: Flexor Digitorum Longus | Course or Site Assessor Environment | | Test 1 | | Test 2 | | Test 3 | |
|---|---|---|---|---|---|---|---|---|
| **Tester places patient and limb in appropriate position** | | | **Y** | **N** | **Y** | **N** | **Y** | **N** |
| Supine or seated – if gastrocnemius tightness is present, then the knee should be flexed | | | ○ | ○ | ○ | ○ | ○ | ○ |
| **Tester placed in proper position** | | | **Y** | **N** | **Y** | **N** | **Y** | **N** |
| Stabilizes the metatarsals and maintains a neutral foot position | | | ○ | ○ | ○ | ○ | ○ | ○ |
| **Tester performs test according to accepted guidelines** | | | **Y** | **N** | **Y** | **N** | **Y** | **N** |
| Instructs the patient to actively flex the DIP joints of the second to fifth digits | | | ○ | ○ | ○ | ○ | ○ | ○ |
| Applies resistance to the plantar surface of the distal phalanx of the four toes (direction of extension) | | | ○ | ○ | ○ | ○ | ○ | ○ |
| Holds resistance for 5 seconds | | | ○ | ○ | ○ | ○ | ○ | ○ |
| Performs assessment bilaterally | | | ○ | ○ | ○ | ○ | ○ | ○ |
| **Identifies implications** | | | **Y** | **N** | **Y** | **N** | **Y** | **N** |
| Correctly grades the MMT | | | ○ | ○ | ○ | ○ | ○ | ○ |
| Total | | | ___/7 | | ___/7 | | ___/7 | |
| Must achieve >4 to pass this examination | | | Ⓟ | Ⓕ | Ⓟ | Ⓕ | Ⓟ | Ⓕ |
| Assessor: Date: | Test 1 Comments: | | | | | | | |
| Assessor: Date: | Test 2 Comments: | | | | | | | |
| Assessor: Date: | Test 3 Comments: | | | | | | | |

**TEST ENVIRONMENTS**
**L:** Laboratory/Classroom
**C:** Clinical/Field Testing
**P:** Practicum
**A:** Assessment/Mock Exam

**TEST INFORMATION**
**Test Statistics:** N/A
**Reference(s):** Kendall et al. (2005)

# MANUAL MUSCLE TESTING

| NATA EC 5th | BOC RD6 | SKILL |
|---|---|---|
| CE-21c | D2-0203 | MMT: Flexor Hallucis Brevis |

**Supplies Needed:** Table

*This problem allows you the opportunity to demonstrate a* **manual muscle test** *for the* **flexor hallucis brevis muscle**. *You have 2 minutes to complete this task.*

| MMT: Flexor Hallucis Brevis | Course or Site Assessor Environment | Test 1 | | Test 2 | | Test 3 | |
|---|---|---|---|---|---|---|---|
| **Tester places patient and limb in appropriate position** | | **Y** | **N** | **Y** | **N** | **Y** | **N** |
| Supine or seated – foot and ankle should be off the table | | O | O | O | O | O | O |
| **Tester placed in proper position** | | **Y** | **N** | **Y** | **N** | **Y** | **N** |
| Stabilizes the foot proximal to the MTP joint and maintains neutral position of the foot and ankle | | O | O | O | O | O | O |
| **Tester performs test according to accepted guidelines** | | **Y** | **N** | **Y** | **N** | **Y** | **N** |
| Instructs the patient to actively flex the MTP joint of the great toe | | O | O | O | O | O | O |
| Applies resistance to the plantar surface of the proximal phalanx of the great toe (direction of extension) | | O | O | O | O | O | O |
| Holds resistance for 5 seconds | | O | O | O | O | O | O |
| Performs assessment bilaterally | | O | O | O | O | O | O |
| **Identifies implications** | | **Y** | **N** | **Y** | **N** | **Y** | **N** |
| Correctly grades the MMT | | O | O | O | O | O | O |
| Total | | ___/7 | | ___/7 | | ___/7 | |
| Must achieve >4 to pass this examination | | Ⓟ | Ⓕ | Ⓟ | Ⓕ | Ⓟ | Ⓕ |

| Assessor: Date: | Test 1 Comments: |
|---|---|
| Assessor: Date: | Test 2 Comments: |
| Assessor: Date: | Test 3 Comments: |

**TEST ENVIRONMENTS**
**L:** Laboratory/Classroom
**C:** Clinical/Field Testing
**P:** Practicum
**A:** Assessment/Mock Exam

**TEST INFORMATION**
**Test Statistics:** N/A
**Reference(s):** Kendall et al. (2005)

## MUSCULOSKELETAL SYSTEM—REGION 1: FOOT AND TOES
# MANUAL MUSCLE TESTING

| NATA EC 5th | BOC RD6 | SKILL |
|---|---|---|
| CE-21c | D2-0203 | MMT: Flexor Hallucis Longus |

**Supplies Needed:** Table

*This problem allows you the opportunity to demonstrate a* **manual muscle test** *for the* **flexor hallucis longus muscle.** *You have 2 minutes to complete this task.*

| MMT: Flexor Hallucis Longus | Course or Site Assessor Environment | | Test 1 | | Test 2 | | Test 3 | |
|---|---|---|---|---|---|---|---|---|
| **Tester places patient and limb in appropriate position** | | | Y | N | Y | N | Y | N |
| Supine or seated – foot and ankle should be off the table | | | O | O | O | O | O | O |
| **Tester placed in proper position** | | | Y | N | Y | N | Y | N |
| Stabilizes the foot proximal to the MTP joint and maintains neutral position of the foot and ankle | | | O | O | O | O | O | O |
| **Tester performs test according to accepted guidelines** | | | Y | N | Y | N | Y | N |
| Instructs the patient to actively flex the IP joint of the great toe | | | O | O | O | O | O | O |
| Applies resistance to the plantar surface of the distal phalanx of the great toe (direction of extension) | | | O | O | O | O | O | O |
| Holds resistance for 5 seconds | | | O | O | O | O | O | O |
| Performs assessment bilaterally | | | O | O | O | O | O | O |
| **Identifies implications** | | | Y | N | Y | N | Y | N |
| Correctly grades the MMT | | | O | O | O | O | O | O |
| Total | | | ___/7 | | ___/7 | | ___/7 | |
| Must achieve >4 to pass this examination | | | Ⓟ | Ⓕ | Ⓟ | Ⓕ | Ⓟ | Ⓕ |

| Assessor: Date: | Test 1 Comments: |
|---|---|
| Assessor: Date: | Test 2 Comments: |
| Assessor: Date: | Test 3 Comments: |

**TEST ENVIRONMENTS**
**L:** Laboratory/Classroom
**C:** Clinical/Field Testing
**P:** Practicum
**A:** Assessment/Mock Exam

**TEST INFORMATION**
**Test Statistics:** N/A
**Reference(s):** Kendall et al. (2005)

# OSTEOKINEMATIC JOINT MOTION

| NATA EC 5th | BOC RD6 | SKILL |
|---|---|---|
| CE-21d | D2-0203 | Goniometric Assessment: Metatarsophalangeal Joint Great Toe (Flexion/Extension) |

**Supplies Needed:** Table, small goniometer

*This problem allows you the opportunity to demonstrate a* **goniometric assessment** *for the* **first MTP joint (flexion/extension)**. *You have 2 minutes to complete this task.*

| Goniometric Assessment: Metatarsophalangeal Joint Great Toe (Flexion/Extension) | Course or Site Assessor Environment | | Test 1 | | Test 2 | | Test 3 |
|---|---|---|---|---|---|---|---|
| **Tester places patient and limb in appropriate position** | | **Y** | **N** | **Y** | **N** | **Y** | **N** |
| Supine or seated with the ankle and foot in neutral | | O | O | O | O | O | O |
| **Tester and goniometer placed in proper position** | | **Y** | **N** | **Y** | **N** | **Y** | **N** |
| Stabilizes the metatarsal (stationary arm over dorsal midline of the metatarsal) | | O | O | O | O | O | O |
| Places the fulcrum over dorsal aspect of the MTP joint | | O | O | O | O | O | O |
| Moves arm over the dorsal midline of the proximal phalanx | | O | O | O | O | O | O |
| **Tester performs test according to accepted guidelines** | | **Y** | **N** | **Y** | **N** | **Y** | **N** |
| Passively flexes or extends the MTP joint in the neutral foot | | O | O | O | O | O | O |
| Takes proper goniometric measurement | | O | O | O | O | O | O |
| Performs assessment bilaterally | | O | O | O | O | O | O |
| **Identifies implications** | | **Y** | **N** | **Y** | **N** | **Y** | **N** |
| Identifies normal ranges (flexion = 30 to 45 degrees; extension = 50 to 70 degrees) | | O | O | O | O | O | O |
| Total | | ___/8 | | ___/8 | | ___/8 | |
| Must achieve >5 to pass this examination | | Ⓟ | Ⓕ | Ⓟ | Ⓕ | Ⓟ | Ⓕ |

| Assessor: Date: | Test 1 Comments: |
|---|---|
| Assessor: Date: | Test 2 Comments: |
| Assessor: Date: | Test 3 Comments: |

**TEST ENVIRONMENTS**
**L:** Laboratory/Classroom
**C:** Clinical/Field Testing
**P:** Practicum
**A:** Assessment/Mock Exam

**TEST INFORMATION**
**Test Statistics:** N/A
**Reference(s):** Norkin & White (2009)

## MUSCULOSKELETAL SYSTEM—REGION 1: FOOT AND TOES
# OSTEOKINEMATIC JOINT MOTION

| NATA EC 5th | BOC RD6 | SKILL |
|---|---|---|
| CE-21d | D2-0203 | Goniometric Assessment: Tarsal Inversion |

**Supplies Needed:** Table, small goniometer

*This problem allows you the opportunity to demonstrate a* **goniometric assessment** *for* **tarsal inversion**. *You have 2 minutes to complete this task.*

| Goniometric Assessment: Tarsal Inversion | Course or Site Assessor Environment | | Test 1 | | Test 2 | | Test 3 |
|---|---|---|---|---|---|---|---|
| **Tester places patient and limb in appropriate position** | | **Y** | **N** | **Y** | **N** | **Y** | **N** |
| Seated, knee flexed to 90 degrees | | O | O | O | O | O | O |
| **Tester and goniometer placed in proper position** | | **Y** | **N** | **Y** | **N** | **Y** | **N** |
| Stabilizes the tibia and fibula (stationary arm over anterior midline of the lower leg) | | O | O | O | O | O | O |
| Places the fulcrum over the anterior aspect of ankle midway between malleoli | | O | O | O | O | O | O |
| Moves arm over the dorsal midline of the second metatarsal | | O | O | O | O | O | O |
| **Tester performs test according to accepted guidelines** | | **Y** | **N** | **Y** | **N** | **Y** | **N** |
| Passively moves the foot downward into plantar flexion, medially into adduction, and supination | | O | O | O | O | O | O |
| Takes proper goniometric measurement | | O | O | O | O | O | O |
| Performs assessment bilaterally | | O | O | O | O | O | O |
| **Identifies implications** | | **Y** | **N** | **Y** | **N** | **Y** | **N** |
| Identifies normal ranges (inversion = 30 to 35 degrees) | | O | O | O | O | O | O |
| Total | | ___/8 | | ___/8 | | ___/8 | |
| Must achieve >5 to pass this examination | | Ⓟ | Ⓕ | Ⓟ | Ⓕ | Ⓟ | Ⓕ |

| Assessor: Date: | Test 1 Comments: |
|---|---|
| Assessor: Date: | Test 2 Comments: |
| Assessor: Date: | Test 3 Comments: |

**TEST ENVIRONMENTS**
**L:** Laboratory/Classroom
**C:** Clinical/Field Testing
**P:** Practicum
**A:** Assessment/Mock Exam

**TEST INFORMATION**
**Test Statistics:** N/A
**Reference(s):**   Norkin & White (2009)

## MUSCULOSKELETAL SYSTEM—REGION 1: FOOT AND TOES
# OSTEOKINEMATIC JOINT MOTION

| NATA EC 5th | BOC RD6 | SKILL |
|---|---|---|
| CE-21d | D2-0203 | Goniometric Assessment: Tarsal Eversion |

**Supplies Needed:** Table, small goniometer

*This problem allows you the opportunity to demonstrate a* **goniometric assessment** *for* **tarsal eversion.** *You have 2 minutes to complete this task.*

| Goniometric Assessment: Tarsal Eversion | Course or Site Assessor Environment | | Test 1 | | Test 2 | | Test 3 | |
|---|---|---|---|---|---|---|---|---|
| | | **Y** | **N** | **Y** | **N** | **Y** | **N** | |
| **Tester places patient and limb in appropriate position** | | Y | N | Y | N | Y | N |
| Seated, knee flexed to 90 degrees | | O | O | O | O | O | O |
| **Tester and goniometer placed in proper position** | | Y | N | Y | N | Y | N |
| Stabilizes the tibia and fibula (stationary arm over anterior midline of the lower leg) | | O | O | O | O | O | O |
| Places the fulcrum over the anterior aspect of ankle midway between malleoli | | O | O | O | O | O | O |
| Moves the arm over the dorsal midline of the second metatarsal | | O | O | O | O | O | O |
| **Tester performs test according to accepted guidelines** | | Y | N | Y | N | Y | N |
| Passively moves the foot upward into dorsiflexion, laterally into abduction, and pronation | | O | O | O | O | O | O |
| Takes proper goniometric measurement | | O | O | O | O | O | O |
| Performs assessment bilaterally | | O | O | O | O | O | O |
| **Identifies implications** | | Y | N | Y | N | Y | N |
| Identifies normal ranges (eversion = 10 to 12 degrees) | | O | O | O | O | O | O |
| **Total** | | __/8 | | __/8 | | __/8 | |
| **Must achieve >5 to pass this examination** | | P | F | P | F | P | F |

| Assessor:<br>Date: | Test 1 Comments: |
|---|---|
| Assessor:<br>Date: | Test 2 Comments: |
| Assessor:<br>Date: | Test 3 Comments: |

**TEST ENVIRONMENTS**
**L:** Laboratory/Classroom
**C:** Clinical/Field Testing
**P:** Practicum
**A:** Assessment/Mock Exam

**TEST INFORMATION**
**Test Statistics:** N/A
**Reference(s):** Norkin & White (2009)

MUSCULOSKELETAL SYSTEM—REGION 1: FOOT AND TOES
# CAPSULAR AND LIGAMENTOUS STRESS TESTING

| NATA EC 5th | BOC RD6 | SKILL |
|---|---|---|
| CE-21e | D2-0203 | Valgus Stress Test for the Metatarsophalangeal and Interphalangeal Joints |

**Supplies Needed:** Table

*This problem allows you the opportunity to demonstrate an* **orthopedic test** *known as the* **valgus stress test for the MTP and IP joints**. *You have 2 minutes to complete this task.*

| Valgus Stress Test for the Metatarsophalangeal and Interphalangeal Joints | Course or Site Assessor Environment | | Test 1 | | Test 2 | | Test 3 | |
|---|---|---|---|---|---|---|---|---|
| **Tester places patient and limb in appropriate position** | | | **Y** | **N** | **Y** | **N** | **Y** | **N** |
| Supine or seated – foot and ankle off the table | | | ◯ | ◯ | ◯ | ◯ | ◯ | ◯ |
| Foot placed in a neutral position | | | ◯ | ◯ | ◯ | ◯ | ◯ | ◯ |
| **Tester placed in proper position** | | | **Y** | **N** | **Y** | **N** | **Y** | **N** |
| Stabilizes proximal bone close to the joint being tested | | | ◯ | ◯ | ◯ | ◯ | ◯ | ◯ |
| Grasps bone distal to the joint being tested near the middle of its shaft | | | ◯ | ◯ | ◯ | ◯ | ◯ | ◯ |
| **Tester performs test according to accepted guidelines** | | | **Y** | **N** | **Y** | **N** | **Y** | **N** |
| Maintains relaxation of the limb | | | ◯ | ◯ | ◯ | ◯ | ◯ | ◯ |
| Moves distal bone laterally, attempting to open the joint on the medial side | | | ◯ | ◯ | ◯ | ◯ | ◯ | ◯ |
| Performs assessment bilaterally | | | ◯ | ◯ | ◯ | ◯ | ◯ | ◯ |
| **Identifies positive findings and implications** | | | **Y** | **N** | **Y** | **N** | **Y** | **N** |
| Pain or increased laxity when compared bilaterally | | | ◯ | ◯ | ◯ | ◯ | ◯ | ◯ |
| MCL sprain or avulsion fracture | | | ◯ | ◯ | ◯ | ◯ | ◯ | ◯ |
| **Total** | | | ___/9 | | ___/9 | | ___/9 | |
| **Must achieve >6 to pass this examination** | | | Ⓟ | Ⓕ | Ⓟ | Ⓕ | Ⓟ | Ⓕ |
| **Assessor: Date:** | **Test 1 Comments:** | | | | | | | |
| **Assessor: Date:** | **Test 2 Comments:** | | | | | | | |
| **Assessor: Date:** | **Test 3 Comments:** | | | | | | | |

**TEST ENVIRONMENTS**
**L:** Laboratory/Classroom
**C:** Clinical/Field Testing
**P:** Practicum
**A:** Assessment/Mock Exam

**TEST INFORMATION**
**Test Statistics:** No data available
**Reference(s):** Starkey & Brown (2015)

# CAPSULAR AND LIGAMENTOUS STRESS TESTING

| NATA EC 5th | BOC RD6 | SKILL |
|---|---|---|
| CE-21e | D2-0203 | Varus Stress Test for the Metatarsophalangeal and Interphalangeal Joints |

**Supplies Needed:** Table

*This problem allows you the opportunity to demonstrate an* **orthopedic test** *known as the* **varus stress test for the MTP and IP joints.** *You have 2 minutes to complete this task.*

| Varus Stress Test for the Metatarsophalangeal and Interphalangeal Joints | Course or Site Assessor Environment | | Test 1 | | Test 2 | | Test 3 |
|---|---|---|---|---|---|---|---|
| **Tester places patient and limb in appropriate position** | | Y | N | Y | N | Y | N |
| Supine or seated – foot and ankle off the table | | O | O | O | O | O | O |
| Foot placed in a neutral position | | O | O | O | O | O | O |
| **Tester placed in proper position** | | Y | N | Y | N | Y | N |
| Stabilizes proximal bone close to the joint being tested | | O | O | O | O | O | O |
| Grasps bone distal to the joint being tested near the middle of its shaft | | O | O | O | O | O | O |
| **Tester performs test according to accepted guidelines** | | Y | N | Y | N | Y | N |
| Maintains relaxation of the limb | | O | O | O | O | O | O |
| Moves distal bone medially, attempting to open the joint on the lateral side | | O | O | O | O | O | O |
| Performs assessment bilaterally | | O | O | O | O | O | O |
| **Identifies positive findings and implications** | | Y | N | Y | N | Y | N |
| Pain or increased laxity when compared bilaterally | | O | O | O | O | O | O |
| LCL sprain or avulsion fracture | | O | O | O | O | O | O |
| **Total** | | /9 | | /9 | | /9 | |
| **Must achieve >6 to pass this examination** | | P | F | P | F | P | F |

| Assessor: Date: | Test 1 Comments: |
|---|---|
| Assessor: Date: | Test 2 Comments: |
| Assessor: Date: | Test 3 Comments: |

**TEST ENVIRONMENTS**
**L:** Laboratory/Classroom
**C:** Clinical/Field Testing
**P:** Practicum
**A:** Assessment/Mock Exam

**TEST INFORMATION**
**Test Statistics:** No data available
**Reference(s):** Starkey & Brown (2015)

MUSCULOSKELETAL SYSTEM—REGION 1: FOOT AND TOES

# JOINT PLAY (ARTHROKINEMATICS)

| NATA EC 5th | BOC RD6 | SKILL |
|---|---|---|
| CE-21f | D2-0203 | Intermetatarsal Glide Assessment |

**Supplies Needed:** Table

*This problem allows you the opportunity to demonstrate an* **orthopedic test** *known as the* **intermetatarsal glide assessment**. *You have 2 minutes to complete this task.*

| Intermetatarsal Glide Assessment | Course or Site Assessor Environment | | Test 1 | | Test 2 | | Test 3 | |
|---|---|---|---|---|---|---|---|---|
| | | | Y | N | Y | N | Y | N |
| **Tester places patient and limb in appropriate position** | | | Y | N | Y | N | Y | N |
| Supine or seated on table with knees extended | | | ○ | ○ | ○ | ○ | ○ | ○ |
| **Tester placed in proper position** | | | Y | N | Y | N | Y | N |
| Grasps the first metatarsal head with one hand | | | ○ | ○ | ○ | ○ | ○ | ○ |
| Grasps the second metatarsal head with the other hand | | | ○ | ○ | ○ | ○ | ○ | ○ |
| **Tester performs test according to accepted guidelines** | | | Y | N | Y | N | Y | N |
| Stabilizes one metatarsal head | | | ○ | ○ | ○ | ○ | ○ | ○ |
| Applies force to move the second metatarsal head in a plantar and dorsal direction | | | ○ | ○ | ○ | ○ | ○ | ○ |
| Repeats procedure until all intermetatarsal joints are evaluated | | | ○ | ○ | ○ | ○ | ○ | ○ |
| **Identifies positive findings and implications** | | | Y | N | Y | N | Y | N |
| Pain or increased glide or decreased glide compared with the opposite extremity | | | ○ | ○ | ○ | ○ | ○ | ○ |
| Trauma to or adhesions in the deep transverse metatarsal ligament, interosseous ligament, or both | | | ○ | ○ | ○ | ○ | ○ | ○ |
| Total | | | __/8 | | __/8 | | __/8 | |
| **Must achieve >5 to pass this examination** | | | Ⓟ | Ⓕ | Ⓟ | Ⓕ | Ⓟ | Ⓕ |

| Assessor: Date: | Test 1 Comments: |
|---|---|
| Assessor: Date: | Test 2 Comments: |
| Assessor: Date: | Test 3 Comments: |

**TEST ENVIRONMENTS**
**L:** Laboratory/Classroom
**C:** Clinical/Field Testing
**P:** Practicum
**A:** Assessment/Mock Exam

**TEST INFORMATION**
**Test Statistics:** No data available
**Reference(s):** Starkey & Brown (2015)

## MUSCULOSKELETAL SYSTEM—REGION 1: FOOT AND TOES
# JOINT PLAY (ARTHROKINEMATICS)

| NATA EC 5th | BOC RD6 | SKILL |
|---|---|---|
| CE-21f | D2-0203 | Midtarsal Joint Play |

**Supplies Needed:** Table

*This problem allows you the opportunity to demonstrate an* **orthopedic test** *known as* **midtarsal joint play.** *You have 2 minutes to complete this task.*

| Midtarsal Joint Play | Course or Site<br>Assessor<br>Environment | | Test 1 | | Test 2 | | Test 3 | |
|---|---|---|---|---|---|---|---|---|
| **Tester places patient and limb in appropriate position** | | Y | N | Y | N | Y | N | |
| Supine or seated | | ○ | ○ | ○ | ○ | ○ | ○ | |
| Knee flexed and the heel stabilized by the edge of the table | | ○ | ○ | ○ | ○ | ○ | ○ | |
| **Tester placed in proper position** | | Y | N | Y | N | Y | N | |
| Grasps the plantar and dorsal aspect of one tarsal with one hand | | ○ | ○ | ○ | ○ | ○ | ○ | |
| Grasps the adjacent tarsal in a similar manner with the other hand | | ○ | ○ | ○ | ○ | ○ | ○ | |
| **Tester performs test according to accepted guidelines** | | Y | N | Y | N | Y | N | |
| Stabilizes one tarsal | | ○ | ○ | ○ | ○ | ○ | ○ | |
| Applies force to move the second tarsal head in a plantar and dorsal direction | | ○ | ○ | ○ | ○ | ○ | ○ | |
| Repeats for each tarsal | | ○ | ○ | ○ | ○ | ○ | ○ | |
| **Identifies positive findings and implications** | | Y | N | Y | N | Y | N | |
| Pain or increased or decreased glide with movement | | ○ | ○ | ○ | ○ | ○ | ○ | |
| Increased glide: ligamentous laxity; decreased glide: joint adhesions or articular changes causing coalition of the joint | | ○ | ○ | ○ | ○ | ○ | ○ | |
| **Total** | | ___/9 | | ___/9 | | ___/9 | | |
| **Must achieve >6 to pass this examination** | | ℗ | Ⓕ | ℗ | Ⓕ | ℗ | Ⓕ | |

| Assessor:<br>Date: | Test 1 Comments: |
|---|---|
| Assessor:<br>Date: | Test 2 Comments: |
| Assessor:<br>Date: | Test 3 Comments: |

**TEST ENVIRONMENTS**
**L:** Laboratory/Classroom
**C:** Clinical/Field Testing
**P:** Practicum
**A:** Assessment/Mock Exam

**TEST INFORMATION**
**Test Statistics:** No data available
**Reference(s):** Starkey & Brown (2015)

## MUSCULOSKELETAL SYSTEM—REGION 1: FOOT AND TOES
# JOINT PLAY (ARTHROKINEMATICS)

| NATA EC 5th | BOC RD6 | SKILL |
|---|---|---|
| CE-21f | D2-0203 | Tarsometatarsal Joint Play |

**Supplies Needed:** Table

*This problem allows you the opportunity to demonstrate an* **orthopedic test** *known as* **tarsometatarsal joint play.** *You have 2 minutes to complete this task.*

| Tarsometatarsal Joint Play | Course or Site Assessor Environment | | | | | |
|---|---|---|---|---|---|---|
| | Test 1 | | Test 2 | | Test 3 | |
| **Tester places patient and limb in appropriate position** | Y | N | Y | N | Y | N |
| Supine or seated – foot in pronation | O | O | O | O | O | O |
| Knee flexed and heel stabilized by the edge of the table | O | O | O | O | O | O |
| **Tester placed in proper position** | Y | N | Y | N | Y | N |
| Grasps the proximal tarsal on the plantar and dorsal surfaces with one hand | O | O | O | O | O | O |
| Grasps the adjacent metatarsal in a similar manner with the second hand | O | O | O | O | O | O |
| **Tester performs test according to accepted guidelines** | Y | N | Y | N | Y | N |
| Stabilizes the tarsal | O | O | O | O | O | O |
| Applies force to move the metatarsal in a plantar and dorsal direction | O | O | O | O | O | O |
| Repeats for each joint | O | O | O | O | O | O |
| **Identifies positive findings and implications** | Y | N | Y | N | Y | N |
| Pain or increased or decreased glide with movement | O | O | O | O | O | O |
| Increased glide: ligamentous laxity; decreased glide: joint adhesions or articular changes causing coalition of the joint | O | O | O | O | O | O |
| **Total** | ___/9 | | ___/9 | | ___/9 | |
| **Must achieve >6 to pass this examination** | Ⓟ | Ⓕ | Ⓟ | Ⓕ | Ⓟ | Ⓕ |

| Assessor: Date: | Test 1 Comments: |
|---|---|
| Assessor: Date: | Test 2 Comments: |
| Assessor: Date: | Test 3 Comments: |

**TEST ENVIRONMENTS**
**L:** Laboratory/Classroom
**C:** Clinical/Field Testing
**P:** Practicum
**A:** Assessment/Mock Exam

**TEST INFORMATION**
**Test Statistics:** No data available
**Reference(s):** Starkey & Brown (2015)

## MUSCULOSKELETAL SYSTEM—REGION 1: FOOT AND TOES
# SPECIAL TESTS

| NATA EC 5th | BOC RD6 | SKILL |
|---|---|---|
| CE-21g, CE-20e | D2-0203 | Dorsiflexion-Eversion Test |

**Supplies Needed:** Table

*This problem allows you the opportunity to demonstrate an* **orthopedic test** *known as the* **dorsiflexion-eversion test** *to rule out* **tarsal tunnel syndrome**. *You have 2 minutes to complete this task.*

| Dorsiflexion-Eversion Test | Course or Site Assessor Environment | | Test 1 | | Test 2 | | Test 3 | |
|---|---|---|---|---|---|---|---|---|
| **Tester places patient and limb in appropriate position** | | | Y | N | Y | N | Y | N |
| Seated with the legs off the table | | | O | O | O | O | O | O |
| **Tester placed in proper position** | | | Y | N | Y | N | Y | N |
| Stands at the patient's feet | | | O | O | O | O | O | O |
| Cups the calcaneus with one hand | | | O | O | O | O | O | O |
| Grasps the distal foot (palm on plantar aspect) with the other hand | | | O | O | O | O | O | O |
| **Tester performs test according to accepted guidelines** | | | Y | N | Y | N | Y | N |
| Passively everts the heel (holds position for 5 seconds) | | | O | O | O | O | O | O |
| Passively dorsiflexes the foot and toes (holds position for 5 seconds) | | | O | O | O | O | O | O |
| Performs assessment bilaterally | | | O | O | O | O | O | O |
| **Identifies positive findings and implications** | | | Y | N | Y | N | Y | N |
| Provocation of pain and/or paresthesia radiating into the foot | | | O | O | O | O | O | O |
| Posterior tibial nerve dysfunction | | | O | O | O | O | O | O |
| | | Total | \_\_\_\_/9 | | \_\_\_\_/9 | | \_\_\_\_/9 | |
| | Must achieve >6 to pass this examination | | Ⓟ | Ⓕ | Ⓟ | Ⓕ | Ⓟ | Ⓕ |

| Assessor:<br>Date: | Test 1 Comments: |
|---|---|
| Assessor:<br>Date: | Test 2 Comments: |
| Assessor:<br>Date: | Test 3 Comments: |

**TEST ENVIRONMENTS**
**L:** Laboratory/Classroom
**C:** Clinical/Field Testing
**P:** Practicum
**A:** Assessment/Mock Exam

**TEST INFORMATION**
**Test Statistics:** No data available
**Reference(s):** Starkey & Brown (2015)

## MUSCULOSKELETAL SYSTEM—REGION 1: FOOT AND TOES
# SPECIAL TESTS

| NATA EC 5th | BOC RD6 | SKILL |
|---|---|---|
| CE-21g, CE-20e | D2-0203 | Long Bone Compression Test |

**Supplies Needed:** Table

*This problem allows you the opportunity to demonstrate an* **orthopedic test** *known as the* **long bone compression test**. *You have 2 minutes to complete this task.*

| Long Bone Compression Test | Course or Site Assessor Environment | Test 1 | | Test 2 | | Test 3 | |
|---|---|---|---|---|---|---|---|
| **Tester places patient and limb in appropriate position** | | **Y** | **N** | **Y** | **N** | **Y** | **N** |
| Supine with foot on the table | | ○ | ○ | ○ | ○ | ○ | ○ |
| Heel stabilized by the table | | ○ | ○ | ○ | ○ | ○ | ○ |
| **Tester placed in proper position** | | **Y** | **N** | **Y** | **N** | **Y** | **N** |
| Stands to the side of the patient | | ○ | ○ | ○ | ○ | ○ | ○ |
| One hand stabilizes the bone proximal to the suspected fracture | | ○ | ○ | ○ | ○ | ○ | ○ |
| Places other hand on the bone distal to the suspected fracture | | ○ | ○ | ○ | ○ | ○ | ○ |
| **Tester performs test according to accepted guidelines** | | **Y** | **N** | **Y** | **N** | **Y** | **N** |
| Hand distal to the suspected fracture applies a longitudinally directed force to the long bone | | ○ | ○ | ○ | ○ | ○ | ○ |
| Performs assessment bilaterally | | ○ | ○ | ○ | ○ | ○ | ○ |
| **Identifies positive findings and implications** | | **Y** | **N** | **Y** | **N** | **Y** | **N** |
| Pain in the area of the suspected fracture | | ○ | ○ | ○ | ○ | ○ | ○ |
| Possible fracture | | ○ | ○ | ○ | ○ | ○ | ○ |
| Total | | ___/9 | | ___/9 | | ___/9 | |
| Must achieve >6 to pass this examination | | Ⓟ | Ⓕ | Ⓟ | Ⓕ | Ⓟ | Ⓕ |

| Assessor:
Date: | Test 1 Comments: |
|---|---|
| Assessor:
Date: | Test 2 Comments: |
| Assessor:
Date: | Test 3 Comments: |

**TEST ENVIRONMENTS**
**L:** Laboratory/Classroom
**C:** Clinical/Field Testing
**P:** Practicum
**A:** Assessment/Mock Exam

**TEST INFORMATION**
**Test Statistics:** No data available
**Reference(s):** Konin et al. (2016)
Starkey & Brown (2015)

## MUSCULOSKELETAL SYSTEM—REGION 1: FOOT AND TOES
# SPECIAL TESTS

| NATA EC 5th | BOC RD6 | SKILL |
|---|---|---|
| CE-21g, CE-20e | D2-0203 | Mulder Sign for Intermetatarsal Neuroma |

**Supplies Needed:** Table

*This problem allows you the opportunity to demonstrate an* **orthopedic test** *known as the* **Mulder sign for intermetatarsal neuroma**. *You have 2 minutes to complete this task.*

| Mulder Sign for Intermetatarsal Neuroma | Course or Site Assessor Environment | | | | | | |
|---|---|---|---|---|---|---|---|
| | | Test 1 | | Test 2 | | Test 3 | |
| **Tester places patient and limb in appropriate position** | | Y | N | Y | N | Y | N |
| Long or short sitting on table | | O | O | O | O | O | O |
| **Tester placed in proper position** | | Y | N | Y | N | Y | N |
| Stands at the patient's feet | | O | O | O | O | O | O |
| Places one hand along the distal fifth metatarsal | | O | O | O | O | O | O |
| Places the other hand along the distal first metatarsal | | O | O | O | O | O | O |
| **Tester performs test according to accepted guidelines** | | Y | N | Y | N | Y | N |
| Applies pressure to compress the transverse arch | | O | O | O | O | O | O |
| Uses the thumb and forefinger to apply pressure over the symptomatic interspace between the metatarsals | | O | O | O | O | O | O |
| Performs assessment bilaterally | | O | O | O | O | O | O |
| **Identifies positive findings and implications** | | Y | N | Y | N | Y | N |
| A click, pain, or reproduction of symptoms | | O | O | O | O | O | O |
| Intermetatarsal neuroma | | O | O | O | O | O | O |
| Total | | ___/9 | | ___/9 | | ___/9 | |
| Must achieve >6 to pass this examination | | P | F | P | F | P | F |

| Assessor: Date: | Test 1 Comments: |
|---|---|
| Assessor: Date: | Test 2 Comments: |
| Assessor: Date: | Test 3 Comments: |

**TEST ENVIRONMENTS**
**L:** Laboratory/Classroom
**C:** Clinical/Field Testing
**P:** Practicum
**A:** Assessment/Mock Exam

**TEST INFORMATION**
**Test Statistics:** No data available
**Reference(s):** Starkey & Brown (2015)

## MUSCULOSKELETAL SYSTEM—REGION 1: FOOT AND TOES
# SPECIAL TESTS

| NATA EC 5th | BOC RD6 | SKILL |
|---|---|---|
| CE-21g, CE-20e | D2-0203 | Navicular Drop Test |

**Supplies Needed:** Table

*This problem allows you the opportunity to demonstrate an* **orthopedic test** *known as the* **navicular drop test**. *You have 2 minutes to complete this task.*

| Navicular Drop Test | Course or Site Assessor Environment | | Test 1 | | Test 2 | | Test 3 | |
|---|---|---|---|---|---|---|---|---|
| | | | Y | N | Y | N | Y | N |
| **Tester places patient and limb in appropriate position** | | | Y | N | Y | N | Y | N |
| Seated with both feet on a noncarpeted floor | | | ○ | ○ | ○ | ○ | ○ | ○ |
| Subtalar joint is placed in a neutral position with the patient's foot flat against the ground but nonweightbearing | | | ○ | ○ | ○ | ○ | ○ | ○ |
| **Tester placed in proper position** | | | Y | N | Y | N | Y | N |
| Kneels in front of the patient | | | ○ | ○ | ○ | ○ | ○ | ○ |
| Places a dot over the patient's navicular tuberosity | | | ○ | ○ | ○ | ○ | ○ | ○ |
| **Tester performs test according to accepted guidelines** | | | Y | N | Y | N | Y | N |
| While foot is in contact with ground but nonweightbearing, an index card is positioned next to the medial longitudinal arch. A mark is made on the card corresponding to the level of the navicular tuberosity. | | | ○ | ○ | ○ | ○ | ○ | ○ |
| The patient stands with body weight evenly distributed. Foot is allowed to relax into pronation. New level of navicular is identified and marked on note card. | | | ○ | ○ | ○ | ○ | ○ | ○ |
| **Identifies positive findings and implications** | | | Y | N | Y | N | Y | N |
| The navicular drops greater than 10 mm | | | ○ | ○ | ○ | ○ | ○ | ○ |
| Excessive pronation | | | ○ | ○ | ○ | ○ | ○ | ○ |
| **Total** | | | __/8 | | __/8 | | __/8 | |
| **Must achieve >5 to pass this examination** | | | Ⓟ | Ⓕ | Ⓟ | Ⓕ | Ⓟ | Ⓕ |

| Assessor: Date: | Test 1 Comments: |
|---|---|
| Assessor: Date: | Test 2 Comments: |
| Assessor: Date: | Test 3 Comments: |

**TEST ENVIRONMENTS**
**L:** Laboratory/Classroom
**C:** Clinical/Field Testing
**P:** Practicum
**A:** Assessment/Mock Exam

**TEST INFORMATION**
**Test Statistics:** No data available
**Reference(s):** Starkey & Brown (2015)

## MUSCULOSKELETAL SYSTEM—REGION 1: FOOT AND TOES
# SPECIAL TESTS

| NATA EC 5th | BOC RD6 | SKILL |
|---|---|---|
| CE-21g, CE-20e | D2-0203 | Test for Supple Pes Planus (Windlass Test) |

**Supplies Needed:** Table

*This problem allows you the opportunity to demonstrate an* **orthopedic test** *known as the* **test for supple pes planus (Windlass test)**. *You have 2 minutes to complete this task.*

| Test for Supple Pes Planus (Windlass Test) | Course or Site _____ Assessor _____ Environment _____ | | | | | |
|---|---|---|---|---|---|---|
| | | Test 1 | | Test 2 | | Test 3 |
| **Tester places patient and limb in appropriate position** | | Y | N | Y | N | Y | N |
| Seated on the edge of the table | | ○ | ○ | ○ | ○ | ○ | ○ |
| **Tester placed in proper position** | | Y | N | Y | N | Y | N |
| Positioned at the patient's foot | | ○ | ○ | ○ | ○ | ○ | ○ |
| **Tester performs test according to accepted guidelines** | | Y | N | Y | N | Y | N |
| With the patient in a nonweightbearing position, the tester notes the presence of a medial longitudinal arch | | ○ | ○ | ○ | ○ | ○ | ○ |
| Instructs the patient to stand so body weight is evenly distributed | | ○ | ○ | ○ | ○ | ○ | ○ |
| Instructs the patient to perform a single-leg heel raise on the limb being tested | | ○ | ○ | ○ | ○ | ○ | ○ |
| **Identifies positive findings and implications** | | Y | N | Y | N | Y | N |
| If the presence of a medial arch when nonweightbearing disappears when weightbearing, the Windlass test is positive if pain reproduced during single-leg heel raise | | ○ | ○ | ○ | ○ | ○ | ○ |
| If medial arch disappears when weightbearing, a supple pes planus is present | | ○ | ○ | ○ | ○ | ○ | ○ |
| If no arch is present when nonweightbearing, a rigid pes planus is present | | ○ | ○ | ○ | ○ | ○ | ○ |
| Windlass test: Pain during the single-leg heel raise is indicative of plantar fasciitis | | ○ | ○ | ○ | ○ | ○ | ○ |
| **Total** | | ___/9 | | ___/9 | | ___/9 | |
| **Must achieve >6 to pass this examination** | | Ⓟ | Ⓕ | Ⓟ | Ⓕ | Ⓟ | Ⓕ |
| **Assessor:** **Date:** | **Test 1 Comments:** | | | | | | |
| **Assessor:** **Date:** | **Test 2 Comments:** | | | | | | |
| **Assessor:** **Date:** | **Test 3 Comments:** | | | | | | |

**TEST ENVIRONMENTS**
**L:** Laboratory/Classroom
**C:** Clinical/Field Testing
**P:** Practicum
**A:** Assessment/Mock Exam

**TEST INFORMATION**
**Test Statistics:** Sensitivity .24
Specificity 1.00
**Reference(s):** Starkey & Brown (2015)

# 5

# MUSCULOSKELETAL SYSTEM— REGION 2: ANKLE AND LOWER LEG

Hauth, J. M., Gloyeske, B. M., & Amato, H. K.
*Clinical Skills Documentation Guide for Athletic Training, Third Edition* (pp. 92-116).
© 2016 SLACK Incorporated.

## MUSCULOSKELETAL SYSTEM—REGION 2: ANKLE AND LOWER LEG
# KNOWLEDGE AND SKILLS

| NATA EC 5th | BOC RD6 | Musculoskeletal System—Region 2: Ankle and Lower Leg | | *Skill: Acquisition, Reinforcement, Proficiency* | | |
|---|---|---|---|---|---|---|
| **NATA EC 5th** | **BOC RD6** | **Palpation** | **Page #** | | | |
| CE-21b, CE-20c | D2-0202 | Palpation: Ankle and Lower Leg – 01 | 94 | | | |
| CE-21b, CE-20c | D2-0202 | Palpation: Ankle and Lower Leg – 02 | 95 | | | |
| CE-21b, CE-20c | D2-0202 | Palpation: Ankle and Lower Leg – 03 | 96 | | | |
| **NATA EC 5th** | **BOC RD6** | **Manual Muscle Testing** | **Page #** | | | |
| CE-21c | D2-0203 | MMT: Gastrocnemius | 97 | | | |
| CE-21c | D2-0203 | MMT: Peroneus Longus/Brevis | 98 | | | |
| CE-21c | D2-0203 | MMT: Peroneus Tertius | 99 | | | |
| CE-21c | D2-0203 | MMT: Soleus | 100 | | | |
| CE-21c | D2-0203 | MMT: Tibialis Anterior | 101 | | | |
| CE-21c | D2-0203 | MMT: Tibialis Posterior | 102 | | | |
| **NATA EC 5th** | **BOC RD6** | **Osteokinematic Joint Motion** | **Page #** | | | |
| CE-21d | D2-0203 | Goniometric Assessment: Subtalar Joint (Inversion/Eversion) | 103 | | | |
| CE-21d | D2-0203 | Goniometric Assessment: Talocrural Joint (Plantar Flexion/Dorsiflexion) | 104 | | | |
| **NATA EC 5th** | **BOC RD6** | **Capsular and Ligamentous Stress Testing** | **Page #** | | | |
| CE-21e | D2-0203 | Anterior Drawer Test for the Ankle | 105 | | | |
| CE-21e | D2-0203 | Cotton Test (Lateral Talar Glide Test) | 106 | | | |
| CE-21e | D2-0203 | Kleiger Test (External Rotation Test) | 107 | | | |
| CE-21e | D2-0203 | Talar Tilt (Eversion Stress Test) | 108 | | | |
| CE-21e | D2-0203 | Talar Tilt (Inversion Stress Test) | 109 | | | |
| **NATA EC 5th** | **BOC RD6** | **Joint Play (Arthrokinematics)** | **Page #** | | | |
| CE-21f | D2-0203 | Subtalar Joint Play | 110 | | | |
| CE-21f | D2-0203 | Distal Tibiofibular Joint Play | 111 | | | |
| **NATA EC 5th** | **BOC RD6** | **Special Tests** | **Page #** | | | |
| CE-21g, CE-20e | D2-0203 | Bump Test for Leg Stress Fractures | 112 | | | |
| CE-21g, CE-20e | D2-0203 | Compression Test (Squeeze Test) | 113 | | | |
| CE-21g, CE-20e | D2-0203 | Homans' Sign | 114 | | | |
| CE-21g, CE-20e | D2-0203 | Thompson's Test (Simmonds' Test) | 115 | | | |
| CE-21g, CE-20e | D2-0203 | Tinel's Sign | 116 | | | |

## MUSCULOSKELETAL SYSTEM—REGION 2: ANKLE AND LOWER LEG
# PALPATION

| NATA EC 5th | BOC RD6 | SKILL |
|---|---|---|
| CE-21b, CE-20c | D2-0202 | Palpation: Ankle and Lower Leg – 01 |

**Supplies Needed:** Table

*This problem allows you the opportunity to demonstrate your ability to* **palpate** *the* **ankle and lower leg.** *You have 2 minutes to complete this task.*

| Palpation: Ankle and Lower Leg – 01 | Course or Site Assessor Environment | Test 1 | | Test 2 | | Test 3 | |
|---|---|---|---|---|---|---|---|
| | | Y | N | Y | N | Y | N |
| Anterior tibiofibular ligament | | ○ | ○ | ○ | ○ | ○ | ○ |
| Posterior talofibular ligament | | ○ | ○ | ○ | ○ | ○ | ○ |
| Posterior medial tibial shaft | | ○ | ○ | ○ | ○ | ○ | ○ |
| Base of the fifth metatarsal | | ○ | ○ | ○ | ○ | ○ | ○ |
| Inferior peroneal retinaculum | | ○ | ○ | ○ | ○ | ○ | ○ |
| Lateral malleolus | | ○ | ○ | ○ | ○ | ○ | ○ |
| Extensor hallucis longus | | ○ | ○ | ○ | ○ | ○ | ○ |
| Total | | ___/7 | | ___/7 | | ___/7 | |
| Must achieve >4 to pass this examination | | Ⓟ | Ⓕ | Ⓟ | Ⓕ | Ⓟ | Ⓕ |

| Assessor: Date: | Test 1 Comments: |
|---|---|
| Assessor: Date: | Test 2 Comments: |
| Assessor: Date: | Test 3 Comments: |

**TEST ENVIRONMENTS**
**L:** Laboratory/Classroom
**C:** Clinical/Field Testing
**P:** Practicum
**A:** Assessment/Mock Exam

**TEST INFORMATION**
**Test Statistics:** N/A
**Reference(s):**  Starkey & Brown (2015)

## MUSCULOSKELETAL SYSTEM—REGION 2: ANKLE AND LOWER LEG
# PALPATION

| NATA EC 5th | BOC RD6 | SKILL |
|---|---|---|
| CE-21b, CE-20c | D2-0202 | Palpation: Ankle and Lower Leg – 02 |

**Supplies Needed:** Table

*This problem allows you the opportunity to demonstrate your ability to* **palpate** *the* **ankle and lower leg**. *You have 2 minutes to complete this task.*

| Palpation: Ankle and Lower Leg – 02 | Course or Site Assessor Environment | | | | | |
|---|---|---|---|---|---|---|
| | | Test 1 | | Test 2 | | Test 3 |
| | | Y | N | Y | N | Y | N |
| Posterior tibiofibular ligament | | ○ | ○ | ○ | ○ | ○ | ○ |
| Anterior talofibular ligament | | ○ | ○ | ○ | ○ | ○ | ○ |
| Anterior tibial shaft | | ○ | ○ | ○ | ○ | ○ | ○ |
| Extensor retinacula | | ○ | ○ | ○ | ○ | ○ | ○ |
| Sinus tarsi | | ○ | ○ | ○ | ○ | ○ | ○ |
| Deltoid ligament | | ○ | ○ | ○ | ○ | ○ | ○ |
| Tibialis anterior | | ○ | ○ | ○ | ○ | ○ | ○ |
| **Total** | | ___/7 | | ___/7 | | ___/7 | |
| **Must achieve >4 to pass this examination** | | Ⓟ | Ⓕ | Ⓟ | Ⓕ | Ⓟ | Ⓕ |
| **Assessor:** **Date:** | **Test 1 Comments:** | | | | | | |
| **Assessor:** **Date:** | **Test 2 Comments:** | | | | | | |
| **Assessor:** **Date:** | **Test 3 Comments:** | | | | | | |

**TEST ENVIRONMENTS**
**L:** Laboratory/Classroom
**C:** Clinical/Field Testing
**P:** Practicum
**A:** Assessment/Mock Exam

**TEST INFORMATION**
**Test Statistics:** N/A
**Reference(s):** Starkey & Brown (2015)

## MUSCULOSKELETAL SYSTEM—REGION 2: ANKLE AND LOWER LEG
# PALPATION

| NATA EC 5th | BOC RD6 | SKILL |
|---|---|---|
| CE-21b, CE-20c | D2-0202 | Palpation: Ankle and Lower Leg – 03 |

**Supplies Needed:** Table

*This problem allows you the opportunity to demonstrate your ability to* **palpate** *the* **ankle and lower leg**. *You have 2 minutes to complete this task.*

| Palpation: Ankle and Lower Leg – 03 | Course or Site Assessor Environment | | Test 1 | | Test 2 | | Test 3 | |
|---|---|---|---|---|---|---|---|---|
| | | | Y | N | Y | N | Y | N |
| Subtendinous calcaneal bursa | | | ○ | ○ | ○ | ○ | ○ | ○ |
| Calcaneofibular ligament | | | ○ | ○ | ○ | ○ | ○ | ○ |
| Fibular shat | | | ○ | ○ | ○ | ○ | ○ | ○ |
| Gastrocnemius-soleus complex | | | ○ | ○ | ○ | ○ | ○ | ○ |
| Posterior tibial pulse | | | ○ | ○ | ○ | ○ | ○ | ○ |
| Dome of the talus | | | ○ | ○ | ○ | ○ | ○ | ○ |
| Medial malleolus | | | ○ | ○ | ○ | ○ | ○ | ○ |
| **Total** | | | __/7 | | __/7 | | __/7 | |
| **Must achieve >4 to pass this examination** | | | Ⓟ | Ⓕ | Ⓟ | Ⓕ | Ⓟ | Ⓕ |
| **Assessor:** **Date:** | **Test 1 Comments:** | | | | | | | |
| **Assessor:** **Date:** | **Test 2 Comments:** | | | | | | | |
| **Assessor:** **Date:** | **Test 3 Comments:** | | | | | | | |

**TEST ENVIRONMENTS**
**L:** Laboratory/Classroom
**C:** Clinical/Field Testing
**P:** Practicum
**A:** Assessment/Mock Exam

**TEST INFORMATION**
**Test Statistics:** N/A
**Reference(s):** Starkey & Brown (2015)

## MUSCULOSKELETAL SYSTEM—REGION 2: ANKLE AND LOWER LEG
# MANUAL MUSCLE TESTING

| NATA EC 5th | BOC RD6 | SKILL |
|---|---|---|
| CE-21c | D2-0203 | MMT: Gastrocnemius |

**Supplies Needed:** Table

*This problem allows you the opportunity to demonstrate a* **manual muscle test** *for the* **gastrocnemius.** *You have 2 minutes to complete this task.*

| MMT: Gastrocnemius | Course or Site Assessor Environment | | Test 1 | | Test 2 | | Test 3 | |
|---|---|---|---|---|---|---|---|---|
| **Tester places patient and limb in appropriate position** | | Y | N | Y | N | Y | N |
| Prone, knee extended (ankle off edge of table) | | ○ | ○ | ○ | ○ | ○ | ○ |
| **Tester placed in proper position** | | Y | N | Y | N | Y | N |
| Stabilizes the leg just above the ankle joint (to prevent knee flexion) | | ○ | ○ | ○ | ○ | ○ | ○ |
| **Tester performs test according to accepted guidelines** | | Y | N | Y | N | Y | N |
| Instructs the patient to actively plantar flex the foot | | ○ | ○ | ○ | ○ | ○ | ○ |
| Applies resistance to the plantar surface of metatarsals (direction of dorsiflexion) | | ○ | ○ | ○ | ○ | ○ | ○ |
| Holds resistance for 5 seconds | | ○ | ○ | ○ | ○ | ○ | ○ |
| Performs assessment bilaterally | | ○ | ○ | ○ | ○ | ○ | ○ |
| **Identifies implications** | | Y | N | Y | N | Y | N |
| Correctly grades the MMT | | ○ | ○ | ○ | ○ | ○ | ○ |
| | Total | ___/7 | | ___/7 | | ___/7 | |
| | Must achieve >4 to pass this examination | Ⓟ | Ⓕ | Ⓟ | Ⓕ | Ⓟ | Ⓕ |

| Assessor: Date: | Test 1 Comments: |
|---|---|
| Assessor: Date: | Test 2 Comments: |
| Assessor: Date: | Test 3 Comments: |

**TEST ENVIRONMENTS**
**L:** Laboratory/Classroom
**C:** Clinical/Field Testing
**P:** Practicum
**A:** Assessment/Mock Exam

**TEST INFORMATION**
**Test Statistics:** N/A
**Reference(s):** Kendall et al. (2005)

## MUSCULOSKELETAL SYSTEM—REGION 2: ANKLE AND LOWER LEG
# MANUAL MUSCLE TESTING

| NATA EC 5th | BOC RD6 | SKILL |
|---|---|---|
| CE-21c | D2-0203 | MMT: Peroneus Longus/Brevis |

**Supplies Needed:** Table

*This problem allows you the opportunity to demonstrate a* **manual muscle test** *for the* **peroneus longus/brevis muscles***. You have 2 minutes to complete this task.*

| MMT: Peroneus Longus/Brevis | Course or Site<br>Assessor<br>Environment | | | | | |
|---|---|---|---|---|---|---|
| | | Test 1 | | Test 2 | | Test 3 | |
| | | Y | N | Y | N | Y | N |
| **Tester places patient and limb in appropriate position** | | Y | N | Y | N | Y | N |
| Supine or side lying (lower leg internally rotated) | | ○ | ○ | ○ | ○ | ○ | ○ |
| **Tester placed in proper position** | | Y | N | Y | N | Y | N |
| Stabilizes the leg just above the ankle joint | | ○ | ○ | ○ | ○ | ○ | ○ |
| **Tester performs test according to accepted guidelines** | | Y | N | Y | N | Y | N |
| Instructs the patient to actively evert the foot | | ○ | ○ | ○ | ○ | ○ | ○ |
| Applies resistance to the lateral aspect of metatarsals (direction of inversion and dorsiflexion) | | ○ | ○ | ○ | ○ | ○ | ○ |
| Holds resistance for 5 seconds | | ○ | ○ | ○ | ○ | ○ | ○ |
| Performs assessment bilaterally | | ○ | ○ | ○ | ○ | ○ | ○ |
| **Identifies implications** | | Y | N | Y | N | Y | N |
| Correctly grades the MMT | | ○ | ○ | ○ | ○ | ○ | ○ |
| Total | | ___/7 | | ___/7 | | ___/7 | |
| Must achieve >4 to pass this examination | | Ⓟ | Ⓕ | Ⓟ | Ⓕ | Ⓟ | Ⓕ |

| Assessor:<br>Date: | Test 1 Comments: |
|---|---|
| Assessor:<br>Date: | Test 2 Comments: |
| Assessor:<br>Date: | Test 3 Comments: |

**TEST ENVIRONMENTS**
**L:** Laboratory/Classroom
**C:** Clinical/Field Testing
**P:** Practicum
**A:** Assessment/Mock Exam

**TEST INFORMATION**
**Test Statistics:** N/A
**Reference(s):** Kendall et al. (2005)

## MUSCULOSKELETAL SYSTEM—REGION 2: ANKLE AND LOWER LEG
# MANUAL MUSCLE TESTING

| NATA EC 5th | BOC RD6 | SKILL |
|---|---|---|
| CE-21c | D2-0203 | MMT: Peroneus Tertius |

**Supplies Needed:** Table

*This problem allows you the opportunity to demonstrate a* **manual muscle test** *for the* **peroneus tertius muscle**. *You have 2 minutes to complete this task.*

| MMT: Peroneus Tertius | Course or Site Assessor Environment | Test 1 | | Test 2 | | Test 3 | |
|---|---|---|---|---|---|---|---|
| | | Y | N | Y | N | Y | N |
| **Tester places patient and limb in appropriate position** | | Y | N | Y | N | Y | N |
| Supine or seated | | O | O | O | O | O | O |
| **Tester placed in proper position** | | Y | N | Y | N | Y | N |
| Supports the leg just above the ankle joint | | O | O | O | O | O | O |
| **Tester performs test according to accepted guidelines** | | Y | N | Y | N | Y | N |
| Instructs the patient to actively dorsiflex ankle and evert foot | | O | O | O | O | O | O |
| Applies resistance to the lateral dorsal surface of the foot (direction of plantar flexion and inversion) | | O | O | O | O | O | O |
| Holds resistance for 5 seconds | | O | O | O | O | O | O |
| Performs assessment bilaterally | | O | O | O | O | O | O |
| **Identifies implications** | | Y | N | Y | N | Y | N |
| Correctly grades the MMT | | O | O | O | O | O | O |
| | Total | __/7 | | __/7 | | __/7 | |
| | Must achieve >4 to pass this examination | (P) | (F) | (P) | (F) | (P) | (F) |

| Assessor: Date: | Test 1 Comments: |
|---|---|
| Assessor: Date: | Test 2 Comments: |
| Assessor: Date: | Test 3 Comments: |

**TEST ENVIRONMENTS**
**L:** Laboratory/Classroom
**C:** Clinical/Field Testing
**P:** Practicum
**A:** Assessment/Mock Exam

**TEST INFORMATION**
**Test Statistics:** N/A
**Reference(s):** Kendall et al. (2005)

## MUSCULOSKELETAL SYSTEM—REGION 2: ANKLE AND LOWER LEG
# MANUAL MUSCLE TESTING

| NATA EC 5th | BOC RD6 | SKILL |
|---|---|---|
| CE-21c | D2-0203 | MMT: Soleus |

**Supplies Needed:** Table

*This problem allows you the opportunity to demonstrate a* **manual muscle test** *for the* **soleus muscle**.
*You have 2 minutes to complete this task.*

| MMT: Soleus | Course or Site<br>Assessor<br>Environment | | Test 1 | | Test 2 | | Test 3 |
|---|---|---|---|---|---|---|---|
| | | **Y** | **N** | **Y** | **N** | **Y** | **N** |
| **Tester places patient and limb in appropriate position** | | **Y** | **N** | **Y** | **N** | **Y** | **N** |
| Prone, knee flexed to 90 degrees | | O | O | O | O | O | O |
| **Tester placed in proper position** | | **Y** | **N** | **Y** | **N** | **Y** | **N** |
| Stabilizes the leg proximal to ankle joint | | O | O | O | O | O | O |
| **Tester performs test according to accepted guidelines** | | **Y** | **N** | **Y** | **N** | **Y** | **N** |
| Instructs the patient to actively plantar flex the foot | | O | O | O | O | O | O |
| Applies resistance to the plantar surface of metatarsals (direction of dorsiflexion) | | O | O | O | O | O | O |
| Holds resistance for 5 seconds | | O | O | O | O | O | O |
| Performs assessment bilaterally | | O | O | O | O | O | O |
| **Identifies implications** | | **Y** | **N** | **Y** | **N** | **Y** | **N** |
| Correctly grades the MMT | | O | O | O | O | O | O |
| **Total** | | ___/7 | | ___/7 | | ___/7 | |
| **Must achieve >4 to pass this examination** | | Ⓟ | Ⓕ | Ⓟ | Ⓕ | Ⓟ | Ⓕ |

| Assessor:<br>Date: | Test 1 Comments: |
|---|---|
| Assessor:<br>Date: | Test 2 Comments: |
| Assessor:<br>Date: | Test 3 Comments: |

**TEST ENVIRONMENTS**
**L:** Laboratory/Classroom
**C:** Clinical/Field Testing
**P:** Practicum
**A:** Assessment/Mock Exam

**TEST INFORMATION**
**Test Statistics:** N/A
**Reference(s):** Kendall et al. (2005)

## MUSCULOSKELETAL SYSTEM—REGION 2: ANKLE AND LOWER LEG
# MANUAL MUSCLE TESTING

| NATA EC 5th | BOC RD6 | SKILL |
|---|---|---|
| CE-21c | D2-0203 | MMT: Tibialis Anterior |

**Supplies Needed:** Table

*This problem allows you the opportunity to demonstrate a* **manual muscle test** *for the* **tibialis anterior muscle**. *You have 2 minutes to complete this task.*

| MMT: Tibialis Anterior | Course or Site Assessor Environment | | Test 1 | | Test 2 | | Test 3 | |
|---|---|---|---|---|---|---|---|---|
| **Tester places patient and limb in appropriate position** | | **Y** | **N** | **Y** | **N** | **Y** | **N** |
| Supine or seated (knee flexed if gastrocnemius tightness present) | | ○ | ○ | ○ | ○ | ○ | ○ |
| **Tester placed in proper position** | | **Y** | **N** | **Y** | **N** | **Y** | **N** |
| Supports the leg just above the ankle joint | | ○ | ○ | ○ | ○ | ○ | ○ |
| **Tester performs test according to accepted guidelines** | | **Y** | **N** | **Y** | **N** | **Y** | **N** |
| Instructs the patient to actively dorsiflex the ankle joint and invert the foot (without extension of the great toe) | | ○ | ○ | ○ | ○ | ○ | ○ |
| Applies resistance to the medial dorsal surface of the foot (direction of plantar flexion and eversion) | | ○ | ○ | ○ | ○ | ○ | ○ |
| Holds resistance for 5 seconds | | ○ | ○ | ○ | ○ | ○ | ○ |
| Performs assessment bilaterally | | ○ | ○ | ○ | ○ | ○ | ○ |
| **Identifies implications** | | **Y** | **N** | **Y** | **N** | **Y** | **N** |
| Correctly grades the MMT | | ○ | ○ | ○ | ○ | ○ | ○ |
| **Total** | | ___/7 | | ___/7 | | ___/7 | |
| **Must achieve >4 to pass this examination** | | Ⓟ | Ⓕ | Ⓟ | Ⓕ | Ⓟ | Ⓕ |
| **Assessor:** **Date:** | **Test 1 Comments:** | | | | | | |
| **Assessor:** **Date:** | **Test 2 Comments:** | | | | | | |
| **Assessor:** **Date:** | **Test 3 Comments:** | | | | | | |

**TEST ENVIRONMENTS**
**L:** Laboratory/Classroom
**C:** Clinical/Field Testing
**P:** Practicum
**A:** Assessment/Mock Exam

**TEST INFORMATION**
**Test Statistics:** N/A
**Reference(s):** Kendall et al. (2005)

## MUSCULOSKELETAL SYSTEM—REGION 2: ANKLE AND LOWER LEG
# MANUAL MUSCLE TESTING

| NATA EC 5th | BOC RD6 | SKILL |
|---|---|---|
| CE-21c | D2-0203 | MMT: Tibialis Posterior |

**Supplies Needed:** Table

*This problem allows you the opportunity to demonstrate a* **manual muscle test** *for the* **tibialis posterior muscle**. *You have 2 minutes to complete this task.*

| MMT: Tibialis Posterior | Course or Site Assessor Environment | Test 1 | | Test 2 | | Test 3 | |
|---|---|---|---|---|---|---|---|
| | | Y | N | Y | N | Y | N |
| **Tester places patient and limb in appropriate position** | | **Y** | **N** | **Y** | **N** | **Y** | **N** |
| Supine or with involved extremity in lateral rotation | | ○ | ○ | ○ | ○ | ○ | ○ |
| **Tester placed in proper position** | | **Y** | **N** | **Y** | **N** | **Y** | **N** |
| Supports the leg just above the ankle joint | | ○ | ○ | ○ | ○ | ○ | ○ |
| **Tester performs test according to accepted guidelines** | | **Y** | **N** | **Y** | **N** | **Y** | **N** |
| Instructs the patient to actively invert foot and plantar flex ankle | | ○ | ○ | ○ | ○ | ○ | ○ |
| Applies resistance to the medial plantar surface of the foot (direction of dorsiflexion and eversion) | | ○ | ○ | ○ | ○ | ○ | ○ |
| Holds resistance for 5 seconds | | ○ | ○ | ○ | ○ | ○ | ○ |
| Performs assessment bilaterally | | ○ | ○ | ○ | ○ | ○ | ○ |
| **Identifies implications** | | **Y** | **N** | **Y** | **N** | **Y** | **N** |
| Correctly grades the MMT | | ○ | ○ | ○ | ○ | ○ | ○ |
| | Total | ___/7 | | ___/7 | | ___/7 | |
| | **Must achieve >4 to pass this examination** | Ⓟ | Ⓕ | Ⓟ | Ⓕ | Ⓟ | Ⓕ |
| **Assessor:** **Date:** | **Test 1 Comments:** | | | | | | |
| **Assessor:** **Date:** | **Test 2 Comments:** | | | | | | |
| **Assessor:** **Date:** | **Test 3 Comments:** | | | | | | |

**TEST ENVIRONMENTS**
**L:** Laboratory/Classroom
**C:** Clinical/Field Testing
**P:** Practicum
**A:** Assessment/Mock Exam

**TEST INFORMATION**
**Test Statistics:** N/A
**Reference(s):**   Kendall et al. (2005)

MUSCULOSKELETAL SYSTEM—REGION 2: ANKLE AND LOWER LEG
# OSTEOKINEMATIC JOINT MOTION

| NATA EC 5th | BOC RD6 | SKILL |
|---|---|---|
| CE-21d | D2-0203 | Goniometric Assessment: Subtalar Joint (Inversion/Eversion) |

**Supplies Needed:** Table, large or small goniometer

*This problem allows you the opportunity to demonstrate a* **goniometric assessment** *for the* **subtalar joint (inversion/eversion)**. *You have 2 minutes to complete this task.*

| Goniometric Assessment: Subtalar Joint (Inversion/Eversion) | Course or Site Assessor Environment | | Test 1 | | Test 2 | | Test 3 |
|---|---|---|---|---|---|---|---|
| | | Y | N | Y | N | Y | N |
| **Tester places patient and limb in appropriate position** | | Y | N | Y | N | Y | N |
| Prone with the hip and knee in neutral | | ○ | ○ | ○ | ○ | ○ | ○ |
| Ankle and lower leg off table, talocrural joint in neutral | | ○ | ○ | ○ | ○ | ○ | ○ |
| **Tester and goniometer placed in proper position** | | Y | N | Y | N | Y | N |
| Places hand over lower leg stabilizing goniometer (stationary arm in line with the Achilles tendon) | | ○ | ○ | ○ | ○ | ○ | ○ |
| Places fulcrum over Achilles tendon between malleoli | | ○ | ○ | ○ | ○ | ○ | ○ |
| Hand placed over calcaneus (moving arm in line with calcaneus) | | ○ | ○ | ○ | ○ | ○ | ○ |
| **Tester performs test according to accepted guidelines** | | Y | N | Y | N | Y | N |
| Passively inverts or everts calcaneus while maintaining neutral talocrural joint | | ○ | ○ | ○ | ○ | ○ | ○ |
| Takes proper goniometric measurement | | ○ | ○ | ○ | ○ | ○ | ○ |
| Performs assessment bilaterally | | ○ | ○ | ○ | ○ | ○ | ○ |
| **Identifies implications** | | Y | N | Y | N | Y | N |
| Identifies normal ranges (inversion = 5 degrees; eversion = 5 degrees) | | ○ | ○ | ○ | ○ | ○ | ○ |
| Total | | /9 | | /9 | | /9 | |
| Must achieve >6 to pass this examination | | Ⓟ | Ⓕ | Ⓟ | Ⓕ | Ⓟ | Ⓕ |

| Assessor: Date: | Test 1 Comments: |
|---|---|
| Assessor: Date: | Test 2 Comments: |
| Assessor: Date: | Test 3 Comments: |

**TEST ENVIRONMENTS**
**L:** Laboratory/Classroom
**C:** Clinical/Field Testing
**P:** Practicum
**A:** Assessment/Mock Exam

**TEST INFORMATION**
**Test Statistics:** N/A
**Reference(s):** Norkin & White (2009)

## MUSCULOSKELETAL SYSTEM—REGION 2: ANKLE AND LOWER LEG
# OSTEOKINEMATIC JOINT MOTION

| NATA EC 5th | BOC RD6 | SKILL |
|---|---|---|
| CE-21d | D2-0203 | Goniometric Assessment: Talocrural Joint (Plantar Flexion/Dorsiflexion) |

**Supplies Needed:** Table, large or small goniometer

*This problem allows you the opportunity to demonstrate a* **goniometric assessment** *for the* **talocrural joint (plantar flexion/dorsiflexion)**. *You have 2 minutes to complete this task.*

| Goniometric Assessment: Talocrural Joint (Plantar Flexion/Dorsiflexion) | Course or Site Assessor Environment _____ _____ _____ | | | | | |
|---|---|---|---|---|---|---|
| | | Test 1 | | Test 2 | | Test 3 |
| **Tester places patient and limb in appropriate position** | | **Y** | **N** | **Y** | **N** | **Y** | **N** |
| Seated with knee flexed to 90 degrees and foot in neutral | | O | O | O | O | O | O |
| **Tester and goniometer placed in proper position** | | **Y** | **N** | **Y** | **N** | **Y** | **N** |
| Stabilizing hand placed on posterior lower leg (stationary arm in line with fibula) | | O | O | O | O | O | O |
| Fulcrum placed at apex of lateral malleolus | | O | O | O | O | O | O |
| Moving hand cups the lateral aspect of the foot (bottom edge of moving arm in line with the fifth metatarsal) | | O | O | O | O | O | O |
| **Tester performs test according to accepted guidelines** | | **Y** | **N** | **Y** | **N** | **Y** | **N** |
| Passively plantar flex or dorsiflex the foot while maintaining subtalar neutral | | O | O | O | O | O | O |
| Takes proper goniometric measurement | | O | O | O | O | O | O |
| Performs assessment bilaterally | | O | O | O | O | O | O |
| **Identifies implications** | | **Y** | **N** | **Y** | **N** | **Y** | **N** |
| Identifies normal ranges (dorsiflexion = 20 degrees; plantar flexion = 40 to 50 degrees) | | O | O | O | O | O | O |
| Total | | ____/8 | | ____/8 | | ____/8 | |
| **Must achieve >5 to pass this examination** | | Ⓟ | Ⓕ | Ⓟ | Ⓕ | Ⓟ | Ⓕ |

| Assessor: Date: | Test 1 Comments: |
|---|---|
| Assessor: Date: | Test 2 Comments: |
| Assessor: Date: | Test 3 Comments: |

**TEST ENVIRONMENTS**
**L:** Laboratory/Classroom
**C:** Clinical/Field Testing
**P:** Practicum
**A:** Assessment/Mock Exam

**TEST INFORMATION**
**Test Statistics:** N/A
**Reference(s):** Norkin & White (2009)

# CAPSULAR AND LIGAMENTOUS STRESS TESTING

| NATA EC 5th | BOC RD6 | SKILL |
|---|---|---|
| CE-21e | D2-0203 | Anterior Drawer Test for the Ankle |

**Supplies Needed:** Table

*This problem allows you the opportunity to demonstrate an* **orthopedic test** *known as the* **anterior drawer test for the ankle***. You have 2 minutes to complete this task.*

| Anterior Drawer Test for the Ankle | Course or Site Assessor Environment | | Test 1 | | Test 2 | | Test 3 |
|---|---|---|---|---|---|---|---|
| **Tester places patient and limb in appropriate position** | | Y | N | Y | N | Y | N |
| Supine or seated with feet relaxed over edge of table | | O | O | O | O | O | O |
| Knee flexed to 90 degrees | | O | O | O | O | O | O |
| **Tester placed in proper position** | | Y | N | Y | N | Y | N |
| Stabilizes tibia and fibula with one hand | | O | O | O | O | O | O |
| Hand grasps calcaneus and holds foot in slight plantar flexion | | O | O | O | O | O | O |
| **Tester performs test according to accepted guidelines** | | Y | N | Y | N | Y | N |
| Maintains relaxation of the limb | | O | O | O | O | O | O |
| Draws talus forward (anterior displacement) on lower leg | | O | O | O | O | O | O |
| Performs assessment bilaterally | | O | O | O | O | O | O |
| **Identifies positive findings and implications** | | Y | N | Y | N | Y | N |
| Excessive anterior translation; clunk | | O | O | O | O | O | O |
| Anterior talofibular ligament sprain | | O | O | O | O | O | O |
| **Total** | | | /9 | | /9 | | /9 |
| **Must achieve >6 to pass this examination** | | P | F | P | F | P | F |

| Assessor: Date: | Test 1 Comments: |
|---|---|
| Assessor: Date: | Test 2 Comments: |
| Assessor: Date: | Test 3 Comments: |

**TEST ENVIRONMENTS**
L: Laboratory/Classroom
C: Clinical/Field Testing
P: Practicum
A: Assessment/Mock Exam

**TEST INFORMATION**
**Test Statistics:** No data available
**Reference(s):** Konin et al. (2016)

# CAPSULAR AND LIGAMENTOUS STRESS TESTING

| NATA EC 5th | BOC RD6 | SKILL |
|---|---|---|
| CE-21e | D2-0203 | Cotton Test (Lateral Talar Glide Test) |

**Supplies Needed:** Table

*This problem allows you the opportunity to demonstrate an* **orthopedic test** *known as the* **cotton test (lateral talar glide test)**. *You have 2 minutes to complete this task.*

| Cotton Test (Lateral Talar Glide Test) | Course or Site Assessor Environment | Test 1 | | Test 2 | | Test 3 | |
|---|---|---|---|---|---|---|---|
| **Tester places patient and limb in appropriate position** | | **Y** | **N** | **Y** | **N** | **Y** | **N** |
| Supine | | ○ | ○ | ○ | ○ | ○ | ○ |
| Foot placed in a neutral position (0 degrees dorsiflexion) | | ○ | ○ | ○ | ○ | ○ | ○ |
| **Tester placed in proper position** | | **Y** | **N** | **Y** | **N** | **Y** | **N** |
| Stabilizes tibia (do not compress the fibula) with one hand | | ○ | ○ | ○ | ○ | ○ | ○ |
| Grasps the ankle mortise (cup calcaneus) just proximal to the tibiotalar joint line | | ○ | ○ | ○ | ○ | ○ | ○ |
| **Tester performs test according to accepted guidelines** | | **Y** | **N** | **Y** | **N** | **Y** | **N** |
| Maintains relaxation of the limb | | ○ | ○ | ○ | ○ | ○ | ○ |
| Passively moves calcaneus and talus laterally | | ○ | ○ | ○ | ○ | ○ | ○ |
| Performs assessment bilaterally | | ○ | ○ | ○ | ○ | ○ | ○ |
| **Identifies positive findings and implications** | | **Y** | **N** | **Y** | **N** | **Y** | **N** |
| Excessive talar translation in involved limb | | ○ | ○ | ○ | ○ | ○ | ○ |
| Distal tibiofibular syndesmosis sprain | | ○ | ○ | ○ | ○ | ○ | ○ |
| | **Total** | \_\_\_\_/9 | | \_\_\_\_/9 | | \_\_\_\_/9 | |
| | **Must achieve >6 to pass this examination** | Ⓟ | Ⓕ | Ⓟ | Ⓕ | Ⓟ | Ⓕ |

| Assessor: Date: | Test 1 Comments: |
|---|---|
| Assessor: Date: | Test 2 Comments: |
| Assessor: Date: | Test 3 Comments: |

**TEST ENVIRONMENTS**
**L:** Laboratory/Classroom
**C:** Clinical/Field Testing
**P:** Practicum
**A:** Assessment/Mock Exam

**TEST INFORMATION**
**Test Statistics:** Sensitivity .12–.55
Specificity .36–.92
(+) LR .24–4.20
(-) LR .56–1.78
**Reference(s):** Sman et al. (2012)
Starkey & Brown (2015)

## MUSCULOSKELETAL SYSTEM—REGION 2: ANKLE AND LOWER LEG
# CAPSULAR AND LIGAMENTOUS STRESS TESTING

| NATA EC 5th | BOC RD6 | SKILL |
|---|---|---|
| CE-21e | D2-0203 | Kleiger Test (External Rotation Test) |

**Supplies Needed:** Table or chair

*This problem allows you the opportunity to demonstrate an* **orthopedic test** *known as the* **Kleiger test (external rotation test)**. *You have 2 minutes to complete this task.*

| Kleiger Test (External Rotation Test) | Course or Site / Assessor / Environment | Test 1 | | Test 2 | | Test 3 | |
|---|---|---|---|---|---|---|---|
| **Tester places patient and limb in appropriate position** | | **Y** | **N** | **Y** | **N** | **Y** | **N** |
| Seated | | ○ | ○ | ○ | ○ | ○ | ○ |
| Knee flexed to 90 degrees (knee over edge of table) | | ○ | ○ | ○ | ○ | ○ | ○ |
| Foot placed in a neutral position (0 degrees dorsiflexion) | | ○ | ○ | ○ | ○ | ○ | ○ |
| **Tester placed in proper position** | | **Y** | **N** | **Y** | **N** | **Y** | **N** |
| Stabilizes tibia (do not compress fibula) with one hand | | ○ | ○ | ○ | ○ | ○ | ○ |
| Grasps the medial aspect of foot while supporting ankle with forearm | | ○ | ○ | ○ | ○ | ○ | ○ |
| **Tester performs test according to accepted guidelines** | | **Y** | **N** | **Y** | **N** | **Y** | **N** |
| Maintains relaxation of the limb | | ○ | ○ | ○ | ○ | ○ | ○ |
| Externally rotates the foot and talus while maintaining stable leg (foot placed in dorsiflexion to stress syndesmosis, plantar flexion to stress deltoid) | | ○ | ○ | ○ | ○ | ○ | ○ |
| Performs assessment bilaterally | | ○ | ○ | ○ | ○ | ○ | ○ |
| **Identifies positive findings and implications** | | **Y** | **N** | **Y** | **N** | **Y** | **N** |
| Medial joint pain, displacement of talus from medial malleolus (deltoid ligament) | | ○ | ○ | ○ | ○ | ○ | ○ |
| Anterolateral ankle pain (syndesmotic pathology) | | ○ | ○ | ○ | ○ | ○ | ○ |
| Total | | ___/10 | | ___/10 | | ___/10 | |
| **Must achieve >6 to pass this examination** | | Ⓟ | Ⓕ | Ⓟ | Ⓕ | Ⓟ | Ⓕ |

| Assessor:<br>Date: | Test 1 Comments: |
|---|---|
| Assessor:<br>Date: | Test 2 Comments: |
| Assessor:<br>Date: | Test 3 Comments: |

**TEST ENVIRONMENTS**
**L:** Laboratory/Classroom
**C:** Clinical/Field Testing
**P:** Practicum
**A:** Assessment/Mock Exam

**TEST INFORMATION**
**Test Statistics:** Sensitivity .27–.73
Specificity 0–.35
**Reference(s):** Konin et al. (2016)
Sman et al. (2012)

## MUSCULOSKELETAL SYSTEM—REGION 2: ANKLE AND LOWER LEG
# CAPSULAR AND LIGAMENTOUS STRESS TESTING

| NATA EC 5th | BOC RD6 | SKILL |
|---|---|---|
| CE-21e | D2-0203 | Talar Tilt (Eversion Stress Test) |

**Supplies Needed:** Table or chair

*This problem allows you the opportunity to demonstrate an* **orthopedic test** *known as the* **talar tilt (eversion stress test)***. You have 2 minutes to complete this task.*

| Talar Tilt (Eversion Stress Test) | Course or Site Assessor Environment | Test 1 | | Test 2 | | Test 3 | |
|---|---|---|---|---|---|---|---|
| **Tester places patient and limb in appropriate position** | | **Y** | **N** | **Y** | **N** | **Y** | **N** |
| Seated or supine (may be done side lying on uninvolved side) | | ○ | ○ | ○ | ○ | ○ | ○ |
| Knee flexed to 90 degrees (knee over edge of table) | | ○ | ○ | ○ | ○ | ○ | ○ |
| Foot placed in a neutral position (0 degrees dorsiflexion) | | ○ | ○ | ○ | ○ | ○ | ○ |
| **Tester placed in proper position** | | **Y** | **N** | **Y** | **N** | **Y** | **N** |
| Stabilizes tibia and fibula with one hand | | ○ | ○ | ○ | ○ | ○ | ○ |
| Grasps the calcaneus and holds foot in neutral position | | ○ | ○ | ○ | ○ | ○ | ○ |
| **Tester performs test according to accepted guidelines** | | **Y** | **N** | **Y** | **N** | **Y** | **N** |
| Maintains relaxation of the limb | | ○ | ○ | ○ | ○ | ○ | ○ |
| Passively everts calcaneus and talus | | ○ | ○ | ○ | ○ | ○ | ○ |
| Performs assessment bilaterally | | ○ | ○ | ○ | ○ | ○ | ○ |
| **Identifies positive findings and implications** | | **Y** | **N** | **Y** | **N** | **Y** | **N** |
| Excessive eversion in involved limb, medial joint pain | | ○ | ○ | ○ | ○ | ○ | ○ |
| Deltoid ligament sprain | | ○ | ○ | ○ | ○ | ○ | ○ |
| | Total | __/10 | | __/10 | | __/10 | |
| | **Must achieve >6 to pass this examination** | Ⓟ | Ⓕ | Ⓟ | Ⓕ | Ⓟ | Ⓕ |

| Assessor: Date: | Test 1 Comments: |
|---|---|
| Assessor: Date: | Test 2 Comments: |
| Assessor: Date: | Test 3 Comments: |

**TEST ENVIRONMENTS**
**L:** Laboratory/Classroom
**C:** Clinical/Field Testing
**P:** Practicum
**A:** Assessment/Mock Exam

**TEST INFORMATION**
**Test Statistics:** No data available
**Reference(s):** Konin et al. (2016)
Starkey & Brown (2015)

## MUSCULOSKELETAL SYSTEM—REGION 2: ANKLE AND LOWER LEG
# CAPSULAR AND LIGAMENTOUS STRESS TESTING

| NATA EC 5th | BOC RD6 | SKILL |
|---|---|---|
| CE-21e | D2-0203 | Talar Tilt (Inversion Stress Test) |

**Supplies Needed:** Table or chair

*This problem allows you the opportunity to demonstrate an* **orthopedic test** *known as the* **talar tilt (inversion stress test)**. *You have 2 minutes to complete this task.*

| Talar Tilt (Inversion Stress Test) | Course or Site / Assessor / Environment _____ | | Test 1 | | Test 2 | | Test 3 | |
|---|---|---|---|---|---|---|---|---|
| **Tester places patient and limb in appropriate position** | | **Y** | **N** | **Y** | **N** | **Y** | **N** | |
| Seated or supine (may be done side lying on uninvolved side) | | O | O | O | O | O | O |
| Knee flexed to 90 degrees (knee over edge of table) | | O | O | O | O | O | O |
| Foot placed in a neutral position (0 degrees dorsiflexion) | | O | O | O | O | O | O |
| **Tester placed in proper position** | | **Y** | **N** | **Y** | **N** | **Y** | **N** |
| Stabilizes tibia and fibula with one hand | | O | O | O | O | O | O |
| Grasps the calcaneus and holds foot in neutral position | | O | O | O | O | O | O |
| **Tester performs test according to accepted guidelines** | | **Y** | **N** | **Y** | **N** | **Y** | **N** |
| Maintains relaxation of the limb | | O | O | O | O | O | O |
| Calcaneus and talus are passively inverted | | O | O | O | O | O | O |
| Performs assessment bilaterally | | O | O | O | O | O | O |
| **Identifies positive findings and implications** | | **Y** | **N** | **Y** | **N** | **Y** | **N** |
| Excessive inversion in involved limb | | O | O | O | O | O | O |
| Calcaneofibular ligament sprain | | O | O | O | O | O | O |
| **Total** | | ___ /10 | | ___ /10 | | ___ /10 | |
| **Must achieve >6 to pass this examination** | | Ⓟ | Ⓕ | Ⓟ | Ⓕ | Ⓟ | Ⓕ |

| Assessor: Date: | Test 1 Comments: |
|---|---|
| Assessor: Date: | Test 2 Comments: |
| Assessor: Date: | Test 3 Comments: |

**TEST ENVIRONMENTS**
**L:** Laboratory/Classroom
**C:** Clinical/Field Testing
**P:** Practicum
**A:** Assessment/Mock Exam

**TEST INFORMATION**
**Test Statistics:** No data available
**Reference(s):** Konin et al. (2016)
Starkey & Brown (2015)

## MUSCULOSKELETAL SYSTEM—REGION 2: ANKLE AND LOWER LEG
# JOINT PLAY (ARTHROKINEMATICS)

| NATA EC 5th | BOC RD6 | SKILL |
|:---:|:---:|:---:|
| CE-21f | D2-0203 | Subtalar Joint Play |

**Supplies Needed:** Table

*This problem allows you the opportunity to demonstrate an* **orthopedic test** *known as* **subtalar joint play**. *You have 2 minutes to complete this task.*

| Subtalar Joint Play | Course or Site / Assessor / Environment | | Test 1 | | Test 2 | | Test 3 |
|---|---|:---:|:---:|:---:|:---:|:---:|:---:|
| | | Y | N | Y | N | Y | N |
| **Tester places patient and limb in appropriate position** | | **Y** | **N** | **Y** | **N** | **Y** | **N** |
| Side lying on uninvolved side | | ○ | ○ | ○ | ○ | ○ | ○ |
| Foot placed in a neutral position (0 degrees dorsiflexion) | | ○ | ○ | ○ | ○ | ○ | ○ |
| **Tester placed in proper position** | | **Y** | **N** | **Y** | **N** | **Y** | **N** |
| Stabilizes talus in the mortise | | ○ | ○ | ○ | ○ | ○ | ○ |
| Cups the calcaneus and holds foot in neutral position | | ○ | ○ | ○ | ○ | ○ | ○ |
| **Tester performs test according to accepted guidelines** | | **Y** | **N** | **Y** | **N** | **Y** | **N** |
| Applies force to move the talus medially | | ○ | ○ | ○ | ○ | ○ | ○ |
| Applies force to move the talus laterally | | ○ | ○ | ○ | ○ | ○ | ○ |
| Performs assessment bilaterally | | ○ | ○ | ○ | ○ | ○ | ○ |
| **Identifies positive findings and implications** | | **Y** | **N** | **Y** | **N** | **Y** | **N** |
| Hypomobile medial glide is associated with decreased pronation/calcaneal eversion | | ○ | ○ | ○ | ○ | ○ | ○ |
| Hypomobile lateral glide is associated with decreased supination/calcaneal inversion | | ○ | ○ | ○ | ○ | ○ | ○ |
| Hypermobile medial glide is associated with lateral ankle sprains | | ○ | ○ | ○ | ○ | ○ | ○ |
| **Total** | | ___/10 | | ___/10 | | ___/10 | |
| **Must achieve >6 to pass this examination** | | Ⓟ | Ⓕ | Ⓟ | Ⓕ | Ⓟ | Ⓕ |

| Assessor: Date: | Test 1 Comments: |
|---|---|
| Assessor: Date: | Test 2 Comments: |
| Assessor: Date: | Test 3 Comments: |

**TEST ENVIRONMENTS**
**L:** Laboratory/Classroom
**C:** Clinical/Field Testing
**P:** Practicum
**A:** Assessment/Mock Exam

**TEST INFORMATION**
**Test Statistics:** No data available
**Reference(s):** Starkey & Brown (2015)

## MUSCULOSKELETAL SYSTEM—REGION 2: ANKLE AND LOWER LEG
# JOINT PLAY (ARTHROKINEMATICS)

| NATA EC 5th | BOC RD6 | SKILL |
|---|---|---|
| CE-21f | D2-0203 | Distal Tibiofibular Joint Play |

**Supplies Needed:** Table or chair

*This problem allows you the opportunity to demonstrate an* **orthopedic test** *known as* **distal tibiofibular joint play**. *You have 2 minutes to complete this task.*

| Distal Tibiofibular Joint Play | Course or Site Assessor Environment | | Test 1 | | Test 2 | | Test 3 | |
|---|---|---|---|---|---|---|---|---|
| **Tester places patient and limb in appropriate position** | | **Y** | **N** | **Y** | **N** | **Y** | **N** | |
| Supine or short sitting with ankle relaxed into plantar flexion | | O | O | O | O | O | O | |
| **Tester placed in proper position** | | **Y** | **N** | **Y** | **N** | **Y** | **N** | |
| Stabilizes the tibia | | O | O | O | O | O | O | |
| Grasps the fibula at the lateral malleolus | | O | O | O | O | O | O | |
| **Tester performs test according to accepted guidelines** | | **Y** | **N** | **Y** | **N** | **Y** | **N** | |
| Applies force to move the fibula posteriorly | | O | O | O | O | O | O | |
| Applies force to move the fibula anteriorly | | O | O | O | O | O | O | |
| Performs assessment bilaterally | | O | O | O | O | O | O | |
| **Identifies positive findings and implications** | | **Y** | **N** | **Y** | **N** | **Y** | **N** | |
| Pain arising from the syndesmosis or increased motion relative to the uninvolved side | | O | O | O | O | O | O | |
| Sprain of the distal tibiofibular syndesmosis | | O | O | O | O | O | O | |
| **Total** | | /8 | | /8 | | /8 | | |
| **Must achieve >5 to pass this examination** | | Ⓟ | Ⓕ | Ⓟ | Ⓕ | Ⓟ | Ⓕ | |

| Assessor: Date: | Test 1 Comments: |
|---|---|
| Assessor: Date: | Test 2 Comments: |
| Assessor: Date: | Test 3 Comments: |

**TEST ENVIRONMENTS**
**L:** Laboratory/Classroom
**C:** Clinical/Field Testing
**P:** Practicum
**A:** Assessment/Mock Exam

**TEST INFORMATION**
**Test Statistics:** No data available
**Reference(s):** Starkey & Brown (2015)

## MUSCULOSKELETAL SYSTEM—REGION 2: ANKLE AND LOWER LEG
# SPECIAL TESTS

| NATA EC 5th | BOC RD6 | SKILL |
|---|---|---|
| CE-21g, CE-20e | D2-0203 | Bump Test for Leg Stress Fractures |

**Supplies Needed:** Table or chair

*This problem allows you the opportunity to demonstrate an* **orthopedic test** *known as the* **bump test** *to rule out a possible advanced* **stress fracture**. *You have 2 minutes to complete this task.*

| Bump Test for Leg Stress Fractures | Course or Site Assessor Environment | Test 1 | | Test 2 | | Test 3 | |
|---|---|---|---|---|---|---|---|
| **Tester places patient and limb in appropriate position** | | Y | N | Y | N | Y | N |
| Supine or seated (with leg off the end of table) | | ○ | ○ | ○ | ○ | ○ | ○ |
| Ankle placed in a neutral position (0 degrees dorsiflexion) | | ○ | ○ | ○ | ○ | ○ | ○ |
| **Tester placed in proper position** | | Y | N | Y | N | Y | N |
| Standing in front of the heel of the involved leg | | ○ | ○ | ○ | ○ | ○ | ○ |
| Stabilizes the posterior portion of the leg with nondominant hand | | ○ | ○ | ○ | ○ | ○ | ○ |
| **Tester performs test according to accepted guidelines** | | Y | N | Y | N | Y | N |
| Bumps the calcaneus using the palm of the dominant hand | | ○ | ○ | ○ | ○ | ○ | ○ |
| Performs assessment bilaterally | | ○ | ○ | ○ | ○ | ○ | ○ |
| **Identifies positive findings and implications** | | Y | N | Y | N | Y | N |
| Pain emanating from fracture of calcaneus, talus, fibula, or tibia | | ○ | ○ | ○ | ○ | ○ | ○ |
| Possible advanced stress fracture | | ○ | ○ | ○ | ○ | ○ | ○ |
| **Total** | | __/8 | | __/8 | | __/8 | |
| **Must achieve >5 to pass this examination** | | Ⓟ | Ⓕ | Ⓟ | Ⓕ | Ⓟ | Ⓕ |

| Assessor: Date: | Test 1 Comments: |
|---|---|
| Assessor: Date: | Test 2 Comments: |
| Assessor: Date: | Test 3 Comments: |

**TEST ENVIRONMENTS**
L:  Laboratory/Classroom
C:  Clinical/Field Testing
P:  Practicum
A:  Assessment/Mock Exam

**TEST INFORMATION**
**Test Statistics:**  No data available
**Reference(s):**  Starkey & Brown (2015)

## MUSCULOSKELETAL SYSTEM—REGION 2: ANKLE AND LOWER LEG
# SPECIAL TESTS

| NATA EC 5th | BOC RD6 | SKILL |
|---|---|---|
| CE-21g, CE-20e | D2-0203 | Compression Test (Squeeze Test) |

**Supplies Needed:** Table

*This problem allows you the opportunity to demonstrate an* **orthopedic test** *known as the* **compression test (squeeze test)** *to rule out a* **fibular fracture** *or* **syndesmosis sprain**. *You have 2 minutes to complete this task.*

| Compression Test (Squeeze Test) | Course or Site Assessor Environment | | Test 1 | | Test 2 | | Test 3 | |
|---|---|---|---|---|---|---|---|---|
| **Tester places patient and limb in appropriate position** | | | **Y** | **N** | **Y** | **N** | **Y** | **N** |
| Supine with foot off the end of table | | | ○ | ○ | ○ | ○ | ○ | ○ |
| Knee placed in full extension | | | ○ | ○ | ○ | ○ | ○ | ○ |
| **Tester placed in proper position** | | | **Y** | **N** | **Y** | **N** | **Y** | **N** |
| Stands to the side of the patient | | | ○ | ○ | ○ | ○ | ○ | ○ |
| Places both hands around the lower leg (tibia/fibula) | | | ○ | ○ | ○ | ○ | ○ | ○ |
| **Tester performs test according to accepted guidelines** | | | **Y** | **N** | **Y** | **N** | **Y** | **N** |
| Squeezes the tibia and fibula together (proximal to injury site) | | | ○ | ○ | ○ | ○ | ○ | ○ |
| Squeezes the tibia and fibula together (distal to injury site) | | | ○ | ○ | ○ | ○ | ○ | ○ |
| Performs assessment bilaterally | | | ○ | ○ | ○ | ○ | ○ | ○ |
| **Identifies positive findings and implications** | | | **Y** | **N** | **Y** | **N** | **Y** | **N** |
| Pain emanating from site of injury (bony) (fibular fracture) | | | ○ | ○ | ○ | ○ | ○ | ○ |
| Pain emanating from distal tibiofibular joint (syndesmotic sprain) | | | ○ | ○ | ○ | ○ | ○ | ○ |
| Total | | | ___/9 | | ___/9 | | ___/9 | |
| Must achieve >6 to pass this examination | | | Ⓟ | Ⓕ | Ⓟ | Ⓕ | Ⓟ | Ⓕ |

| Assessor:<br>Date: | Test 1 Comments: |
|---|---|
| Assessor:<br>Date: | Test 2 Comments: |
| Assessor:<br>Date: | Test 3 Comments: |

**TEST ENVIRONMENTS**
**L:** Laboratory/Classroom
**C:** Clinical/Field Testing
**P:** Practicum
**A:** Assessment/Mock Exam

**TEST INFORMATION**
**Test Statistics:** No data available
**Reference(s):** Konin et al. (2016)
Starkey & Brown (2015)

## MUSCULOSKELETAL SYSTEM—REGION 2: ANKLE AND LOWER LEG
# SPECIAL TESTS

| NATA EC 5th | BOC RD6 | SKILL |
|---|---|---|
| CE-21g, CE-20e | D2-0203 | Homans' Sign |

**Supplies Needed:** Table

*This problem allows you the opportunity to demonstrate an* **orthopedic test** *known as* **Homans' sign.**
*You have 2 minutes to complete this task.*

| Homans' Sign | Course or Site Assessor Environment | Test 1 | | Test 2 | | Test 3 | |
|---|---|---|---|---|---|---|---|
| | | **Y** | **N** | **Y** | **N** | **Y** | **N** |
| **Tester places patient and limb in appropriate position** | | **Y** | **N** | **Y** | **N** | **Y** | **N** |
| Supine | | ○ | ○ | ○ | ○ | ○ | ○ |
| Knee of involved side in full extension | | ○ | ○ | ○ | ○ | ○ | ○ |
| **Tester placed in proper position** | | **Y** | **N** | **Y** | **N** | **Y** | **N** |
| Stands to the side of the patient | | ○ | ○ | ○ | ○ | ○ | ○ |
| Places one hand over the lower leg to support the limb | | ○ | ○ | ○ | ○ | ○ | ○ |
| Places the other hand on the plantar surface of the foot | | ○ | ○ | ○ | ○ | ○ | ○ |
| **Tester performs test according to accepted guidelines** | | **Y** | **N** | **Y** | **N** | **Y** | **N** |
| Passively dorsiflexes the foot | | ○ | ○ | ○ | ○ | ○ | ○ |
| Maintains relaxation of the limb | | ○ | ○ | ○ | ○ | ○ | ○ |
| Performs assessment bilaterally | | ○ | ○ | ○ | ○ | ○ | ○ |
| **Identifies positive findings and implications** | | **Y** | **N** | **Y** | **N** | **Y** | **N** |
| Pain in the calf area upon passive dorsiflexion | | ○ | ○ | ○ | ○ | ○ | ○ |
| Possible thrombophlebitis from deep vein thrombosis | | ○ | ○ | ○ | ○ | ○ | ○ |
| Total | | ___/10 | | ___/10 | | ___/10 | |
| Must achieve >6 to pass this examination | | Ⓟ | Ⓕ | Ⓟ | Ⓕ | Ⓟ | Ⓕ |
| **Assessor:** **Date:** | **Test 1 Comments:** | | | | | | |
| **Assessor:** **Date:** | **Test 2 Comments:** | | | | | | |
| **Assessor:** **Date:** | **Test 3 Comments:** | | | | | | |

**TEST ENVIRONMENTS**
**L:** Laboratory/Classroom
**C:** Clinical/Field Testing
**P:** Practicum
**A:** Assessment/Mock Exam

**TEST INFORMATION**
**Test Statistics:** No data available
**Reference(s):** Konin et al. (2016)

## MUSCULOSKELETAL SYSTEM—REGION 2: ANKLE AND LOWER LEG
# SPECIAL TESTS

| NATA EC 5th | BOC RD6 | SKILL |
|---|---|---|
| CE-21g, CE-20e | D2-0203 | Thompson's Test (Simmonds' Test) |

**Supplies Needed:** Table

*This problem allows you the opportunity to demonstrate an* **orthopedic test** *known as* **Thompson's test (Simmonds' test)**. *You have 2 minutes to complete this task.*

| Thompson's Test (Simmonds' Test) | Course or Site Assessor Environment | | Test 1 | | Test 2 | | Test 3 | |
|---|---|---|---|---|---|---|---|---|
| | | | Y | N | Y | N | Y | N |
| **Tester places patient and limb in appropriate position** | | | Y | N | Y | N | Y | N |
| Prone with foot off the end of table | | | O | O | O | O | O | O |
| **Tester placed in proper position** | | | Y | N | Y | N | Y | N |
| Stands to the side of the patient | | | O | O | O | O | O | O |
| **Tester performs test according to accepted guidelines** | | | Y | N | Y | N | Y | N |
| Squeezes the belly of the calf (gastrocnemius/soleus) | | | O | O | O | O | O | O |
| Maintains relaxation of the limb | | | O | O | O | O | O | O |
| Performs assessment bilaterally | | | O | O | O | O | O | O |
| **Identifies positive findings and implications** | | | Y | N | Y | N | Y | N |
| When calf is squeezed, the foot does not plantar flex | | | O | O | O | O | O | O |
| Ruptured Achilles tendon | | | O | O | O | O | O | O |
| **Total** | | | ___/7 | | ___/7 | | ___/7 | |
| **Must achieve >4 to pass this examination** | | | Ⓟ | Ⓕ | Ⓟ | Ⓕ | Ⓟ | Ⓕ |

| Assessor:<br>Date: | Test 1 Comments: |
|---|---|
| Assessor:<br>Date: | Test 2 Comments: |
| Assessor:<br>Date: | Test 3 Comments: |

**TEST ENVIRONMENTS**
**L:** Laboratory/Classroom
**C:** Clinical/Field Testing
**P:** Practicum
**A:** Assessment/Mock Exam

**TEST INFORMATION**
**Test Statistics:** No data available
**Reference(s):** Konin et al. (2016)
Starkey & Brown (2015)

## MUSCULOSKELETAL SYSTEM—REGION 2: ANKLE AND LOWER LEG
# SPECIAL TESTS

| NATA EC 5th | BOC RD6 | SKILL |
|---|---|---|
| CE-21g, CE-20e | D2-0203 | Tinel's Sign |

**Supplies Needed:** Table

*This problem allows you the opportunity to demonstrate an* **orthopedic test** *known as* **Tinel's sign**. *You have 2 minutes to complete this task.*

| Tinel's Sign | Course or Site / Assessor / Environment | | Test 1 | | Test 2 | | Test 3 | |
|---|---|---|---|---|---|---|---|---|
| **Tester places patient and limb in appropriate position** | | | Y | N | Y | N | Y | N |
| The patient is positioned in supine, long sitting, or seated | | | ○ | ○ | ○ | ○ | ○ | ○ |
| Foot placed in a stable position | | | ○ | ○ | ○ | ○ | ○ | ○ |
| **Tester placed in proper position** | | | Y | N | Y | N | Y | N |
| Stands to the side of the limb | | | ○ | ○ | ○ | ○ | ○ | ○ |
| Places one hand over the lower leg to support the limb | | | ○ | ○ | ○ | ○ | ○ | ○ |
| Places the other hand in position to tap the area around medial malleolus | | | ○ | ○ | ○ | ○ | ○ | ○ |
| **Tester performs test according to accepted guidelines** | | | Y | N | Y | N | Y | N |
| Taps firmly on the dorsum of the ankle | | | ○ | ○ | ○ | ○ | ○ | ○ |
| Taps firmly behind the medial malleolus | | | ○ | ○ | ○ | ○ | ○ | ○ |
| Performs assessment bilaterally | | | ○ | ○ | ○ | ○ | ○ | ○ |
| **Identifies positive findings and implications** | | | Y | N | Y | N | Y | N |
| Paresthesia on dorsum of ankle (irritation of anterior tibial branch of deep peroneal nerve) | | | ○ | ○ | ○ | ○ | ○ | ○ |
| Paresthesia behind medial malleolus (irritation of posterior tibial nerve) | | | ○ | ○ | ○ | ○ | ○ | ○ |
| **Total** | | | __/10 | | __/10 | | __/10 | |
| **Must achieve >6 to pass this examination** | | | Ⓟ | Ⓕ | Ⓟ | Ⓕ | Ⓟ | Ⓕ |

| Assessor: Date: | Test 1 Comments: |
|---|---|
| Assessor: Date: | Test 2 Comments: |
| Assessor: Date: | Test 3 Comments: |

**TEST ENVIRONMENTS**
**L:** Laboratory/Classroom
**C:** Clinical/Field Testing
**P:** Practicum
**A:** Assessment/Mock Exam

**TEST INFORMATION**
**Test Statistics:** No data available
**Reference(s):** Konin et al. (2016)
Scifers (2008)

# 6

# MUSCULOSKELETAL SYSTEM—
# REGION 3: KNEE

Hauth, J. M., Gloyeske, B. M., & Amato, H. K.
*Clinical Skills Documentation Guide for Athletic Training, Third Edition* (pp. 117-153).
© 2016 SLACK Incorporated.

## Musculoskeletal System—Region 3: Knee
# Knowledge and Skills

| Musculoskeletal System—Region 3: Knee | | | | Skill: Acquisition, Reinforcement, Proficiency | | |
|---|---|---|---|---|---|---|
| **NATA EC 5th** | **BOC RD6** | **Palpation** | **Page #** | | | |
| CE-21b, CE-20c | D2-0202 | Palpation: Knee – 01 | 119 | | | |
| CE-21b, CE-20c | D2-0202 | Palpation: Knee – 02 | 120 | | | |
| CE-21b, CE-20c | D2-0202 | Palpation: Knee – 03 | 121 | | | |
| **NATA EC 5th** | **BOC RD6** | **Manual Muscle Testing** | **Page #** | | | |
| CE-21c | D2-0203 | MMT: Biceps Femoris | 122 | | | |
| CE-21c | D2-0203 | MMT: Semimembranosus | 123 | | | |
| CE-21c | D2-0203 | MMT: Semitendinosus | 124 | | | |
| CE-21c | D2-0203 | MMT: Quadriceps Femoris (Rectus Femoris, Vastus Medialis, Vastus Intermedius, Vastus Lateralis) | 125 | | | |
| CE-21c | D2-0203 | MMT: Sartorius | 126 | | | |
| **NATA EC 5th** | **BOC RD6** | **Osteokinematic Joint Motion** | **Page #** | | | |
| CE-21d | D2-0203 | Goniometric Assessment: Tibiofemoral Joint (Flexion) | 127 | | | |
| CE-21d | D2-0203 | Goniometric Assessment: Tibiofemoral Joint (Extension) | 128 | | | |
| **NATA EC 5th** | **BOC RD6** | **Capsular and Ligamentous Stress Testing** | **Page #** | | | |
| CE-21e | D2-0203 | Anterior Drawer Test for the Knee | 129 | | | |
| CE-21e | D2-0203 | Godfrey Test (Godfrey 90/90 Test) | 130 | | | |
| CE-21e | D2-0203 | Hughston Posterolateral Drawer Test | 131 | | | |
| CE-21e | D2-0203 | Hughston Posteromedial Drawer Test | 132 | | | |
| CE-21e | D2-0203 | Hughston Jerk Test | 133 | | | |
| CE-21e | D2-0203 | Lachman's Test | 134 | | | |
| CE-21e | D2-0203 | Lateral Pivot Shift Test | 135 | | | |
| CE-21e | D2-0203 | Posterior Drawer Test for the Knee | 136 | | | |
| CE-21e | D2-0203 | Posterior Sag Sign | 137 | | | |
| CE-21e | D2-0203 | Quadriceps Active Test | 138 | | | |
| CE-21e | D2-0203 | Slocum Drawer Test (External Tibial Rotation) | 139 | | | |
| CE-21e | D2-0203 | Slocum Drawer Test (Internal Tibial Rotation) | 140 | | | |
| CE-21e | D2-0203 | Valgus Stress Test for the Knee | 141 | | | |
| CE-21e | D2-0203 | Varus Stress Test for the Knee | 142 | | | |
| **NATA EC 5th** | **BOC RD6** | **Special Tests** | **Page #** | | | |
| CE-21g, CE-20e | D2-0203 | Apley's Grind | 143 | | | |
| CE-21g, CE-20e | D2-0203 | Ballotable Patella | 144 | | | |
| CE-21g, CE-20e | D2-0203 | Bounce Home | 145 | | | |
| CE-21g, CE-20e | D2-0203 | External Rotation Test (Dial Test) | 146 | | | |
| CE-21g, CE-20e | D2-0203 | External Rotation Recurvatum Test | 147 | | | |
| CE-21g, CE-20e | D2-0203 | McMurray's Test | 148 | | | |
| CE-21g, CE-20e | D2-0203 | Nobel's Compression Test | 149 | | | |
| CE-21g, CE-20e | D2-0203 | Patellar Apprehension Test | 150 | | | |
| CE-21g, CE-20e | D2-0203 | Sweep Test | 151 | | | |
| CE-21g, CE-20e | D2-0203 | Thessaly's Test | 152 | | | |
| CE-21g, CE-20e | D2-0203 | Wilson's Test | 153 | | | |

## MUSCULOSKELETAL SYSTEM—REGION 3: KNEE
# PALPATION

| NATA EC 5th | BOC RD6 | SKILL |
|---|---|---|
| CE-21b, CE-20c | D2-0202 | Palpation: Knee – 01 |

**Supplies Needed:** Table

*This problem allows you the opportunity to demonstrate your ability to* **palpate** *the* **knee**.
*You have 2 minutes to complete this task.*

| Palpation: Knee – 01 | Course or Site<br>Assessor<br>Environment | | | | | | |
|---|---|---|---|---|---|---|---|
| | | Test 1 | | Test 2 | | Test 3 | |
| | | Y | N | Y | N | Y | N |
| Lateral collateral ligament | | O | O | O | O | O | O |
| Fibular head | | O | O | O | O | O | O |
| Biceps femoris tendon | | O | O | O | O | O | O |
| Iliotibial band | | O | O | O | O | O | O |
| Adductor tubercle | | O | O | O | O | O | O |
| Quadriceps tendon | | O | O | O | O | O | O |
| Medial meniscus and joint line | | O | O | O | O | O | O |
| Total | | ___/7 | | ___/7 | | ___/7 | |
| Must achieve >4 to pass this examination | | P | F | P | F | P | F |

| Assessor:<br>Date: | Test 1 Comments: |
|---|---|
| Assessor:<br>Date: | Test 2 Comments: |
| Assessor:<br>Date: | Test 3 Comments: |

**TEST ENVIRONMENTS**
**L:** Laboratory/Classroom
**C:** Clinical/Field Testing
**P:** Practicum
**A:** Assessment/Mock Exam

**TEST INFORMATION**
**Test Statistics:** N/A
**Reference(s):** Starkey & Brown (2015)

## MUSCULOSKELETAL SYSTEM—REGION 3: KNEE
# PALPATION

| NATA EC 5th | BOC RD6 | SKILL |
|---|---|---|
| CE-21b, CE-20c | D2-0202 | Palpation: Knee – 02 |

**Supplies Needed:** Table

*This problem allows you the opportunity to demonstrate your ability to **palpate** the **knee**.*
*You have 2 minutes to complete this task.*

| Palpation: Knee – 02 | Course or Site<br>Assessor<br>Environment | | | | | | |
|---|---|---|---|---|---|---|---|
| | | Test 1 | | Test 2 | | Test 3 | |
| | | Y | N | Y | N | Y | N |
| Common peroneal nerve | | ○ | ○ | ○ | ○ | ○ | ○ |
| Semimembranosus tendon | | ○ | ○ | ○ | ○ | ○ | ○ |
| Pes anserine tendon and bursa | | ○ | ○ | ○ | ○ | ○ | ○ |
| Superior patellar border | | ○ | ○ | ○ | ○ | ○ | ○ |
| Medial collateral ligament | | ○ | ○ | ○ | ○ | ○ | ○ |
| Lateral meniscus and joint line | | ○ | ○ | ○ | ○ | ○ | ○ |
| Tibial tuberosity | | ○ | ○ | ○ | ○ | ○ | ○ |
| Total | | ___/7 | | ___/7 | | ___/7 | |
| Must achieve >4 to pass this examination | | Ⓟ | Ⓕ | Ⓟ | Ⓕ | Ⓟ | Ⓕ |
| **Assessor:**<br>**Date:** | **Test 1 Comments:** | | | | | | |
| **Assessor:**<br>**Date:** | **Test 2 Comments:** | | | | | | |
| **Assessor:**<br>**Date:** | **Test 3 Comments:** | | | | | | |

**TEST ENVIRONMENTS**
**L:** Laboratory/Classroom
**C:** Clinical/Field Testing
**P:** Practicum
**A:** Assessment/Mock Exam

**TEST INFORMATION**
**Test Statistics:** N/A
**Reference(s):** Starkey & Brown (2015)

**MUSCULOSKELETAL SYSTEM—REGION 3: KNEE**
# PALPATION

| NATA EC 5th | BOC RD6 | SKILL |
|---|---|---|
| CE-21b, CE-20c | D2-0202 | Palpation: Knee – 03 |

**Supplies Needed:** Table

*This problem allows you the opportunity to demonstrate your ability to* **palpate** *the* **knee**.
*You have 2 minutes to complete this task.*

| Palpation: Knee – 03 | Course or Site / Assessor / Environment | | | | | | |
|---|---|---|---|---|---|---|---|
| | | Test 1 | | Test 2 | | Test 3 | |
| | | Y | N | Y | N | Y | N |
| Patellar tendon | | ○ | ○ | ○ | ○ | ○ | ○ |
| Lateral epicondyle | | ○ | ○ | ○ | ○ | ○ | ○ |
| Popliteal pulse | | ○ | ○ | ○ | ○ | ○ | ○ |
| Gerdy's tubercle | | ○ | ○ | ○ | ○ | ○ | ○ |
| Semitendinosus tendon | | ○ | ○ | ○ | ○ | ○ | ○ |
| Medial tibial plateau | | ○ | ○ | ○ | ○ | ○ | ○ |
| Rectus femoris | | ○ | ○ | ○ | ○ | ○ | ○ |
| Total | | __/7 | | __/7 | | __/7 | |
| Must achieve >4 to pass this examination | | Ⓟ | Ⓕ | Ⓟ | Ⓕ | Ⓟ | Ⓕ |

| Assessor: Date: | Test 1 Comments: |
|---|---|
| Assessor: Date: | Test 2 Comments: |
| Assessor: Date: | Test 3 Comments: |

**TEST ENVIRONMENTS**
**L:** Laboratory/Classroom
**C:** Clinical/Field Testing
**P:** Practicum
**A:** Assessment/Mock Exam

**TEST INFORMATION**
**Test Statistics:** N/A
**Reference(s):** Starkey & Brown (2015)

## MUSCULOSKELETAL SYSTEM—REGION 3: KNEE
# MANUAL MUSCLE TESTING

| NATA EC 5th | BOC RD6 | SKILL |
|---|---|---|
| CE-21c | D2-0203 | MMT: Biceps Femoris |

**Supplies Needed:** Table

*This problem allows you the opportunity to demonstrate a* **manual muscle test** *for the* **biceps femoris**. *You have 2 minutes to complete this task.*

| MMT: Biceps Femoris | Course or Site Assessor Environment | | | | | |
|---|---|---|---|---|---|---|
| | | Test 1 | | Test 2 | | Test 3 |
| | | Y | N | Y | N | Y | N |
| **Tester places patient and limb in appropriate position** | | Y | N | Y | N | Y | N |
| Prone, flexion of the knee between 50 and 70 degrees | | ○ | ○ | ○ | ○ | ○ | ○ |
| Knee and hip placed in slight lateral rotation | | ○ | ○ | ○ | ○ | ○ | ○ |
| **Tester placed in proper position** | | Y | N | Y | N | Y | N |
| Stabilizes the lower leg at the lateral malleolus and femur at the greater trochanter | | ○ | ○ | ○ | ○ | ○ | ○ |
| **Tester performs test according to accepted guidelines** | | Y | N | Y | N | Y | N |
| Instructs the patient to actively flex the knee | | ○ | ○ | ○ | ○ | ○ | ○ |
| Applies resistance to the posterior surface of lower leg (direction of knee extension) | | ○ | ○ | ○ | ○ | ○ | ○ |
| Holds resistance for 5 seconds | | ○ | ○ | ○ | ○ | ○ | ○ |
| Performs assessment bilaterally | | ○ | ○ | ○ | ○ | ○ | ○ |
| **Identifies implications** | | Y | N | Y | N | Y | N |
| Correctly grades the MMT | | ○ | ○ | ○ | ○ | ○ | ○ |
| **Total** | | ___/8 | | ___/8 | | ___/8 | |
| **Must achieve >5 to pass this examination** | | Ⓟ | Ⓕ | Ⓟ | Ⓕ | Ⓟ | Ⓕ |

| Assessor: Date: | Test 1 Comments: |
|---|---|
| Assessor: Date: | Test 2 Comments: |
| Assessor: Date: | Test 3 Comments: |

**TEST ENVIRONMENTS**
**L:** Laboratory/Classroom
**C:** Clinical/Field Testing
**P:** Practicum
**A:** Assessment/Mock Exam

**TEST INFORMATION**
**Test Statistics:** N/A
**Reference(s):** Kendall et al. (2005)

## MUSCULOSKELETAL SYSTEM—REGION 3: KNEE
# MANUAL MUSCLE TESTING

| NATA EC 5th | BOC RD6 | SKILL |
|---|---|---|
| CE-21c | D2-0203 | MMT: Semimembranosus |

**Supplies Needed:** Table

*This problem allows you the opportunity to demonstrate a* **manual muscle test** *for the* **semimembranosus**. *You have 2 minutes to complete this task.*

| MMT: Semimembranosus | Course or Site Assessor Environment | | Test 1 | | Test 2 | | Test 3 | |
|---|---|---|---|---|---|---|---|---|
| **Tester places patient and limb in appropriate position** | | **Y** | **N** | **Y** | **N** | **Y** | **N** | |
| Prone, flexion of the knee between 50 and 70 degrees | | ○ | ○ | ○ | ○ | ○ | ○ | |
| Knee and hip placed in slight medial rotation | | ○ | ○ | ○ | ○ | ○ | ○ | |
| **Tester placed in proper position** | | **Y** | **N** | **Y** | **N** | **Y** | **N** | |
| Stabilizes the lower leg at the lateral malleolus and femur at the greater trochanter | | ○ | ○ | ○ | ○ | ○ | ○ | |
| **Tester performs test according to accepted guidelines** | | **Y** | **N** | **Y** | **N** | **Y** | **N** | |
| Instructs the patient to actively flex the knee | | ○ | ○ | ○ | ○ | ○ | ○ | |
| Applies resistance to posterior surface of the lower leg (direction of knee extension) | | ○ | ○ | ○ | ○ | ○ | ○ | |
| Holds resistance for 5 seconds | | ○ | ○ | ○ | ○ | ○ | ○ | |
| Performs assessment bilaterally | | ○ | ○ | ○ | ○ | ○ | ○ | |
| **Identifies implications** | | **Y** | **N** | **Y** | **N** | **Y** | **N** | |
| Correctly grades the MMT | | ○ | ○ | ○ | ○ | ○ | ○ | |
| Total | | ___/8 | | ___/8 | | ___/8 | | |
| **Must achieve >5 to pass this examination** | | Ⓟ | Ⓕ | Ⓟ | Ⓕ | Ⓟ | Ⓕ | |

| Assessor:<br>Date: | Test 1 Comments: |
|---|---|
| Assessor:<br>Date: | Test 2 Comments: |
| Assessor:<br>Date: | Test 3 Comments: |

**TEST ENVIRONMENTS**
**L:** Laboratory/Classroom
**C:** Clinical/Field Testing
**P:** Practicum
**A:** Assessment/Mock Exam

**TEST INFORMATION**
**Test Statistics:** N/A
**Reference(s):** Kendall et al. (2005)

MUSCULOSKELETAL SYSTEM—REGION 3: KNEE
# MANUAL MUSCLE TESTING

| NATA EC 5th | BOC RD6 | SKILL |
|---|---|---|
| CE-21c | D2-0203 | MMT: Semitendinosus |

**Supplies Needed:** Table

*This problem allows you the opportunity to demonstrate a* **manual muscle test** *for the* **semitendinosus**. *You have 2 minutes to complete this task.*

| MMT: Semitendinosus | Course or Site Assessor Environment | Test 1 | | Test 2 | | Test 3 | |
|---|---|---|---|---|---|---|---|
| **Tester places patient and limb in appropriate position** | | **Y** | **N** | **Y** | **N** | **Y** | **N** |
| Prone, flexion of the knee between 50 and 70 degrees | | ○ | ○ | ○ | ○ | ○ | ○ |
| Knee and hip placed in slight medial rotation | | ○ | ○ | ○ | ○ | ○ | ○ |
| **Tester placed in proper position** | | **Y** | **N** | **Y** | **N** | **Y** | **N** |
| Stabilizes the lower leg at the lateral malleolus and femur at the greater trochanter | | ○ | ○ | ○ | ○ | ○ | ○ |
| **Tester performs test according to accepted guidelines** | | **Y** | **N** | **Y** | **N** | **Y** | **N** |
| Instructs the patient to actively flex the knee | | ○ | ○ | ○ | ○ | ○ | ○ |
| Applies resistance to posterior surface of the lower leg (direction of knee extension) | | ○ | ○ | ○ | ○ | ○ | ○ |
| Holds resistance for 5 seconds | | ○ | ○ | ○ | ○ | ○ | ○ |
| Performs assessment bilaterally | | ○ | ○ | ○ | ○ | ○ | ○ |
| **Identifies implications** | | **Y** | **N** | **Y** | **N** | **Y** | **N** |
| Correctly grades the MMT | | ○ | ○ | ○ | ○ | ○ | ○ |
| **Total** | | ___/8 | | ___/8 | | ___/8 | |
| **Must achieve >5 to pass this examination** | | Ⓟ | Ⓕ | Ⓟ | Ⓕ | Ⓟ | Ⓕ |
| **Assessor:** **Date:** | **Test 1 Comments:** | | | | | | |
| **Assessor:** **Date:** | **Test 2 Comments:** | | | | | | |
| **Assessor:** **Date:** | **Test 3 Comments:** | | | | | | |

**TEST ENVIRONMENTS**
**L:** Laboratory/Classroom
**C:** Clinical/Field Testing
**P:** Practicum
**A:** Assessment/Mock Exam

**TEST INFORMATION**
**Test Statistics:** N/A
**Reference(s):**  Kendall et al. (2005)

MUSCULOSKELETAL SYSTEM—REGION 3: KNEE
# MANUAL MUSCLE TESTING

| NATA EC 5th | BOC RD6 | SKILL |
|:---:|:---:|:---:|
| CE-21c | D2-0203 | MMT: Quadriceps Femoris (Rectus Femoris, Vastus Medialis, Vastus Intermedius, Vastus Lateralis) |

**Supplies Needed:** Table

*This problem allows you the opportunity to demonstrate a* **manual muscle test** *for the* **quadriceps femoris.** *You have 2 minutes to complete this task.*

| MMT: Quadriceps Femoris (Rectus Femoris, Vastus Medialis, Vastus Intermedius, Vastus Lateralis) | Course or Site Assessor Environment | | Test 1 | | Test 2 | | Test 3 | |
|:---|:---:|:---:|:---:|:---:|:---:|:---:|:---:|:---:|
| **Tester places patient and limb in appropriate position** | | **Y** | **N** | **Y** | **N** | **Y** | **N** | |
| Seated, with the knee over the edge of the table and holding on to the table | | ○ | ○ | ○ | ○ | ○ | ○ | |
| **Tester placed in proper position** | | **Y** | **N** | **Y** | **N** | **Y** | **N** | |
| Stabilizes the femur superiorly to the patella and lower leg proximal to the malleoli | | ○ | ○ | ○ | ○ | ○ | ○ | |
| **Tester performs test according to accepted guidelines** | | **Y** | **N** | **Y** | **N** | **Y** | **N** | |
| Instructs the patient to actively extend the knee | | ○ | ○ | ○ | ○ | ○ | ○ | |
| Applies resistance to the anterior portion of the lower leg (direction of knee flexion) | | ○ | ○ | ○ | ○ | ○ | ○ | |
| Holds resistance for 5 seconds | | ○ | ○ | ○ | ○ | ○ | ○ | |
| Performs assessment bilaterally | | ○ | ○ | ○ | ○ | ○ | ○ | |
| **Identifies implications** | | **Y** | **N** | **Y** | **N** | **Y** | **N** | |
| Correctly grades the MMT | | ○ | ○ | ○ | ○ | ○ | ○ | |
| Total | | __/7 | | __/7 | | __/7 | | |
| **Must achieve >4 to pass this examination** | | Ⓟ | Ⓕ | Ⓟ | Ⓕ | Ⓟ | Ⓕ | |

| Assessor: Date: | Test 1 Comments: |
|:---|:---|
| Assessor: Date: | Test 2 Comments: |
| Assessor: Date: | Test 3 Comments: |

**TEST ENVIRONMENTS**
**L:** Laboratory/Classroom
**C:** Clinical/Field Testing
**P:** Practicum
**A:** Assessment/Mock Exam

**TEST INFORMATION**
**Test Statistics:** N/A
**Reference(s):** Kendall et al. (2005)

## MUSCULOSKELETAL SYSTEM—REGION 3: KNEE
# MANUAL MUSCLE TESTING

| NATA EC 5th | BOC RD6 | SKILL |
|---|---|---|
| CE-21c | D2-0203 | MMT: Sartorius |

**Supplies Needed:** Table

*This problem allows you the opportunity to demonstrate a* **manual muscle test** *for the* **sartorius.** *You have 2 minutes to complete this task.*

| MMT: Sartorius | Course or Site Assessor Environment | | | | | |
|---|---|---|---|---|---|---|
| | | Test 1 | | Test 2 | | Test 3 |
| **Tester places patient and limb in appropriate position** | | Y | N | Y | N | Y | N |
| Supine, lateral rotation, abduction, and flexion of the thigh; flexion of the knee to 90 degrees | | O | O | O | O | O | O |
| **Tester placed in proper position** | | Y | N | Y | N | Y | N |
| Stabilizes the femur superiorly to the patella, stabilizes the lower leg inferiorly to the medial malleoli | | O | O | O | O | O | O |
| **Tester performs test according to accepted guidelines** | | Y | N | Y | N | Y | N |
| Instructs the patient to maintain position | | O | O | O | O | O | O |
| Applies a downward and inward force at the knee | | O | O | O | O | O | O |
| Applies a lateral force at the ankle | | O | O | O | O | O | O |
| Holds resistance for 5 seconds | | O | O | O | O | O | O |
| Performs assessment bilaterally | | O | O | O | O | O | O |
| **Identifies implications** | | Y | N | Y | N | Y | N |
| Correctly grades the MMT | | O | O | O | O | O | O |
| **Total** | | ___/8 | | ___/8 | | ___/8 | |
| **Must achieve >5 to pass this examination** | | Ⓟ | Ⓕ | Ⓟ | Ⓕ | Ⓟ | Ⓕ |

| Assessor: Date: | Test 1 Comments: |
|---|---|
| Assessor: Date: | Test 2 Comments: |
| Assessor: Date: | Test 3 Comments: |

**TEST ENVIRONMENTS**
**L:** Laboratory/Classroom
**C:** Clinical/Field Testing
**P:** Practicum
**A:** Assessment/Mock Exam

**TEST INFORMATION**
**Test Statistics:** N/A
**Reference(s):** Kendall et al. (2005)

**MUSCULOSKELETAL SYSTEM—REGION 3: KNEE**
# OSTEOKINEMATIC JOINT MOTION

| NATA EC 5th | BOC RD6 | SKILL |
|---|---|---|
| CE-21d | D2-0203 | Goniometric Assessment: Tibiofemoral Joint (Flexion) |

**Supplies Needed:** Table, large goniometer

*This problem allows you the opportunity to demonstrate a* **goniometric assessment** *for the* **tibiofemoral joint (flexion)**. *You have 2 minutes to complete this task.*

| Goniometric Assessment: Tibiofemoral Joint (Flexion) | Course or Site Assessor Environment _____ _____ _____ | | Test 1 | | Test 2 | | Test 3 |
|---|---|---|---|---|---|---|---|
| **Tester places patient and limb in appropriate position** | | Y | N | Y | N | Y | N |
| Supine, with knee in extension, and hip in 0 degrees of extension, abduction, and adduction | | ○ | ○ | ○ | ○ | ○ | ○ |
| **Tester and goniometer placed in proper position** | | Y | N | Y | N | Y | N |
| Stabilizes the femur to prevent rotation, abduction, and adduction of the hip | | ○ | ○ | ○ | ○ | ○ | ○ |
| Places the fulcrum over the lateral epicondyle of the femur, stationary arm in line with greater trochanter | | ○ | ○ | ○ | ○ | ○ | ○ |
| Moving arm aligned with lateral malleolus | | ○ | ○ | ○ | ○ | ○ | ○ |
| **Tester performs test according to accepted guidelines** | | Y | N | Y | N | Y | N |
| Passively flexes the hip to 90 degrees and the knee to the end-feel, while stabilizing thigh to prevent further hip motion | | ○ | ○ | ○ | ○ | ○ | ○ |
| Takes proper goniometric measurement | | ○ | ○ | ○ | ○ | ○ | ○ |
| Performs assessment bilaterally | | ○ | ○ | ○ | ○ | ○ | ○ |
| **Identifies implications** | | Y | N | Y | N | Y | N |
| Identifies normal ranges (flexion = 150 degrees) | | ○ | ○ | ○ | ○ | ○ | ○ |
| Total | | ___/8 | | ___/8 | | ___/8 | |
| **Must achieve >5 to pass this examination** | | Ⓟ | Ⓕ | Ⓟ | Ⓕ | Ⓟ | Ⓕ |

| Assessor: Date: | Test 1 Comments: |
|---|---|
| Assessor: Date: | Test 2 Comments: |
| Assessor: Date: | Test 3 Comments: |

**TEST ENVIRONMENTS**
**L:** Laboratory/Classroom
**C:** Clinical/Field Testing
**P:** Practicum
**A:** Assessment/Mock Exam

**TEST INFORMATION**
**Test Statistics:** N/A
**Reference(s):** Norkin & White (2009)

MUSCULOSKELETAL SYSTEM—REGION 3: KNEE
# OSTEOKINEMATIC JOINT MOTION

| NATA EC 5th | BOC RD6 | SKILL |
|---|---|---|
| CE-21d | D2-0203 | Goniometric Assessment: Tibiofemoral Joint (Extension) |

**Supplies Needed:** Table, large goniometer, small towel

*This problem allows you the opportunity to demonstrate a* **goniometric assessment** *for the* **tibiofemoral joint (extension)***. You have 2 minutes to complete this task.*

| Goniometric Assessment: Tibiofemoral Joint (Extension) | Course or Site Assessor Environment | | Test 1 | | Test 2 | | Test 3 | |
|---|---|---|---|---|---|---|---|---|
| **Tester places patient and limb in appropriate position** | | | **Y** | **N** | **Y** | **N** | **Y** | **N** |
| Supine with hip and knee in 0 degrees flexion, with towel roll placed under heel to allow for knee extension | | | ○ | ○ | ○ | ○ | ○ | ○ |
| **Tester and goniometer placed in proper position** | | | **Y** | **N** | **Y** | **N** | **Y** | **N** |
| Stabilizes the femur to prevent rotation, abduction, and adduction of the hip | | | ○ | ○ | ○ | ○ | ○ | ○ |
| Places the fulcrum over the lateral epicondyle of the femur, stationary arm in line with greater trochanter | | | ○ | ○ | ○ | ○ | ○ | ○ |
| Moving arm aligned with lateral malleolus | | | ○ | ○ | ○ | ○ | ○ | ○ |
| **Tester performs test according to accepted guidelines** | | | **Y** | **N** | **Y** | **N** | **Y** | **N** |
| Provides passive extension | | | ○ | ○ | ○ | ○ | ○ | ○ |
| Takes proper goniometric measurement | | | ○ | ○ | ○ | ○ | ○ | ○ |
| Performs assessment bilaterally | | | ○ | ○ | ○ | ○ | ○ | ○ |
| **Identifies implications** | | | **Y** | **N** | **Y** | **N** | **Y** | **N** |
| Identifies normal ranges (extension = 0 to 5 degrees) | | | ○ | ○ | ○ | ○ | ○ | ○ |
| **Total** | | | ___/8 | | ___/8 | | ___/8 | |
| **Must achieve >5 to pass this examination** | | | Ⓟ | Ⓕ | Ⓟ | Ⓕ | Ⓟ | Ⓕ |

| Assessor: Date: | Test 1 Comments: |
|---|---|
| Assessor: Date: | Test 2 Comments: |
| Assessor: Date: | Test 3 Comments: |

**TEST ENVIRONMENTS**
**L:** Laboratory/Classroom
**C:** Clinical/Field Testing
**P:** Practicum
**A:** Assessment/Mock Exam

**TEST INFORMATION**
**Test Statistics:** N/A
**Reference(s):** Norkin & White (2009)

# CAPSULAR AND LIGAMENTOUS STRESS TESTING

| NATA EC 5th | BOC RD6 | SKILL |
|---|---|---|
| CE-21e | D2-0203 | Anterior Drawer Test for the Knee |

**Supplies Needed:** Table

*This problem allows you the opportunity to demonstrate an* **orthopedic test** *known as the* **anterior drawer test for the knee**. *You have 2 minutes to complete this task.*

| Anterior Drawer Test for the Knee | Course or Site / Assessor / Environment | | Test 1 | | Test 2 | | Test 3 |
|---|---|---|---|---|---|---|---|
| **Tester places patient and limb in appropriate position** | | Y | N | Y | N | Y | N |
| Supine on the table | | O | O | O | O | O | O |
| Hip flexed to 45 degrees and knee flexed to 90 degrees | | O | O | O | O | O | O |
| **Tester placed in proper position** | | Y | N | Y | N | Y | N |
| Sits on the examination table in front of the involved knee, grasping the tibia just below the joint line | | O | O | O | O | O | O |
| Places thumb along joint line on either side of the patellar tendon | | O | O | O | O | O | O |
| Wraps index fingers around knee to ensure hamstrings are relaxed | | O | O | O | O | O | O |
| **Tester performs test according to accepted guidelines** | | Y | N | Y | N | Y | N |
| Maintains relaxation of the limb | | O | O | O | O | O | O |
| Draws tibia forward (anterior displacement) on lower leg | | O | O | O | O | O | O |
| Performs assessment bilaterally | | O | O | O | O | O | O |
| **Identifies positive findings and implications** | | Y | N | Y | N | Y | N |
| Excessive anterior translation; clunk | | O | O | O | O | O | O |
| ACL sprain | | O | O | O | O | O | O |
| **Total** | | /10 | | /10 | | 10 | |
| **Must achieve >6 to pass this examination** | | P | F | P | F | P | F |

| Assessor: Date: | Test 1 Comments: |
|---|---|
| Assessor: Date: | Test 2 Comments: |
| Assessor: Date: | Test 3 Comments: |

**TEST ENVIRONMENTS**
L: Laboratory/Classroom
C: Clinical/Field Testing
P: Practicum
A: Assessment/Mock Exam

**TEST INFORMATION**
**Test Statistics:** Sensitivity .63–.99
Specificity .42–1.00
(+) LR 2.15–11.30
(-) LR .23–.41
**Reference(s):** Cook & Hegedus (2013)
Makhmalbaf et al. (2013)
Starkey & Brown (2015)

MUSCULOSKELETAL SYSTEM—REGION 3: KNEE
# CAPSULAR AND LIGAMENTOUS STRESS TESTING

| NATA EC 5th | BOC RD6 | SKILL |
|---|---|---|
| CE-21e | D2-0203 | Godfrey Test (Godfrey 90/90 Test) |

**Supplies Needed:** Table

*This problem allows you the opportunity to demonstrate an* **orthopedic test** *known as the* **Godfrey test (Godfrey 90/90 test)***. You have 2 minutes to complete this task.*

| Godfrey Test (Godfrey 90/90 Test) | Course or Site Assessor Environment | | Test 1 | | Test 2 | | Test 3 | |
|---|---|---|---|---|---|---|---|---|
| **Tester places patient and limb in appropriate position** | | | **Y** | **N** | **Y** | **N** | **Y** | **N** |
| Supine on the table | | | ○ | ○ | ○ | ○ | ○ | ○ |
| Knees extended and legs together | | | ○ | ○ | ○ | ○ | ○ | ○ |
| **Tester placed in proper position** | | | **Y** | **N** | **Y** | **N** | **Y** | **N** |
| Stands next to the patient | | | ○ | ○ | ○ | ○ | ○ | ○ |
| **Tester performs test according to accepted guidelines** | | | **Y** | **N** | **Y** | **N** | **Y** | **N** |
| Maintains relaxation of the limb | | | ○ | ○ | ○ | ○ | ○ | ○ |
| Lifts the patient's lower legs to 90 degrees H' and K' flexion | | | ○ | ○ | ○ | ○ | ○ | ○ |
| Examiner observes the level of the tibial tuberosities | | | ○ | ○ | ○ | ○ | ○ | ○ |
| **Identifies positive findings and implications** | | | **Y** | **N** | **Y** | **N** | **Y** | **N** |
| Excessive unilateral posterior displacement of the tibial tuberosity | | | ○ | ○ | ○ | ○ | ○ | ○ |
| Sprain of the PCL | | | ○ | ○ | ○ | ○ | ○ | ○ |
| **Total** | | | ___/8 | | ___/8 | | ___/8 | |
| **Must achieve >5 to pass this examination** | | | Ⓟ | Ⓕ | Ⓟ | Ⓕ | Ⓟ | Ⓕ |

| Assessor: Date: | Test 1 Comments: |
|---|---|
| Assessor: Date: | Test 2 Comments: |
| Assessor: Date: | Test 3 Comments: |

**TEST ENVIRONMENTS**
**L:** Laboratory/Classroom
**C:** Clinical/Field Testing
**P:** Practicum
**A:** Assessment/Mock Exam

**TEST INFORMATION**
**Test Statistics:** Sensitivity .46–1.00
Specificity 1.00
**Reference(s):** Cook & Hegedus (2013)
Starkey & Brown (2015)

# CAPSULAR AND LIGAMENTOUS STRESS TESTING

| NATA EC 5th | BOC RD6 | SKILL |
|:---:|:---:|:---:|
| CE-21e | D2-0203 | Hughston Posterolateral Drawer Test |

**Supplies Needed:** Table

*This problem allows you the opportunity to demonstrate an* **orthopedic test** *known as the* **Hughston posterolateral drawer test** *for* **posterolateral instability**. *You have 2 minutes to complete this task.*

| Hughston Posterolateral Drawer Test | Course or Site / Assessor / Environment | | Test 1 | | Test 2 | | Test 3 | |
|---|---|---|:---:|:---:|:---:|:---:|:---:|:---:|
| | | | Y | N | Y | N | Y | N |
| **Tester places patient and limb in appropriate position** | | | Y | N | Y | N | Y | N |
| Supine with the hip flexed to 45 degrees and knee flexed to 80 degrees | | | ○ | ○ | ○ | ○ | ○ | ○ |
| Tibia is externally rotated 15 degrees | | | ○ | ○ | ○ | ○ | ○ | ○ |
| **Tester placed in proper position** | | | Y | N | Y | N | Y | N |
| Sits on the foot of the limb being tested | | | ○ | ○ | ○ | ○ | ○ | ○ |
| Hands grasp the proximal tibia | | | ○ | ○ | ○ | ○ | ○ | ○ |
| **Tester performs test according to accepted guidelines** | | | Y | N | Y | N | Y | N |
| Maintains relaxation of the limb | | | ○ | ○ | ○ | ○ | ○ | ○ |
| Applies a posterior force to the proximal tibia | | | ○ | ○ | ○ | ○ | ○ | ○ |
| Performs assessment bilaterally | | | ○ | ○ | ○ | ○ | ○ | ○ |
| **Identifies positive findings and implications** | | | Y | N | Y | N | Y | N |
| Increased external rotation of the lateral tibial condyle relative to the lateral femoral condyle relative to the uninvolved side | | | ○ | ○ | ○ | ○ | ○ | ○ |
| Total | | | ___/8 | | ___/8 | | ___/8 | |
| Must achieve >5 to pass this examination | | | Ⓟ | Ⓕ | Ⓟ | Ⓕ | Ⓟ | Ⓕ |
| Assessor: Date: | Test 1 Comments: | | | | | | | |
| Assessor: Date: | Test 2 Comments: | | | | | | | |
| Assessor: Date: | Test 3 Comments: | | | | | | | |

**TEST ENVIRONMENTS**
**L:** Laboratory/Classroom
**C:** Clinical/Field Testing
**P:** Practicum
**A:** Assessment/Mock Exam

**TEST INFORMATION**
**Test Statistics:** No data available
**Reference(s):** Starkey & Brown (2015)

MUSCULOSKELETAL SYSTEM—REGION 3: KNEE
# CAPSULAR AND LIGAMENTOUS STRESS TESTING

| NATA EC 5th | BOC RD6 | SKILL |
|---|---|---|
| CE-21e | D2-0203 | Hughston Posteromedial Drawer Test |

**Supplies Needed:** Table

*This problem allows you the opportunity to demonstrate an* **orthopedic test** *known as the* **Hughston posteromedial drawer test** *for* **posterior medial instability.** *You have 2 minutes to complete this task.*

| Hughston Posteromedial Drawer Test | Course or Site Assessor Environment | | Test 1 | | Test 2 | | Test 3 | |
|---|---|---|---|---|---|---|---|---|
| **Tester places patient and limb in appropriate position** | | | **Y** | **N** | **Y** | **N** | **Y** | **N** |
| Supine with the hip flexed to 45 degrees and knee flexed to 80 degrees | | | O | O | O | O | O | O |
| Tibia is internally rotated 15 degrees | | | O | O | O | O | O | O |
| **Tester placed in proper position** | | | **Y** | **N** | **Y** | **N** | **Y** | **N** |
| Sits on the foot of the limb being tested | | | O | O | O | O | O | O |
| Hands grasp the proximal tibia | | | O | O | O | O | O | O |
| **Tester performs test according to accepted guidelines** | | | **Y** | **N** | **Y** | **N** | **Y** | **N** |
| Maintains relaxation of the limb | | | O | O | O | O | O | O |
| Applies a posterior force to the proximal tibia | | | O | O | O | O | O | O |
| Performs assessment bilaterally | | | O | O | O | O | O | O |
| **Identifies positive findings and implications** | | | **Y** | **N** | **Y** | **N** | **Y** | **N** |
| Increased external rotation of the lateral tibial condyle relative to the lateral femoral condyle relative to the uninvolved side | | | O | O | O | O | O | O |
| **Total** | | | ___/8 | | ___/8 | | ___/8 | |
| **Must achieve >5 to pass this examination** | | | Ⓟ | Ⓕ | Ⓟ | Ⓕ | Ⓟ | Ⓕ |

| Assessor:<br>Date: | Test 1 Comments: |
|---|---|
| Assessor:<br>Date: | Test 2 Comments: |
| Assessor:<br>Date: | Test 3 Comments: |

**TEST ENVIRONMENTS**
**L:** Laboratory/Classroom
**C:** Clinical/Field Testing
**P:** Practicum
**A:** Assessment/Mock Exam

**TEST INFORMATION**
**Test Statistics:** No data available
**Reference(s):** Starkey & Brown (2015)

## MUSCULOSKELETAL SYSTEM—REGION 3: KNEE
# CAPSULAR AND LIGAMENTOUS STRESS TESTING

| NATA EC 5th | BOC RD6 | SKILL |
|:---:|:---:|:---:|
| CE-21e | D2-0203 | Hughston Jerk Test |

**Supplies Needed:** Table

*This problem allows you the opportunity to demonstrate an* **orthopedic test** *known as the* **Hughston jerk test** *for* **anterolateral knee stability.** *You have 2 minutes to complete this task.*

| Hughston Jerk Test | Course or Site Assessor Environment | | Test 1 | | Test 2 | | Test 3 | |
|---|---|---|:---:|:---:|:---:|:---:|:---:|:---:|
| **Tester places patient and limb in appropriate position** | | | Y | N | Y | N | Y | N |
| Supine on the table | | | ○ | ○ | ○ | ○ | ○ | ○ |
| **Tester placed in proper position** | | | Y | N | Y | N | Y | N |
| Grasps the lateral knee and lateral ankle | | | ○ | ○ | ○ | ○ | ○ | ○ |
| Flexes the hip to 45 degrees and flexes the knee to 90 degrees | | | ○ | ○ | ○ | ○ | ○ | ○ |
| **Tester performs test according to accepted guidelines** | | | Y | N | Y | N | Y | N |
| Applies a valgus and internal rotation force to the tibia | | | ○ | ○ | ○ | ○ | ○ | ○ |
| Passively moves the patient's knee into extension | | | ○ | ○ | ○ | ○ | ○ | ○ |
| Performs assessment bilaterally | | | ○ | ○ | ○ | ○ | ○ | ○ |
| **Identifies positive findings and implications** | | | Y | N | Y | N | Y | N |
| Subluxation of the tibia on the femur is felt between 30 to 40 degrees | | | ○ | ○ | ○ | ○ | ○ | ○ |
| Anterolateral instability (ACL, capsule, LCL) | | | ○ | ○ | ○ | ○ | ○ | ○ |
| | | Total | ___/8 | | ___/8 | | ___/8 | |
| | Must achieve >5 to pass this examination | | Ⓟ | Ⓕ | Ⓟ | Ⓕ | Ⓟ | Ⓕ |
| **Assessor:** **Date:** | **Test 1 Comments:** | | | | | | | |
| **Assessor:** **Date:** | **Test 2 Comments:** | | | | | | | |
| **Assessor:** **Date:** | **Test 3 Comments:** | | | | | | | |

**TEST ENVIRONMENTS**
**L:** Laboratory/Classroom
**C:** Clinical/Field Testing
**P:** Practicum
**A:** Assessment/Mock Exam

**TEST INFORMATION**
**Test Statistics:** No data available
**Reference(s):** Starkey & Brown (2015)

MUSCULOSKELETAL SYSTEM—REGION 3: KNEE
# CAPSULAR AND LIGAMENTOUS STRESS TESTING

| NATA EC 5th | BOC RD6 | SKILL |
|---|---|---|
| CE-21e | D2-0203 | Lachman's Test |

**Supplies Needed:** Table

*This problem allows you the opportunity to demonstrate an* **orthopedic test** *known as* **Lachman's test** *for* **anterior cruciate ligament injury**. *You have 2 minutes to complete this task.*

| Lachman's Test | Course or Site<br>Assessor<br>Environment | | | | | |
|---|---|---|---|---|---|---|
| | | Test 1 | | Test 2 | | Test 3 |
| **Tester places patient and limb in appropriate position** | | Y | N | Y | N | Y | N |
| Supine on the table | | O | O | O | O | O | O |
| Knee passively flexed to 20 to 25 degrees | | O | O | O | O | O | O |
| **Tester placed in proper position** | | Y | N | Y | N | Y | N |
| One hand grasps the tibia around the level of the tibial tuberosity | | O | O | O | O | O | O |
| Opposite hand grasps the femur just above the condyles | | O | O | O | O | O | O |
| **Tester performs test according to accepted guidelines** | | Y | N | Y | N | Y | N |
| Supports the weight of the leg | | O | O | O | O | O | O |
| Draws the tibia anteriorly while a posterior pressure is applied to stabilize the femur | | O | O | O | O | O | O |
| Performs assessment bilaterally | | O | O | O | O | O | O |
| **Identifies positive findings and implications** | | Y | N | Y | N | Y | N |
| An increased amount of anterior tibial translation compared with the opposite limb or lack of a firm end-feel | | O | O | O | O | O | O |
| Spring of the ACL or posterolateral bundle of the ACL | | O | O | O | O | O | O |
| **Total** | | ___/9 | | ___/9 | | ___/9 |
| **Must achieve >6 to pass this examination** | | Ⓟ | Ⓕ | Ⓟ | Ⓕ | Ⓟ | Ⓕ |

| Assessor:<br>Date: | Test 1 Comments: |
|---|---|
| Assessor:<br>Date: | Test 2 Comments: |
| Assessor:<br>Date: | Test 3 Comments: |

**TEST ENVIRONMENTS**
**L:** Laboratory/Classroom
**C:** Clinical/Field Testing
**P:** Practicum
**A:** Assessment/Mock Exam

**TEST INFORMATION**
**Test Statistics:** Sensitivity .63–.99
Specificity .55–.99
(+) LR 9.56
(-) LR .43
**Reference(s):** Ostrowski (2006)
Starkey & Brown (2015)

# CAPSULAR AND LIGAMENTOUS STRESS TESTING

| NATA EC 5th | BOC RD6 | SKILL |
|---|---|---|
| CE-21e | D2-0203 | Lateral Pivot Shift Test |

**Supplies Needed:** Table

*This problem allows you the opportunity to demonstrate an* **orthopedic test** *known as the* **lateral pivot shift test** *to rule out an* **anterior cruciate ligament injury**. *You have 2 minutes to complete this task.*

| Lateral Pivot Shift Test | Course or Site / Assessor / Environment | | Test 1 | | Test 2 | | Test 3 | |
|---|---|---|---|---|---|---|---|---|
| **Tester places patient and limb in appropriate position** | | | Y | N | Y | N | Y | N |
| Supine with hip passively flexed to 30 degrees | | | O | O | O | O | O | O |
| **Tester placed in proper position** | | | Y | N | Y | N | Y | N |
| Stands to the side of the patient | | | O | O | O | O | O | O |
| Places the supinated cephalic hand underneath the knee | | | O | O | O | O | O | O |
| Grasps the lower leg or ankle with the caudal hand and passively internally rotates the tibia to 20 degrees | | | O | O | O | O | O | O |
| While maintaining tibial internal rotation, allows the knee to sag into extension | | | O | O | O | O | O | O |
| **Tester performs test according to accepted guidelines** | | | Y | N | Y | N | Y | N |
| While maintaining internal rotation, a valgus force is applied to the knee while it is slowly flexed | | | O | O | O | O | O | O |
| **Identifies positive findings and implications** | | | Y | N | Y | N | Y | N |
| Subluxation of the tibia on the femur is felt between 30 to 40 degrees | | | O | O | O | O | O | O |
| Anterolateral instability (ACL, capsule, LCL) | | | O | O | O | O | O | O |
| **Total** | | | __/8 | | __/8 | | __/8 | |
| **Must achieve >5 to pass this examination** | | | P | F | P | F | P | F |

| Assessor: Date: | Test 1 Comments: |
|---|---|
| Assessor: Date: | Test 2 Comments: |
| Assessor: Date: | Test 3 Comments: |

**TEST ENVIRONMENTS**
**L:** Laboratory/Classroom
**C:** Clinical/Field Testing
**P:** Practicum
**A:** Assessment/Mock Exam

**TEST INFORMATION**
**Test Statistics:** Sensitivity .18–.48
Specificity .97–.99
(+) LR 16.5
(-) LR .68
**Reference(s):** Ostrowski (2006)
Starkey & Brown (2015)

# CAPSULAR AND LIGAMENTOUS STRESS TESTING

| NATA EC 5th | BOC RD6 | SKILL |
|---|---|---|
| CE-21e | D2-0203 | Posterior Drawer Test for the Knee |

**Supplies Needed:** Table

*This problem allows you the opportunity to demonstrate an* **orthopedic test** *known as the* **posterior drawer test for the knee**. *You have 2 minutes to complete this task.*

| Posterior Drawer Test for the Knee | Course or Site / Assessor / Environment | Test 1 | | Test 2 | | Test 3 | |
|---|---|---|---|---|---|---|---|
| **Tester places patient and limb in appropriate position** | | Y | N | Y | N | Y | N |
| Supine | | ○ | ○ | ○ | ○ | ○ | ○ |
| Hip flexed to 45 degrees and knee flexed to 90 degrees | | ○ | ○ | ○ | ○ | ○ | ○ |
| **Tester placed in proper position** | | Y | N | Y | N | Y | N |
| Sits on examination table in front of involved knee | | ○ | ○ | ○ | ○ | ○ | ○ |
| The patient's tibia is stabilized in the neutral position | | ○ | ○ | ○ | ○ | ○ | ○ |
| **Tester performs test according to accepted guidelines** | | Y | N | Y | N | Y | N |
| Grasps the tibia just below the joint line of the knee with fingertips placed along the joint line on either side of the patellar tendon | | ○ | ○ | ○ | ○ | ○ | ○ |
| Pushes proximal tibia posteriorly | | ○ | ○ | ○ | ○ | ○ | ○ |
| Performs assessment bilaterally | | ○ | ○ | ○ | ○ | ○ | ○ |
| **Identifies positive findings and implications** | | Y | N | Y | N | Y | N |
| Excessive posterior tibial translation | | ○ | ○ | ○ | ○ | ○ | ○ |
| PCL sprain | | ○ | ○ | ○ | ○ | ○ | ○ |
| **Total** | | __/9 | | __/9 | | __/9 | |
| **Must achieve >6 to pass this examination** | | Ⓟ | Ⓕ | Ⓟ | Ⓕ | Ⓟ | Ⓕ |

| Assessor: Date: | Test 1 Comments: |
|---|---|
| Assessor: Date: | Test 2 Comments: |
| Assessor: Date: | Test 3 Comments: |

**TEST ENVIRONMENTS**
**L:** Laboratory/Classroom
**C:** Clinical/Field Testing
**P:** Practicum
**A:** Assessment/Mock Exam

**TEST INFORMATION**
**Test Statistics:** Sensitivity .51–1.0
Specificity .99
(+) LR 5.1–10
(-) LR 0–.49
**Reference(s):** Malanga, Andrus, et al. (2003)
Starkey & Brown (2015)

# CAPSULAR AND LIGAMENTOUS STRESS TESTING

| NATA EC 5th | BOC RD6 | SKILL |
|---|---|---|
| CE-21e | D2-0203 | Posterior Sag Sign |

**Supplies Needed:** Table

*This problem allows you the opportunity to demonstrate an* **orthopedic test** *known as the* **posterior sag sign**. *You have 2 minutes to complete this task.*

| Posterior Sag Sign | Course or Site / Assessor / Environment | Test 1 | | Test 2 | | Test 3 | |
|---|---|---|---|---|---|---|---|
| | | **Y** | **N** | **Y** | **N** | **Y** | **N** |
| **Tester places patient and limb in appropriate position** | | Y | N | Y | N | Y | N |
| Supine | | ○ | ○ | ○ | ○ | ○ | ○ |
| Hips flexed to 45 degrees and knees flexed to 90 degrees | | ○ | ○ | ○ | ○ | ○ | ○ |
| **Tester placed in proper position** | | Y | N | Y | N | Y | N |
| Stands next to the patient | | ○ | ○ | ○ | ○ | ○ | ○ |
| Holds lower legs just proximal to the ankle | | ○ | ○ | ○ | ○ | ○ | ○ |
| **Tester performs test according to accepted guidelines** | | Y | N | Y | N | Y | N |
| Maintains relaxation of the limb | | ○ | ○ | ○ | ○ | ○ | ○ |
| Observes tibial tuberosity | | ○ | ○ | ○ | ○ | ○ | ○ |
| Performs assessment bilaterally | | ○ | ○ | ○ | ○ | ○ | ○ |
| **Identifies positive findings and implications** | | Y | N | Y | N | Y | N |
| Unilateral displacement of the tibia posteriorly | | ○ | ○ | ○ | ○ | ○ | ○ |
| PCL tear | | ○ | ○ | ○ | ○ | ○ | ○ |
| **Total** | | ___/9 | | ___/9 | | ___/9 | |
| **Must achieve >6 to pass this examination** | | Ⓟ | Ⓕ | Ⓟ | Ⓕ | Ⓟ | Ⓕ |

| Assessor: Date: | Test 1 Comments: |
|---|---|
| Assessor: Date: | Test 2 Comments: |
| Assessor: Date: | Test 3 Comments: |

**TEST ENVIRONMENTS**
**L:** Laboratory/Classroom
**C:** Clinical/Field Testing
**P:** Practicum
**A:** Assessment/Mock Exam

**TEST INFORMATION**
**Test Statistics:** Sensitivity .79
Specificity 1.0
**Reference(s):** Malanga, Andrus, et al. (2003)
Starkey & Brown (2015)

## MUSCULOSKELETAL SYSTEM—REGION 3: KNEE
# CAPSULAR AND LIGAMENTOUS STRESS TESTING

| NATA EC 5th | BOC RD6 | SKILL |
|---|---|---|
| CE-21e | D2-0203 | Quadriceps Active Test |

**Supplies Needed:** Table

*This problem allows you the opportunity to demonstrate an* **orthopedic test** *known as the* **quadriceps active test**. *You have 2 minutes to complete this task.*

| Quadriceps Active Test | Course or Site / Assessor / Environment | | Test 1 | | Test 2 | | Test 3 | |
|---|---|---|---|---|---|---|---|---|
| **Tester places patient and limb in appropriate position** | | | Y | N | Y | N | Y | N |
| Supine | | | ○ | ○ | ○ | ○ | ○ | ○ |
| Knee flexed to 90 degrees | | | ○ | ○ | ○ | ○ | ○ | ○ |
| **Tester placed in proper position** | | | Y | N | Y | N | Y | N |
| Positioned at the side of the patient | | | ○ | ○ | ○ | ○ | ○ | ○ |
| One hand stabilizes distal tibia and the other stabilizes distal femur | | | ○ | ○ | ○ | ○ | ○ | ○ |
| **Tester performs test according to accepted guidelines** | | | Y | N | Y | N | Y | N |
| While resisting knee extension, the patient is asked to slide the foot forward by contracting the quadriceps | | | ○ | ○ | ○ | ○ | ○ | ○ |
| Observes for anterior translation of the tibia | | | ○ | ○ | ○ | ○ | ○ | ○ |
| Performs assessment bilaterally | | | ○ | ○ | ○ | ○ | ○ | ○ |
| **Identifies positive findings and implications** | | | Y | N | Y | N | Y | N |
| Excessive unilateral anterior translation of the tibia on the femur | | | ○ | ○ | ○ | ○ | ○ | ○ |
| Grade II or III PCL sprain | | | ○ | ○ | ○ | ○ | ○ | ○ |
| Total | | | __/9 | | __/9 | | __/9 | |
| Must achieve >6 to pass this examination | | | ⓅF | | ⓅF | | ⓅF | |

| Assessor: Date: | Test 1 Comments: |
|---|---|
| Assessor: Date: | Test 2 Comments: |
| Assessor: Date: | Test 3 Comments: |

**TEST ENVIRONMENTS**
L: Laboratory/Classroom
C: Clinical/Field Testing
P: Practicum
A: Assessment/Mock Exam

**TEST INFORMATION**
**Test Statistics:** Sensitivity .54–.98
Specificity .97–1.0
(+) LR 18–32.67
(-) LR .02–.47
**Reference(s):** Malanga, Andrus, et al. (2003)
Starkey & Brown (2015)

## MUSCULOSKELETAL SYSTEM—REGION 3: KNEE
# CAPSULAR AND LIGAMENTOUS STRESS TESTING

| NATA EC 5th | BOC RD6 | SKILL |
|---|---|---|
| CE-21e | D2-0203 | Slocum Drawer Test (External Tibial Rotation) |

**Supplies Needed:** Table

*This problem allows you the opportunity to demonstrate an* **orthopedic test** *known as the* **Slocum drawer test (external tibial rotation)** *for the knee. You have 2 minutes to complete this task.*

| Slocum Drawer Test (External Tibial Rotation) | Course or Site Assessor Environment | | Test 1 | | Test 2 | | Test 3 | |
|---|---|---|---|---|---|---|---|---|
| **Tester places patient and limb in appropriate position** | | **Y** | **N** | **Y** | **N** | **Y** | **N** | |
| Supine | | ○ | ○ | ○ | ○ | ○ | ○ | |
| Knee flexed to 90 degrees | | ○ | ○ | ○ | ○ | ○ | ○ | |
| **Tester placed in proper position** | | **Y** | **N** | **Y** | **N** | **Y** | **N** | |
| Sits on the patient's foot | | ○ | ○ | ○ | ○ | ○ | ○ | |
| Tibia is externally rotated 15 degrees to test for anteromedial capsular instability | | ○ | ○ | ○ | ○ | ○ | ○ | |
| **Tester performs test according to accepted guidelines** | | **Y** | **N** | **Y** | **N** | **Y** | **N** | |
| Tibia is drawn anteriorly | | ○ | ○ | ○ | ○ | ○ | ○ | |
| Performs assessment bilaterally | | ○ | ○ | ○ | ○ | ○ | ○ | |
| **Identifies positive findings and implications** | | **Y** | **N** | **Y** | **N** | **Y** | **N** | |
| Increased amount of unilateral anterior tibial translation or lack of a firm end-feel | | ○ | ○ | ○ | ○ | ○ | ○ | |
| Damage to the MCL, anteromedial capsule, ACL, posteromedial capsule, pes anserine, medial meniscus | | ○ | ○ | ○ | ○ | ○ | ○ | |
| **Total** | | __/8 | | __/8 | | __/8 | | |
| **Must achieve >5 to pass this examination** | | Ⓟ | Ⓕ | Ⓟ | Ⓕ | Ⓟ | Ⓕ | |

| Assessor: Date: | Test 1 Comments: |
|---|---|
| Assessor: Date: | Test 2 Comments: |
| Assessor: Date: | Test 3 Comments: |

**TEST ENVIRONMENTS**
**L:** Laboratory/Classroom
**C:** Clinical/Field Testing
**P:** Practicum
**A:** Assessment/Mock Exam

**TEST INFORMATION**
**Test Statistics:** No data available
**Reference(s):** Starkey & Brown (2015)

**MUSCULOSKELETAL SYSTEM—REGION 3: KNEE**
# CAPSULAR AND LIGAMENTOUS STRESS TESTING

| NATA EC 5th | BOC RD6 | SKILL |
|---|---|---|
| CE-21e | D2-0203 | Slocum Drawer Test (Internal Tibial Rotation) |

**Supplies Needed:** Table

*This problem allows you the opportunity to demonstrate an* **orthopedic test** *known as the* **Slocum drawer test (internal tibial rotation)** *for the knee. You have 2 minutes to complete this task.*

| Slocum Drawer Test (Internal Tibial Rotation) | Course or Site Assessor Environment | | Test 1 | | Test 2 | | Test 3 | |
|---|---|---|---|---|---|---|---|---|
| **Tester places patient and limb in appropriate position** | | **Y** | **N** | **Y** | **N** | **Y** | **N** | |
| Supine | | ○ | ○ | ○ | ○ | ○ | ○ | |
| Knee flexed to 90 degrees | | ○ | ○ | ○ | ○ | ○ | ○ | |
| **Tester placed in proper position** | | **Y** | **N** | **Y** | **N** | **Y** | **N** | |
| Sits on the patient's foot | | ○ | ○ | ○ | ○ | ○ | ○ | |
| Tibia is internally rotated 25 degrees to test for anterolateral capsular instability | | ○ | ○ | ○ | ○ | ○ | ○ | |
| **Tester performs test according to accepted guidelines** | | **Y** | **N** | **Y** | **N** | **Y** | **N** | |
| Tibia is drawn anteriorly | | ○ | ○ | ○ | ○ | ○ | ○ | |
| Performs assessment bilaterally | | ○ | ○ | ○ | ○ | ○ | ○ | |
| **Identifies positive findings and implications** | | **Y** | **N** | **Y** | **N** | **Y** | **N** | |
| Increased amount of unilateral anterior tibial translation or lack of a firm end-feel | | ○ | ○ | ○ | ○ | ○ | ○ | |
| Damage to the ACL, anterolateral capsule, LCL, iliotibial band, popliteus tendon, posterolateral complex, lateral meniscus | | ○ | ○ | ○ | ○ | ○ | ○ | |
| **Total** | | ___/8 | | ___/8 | | ___/8 | | |
| **Must achieve >5 to pass this examination** | | Ⓟ | Ⓕ | Ⓟ | Ⓕ | Ⓟ | Ⓕ | |
| **Assessor:** **Date:** | **Test 1 Comments:** | | | | | | | |
| **Assessor:** **Date:** | **Test 2 Comments:** | | | | | | | |
| **Assessor:** **Date:** | **Test 3 Comments:** | | | | | | | |

**TEST ENVIRONMENTS**
**L:** Laboratory/Classroom
**C:** Clinical/Field Testing
**P:** Practicum
**A:** Assessment/Mock Exam

**TEST INFORMATION**
**Test Statistics:** No data available
**Reference(s):** Starkey & Brown (2015)

# CAPSULAR AND LIGAMENTOUS STRESS TESTING

| NATA EC 5th | BOC RD6 | SKILL |
|---|---|---|
| CE-21e | D2-0203 | Valgus Stress Test for the Knee |

**Supplies Needed:** Table

*This problem allows you the opportunity to demonstrate an* **orthopedic test** *known as the* **valgus stress test for the knee.** *You have 2 minutes to complete this task.*

| Valgus Stress Test for the Knee | Course or Site / Assessor / Environment | | Test 1 | | Test 2 | | Test 3 |
|---|---|---|---|---|---|---|---|
| **Tester places patient and limb in appropriate position** | | Y | N | Y | N | Y | N |
| Supine with the involved leg close to the edge of the table | | O | O | O | O | O | O |
| **Tester placed in proper position** | | Y | N | Y | N | Y | N |
| Stands lateral to the involved limb | | O | O | O | O | O | O |
| One hand supports the medial tibia and the other hand is placed along the lateral joint line of the knee | | O | O | O | O | O | O |
| To test medial joint capsule and other medial structures, the knee is kept in complete extension | | O | O | O | O | O | O |
| To isolate the MCL, the knee is flexed to 25 degrees | | O | O | O | O | O | O |
| **Tester performs test according to accepted guidelines** | | Y | N | Y | N | Y | N |
| The tester provides a medial (valgus) force to the knee while the distal tibia is moved laterally | | O | O | O | O | O | O |
| **Identifies positive findings and implications** | | Y | N | Y | N | Y | N |
| Unilateral increased laxity, altered end-feel, and/or pain | | O | O | O | O | O | O |
| In complete extension: MCL sprain, medial joint capsule, cruciate ligaments, distal femoral epiphyseal fracture | | O | O | O | O | O | O |
| In 25 degrees of flexion: MCL sprain | | O | O | O | O | O | O |
| **Total** | | __/9 | | __/9 | | __/9 | |
| **Must achieve >6 to pass this examination** | | ⓟ | Ⓕ | ⓟ | Ⓕ | ⓟ | Ⓕ |

| Assessor: Date: | Test 1 Comments: |
|---|---|
| Assessor: Date: | Test 2 Comments: |
| Assessor: Date: | Test 3 Comments: |

**TEST ENVIRONMENTS**
**L:** Laboratory/Classroom
**C:** Clinical/Field Testing
**P:** Practicum
**A:** Assessment/Mock Exam

**TEST INFORMATION**
**Test Statistics:** Sensitivity .78–1.00
Specificity .49–1.00
(+) LR 1.80–2.30
(-) LR .20–.30
**Reference(s):** Cook & Hegedus (2013)
Starkey & Brown (2015)

**MUSCULOSKELETAL SYSTEM—REGION 3: KNEE**
# CAPSULAR AND LIGAMENTOUS STRESS TESTING

| NATA EC 5th | BOC RD6 | SKILL |
|:---:|:---:|:---:|
| CE-21e | D2-0203 | Varus Stress Test for the Knee |

**Supplies Needed:** Table

*This problem allows you the opportunity to demonstrate an* **orthopedic test** *known as the* **varus stress test for the knee***. You have 2 minutes to complete this task.*

| Varus Stress Test for the Knee | Course or Site Assessor Environment | | Test 1 | | Test 2 | | Test 3 | |
|---|---|---|:---:|:---:|:---:|:---:|:---:|:---:|
| | | | **Y** | **N** | **Y** | **N** | **Y** | **N** |
| **Tester places patient and limb in appropriate position** | | | **Y** | **N** | **Y** | **N** | **Y** | **N** |
| Supine with involved leg close to the edge of the table | | | ○ | ○ | ○ | ○ | ○ | ○ |
| **Tester placed in proper position** | | | **Y** | **N** | **Y** | **N** | **Y** | **N** |
| Sits on the table | | | ○ | ○ | ○ | ○ | ○ | ○ |
| One hand supports the lateral tibia and the other hand is placed along the medial joint line of the knee | | | ○ | ○ | ○ | ○ | ○ | ○ |
| To test lateral joint capsule and other lateral structures, the knee is kept in complete extension | | | ○ | ○ | ○ | ○ | ○ | ○ |
| To isolate the LCL, the knee is flexed to 25 degrees | | | ○ | ○ | ○ | ○ | ○ | ○ |
| **Tester performs test according to accepted guidelines** | | | **Y** | **N** | **Y** | **N** | **Y** | **N** |
| The tester provides a lateral (varus) force to the knee while the distal tibia is moved medially | | | ○ | ○ | ○ | ○ | ○ | ○ |
| **Identifies positive findings and implications** | | | **Y** | **N** | **Y** | **N** | **Y** | **N** |
| Unilateral increased laxity, altered end-feel, and/or pain | | | ○ | ○ | ○ | ○ | ○ | ○ |
| In complete extension: LCL sprain, lateral joint capsule, cruciate ligaments, distal femoral epiphyseal fracture | | | ○ | ○ | ○ | ○ | ○ | ○ |
| In 25 degrees of flexion: LCL sprain | | | ○ | ○ | ○ | ○ | ○ | ○ |
| | | **Total** | \_\_\_\_/9 | | \_\_\_\_/9 | | \_\_\_\_/9 | |
| | **Must achieve >6 to pass this examination** | | Ⓟ | Ⓕ | Ⓟ | Ⓕ | Ⓟ | Ⓕ |

| Assessor: Date: | Test 1 Comments: |
|---|---|
| Assessor: Date: | Test 2 Comments: |
| Assessor: Date: | Test 3 Comments: |

## TEST ENVIRONMENTS
**L:** Laboratory/Classroom
**C:** Clinical/Field Testing
**P:** Practicum
**A:** Assessment/Mock Exam

## TEST INFORMATION
**Test Statistics:** Sensitivity .25
**Reference(s):** Malanga, Andrus, et al. (2003)
Starkey & Brown (2015)

## MUSCULOSKELETAL SYSTEM—REGION 3: KNEE
# SPECIAL TESTS

| NATA EC 5th | BOC RD6 | SKILL |
|---|---|---|
| CE-21g, CE-20e | D2-0203 | Apley's Grind |

**Supplies Needed:** Table

*This problem allows you the opportunity to demonstrate an* **orthopedic test** *known as* **Apley's grind** *to rule out a possible* **meniscal lesion.** *You have 2 minutes to complete this task.*

| Apley's Grind | Course or Site Assessor Environment | | Test 1 | | Test 2 | | Test 3 | |
|---|---|---|---|---|---|---|---|---|
| **Tester places patient and limb in appropriate position** | | **Y** | **N** | **Y** | **N** | **Y** | **N** |
| Prone | | ○ | ○ | ○ | ○ | ○ | ○ |
| Knee flexed to 90 degrees | | ○ | ○ | ○ | ○ | ○ | ○ |
| **Tester placed in proper position** | | **Y** | **N** | **Y** | **N** | **Y** | **N** |
| Stands lateral to the involved side | | ○ | ○ | ○ | ○ | ○ | ○ |
| Stabilizes the posterior portion of the femur with nondominant hand | | ○ | ○ | ○ | ○ | ○ | ○ |
| Stabilizes the plantar aspect of calcaneus with dominant hand | | ○ | ○ | ○ | ○ | ○ | ○ |
| **Tester performs test according to accepted guidelines** | | **Y** | **N** | **Y** | **N** | **Y** | **N** |
| Applies axial pressure to the plantar aspect of the calcaneus while internally and externally rotating the tibia | | ○ | ○ | ○ | ○ | ○ | ○ |
| Grasps the ankle and applies distraction while simultaneously internally and externally rotating the tibia | | ○ | ○ | ○ | ○ | ○ | ○ |
| **Identifies positive findings and implications** | | **Y** | **N** | **Y** | **N** | **Y** | **N** |
| Pain experienced during compression that is relieved during distraction | | ○ | ○ | ○ | ○ | ○ | ○ |
| **Total** | | __/8 | | __/8 | | __/8 | |
| **Must achieve >5 to pass this examination** | | Ⓟ | Ⓕ | Ⓟ | Ⓕ | Ⓟ | Ⓕ |

| Assessor: Date: | Test 1 Comments: |
|---|---|
| Assessor: Date: | Test 2 Comments: |
| Assessor: Date: | Test 3 Comments: |

**TEST ENVIRONMENTS**
**L:** Laboratory/Classroom
**C:** Clinical/Field Testing
**P:** Practicum
**A:** Assessment/Mock Exam

**TEST INFORMATION**
**Test Statistics:** Sensitivity .13–.16
Specificity .80–.90
(+) LR .80–1.3
(-) LR .97–1.05
**Reference(s):** Starkey & Brown (2015)

MUSCULOSKELETAL SYSTEM—REGION 3: KNEE
# SPECIAL TESTS

| NATA EC 5th | BOC RD6 | SKILL |
|---|---|---|
| CE-21g, CE-20e | D2-0203 | Ballotable Patella |

**Supplies Needed:** Table

*This problem allows you the opportunity to demonstrate an* **orthopedic test** *known as the* **ballotable patella** *to rule out* **joint effusion**. *You have 2 minutes to complete this task.*

| Ballotable Patella | Course or Site Assessor Environment | | Test 1 | | Test 2 | | Test 3 | |
|---|---|---|---|---|---|---|---|---|
| **Tester places patient and limb in appropriate position** | | | **Y** | **N** | **Y** | **N** | **Y** | **N** |
| Supine | | | ○ | ○ | ○ | ○ | ○ | ○ |
| Knee is extended and quadriceps are relaxed | | | ○ | ○ | ○ | ○ | ○ | ○ |
| **Tester placed in proper position** | | | **Y** | **N** | **Y** | **N** | **Y** | **N** |
| Stands on the side being tested | | | ○ | ○ | ○ | ○ | ○ | ○ |
| Places one hand on the superior aspect of patella and the other on the inferior aspect of patella | | | ○ | ○ | ○ | ○ | ○ | ○ |
| **Tester performs test according to accepted guidelines** | | | **Y** | **N** | **Y** | **N** | **Y** | **N** |
| The superior hand applies an inferior force | | | ○ | ○ | ○ | ○ | ○ | ○ |
| The inferior hand applies a superior force | | | ○ | ○ | ○ | ○ | ○ | ○ |
| A finger presses the patella down toward the patellar groove | | | ○ | ○ | ○ | ○ | ○ | ○ |
| **Identifies positive findings and implications** | | | **Y** | **N** | **Y** | **N** | **Y** | **N** |
| The patella fails to "bounce back" after being depressed | | | ○ | ○ | ○ | ○ | ○ | ○ |
| | | Total | __/8 | | __/8 | | __/8 | |
| | Must achieve >5 to pass this examination | | Ⓟ | Ⓕ | Ⓟ | Ⓕ | Ⓟ | Ⓕ |
| **Assessor:** **Date:** | **Test 1 Comments:** | | | | | | | |
| **Assessor:** **Date:** | **Test 2 Comments:** | | | | | | | |
| **Assessor:** **Date:** | **Test 3 Comments:** | | | | | | | |

**TEST ENVIRONMENTS**
**L:** Laboratory/Classroom
**C:** Clinical/Field Testing
**P:** Practicum
**A:** Assessment/Mock Exam

**TEST INFORMATION**
**Test Statistics:** Sensitivity .83
Specificity .49
(+) LR 1.60
(-) LR .30
**Reference(s):** Cook & Hegedus (2013)
Konin et al. (2016)
Starkey & Brown (2015)

# MUSCULOSKELETAL SYSTEM—REGION 3: KNEE
## SPECIAL TESTS

| NATA EC 5th | BOC RD6 | SKILL |
|---|---|---|
| CE-21g, CE-20e | D2-0203 | Bounce Home |

**Supplies Needed:** Table

*This problem allows you the opportunity to demonstrate an* **orthopedic test** *known as the* **bounce home** *to rule out a* **meniscal lesion***. You have 2 minutes to complete this task.*

| Bounce Home | Course or Site<br>Assessor<br>Environment | Test 1 | | Test 2 | | Test 3 | |
|---|---|---|---|---|---|---|---|
| | | Y | N | Y | N | Y | N |
| **Tester places patient and limb in appropriate position** | | **Y** | **N** | **Y** | **N** | **Y** | **N** |
| Supine | | ○ | ○ | ○ | ○ | ○ | ○ |
| Knee placed into full flexion | | ○ | ○ | ○ | ○ | ○ | ○ |
| **Tester placed in proper position** | | **Y** | **N** | **Y** | **N** | **Y** | **N** |
| Stands to the side of the patient | | ○ | ○ | ○ | ○ | ○ | ○ |
| Places one hand under the heel of the involved limb | | ○ | ○ | ○ | ○ | ○ | ○ |
| Places other hand under the knee joint | | ○ | ○ | ○ | ○ | ○ | ○ |
| **Tester performs test according to accepted guidelines** | | **Y** | **N** | **Y** | **N** | **Y** | **N** |
| Passively extends the knee | | ○ | ○ | ○ | ○ | ○ | ○ |
| Allows the knee to fall to neutral (gravity) | | ○ | ○ | ○ | ○ | ○ | ○ |
| Maintains relaxation of the limb | | ○ | ○ | ○ | ○ | ○ | ○ |
| Performs assessment bilaterally | | ○ | ○ | ○ | ○ | ○ | ○ |
| **Identifies positive findings and implications** | | **Y** | **N** | **Y** | **N** | **Y** | **N** |
| Pain | | ○ | ○ | ○ | ○ | ○ | ○ |
| Rubbery end-feel | | ○ | ○ | ○ | ○ | ○ | ○ |
| **Total** | | ____/11 | | ____/11 | | ____/11 | |
| **Must achieve >7 to pass this examination** | | Ⓟ | Ⓕ | Ⓟ | Ⓕ | Ⓟ | Ⓕ |

| Assessor:<br>Date: | Test 1 Comments: |
|---|---|
| Assessor:<br>Date: | Test 2 Comments: |
| Assessor:<br>Date: | Test 3 Comments: |

**TEST ENVIRONMENTS**
**L:** Laboratory/Classroom
**C:** Clinical/Field Testing
**P:** Practicum
**A:** Assessment/Mock Exam

**TEST INFORMATION**
**Test Statistics:** Sensitivity .36–.47
Specificity .67–.86
(+) LR 1.20–2.90
(-) LR .66–.93
**Reference(s):** Cook & Hegedus (2013)
Konin et al. (2016)

## MUSCULOSKELETAL SYSTEM—REGION 3: KNEE
# SPECIAL TESTS

| NATA EC 5th | BOC RD6 | SKILL |
|---|---|---|
| CE-21g, CE-20e | D2-0203 | External Rotation Test (Dial Test) |

**Supplies Needed:** Table

*This problem allows you the opportunity to demonstrate an* **orthopedic test** *known as the* **external rotation test (dial test)** *for* **posterolateral knee instability.** *You have 2 minutes to complete this task.*

| External Rotation Test (Dial Test) | Course or Site<br>Assessor<br>Environment<br>Test 1 | | Test 2 | | Test 3 | |
|---|---|---|---|---|---|---|
| **Tester places patient and limb in appropriate position** | Y | N | Y | N | Y | N |
| Supine on table | ○ | ○ | ○ | ○ | ○ | ○ |
| **Tester placed in proper position** | Y | N | Y | N | Y | N |
| Stands at the patient's feet | ○ | ○ | ○ | ○ | ○ | ○ |
| Places each hand on plantar aspect of patient's feet | ○ | ○ | ○ | ○ | ○ | ○ |
| **Tester performs test according to accepted guidelines** | Y | N | Y | N | Y | N |
| Passively flexes the knee to 30 degrees | ○ | ○ | ○ | ○ | ○ | ○ |
| Forcefully externally rotates the patient's lower leg and compares the position of the foot relative to the femur bilaterally | ○ | ○ | ○ | ○ | ○ | ○ |
| The knee is flexed to 90 degrees and the test is repeated | ○ | ○ | ○ | ○ | ○ | ○ |
| Performs assessment bilaterally | ○ | ○ | ○ | ○ | ○ | ○ |
| **Identifies positive findings and implications** | Y | N | Y | N | Y | N |
| An increase in external rotation >10 degrees compared bilaterally | ○ | ○ | ○ | ○ | ○ | ○ |
| 30 degrees = posterolateral corner; 90 degrees = PCL; 30 degrees and 90 degrees = posterolateral corner and PCL | ○ | ○ | ○ | ○ | ○ | ○ |
| **Total** | ___/9 | | ___/9 | | ___/9 | |
| **Must achieve >6 to pass this examination** | Ⓟ | Ⓕ | Ⓟ | Ⓕ | Ⓟ | Ⓕ |

| Assessor:<br>Date: | Test 1 Comments: |
|---|---|
| Assessor:<br>Date: | Test 2 Comments: |
| Assessor:<br>Date: | Test 3 Comments: |

**TEST ENVIRONMENTS**
**L:** Laboratory/Classroom
**C:** Clinical/Field Testing
**P:** Practicum
**A:** Assessment/Mock Exam

**TEST INFORMATION**
**Test Statistics:** Sensitivity .03–.39
Specificity .99
(+) LR 3.00
(-) LR .98
**Reference(s):** Cook & Hegedus (2013)
Starkey & Brown (2015)

## MUSCULOSKELETAL SYSTEM—REGION 3: KNEE
# SPECIAL TESTS

| NATA EC 5th | BOC RD6 | SKILL |
|---|---|---|
| CE-21g, CE-20e | D2-0203 | External Rotation Recurvatum Test |

**Supplies Needed:** Table

*This problem allows you the opportunity to demonstrate an* **orthopedic test** *known as the* **external rotation recurvatum test** *for* **posterolateral knee injury.** *You have 2 minutes to complete this task.*

| External Rotation Recurvatum Test | Course or Site Assessor Environment | Test 1 | | Test 2 | | Test 3 | |
|---|---|---|---|---|---|---|---|
| Tester places patient and limb in appropriate position | | Y | N | Y | N | Y | N |
| Supine | | ○ | ○ | ○ | ○ | ○ | ○ |
| **Tester placed in proper position** | | Y | N | Y | N | Y | N |
| Stands at the patient's feet | | ○ | ○ | ○ | ○ | ○ | ○ |
| Places hands across dorsal surface of feet grasping the great toes with palm along medial arch | | ○ | ○ | ○ | ○ | ○ | ○ |
| **Tester performs test according to accepted guidelines** | | Y | N | Y | N | Y | N |
| Lifts the patient's legs approximately 12 inches off the table | | ○ | ○ | ○ | ○ | ○ | ○ |
| Maintains relaxation of the limb | | ○ | ○ | ○ | ○ | ○ | ○ |
| **Identifies positive findings and implications** | | Y | N | Y | N | Y | N |
| Marked difference in hyperextension, external femoral rotation, or varus alignment between knees | | ○ | ○ | ○ | ○ | ○ | ○ |
| Posterolateral corner trauma or PCL sprain | | ○ | ○ | ○ | ○ | ○ | ○ |
| Total | | ___/7 | | ___/7 | | ___/7 | |
| **Must achieve >4 to pass this examination** | | Ⓟ | Ⓕ | Ⓟ | Ⓕ | Ⓟ | Ⓕ |

| Assessor: Date: | Test 1 Comments: |
|---|---|
| Assessor: Date: | Test 2 Comments: |
| Assessor: Date: | Test 3 Comments: |

**TEST ENVIRONMENTS**
**L:** Laboratory/Classroom
**C:** Clinical/Field Testing
**P:** Practicum
**A:** Assessment/Mock Exam

**TEST INFORMATION**
**Test Statistics:** No data available for nonanesthetized patient
**Reference(s):** Starkey & Brown (2015)

## MUSCULOSKELETAL SYSTEM—REGION 3: KNEE
# SPECIAL TESTS

| NATA EC 5th | BOC RD6 | SKILL |
|---|---|---|
| CE-21g, CE-20e | D2-0203 | McMurray's Test |

**Supplies Needed:** Table

*This problem allows you the opportunity to demonstrate an* **orthopedic test** *known as* **McMurray's test** *for* **meniscal injuries.** *You have 2 minutes to complete this task.*

| McMurray's Test | Course or Site<br>Assessor<br>Environment | Test 1 | | Test 2 | | Test 3 | |
|---|---|---|---|---|---|---|---|
| **Tester places patient and limb in appropriate position** | | Y | N | Y | N | Y | N |
| Supine on the table | | ○ | ○ | ○ | ○ | ○ | ○ |
| **Tester placed in proper position** | | Y | N | Y | N | Y | N |
| Stands lateral to the involved knee | | ○ | ○ | ○ | ○ | ○ | ○ |
| Caudal hand grasps the distal ankle | | ○ | ○ | ○ | ○ | ○ | ○ |
| Cephalic hand is positioned at the knee palpating medial and lateral joint lines | | ○ | ○ | ○ | ○ | ○ | ○ |
| **Tester performs test according to accepted guidelines** | | Y | N | Y | N | Y | N |
| With the tibia maintained in its neutral position, apply a valgus force through full flexion and varus force back through extension | | ○ | ○ | ○ | ○ | ○ | ○ |
| Internally rotates the tibia, applies a valgus force through full flexion and varus force back through extension | | ○ | ○ | ○ | ○ | ○ | ○ |
| Externally rotates the tibia, applies a valgus force through full flexion and varus force back through extension | | ○ | ○ | ○ | ○ | ○ | ○ |
| **Identifies positive findings and implications** | | Y | N | Y | N | Y | N |
| Popping, clicking, or locking of the knee (similar to experienced symptoms) or pain | | ○ | ○ | ○ | ○ | ○ | ○ |
| Meniscal tear on the side of reported symptoms | | ○ | ○ | ○ | ○ | ○ | ○ |
| | Total | ___/9 | | ___/9 | | ___/9 | |
| | **Must achieve >6 to pass this examination** | Ⓟ | Ⓕ | Ⓟ | Ⓕ | Ⓟ | Ⓕ |

| Assessor:<br>Date: | Test 1 Comments: |
|---|---|
| Assessor:<br>Date: | Test 2 Comments: |
| Assessor:<br>Date: | Test 3 Comments: |

**TEST ENVIRONMENTS**
**L:** Laboratory/Classroom
**C:** Clinical/Field Testing
**P:** Practicum
**A:** Assessment/Mock Exam

**TEST INFORMATION**
**Test Statistics:** Sensitivity .55
Specificity .77
(+) LR 1.05–8.00
(-) LR .24–.94
**Reference(s):** Meserve et al. (2008)
Starkey & Brown (2015)

# SPECIAL TESTS

| NATA EC 5th | BOC RD6 | SKILL |
|---|---|---|
| CE-21g, CE-20e | D2-0203 | Nobel's Compression Test |

**Supplies Needed:** Table

*This problem allows you the opportunity to demonstrate an* **orthopedic test** *known as the* **Nobel's compression test** *for* **iliotibial band friction syndrome.** *You have 2 minutes to complete this task.*

| Nobel's Compression Test | Course or Site<br>Assessor<br>Environment | | Test 1 | | Test 2 | | Test 3 | |
|---|---|---|---|---|---|---|---|---|
| **Tester places patient and limb in appropriate position** | | | Y | N | Y | N | Y | N |
| Supine with the involved knee flexed | | | O | O | O | O | O | O |
| **Tester placed in proper position** | | | Y | N | Y | N | Y | N |
| Stands lateral to the side being tested | | | O | O | O | O | O | O |
| Supports the knee above the joint line with the thumb slightly superior to the lateral femoral condyle | | | O | O | O | O | O | O |
| **Tester performs test according to accepted guidelines** | | | Y | N | Y | N | Y | N |
| While applying pressure over the lateral femoral condyle, the knee is passively extended and flexed | | | O | O | O | O | O | O |
| **Identifies positive findings and implications** | | | Y | N | Y | N | Y | N |
| Pain under the thumb (commonly at 30 degrees of extension) | | | O | O | O | O | O | O |
| Inflammation of the iliotibial band, associated bursa, or lateral femoral condyle | | | O | O | O | O | O | O |
| **Total** | | | __/6 | | __/6 | | __/6 | |
| **Must achieve >4 to pass this examination** | | | P | F | P | F | P | F |
| **Assessor:**<br>**Date:** | **Test 1 Comments:** | | | | | | | |
| **Assessor:**<br>**Date:** | **Test 2 Comments:** | | | | | | | |
| **Assessor:**<br>**Date:** | **Test 3 Comments:** | | | | | | | |

**TEST ENVIRONMENTS**
**L:** Laboratory/Classroom
**C:** Clinical/Field Testing
**P:** Practicum
**A:** Assessment/Mock Exam

**TEST INFORMATION**
**Test Statistics:** No data available
**Reference(s):** Starkey & Brown (2015)

## MUSCULOSKELETAL SYSTEM—REGION 3: KNEE
## SPECIAL TESTS

| NATA EC 5th | BOC RD6 | SKILL |
|---|---|---|
| CE-21g, CE-20e | D2-0203 | Patellar Apprehension Test |

**Supplies Needed:** Table, bolster

*This problem allows you the opportunity to demonstrate an* **orthopedic test** *known as the* **patellar apprehension test** *to rule out* **medial patellar retinacular laxity** *of the knee. You have 2 minutes to complete this task.*

| Patellar Apprehension Test | Course or Site Assessor Environment | | Test 1 | | Test 2 | | Test 3 | |
|---|---|---|:---:|:---:|:---:|:---:|:---:|:---:|
| **Tester places patient and limb in appropriate position** | | | **Y** | **N** | **Y** | **N** | **Y** | **N** |
| Supine with the knee extended | | | ○ | ○ | ○ | ○ | ○ | ○ |
| Bolster placed under involved knee | | | ○ | ○ | ○ | ○ | ○ | ○ |
| **Tester placed in proper position** | | | **Y** | **N** | **Y** | **N** | **Y** | **N** |
| Stands lateral to the patient | | | ○ | ○ | ○ | ○ | ○ | ○ |
| **Tester performs test according to accepted guidelines** | | | **Y** | **N** | **Y** | **N** | **Y** | **N** |
| Attempts to push the patella as far laterally as possible, taking care not to cause it to actually dislocate | | | ○ | ○ | ○ | ○ | ○ | ○ |
| **Identifies positive findings and implications** | | | **Y** | **N** | **Y** | **N** | **Y** | **N** |
| Forcible contraction of the quadriceps | | | ○ | ○ | ○ | ○ | ○ | ○ |
| Laxity of the medial patellar retinaculum | | | ○ | ○ | ○ | ○ | ○ | ○ |
| | | **Total** | \_\_\_\_/6 | | \_\_\_\_/6 | | \_\_\_\_/6 | |
| | **Must achieve >4 to pass this examination** | | Ⓟ | Ⓕ | Ⓟ | Ⓕ | Ⓟ | Ⓕ |

| Assessor: Date: | Test 1 Comments: |
|---|---|
| Assessor: Date: | Test 2 Comments: |
| Assessor: Date: | Test 3 Comments: |

**TEST ENVIRONMENTS**
**L:** Laboratory/Classroom
**C:** Clinical/Field Testing
**P:** Practicum
**A:** Assessment/Mock Exam

**TEST INFORMATION**
**Test Statistics:** Sensitivity .07–.37
Specificity .86–.92
(+) LR .87–2.30
(-) LR .79–1.00
**Reference(s):** Cook & Hegedus (2013)
Starkey & Brown (2015)

**MUSCULOSKELETAL SYSTEM—REGION 3: KNEE**
# SPECIAL TESTS

| NATA EC 5th | BOC RD6 | SKILL |
|---|---|---|
| CE-21g, CE-20e | D2-0203 | Sweep Test |

**Supplies Needed:** Table

*This problem allows you the opportunity to demonstrate an* **orthopedic test** *known as the* **sweep test** *to rule out a possible* **joint effusion**. *You have 2 minutes to complete this task.*

| Sweep Test | Course or Site Assessor Environment | | Test 1 | | Test 2 | | Test 3 | |
|---|---|---|---|---|---|---|---|---|
| **Tester places patient and limb in appropriate position** | | Y | N | Y | N | Y | N |
| Supine with knee extended | | ○ | ○ | ○ | ○ | ○ | ○ |
| **Tester placed in proper position** | | Y | N | Y | N | Y | N |
| Stands lateral to involved side | | ○ | ○ | ○ | ○ | ○ | ○ |
| **Tester performs test according to accepted guidelines** | | Y | N | Y | N | Y | N |
| Strokes fluid from the medial side of the knee proximally and laterally | | ○ | ○ | ○ | ○ | ○ | ○ |
| Allows time for the normal contour of the knee to return | | ○ | ○ | ○ | ○ | ○ | ○ |
| With opposite hand, applies pressure to the lateral aspect of the knee | | ○ | ○ | ○ | ○ | ○ | ○ |
| **Identifies positive findings and implications** | | Y | N | Y | N | Y | N |
| Swelling appears on the medial aspect of the knee | | ○ | ○ | ○ | ○ | ○ | ○ |
| Joint effusion, ACL trauma, osteochondral fracture, synovitis, meniscal lesion, or patellar dislocation | | ○ | ○ | ○ | ○ | ○ | ○ |
| Total | | ___/7 | | ___/7 | | ___/7 | |
| **Must achieve >4 to pass this examination** | | Ⓟ | Ⓕ | Ⓟ | Ⓕ | Ⓟ | Ⓕ |

| Assessor:
Date: | Test 1 Comments: |
|---|---|
| Assessor:
Date: | Test 2 Comments: |
| Assessor:
Date: | Test 3 Comments: |

**TEST ENVIRONMENTS**
**L:** Laboratory/Classroom
**C:** Clinical/Field Testing
**P:** Practicum
**A:** Assessment/Mock Exam

**TEST INFORMATION**
**Test Statistics:** No data available
**Reference(s):** Starkey & Brown (2015)

MUSCULOSKELETAL SYSTEM—REGION 3: KNEE
# SPECIAL TESTS

| NATA EC 5th | BOC RD6 | SKILL |
|---|---|---|
| CE-21g, CE-20e | D2-0203 | Thessaly's Test |

**Supplies Needed:** N/A

*This problem allows you the opportunity to demonstrate an* **orthopedic test** *known as* **Thessaly's test** *to identify* **meniscal lesions.** *You have 2 minutes to complete this task.*

| Thessaly's Test | Course or Site<br>Assessor<br>Environment | | Test 1 | | Test 2 | | Test 3 |
|---|---|---|---|---|---|---|---|
| **Tester places patient and limb in appropriate position** | | Y | N | Y | N | Y | N |
| Stands flatfooted on the leg being tested | | ○ | ○ | ○ | ○ | ○ | ○ |
| The knee of the opposite leg is flexed to approximately 45 degrees | | ○ | ○ | ○ | ○ | ○ | ○ |
| **Tester placed in proper position** | | Y | N | Y | N | Y | N |
| Stands facing the patient, supporting the patient's arms | | ○ | ○ | ○ | ○ | ○ | ○ |
| **Tester performs test according to accepted guidelines** | | Y | N | Y | N | Y | N |
| Uninvolved limb is tested first | | ○ | ○ | ○ | ○ | ○ | ○ |
| The patient flexes the knee to 5 degrees | | ○ | ○ | ○ | ○ | ○ | ○ |
| The patient rotates the body three times to internally and externally rotate the femur on the tibia | | ○ | ○ | ○ | ○ | ○ | ○ |
| The patient then flexes the knee to 20 degrees | | ○ | ○ | ○ | ○ | ○ | ○ |
| Internally and externally rotates femur on the tibia three times | | ○ | ○ | ○ | ○ | ○ | ○ |
| **Identifies positive findings and implications** | | Y | N | Y | N | Y | N |
| Joint-line discomfort or complaints of "locking/clicking" | | ○ | ○ | ○ | ○ | ○ | ○ |
| Lesion of the medial or lateral meniscus | | ○ | ○ | ○ | ○ | ○ | ○ |
| **Total** | | ___/10 | | ___/10 | | ___/10 | |
| **Must achieve >6 to pass this examination** | | Ⓟ | Ⓕ | Ⓟ | Ⓕ | Ⓟ | Ⓕ |

| Assessor:<br>Date: | Test 1 Comments: |
|---|---|
| Assessor:<br>Date: | Test 2 Comments: |
| Assessor:<br>Date: | Test 3 Comments: |

**TEST ENVIRONMENTS**
**L:** Laboratory/Classroom
**C:** Clinical/Field Testing
**P:** Practicum
**A:** Assessment/Mock Exam

**TEST INFORMATION**
**Test Statistics:** Sensitivity .66–.92
Specificity .91–.97
(+) LR 7.3–30.67
(-) LR .08–.37
**Reference(s):** Karachalios et al. (2005)
Starkey & Brown (2015)

## MUSCULOSKELETAL SYSTEM—REGION 3: KNEE
# SPECIAL TESTS

| NATA EC 5th | BOC RD6 | SKILL |
|---|---|---|
| CE-21g, CE-20e | D2-0203 | Wilson's Test |

**Supplies Needed:** Table

*This problem allows you the opportunity to demonstrate an* **orthopedic test** *known as* **Wilson's test** *to rule out* **osteochondral defects** *of the knee. You have 2 minutes to complete this task.*

| Wilson's Test | Course or Site Assessor Environment | | Test 1 | | Test 2 | | Test 3 | |
|---|---|---|---|---|---|---|---|---|
| **Tester places patient and limb in appropriate position** | | **Y** | **N** | **Y** | **N** | **Y** | **N** | |
| Seated at the edge of the table with knees over edge | | ○ | ○ | ○ | ○ | ○ | ○ | |
| **Tester placed in proper position** | | **Y** | **N** | **Y** | **N** | **Y** | **N** | |
| Positioned in front of the patient to observe any reactions secondary to pain or discomfort | | ○ | ○ | ○ | ○ | ○ | ○ | |
| **Tester performs test according to accepted guidelines** | | **Y** | **N** | **Y** | **N** | **Y** | **N** | |
| Instructs the patient to actively extend the knee while maintaining tibial internal rotation, stopping at the position pain is experienced | | ○ | ○ | ○ | ○ | ○ | ○ | |
| Instructs the patient to externally rotate the tibia while knee is still in the present position | | ○ | ○ | ○ | ○ | ○ | ○ | |
| **Identifies positive findings and implications** | | **Y** | **N** | **Y** | **N** | **Y** | **N** | |
| Pain experienced during extension that is relieved with external rotation | | ○ | ○ | ○ | ○ | ○ | ○ | |
| Osteochondritis dissecans on the intercondylar area of the medial femoral condyle | | ○ | ○ | ○ | ○ | ○ | ○ | |
| **Total** | | ___/6 | | ___/6 | | ___/6 | | |
| **Must achieve >4 to pass this examination** | | Ⓟ | Ⓕ | Ⓟ | Ⓕ | Ⓟ | Ⓕ | |

| Assessor: Date: | Test 1 Comments: |
|---|---|
| Assessor: Date: | Test 2 Comments: |
| Assessor: Date: | Test 3 Comments: |

**TEST ENVIRONMENTS**
**L:** Laboratory/Classroom
**C:** Clinical/Field Testing
**P:** Practicum
**A:** Assessment/Mock Exam

**TEST INFORMATION**
**Test Statistics:** Sensitivity .65–.67
Specificity .98–.99
(+) LR 33.50–65.00
(-) LR .34–.35
**Reference(s):** Cook & Hegedus (2013)
Starkey & Brown (2015)

# 7

# MUSCULOSKELETAL SYSTEM— REGION 4: HIP AND PELVIS

Hauth, J. M., Gloyeske, B. M., & Amato, H. K.
*Clinical Skills Documentation Guide for Athletic Training, Third Edition* (pp. 154-190).
© 2016 SLACK Incorporated.

MUSCULOSKELETAL SYSTEM—REGION 4: HIP AND PELVIS
# KNOWLEDGE AND SKILLS

| Musculoskeletal System—Region 4: Hip and Pelvis | | | | Skill: Acquisition, Reinforcement, Proficiency | | |
|---|---|---|---|---|---|---|
| **NATA EC 5th** | **BOC RD6** | **Palpation** | **Page #** | | | |
| CE-21b, CE-20c | D2-0202 | Palpation: Hip and Pelvis – 01 | 156 | | | |
| CE-21b, CE-20c | D2-0202 | Palpation: Hip and Pelvis – 02 | 157 | | | |
| CE-21b, CE-20c | D2-0202 | Palpation: Hip and Pelvis – 03 | 158 | | | |
| **NATA EC 5th** | **BOC RD6** | **Manual Muscle Testing** | **Page #** | | | |
| CE-21c | D2-0203 | MMT: Gluteus Medius | 159 | | | |
| CE-21c | D2-0203 | MMT: Gluteus Minimus | 160 | | | |
| CE-21c | D2-0203 | MMT: Gluteus Maximus | 161 | | | |
| CE-21c | D2-0203 | MMT: Hip Adduction | 162 | | | |
| CE-21c | D2-0203 | MMT: Hip External Rotators | 163 | | | |
| CE-21c | D2-0203 | MMT: Hip Internal Rotators | 164 | | | |
| CE-21c | D2-0203 | MMT: Quadratus Lumborum | 165 | | | |
| CE-21c | D2-0203 | MMT: Iliopsoas | 166 | | | |
| CE-21c | D2-0203 | MMT: Tensor Fasciae Latae | 167 | | | |
| **NATA EC 5th** | **BOC RD6** | **Osteokinematic Joint Motion** | **Page #** | | | |
| CE-21d | D2-0203 | Goniometric Assessment: Iliofemoral Joint (Abduction) | 168 | | | |
| CE-21d | D2-0203 | Goniometric Assessment: Iliofemoral Joint (Adduction) | 169 | | | |
| CE-21d | D2-0203 | Goniometric Assessment: Iliofemoral Joint (Internal Rotation) | 170 | | | |
| CE-21d | D2-0203 | Goniometric Assessment: Iliofemoral Joint (Internal Rotation) – Alternate | 171 | | | |
| CE-21d | D2-0203 | Goniometric Assessment: Iliofemoral Joint (External Rotation) | 172 | | | |
| CE-21d | D2-0203 | Goniometric Assessment: Iliofemoral Joint (External Rotation) – Alternate | 173 | | | |
| CE-21d | D2-0203 | Goniometric Assessment: Iliofemoral Joint (Extension) | 174 | | | |
| CE-21d | D2-0203 | Goniometric Assessment: Iliofemoral Joint (Flexion) | 175 | | | |
| **NATA EC 5th** | **BOC RD6** | **Capsular and Ligamentous Stress Testing** | **Page #** | | | |
| CE-21e | D2-0203 | Sacroiliac Compression Test | 176 | | | |
| CE-21e | D2-0203 | Sacroiliac Distraction Test | 177 | | | |
| **NATA EC 5th** | **BOC RD6** | **Special Tests** | **Page #** | | | |
| CE-21g, CE-20e | D2-0203 | Ely's Test | 178 | | | |
| CE-21g, CE-20e | D2-0203 | Flexion-Abduction-External Rotation (FABER) Test (Patrick's Test) | 179 | | | |
| CE-21g, CE-20e | D2-0203 | Flexion-Adduction-Internal Rotation (FADDIR) Test | 180 | | | |
| CE-21g, CE-20e | D2-0203 | Flexion-Adduction-Internal Rotation (FAIR) Test | 181 | | | |
| CE-21g, CE-20e | D2-0203 | Gaenslen's Test | 182 | | | |
| CE-21g, CE-20e | D2-0203 | Hip Scouring | 183 | | | |
| CE-21g, CE-20e | D2-0203 | Ober's Test | 184 | | | |
| CE-21g, CE-20e | D2-0203 | Thomas Test | 185 | | | |
| CE-21g, CE-20e | D2-0203 | Trendelenburg's Sign | 186 | | | |
| CE-21g, CE-20e | D2-0203 | Leg Length Assessment (True) | 187 | | | |
| CE-21g, CE-20e | D2-0203 | Leg Length Assessment (Apparent) | 188 | | | |
| CE-21g, CE-20e | D2-0203 | Girth Measurement (Thigh) | 189 | | | |
| CE-21g, CE-20e | D2-0203 | Postural Measurement (Q-Angle) | 190 | | | |

## MUSCULOSKELETAL SYSTEM—REGION 4: HIP AND PELVIS
# PALPATION

| NATA EC 5th | BOC RD6 | SKILL |
|---|---|---|
| CE-21b, CE-20c | D2-0202 | Palpation: Hip and Pelvis – 01 |

**Supplies Needed:** Table

*This problem allows you the opportunity to demonstrate your ability to* **palpate** *the* **hip and pelvis**.
*You have 2 minutes to complete this task.*

| Palpation: Hip and Pelvis – 01 | Course or Site Assessor Environment | | Test 1 | | Test 2 | | Test 3 | |
|---|---|---|---|---|---|---|---|---|
| | | | Y | N | Y | N | Y | N |
| Anterior superior iliac spine | | | ○ | ○ | ○ | ○ | ○ | ○ |
| Rectus femoris | | | ○ | ○ | ○ | ○ | ○ | ○ |
| Ischial tuberosity | | | ○ | ○ | ○ | ○ | ○ | ○ |
| Iliotibial band | | | ○ | ○ | ○ | ○ | ○ | ○ |
| Adductor magnus | | | ○ | ○ | ○ | ○ | ○ | ○ |
| Adductor longus | | | ○ | ○ | ○ | ○ | ○ | ○ |
| Pubic tubercle | | | ○ | ○ | ○ | ○ | ○ | ○ |
| Total | | | /7 | | /7 | | /7 | |
| Must achieve >4 to pass this examination | | | Ⓟ | Ⓕ | Ⓟ | Ⓕ | Ⓟ | Ⓕ |

| Assessor: Date: | Test 1 Comments: |
|---|---|
| Assessor: Date: | Test 2 Comments: |
| Assessor: Date: | Test 3 Comments: |

**TEST ENVIRONMENTS**
**L:** Laboratory/Classroom
**C:** Clinical/Field Testing
**P:** Practicum
**A:** Assessment/Mock Exam

**TEST INFORMATION**
**Test Statistics:** N/A
**Reference(s):** Starkey & Brown (2015)

## MUSCULOSKELETAL SYSTEM—REGION 4: HIP AND PELVIS
# PALPATION

| NATA EC 5th | BOC RD6 | SKILL |
|---|---|---|
| CE-21b, CE-20c | D2-0202 | Palpation: Hip and Pelvis – 02 |

**Supplies Needed:** Table

*This problem allows you the opportunity to demonstrate your ability to* **palpate** *the* **hip and pelvis**. *You have 2 minutes to complete this task.*

| Palpation: Hip and Pelvis – 02 | Course or Site _____ Assessor _____ Environment _____ | | | | | |
|---|---|---|---|---|---|---|
| | | Test 1 | | Test 2 | | Test 3 |
| | | Y | N | Y | N | Y | N |
| Anterior inferior iliac spine | | ○ | ○ | ○ | ○ | ○ | ○ |
| Iliac crest | | ○ | ○ | ○ | ○ | ○ | ○ |
| Biceps femoris | | ○ | ○ | ○ | ○ | ○ | ○ |
| Semitendinosus | | ○ | ○ | ○ | ○ | ○ | ○ |
| Gracilis | | ○ | ○ | ○ | ○ | ○ | ○ |
| Inguinal lymph node | | ○ | ○ | ○ | ○ | ○ | ○ |
| Piriformis | | ○ | ○ | ○ | ○ | ○ | ○ |
| **Total** | | ____/7 | | ____/7 | | ____/7 | |
| **Must achieve >4 to pass this examination** | | Ⓟ | Ⓕ | Ⓟ | Ⓕ | Ⓟ | Ⓕ |

| Assessor: Date: | Test 1 Comments: |
|---|---|
| Assessor: Date: | Test 2 Comments: |
| Assessor: Date: | Test 3 Comments: |

**TEST ENVIRONMENTS**
**L:** Laboratory/Classroom
**C:** Clinical/Field Testing
**P:** Practicum
**A:** Assessment/Mock Exam

**TEST INFORMATION**
**Test Statistics:** N/A
**Reference(s):** Starkey & Brown (2015)

MUSCULOSKELETAL SYSTEM—REGION 4: HIP AND PELVIS
# PALPATION

| NATA EC 5th | BOC RD6 | SKILL |
|---|---|---|
| CE-21b, CE-20c | D2-0202 | Palpation: Hip and Pelvis – 03 |

**Supplies Needed:** Table

*This problem allows you the opportunity to demonstrate your ability to* **palpate** *the* **hip and pelvis**. *You have 2 minutes to complete this task.*

| Palpation: Hip and Pelvis – 03 | Course or Site Assessor Environment | | Test 1 | | Test 2 | | Test 3 | |
|---|---|---|---|---|---|---|---|---|
| | | | Y | N | Y | N | Y | N |
| Adductor tubercle | | | ○ | ○ | ○ | ○ | ○ | ○ |
| Sacrum | | | ○ | ○ | ○ | ○ | ○ | ○ |
| Inguinal ligament | | | ○ | ○ | ○ | ○ | ○ | ○ |
| Gluteus maximus | | | ○ | ○ | ○ | ○ | ○ | ○ |
| Gluteus medius | | | ○ | ○ | ○ | ○ | ○ | ○ |
| Greater trochanter | | | ○ | ○ | ○ | ○ | ○ | ○ |
| Posterior superior iliac spine | | | ○ | ○ | ○ | ○ | ○ | ○ |
| Total | | | ___/7 | | ___/7 | | ___/7 | |
| Must achieve >4 to pass this examination | | | ⓅP | ⒻF | ⓅP | ⒻF | ⓅP | ⒻF |

| Assessor: Date: | Test 1 Comments: |
|---|---|
| Assessor: Date: | Test 2 Comments: |
| Assessor: Date: | Test 3 Comments: |

**TEST ENVIRONMENTS**
**L:** Laboratory/Classroom
**C:** Clinical/Field Testing
**P:** Practicum
**A:** Assessment/Mock Exam

**TEST INFORMATION**
**Test Statistics:** N/A
**Reference(s):** Starkey & Brown (2015)

# MANUAL MUSCLE TESTING

| NATA EC 5th | BOC RD6 | SKILL |
|---|---|---|
| CE-21c | D2-0203 | MMT: Gluteus Medius |

**Supplies Needed:** Table

*This problem allows you the opportunity to demonstrate a* **manual muscle test** *for the* **gluteus medius**. *You have 2 minutes to complete this task.*

| MMT: Gluteus Medius | Course or Site Assessor Environment | | | | | |
|---|---|---|---|---|---|---|
| | | Test 1 | | Test 2 | | Test 3 |
| **Tester places patient and limb in appropriate position** | | Y | N | Y | N | Y | N |
| Side lying (opposite side being tested) | | O | O | O | O | O | O |
| Inferior leg flexed at hip and knee | | O | O | O | O | O | O |
| Pelvis rotated slightly forward | | O | O | O | O | O | O |
| **Tester placed in proper position** | | Y | N | Y | N | Y | N |
| Stabilizes iliac crest | | O | O | O | O | O | O |
| Stabilizes lateral malleoli of leg being tested | | O | O | O | O | O | O |
| **Tester performs test according to accepted guidelines** | | Y | N | Y | N | Y | N |
| Instructs the patient to actively abduct superior leg | | O | O | O | O | O | O |
| Applies resistance to the lateral portion of lower leg (direction of hip adduction and slight flexion) | | O | O | O | O | O | O |
| Holds resistance for 5 seconds | | O | O | O | O | O | O |
| Performs assessment bilaterally | | O | O | O | O | O | O |
| **Identifies implications** | | Y | N | Y | N | Y | N |
| Correctly grades the MMT | | O | O | O | O | O | O |
| Total | | __/10 | | __/10 | | __/10 |
| Must achieve >6 to pass this examination | | Ⓟ | Ⓕ | Ⓟ | Ⓕ | Ⓟ | Ⓕ |

| Assessor: Date: | Test 1 Comments: |
|---|---|
| Assessor: Date: | Test 2 Comments: |
| Assessor: Date: | Test 3 Comments: |

**TEST ENVIRONMENTS**
**L:** Laboratory/Classroom
**C:** Clinical/Field Testing
**P:** Practicum
**A:** Assessment/Mock Exam

**TEST INFORMATION**
**Test Statistics:** N/A
**Reference(s):** Kendall et al. (2005)

MUSCULOSKELETAL SYSTEM—REGION 4: HIP AND PELVIS
# MANUAL MUSCLE TESTING

| NATA EC 5th | BOC RD6 | SKILL |
|---|---|---|
| CE-21c | D2-0203 | MMT: Gluteus Minimus |

**Supplies Needed:** Table

*This problem allows you the opportunity to demonstrate a* **manual muscle test** *for the* **gluteus minimus***.*
*You have 2 minutes to complete this task.*

| MMT: Gluteus Minimus | Course or Site Assessor Environment | Test 1 | | Test 2 | | Test 3 | |
|---|---|---|---|---|---|---|---|
| | | Y | N | Y | N | Y | N |
| **Tester places patient and limb in appropriate position** | | Y | N | Y | N | Y | N |
| Side lying (opposite side being tested) | | ○ | ○ | ○ | ○ | ○ | ○ |
| Body in a straight line | | ○ | ○ | ○ | ○ | ○ | ○ |
| **Tester placed in proper position** | | Y | N | Y | N | Y | N |
| Stabilizes iliac crest | | ○ | ○ | ○ | ○ | ○ | ○ |
| Stabilizes lateral malleoli of leg being tested | | ○ | ○ | ○ | ○ | ○ | ○ |
| **Tester performs test according to accepted guidelines** | | Y | N | Y | N | Y | N |
| Instructs the patient to actively abduct superior leg | | ○ | ○ | ○ | ○ | ○ | ○ |
| Applies resistance to the lateral portion of lower leg (direction of hip adduction) | | ○ | ○ | ○ | ○ | ○ | ○ |
| Holds resistance for 5 seconds | | ○ | ○ | ○ | ○ | ○ | ○ |
| Performs assessment bilaterally | | ○ | ○ | ○ | ○ | ○ | ○ |
| **Identifies implications** | | Y | N | Y | N | Y | N |
| Correctly grades the MMT | | ○ | ○ | ○ | ○ | ○ | ○ |
| | Total | __/9 | | __/9 | | __/9 | |
| | Must achieve >6 to pass this examination | Ⓟ | Ⓕ | Ⓟ | Ⓕ | Ⓟ | Ⓕ |

| Assessor: Date: | Test 1 Comments: |
|---|---|
| Assessor: Date: | Test 2 Comments: |
| Assessor: Date: | Test 3 Comments: |

**TEST ENVIRONMENTS**
**L:** Laboratory/Classroom
**C:** Clinical/Field Testing
**P:** Practicum
**A:** Assessment/Mock Exam

**TEST INFORMATION**
**Test Statistics:** N/A
**Reference(s):**   Kendall et al. (2005)

# MANUAL MUSCLE TESTING

| NATA EC 5th | BOC RD6 | SKILL |
|---|---|---|
| CE-21c | D2-0203 | MMT: Gluteus Maximus |

**Supplies Needed:** Table

*This problem allows you the opportunity to demonstrate a* **manual muscle test** *for the* **gluteus maximus**. *You have 2 minutes to complete this task.*

| MMT: Gluteus Maximus | Course or Site Assessor Environment | Test 1 | | Test 2 | | Test 3 | |
|---|---|---|---|---|---|---|---|
| **Tester places patient and limb in appropriate position** | | Y | N | Y | N | Y | N |
| Prone | | O | O | O | O | O | O |
| Knee flexed to 90 degrees | | O | O | O | O | O | O |
| **Tester placed in proper position** | | Y | N | Y | N | Y | N |
| Stabilizes PSIS on side being tested | | O | O | O | O | O | O |
| Stabilizes popliteal fossa of side being tested | | O | O | O | O | O | O |
| **Tester performs test according to accepted guidelines** | | Y | N | Y | N | Y | N |
| Instructs the patient to actively extend hip | | O | O | O | O | O | O |
| Applies resistance to the posterior portion of femur (direction of hip flexion) | | O | O | O | O | O | O |
| Holds resistance for 5 seconds | | O | O | O | O | O | O |
| Performs assessment bilaterally | | O | O | O | O | O | O |
| **Identifies implications** | | Y | N | Y | N | Y | N |
| Correctly grades the MMT | | O | O | O | O | O | O |
| **Total** | | /9 | | /9 | | /9 | |
| **Must achieve >6 to pass this examination** | | P | F | P | F | P | F |

| Assessor: Date: | Test 1 Comments: |
|---|---|
| Assessor: Date: | Test 2 Comments: |
| Assessor: Date: | Test 3 Comments: |

**TEST ENVIRONMENTS**
**L:** Laboratory/Classroom
**C:** Clinical/Field Testing
**P:** Practicum
**A:** Assessment/Mock Exam

**TEST INFORMATION**
**Test Statistics:** N/A
**Reference(s):** Kendall et al. (2005)

## MUSCULOSKELETAL SYSTEM—REGION 4: HIP AND PELVIS
# MANUAL MUSCLE TESTING

| NATA EC 5th | BOC RD6 | SKILL |
|:---:|:---:|:---:|
| CE-21c | D2-0203 | MMT: Hip Adduction |

**Supplies Needed:** Table

*This problem allows you the opportunity to demonstrate a* **manual muscle test** *for* **hip adduction**. *You have 2 minutes to complete this task.*

| MMT: Hip Adduction | Course or Site Assessor Environment | | Test 1 | | Test 2 | | Test 3 | |
|:---|:---:|:---:|:---:|:---:|:---:|:---:|:---:|:---:|
| | | | Y | N | Y | N | Y | N |
| **Tester places patient and limb in appropriate position** | | | Y | N | Y | N | Y | N |
| Side lying (side being tested) | | | ○ | ○ | ○ | ○ | ○ | ○ |
| Body in a straight line | | | ○ | ○ | ○ | ○ | ○ | ○ |
| **Tester placed in proper position** | | | Y | N | Y | N | Y | N |
| Stabilizes medial aspect of superior leg | | | ○ | ○ | ○ | ○ | ○ | ○ |
| Stabilizes medial aspect of inferior leg | | | ○ | ○ | ○ | ○ | ○ | ○ |
| **Tester performs test according to accepted guidelines** | | | Y | N | Y | N | Y | N |
| Instructs the patient to actively adduct inferior leg | | | ○ | ○ | ○ | ○ | ○ | ○ |
| Applies resistance to the medial portion of inferior leg (direction of hip abduction) | | | ○ | ○ | ○ | ○ | ○ | ○ |
| Holds resistance for 5 seconds | | | ○ | ○ | ○ | ○ | ○ | ○ |
| Performs assessment bilaterally | | | ○ | ○ | ○ | ○ | ○ | ○ |
| **Identifies implications** | | | Y | N | Y | N | Y | N |
| Correctly grades the MMT | | | ○ | ○ | ○ | ○ | ○ | ○ |
| Total | | | ___/9 | | ___/9 | | ___/9 | |
| **Must achieve >6 to pass this examination** | | | Ⓟ | Ⓕ | Ⓟ | Ⓕ | Ⓟ | Ⓕ |

| Assessor: Date: | Test 1 Comments: |
|:---|:---|
| Assessor: Date: | Test 2 Comments: |
| Assessor: Date: | Test 3 Comments: |

**TEST ENVIRONMENTS**
**L:** Laboratory/Classroom
**C:** Clinical/Field Testing
**P:** Practicum
**A:** Assessment/Mock Exam

**TEST INFORMATION**
**Test Statistics:** N/A
**Reference(s):**   Kendall et al. (2005)

## MUSCULOSKELETAL SYSTEM—REGION 4: HIP AND PELVIS
# MANUAL MUSCLE TESTING

| NATA EC 5th | BOC RD6 | SKILL |
|---|---|---|
| CE-21c | D2-0203 | MMT: Hip External Rotators |

**Supplies Needed:** Table

*This problem allows you the opportunity to demonstrate a* **manual muscle test** *for the* **hip external rotators***. You have 2 minutes to complete this task.*

| MMT: Hip External Rotators | Course or Site Assessor Environment | | Test 1 | | Test 2 | | Test 3 | |
|---|---|---|---|---|---|---|---|---|
| | | | **Y** | **N** | **Y** | **N** | **Y** | **N** |
| **Tester places patient and limb in appropriate position** | | | **Y** | **N** | **Y** | **N** | **Y** | **N** |
| Seated | | | ○ | ○ | ○ | ○ | ○ | ○ |
| Knees bent over edge of table and holding onto side of table | | | ○ | ○ | ○ | ○ | ○ | ○ |
| **Tester placed in proper position** | | | **Y** | **N** | **Y** | **N** | **Y** | **N** |
| Stabilizes medial aspect of knee with dominant hand | | | ○ | ○ | ○ | ○ | ○ | ○ |
| Stabilizes posterolateral aspect of lower leg with nondominant hand | | | ○ | ○ | ○ | ○ | ○ | ○ |
| **Tester performs test according to accepted guidelines** | | | **Y** | **N** | **Y** | **N** | **Y** | **N** |
| Instructs the patient to actively externally rotate the femur | | | ○ | ○ | ○ | ○ | ○ | ○ |
| Applies resistance to the lateral portion of the knee (direction of hip internal rotation) | | | ○ | ○ | ○ | ○ | ○ | ○ |
| Holds resistance for 5 seconds | | | ○ | ○ | ○ | ○ | ○ | ○ |
| Performs assessment bilaterally | | | ○ | ○ | ○ | ○ | ○ | ○ |
| **Identifies implications** | | | **Y** | **N** | **Y** | **N** | **Y** | **N** |
| Correctly grades the MMT | | | ○ | ○ | ○ | ○ | ○ | ○ |
| | **Total** | | ___/9 | | ___/9 | | ___/9 | |
| | **Must achieve >6 to pass this examination** | | Ⓟ | Ⓕ | Ⓟ | Ⓕ | Ⓟ | Ⓕ |

| Assessor:<br>Date: | Test 1 Comments: |
|---|---|
| Assessor:<br>Date: | Test 2 Comments: |
| Assessor:<br>Date: | Test 3 Comments: |

**TEST ENVIRONMENTS**
**L:** Laboratory/Classroom
**C:** Clinical/Field Testing
**P:** Practicum
**A:** Assessment/Mock Exam

**TEST INFORMATION**
**Test Statistics:** N/A
**Reference(s):**  Kendall et al. (2005)

MUSCULOSKELETAL SYSTEM—REGION 4: HIP AND PELVIS
# MANUAL MUSCLE TESTING

| NATA EC 5th | BOC RD6 | SKILL |
|---|---|---|
| CE-21c | D2-0203 | MMT: Hip Internal Rotators |

**Supplies Needed:** Table

*This problem allows you the opportunity to demonstrate a* **manual muscle test** *for the* **hip internal rotators**. *You have 2 minutes to complete this task.*

| MMT: Hip Internal Rotators | Course or Site Assessor Environment | | Test 1 | | Test 2 | | Test 3 | |
|---|---|---|---|---|---|---|---|---|
| **Tester places patient and limb in appropriate position** | | | **Y** | **N** | **Y** | **N** | **Y** | **N** |
| Seated | | | ○ | ○ | ○ | ○ | ○ | ○ |
| Knees bent over edge of table and holding onto side of table | | | ○ | ○ | ○ | ○ | ○ | ○ |
| **Tester placed in proper position** | | | **Y** | **N** | **Y** | **N** | **Y** | **N** |
| Stabilizes medial aspect of knee with dominant hand | | | ○ | ○ | ○ | ○ | ○ | ○ |
| Stabilizes posterolateral aspect of lower leg with nondominant hand | | | ○ | ○ | ○ | ○ | ○ | ○ |
| **Tester performs test according to accepted guidelines** | | | **Y** | **N** | **Y** | **N** | **Y** | **N** |
| Instructs the patient to actively internally rotate the femur | | | ○ | ○ | ○ | ○ | ○ | ○ |
| Applies resistance to medial aspect of knee (direction of hip external rotation) | | | ○ | ○ | ○ | ○ | ○ | ○ |
| Holds resistance for 5 seconds | | | ○ | ○ | ○ | ○ | ○ | ○ |
| Performs assessment bilaterally | | | ○ | ○ | ○ | ○ | ○ | ○ |
| **Identifies implications** | | | **Y** | **N** | **Y** | **N** | **Y** | **N** |
| Correctly grades the MMT | | | ○ | ○ | ○ | ○ | ○ | ○ |
| | | Total | ___/9 | | ___/9 | | ___/9 | |
| | Must achieve >6 to pass this examination | | Ⓟ | Ⓕ | Ⓟ | Ⓕ | Ⓟ | Ⓕ |

| Assessor: Date: | Test 1 Comments: |
|---|---|
| Assessor: Date: | Test 2 Comments: |
| Assessor: Date: | Test 3 Comments: |

**TEST ENVIRONMENTS**
**L:** Laboratory/Classroom
**C:** Clinical/Field Testing
**P:** Practicum
**A:** Assessment/Mock Exam

**TEST INFORMATION**
**Test Statistics:** N/A
**Reference(s):** Kendall et al. (2005)

# MANUAL MUSCLE TESTING

| NATA EC 5th | BOC RD6 | SKILL |
|---|---|---|
| CE-21c | D2-0203 | MMT: Quadratus Lumborum |

**Supplies Needed:** Table

*This problem allows you the opportunity to demonstrate a* **manual muscle test** *for the* **quadratus lumborum**. *You have 2 minutes to complete this task.*

| MMT: Quadratus Lumborum | Course or Site Assessor Environment | | | | | |
|---|---|---|---|---|---|---|
| | | Test 1 | | Test 2 | | Test 3 |
| **Tester places patient and limb in appropriate position** | | Y | N | Y | N | Y | N |
| Supine | | O | O | O | O | O | O |
| Hip and lumbar spine in full extension | | O | O | O | O | O | O |
| **Tester placed in proper position** | | Y | N | Y | N | Y | N |
| Stands at edge of table, holding the affected leg at the ankle | | O | O | O | O | O | O |
| **Tester performs test according to accepted guidelines** | | Y | N | Y | N | Y | N |
| Instructs the patient to actively laterally elevate the pelvis | | O | O | O | O | O | O |
| Applies resistance as traction on the extremity (directly opposing the line of pull of the muscle) | | O | O | O | O | O | O |
| Holds resistance for 5 seconds | | O | O | O | O | O | O |
| Performs assessment bilaterally | | O | O | O | O | O | O |
| **Identifies implications** | | Y | N | Y | N | Y | N |
| Correctly grades the MMT | | O | O | O | O | O | O |
| Total | | ___/8 | | ___/8 | | ___/8 |
| **Must achieve >5 to pass this examination** | | Ⓟ | Ⓕ | Ⓟ | Ⓕ | Ⓟ | Ⓕ |

| Assessor: Date: | Test 1 Comments: |
|---|---|
| Assessor: Date: | Test 2 Comments: |
| Assessor: Date: | Test 3 Comments: |

**TEST ENVIRONMENTS**
**L:** Laboratory/Classroom
**C:** Clinical/Field Testing
**P:** Practicum
**A:** Assessment/Mock Exam

**TEST INFORMATION**
**Test Statistics:** N/A
**Reference(s):** Kendall et al. (2005)

## MUSCULOSKELETAL SYSTEM—REGION 4: HIP AND PELVIS
# MANUAL MUSCLE TESTING

| NATA EC 5th | BOC RD6 | SKILL |
|---|---|---|
| CE-21c | D2-0203 | MMT: Iliopsoas |

**Supplies Needed:** Table

*This problem allows you the opportunity to demonstrate a* **manual muscle test** *for the* **iliopsoas**.
*You have 2 minutes to complete this task.*

| MMT: Iliopsoas | Course or Site Assessor Environment | | Test 1 | | Test 2 | | Test 3 | |
|---|---|---|---|---|---|---|---|---|
| **Tester places patient and limb in appropriate position** | | | Y | N | Y | N | Y | N |
| Supine | | | ○ | ○ | ○ | ○ | ○ | ○ |
| Hip in a position of full extension, slight abduction, slight lateral rotation | | | ○ | ○ | ○ | ○ | ○ | ○ |
| **Tester placed in proper position** | | | Y | N | Y | N | Y | N |
| Places stabilizing hand over opposite ASIS | | | ○ | ○ | ○ | ○ | ○ | ○ |
| Places force hand over anteromedial aspect of contralateral limb | | | ○ | ○ | ○ | ○ | ○ | ○ |
| **Tester performs test according to accepted guidelines** | | | Y | N | Y | N | Y | N |
| Instructs the patient to actively flex the hip | | | ○ | ○ | ○ | ○ | ○ | ○ |
| Applies resistance to the anteromedial aspect of lower leg (direction of hip extension) | | | ○ | ○ | ○ | ○ | ○ | ○ |
| Holds resistance for 5 seconds | | | ○ | ○ | ○ | ○ | ○ | ○ |
| Performs assessment bilaterally | | | ○ | ○ | ○ | ○ | ○ | ○ |
| **Identifies implications** | | | Y | N | Y | N | Y | N |
| Correctly grades the MMT | | | ○ | ○ | ○ | ○ | ○ | ○ |
| | | **Total** | __/9 | | __/9 | | __/9 | |
| | **Must achieve >6 to pass this examination** | | Ⓟ | Ⓕ | Ⓟ | Ⓕ | Ⓟ | Ⓕ |
| **Assessor:** **Date:** | **Test 1 Comments:** | | | | | | | |
| **Assessor:** **Date:** | **Test 2 Comments:** | | | | | | | |
| **Assessor:** **Date:** | **Test 3 Comments:** | | | | | | | |

**TEST ENVIRONMENTS**
**L:** Laboratory/Classroom
**C:** Clinical/Field Testing
**P:** Practicum
**A:** Assessment/Mock Exam

**TEST INFORMATION**
**Test Statistics:** N/A
**Reference(s):** Kendall et al. (2005)

# MANUAL MUSCLE TESTING

| NATA EC 5th | BOC RD6 | SKILL |
|---|---|---|
| CE-21c | D2-0203 | MMT: Tensor Fasciae Latae |

**Supplies Needed:** Table

*This problem allows you the opportunity to demonstrate a* **manual muscle test** *for* **tensor fasciae latae**. *You have 2 minutes to complete this task.*

| MMT: Tensor Fasciae Latae | Course or Site Assessor Environment | | Test 1 | | Test 2 | | Test 3 | |
|---|---|---|---|---|---|---|---|---|
| **Tester places patient and limb in appropriate position** | | **Y** | **N** | **Y** | **N** | **Y** | **N** | |
| Supine | | O | O | O | O | O | O | |
| Knee extension | | O | O | O | O | O | O | |
| Hip abduction, flexion, and medial rotation | | O | O | O | O | O | O | |
| **Tester placed in proper position** | | **Y** | **N** | **Y** | **N** | **Y** | **N** | |
| Places dominant hand on anteromedial aspect of lower leg | | O | O | O | O | O | O | |
| **Tester performs test according to accepted guidelines** | | **Y** | **N** | **Y** | **N** | **Y** | **N** | |
| Instructs the patient to actively hold position | | O | O | O | O | O | O | |
| Applies resistance against leg (direction of extension and adduction) | | O | O | O | O | O | O | |
| Holds resistance for 5 seconds | | O | O | O | O | O | O | |
| Performs assessment bilaterally | | O | O | O | O | O | O | |
| **Identifies implications** | | **Y** | **N** | **Y** | **N** | **Y** | **N** | |
| Correctly grades the MMT | | O | O | O | O | O | O | |
| **Total** | | ___/9 | | ___/9 | | ___/9 | | |
| **Must achieve >6 to pass this examination** | | (P) | (F) | (P) | (F) | (P) | (F) | |

| Assessor:<br>Date: | Test 1 Comments: |
|---|---|
| Assessor:<br>Date: | Test 2 Comments: |
| Assessor:<br>Date: | Test 3 Comments: |

**TEST ENVIRONMENTS**
**L:** Laboratory/Classroom
**C:** Clinical/Field Testing
**P:** Practicum
**A:** Assessment/Mock Exam

**TEST INFORMATION**
**Test Statistics:** N/A
**Reference(s):** Kendall et al. (2005)

## MUSCULOSKELETAL SYSTEM—REGION 4: HIP AND PELVIS
# OSTEOKINEMATIC JOINT MOTION

| NATA EC 5th | BOC RD6 | SKILL |
|:---:|:---:|:---:|
| CE-21d | D2-0203 | Goniometric Assessment: Iliofemoral Joint (Abduction) |

**Supplies Needed:** Table, large goniometer

*This problem allows you the opportunity to demonstrate a* **goniometric assessment** *for the* **iliofemoral joint (abduction)**. *You have 2 minutes to complete this task.*

| Goniometric Assessment: Iliofemoral Joint (Abduction) | Course or Site Assessor Environment | | Test 1 | | Test 2 | | Test 3 | |
|---|---|---|:---:|:---:|:---:|:---:|:---:|:---:|
| **Tester places patient and limb in appropriate position** | | | **Y** | **N** | **Y** | **N** | **Y** | **N** |
| Supine with knees extended | | | ○ | ○ | ○ | ○ | ○ | ○ |
| Hips in neutral position | | | ○ | ○ | ○ | ○ | ○ | ○ |
| **Tester and goniometer placed in proper position** | | | **Y** | **N** | **Y** | **N** | **Y** | **N** |
| Places fulcrum over the ASIS on the side being tested | | | ○ | ○ | ○ | ○ | ○ | ○ |
| Fixed arm is lined up with the opposite ASIS | | | ○ | ○ | ○ | ○ | ○ | ○ |
| Distal arm is placed in line with the anterior midline of the femur, using midline of the patella for reference | | | ○ | ○ | ○ | ○ | ○ | ○ |
| **Tester performs test according to accepted guidelines** | | | **Y** | **N** | **Y** | **N** | **Y** | **N** |
| Abducts the hip with one hand by sliding the lower extremity laterally | | | ○ | ○ | ○ | ○ | ○ | ○ |
| Stabilizes lateral pelvis with opposite hand | | | ○ | ○ | ○ | ○ | ○ | ○ |
| Takes proper goniometric measurement | | | ○ | ○ | ○ | ○ | ○ | ○ |
| Performs assessment bilaterally | | | ○ | ○ | ○ | ○ | ○ | ○ |
| **Identifies implications** | | | **Y** | **N** | **Y** | **N** | **Y** | **N** |
| Identifies normal ranges (abduction = 40 degrees) | | | ○ | ○ | ○ | ○ | ○ | ○ |
| | | Total | \_\_\_\_/10 | | \_\_\_\_/10 | | \_\_\_\_/10 | |
| | Must achieve >6 to pass this examination | | Ⓟ | Ⓕ | Ⓟ | Ⓕ | Ⓟ | Ⓕ |
| **Assessor: Date:** | **Test 1 Comments:** | | | | | | | |
| **Assessor: Date:** | **Test 2 Comments:** | | | | | | | |
| **Assessor: Date:** | **Test 3 Comments:** | | | | | | | |

**TEST ENVIRONMENTS**
**L:** Laboratory/Classroom
**C:** Clinical/Field Testing
**P:** Practicum
**A:** Assessment/Mock Exam

**TEST INFORMATION**
**Test Statistics:** N/A
**Reference(s):** Norkin & White (2009)

# OSTEOKINEMATIC JOINT MOTION

| NATA EC 5th | BOC RD6 | SKILL |
|---|---|---|
| CE-21d | D2-0203 | Goniometric Assessment: Iliofemoral Joint (Adduction) |

**Supplies Needed:** Table, large goniometer

*This problem allows you the opportunity to demonstrate a* **goniometric assessment** *for the* **iliofemoral joint (adduction)**. *You have 2 minutes to complete this task.*

| Goniometric Assessment: Iliofemoral Joint (Adduction) | Course or Site Assessor Environment | | | | | |
|---|---|---|---|---|---|---|
| | Test 1 | | Test 2 | | Test 3 | |
| **Tester places patient and limb in appropriate position** | Y | N | Y | N | Y | N |
| Supine with knees extended | O | O | O | O | O | O |
| Hips in neutral position | O | O | O | O | O | O |
| Contralateral extremity abducted to provide space for full range of motion | O | O | O | O | O | O |
| **Tester and goniometer placed in proper position** | Y | N | Y | N | Y | N |
| Places fulcrum over the ASIS on the side being tested | O | O | O | O | O | O |
| Fixed arm is lined up with the opposite ASIS | O | O | O | O | O | O |
| Moving arm is placed in line with the anterior midline of the femur, using midline of the patella for reference | O | O | O | O | O | O |
| **Tester performs test according to accepted guidelines** | Y | N | Y | N | Y | N |
| Adducts the hip with one hand by sliding the lower extremity medially | O | O | O | O | O | O |
| Stabilizes lateral pelvis with opposite hand | O | O | O | O | O | O |
| Takes proper goniometric measurement | O | O | O | O | O | O |
| Performs assessment bilaterally | O | O | O | O | O | O |
| **Identifies implications** | Y | N | Y | N | Y | N |
| Identifies normal ranges (adduction = 20 degrees) | O | O | O | O | O | O |
| **Total** | ___/11 | | ___/11 | | ___/11 | |
| **Must achieve >7 to pass this examination** | Ⓟ | Ⓕ | Ⓟ | Ⓕ | Ⓟ | Ⓕ |

| Assessor: Date: | Test 1 Comments: |
|---|---|
| Assessor: Date: | Test 2 Comments: |
| Assessor: Date: | Test 3 Comments: |

**TEST ENVIRONMENTS**
**L:** Laboratory/Classroom
**C:** Clinical/Field Testing
**P:** Practicum
**A:** Assessment/Mock Exam

**TEST INFORMATION**
**Test Statistics:** N/A
**Reference(s):** Norkin & White (2009)

## MUSCULOSKELETAL SYSTEM—REGION 4: HIP AND PELVIS
# OSTEOKINEMATIC JOINT MOTION

| NATA EC 5th | BOC RD6 | SKILL |
|---|---|---|
| CE-21d | D2-0203 | Goniometric Assessment: Iliofemoral Joint (Internal Rotation) |

**Supplies Needed:** Table, towel, large goniometer

*This problem allows you the opportunity to demonstrate a* **goniometric assessment** *for the* **iliofemoral joint (internal rotation)***. You have 2 minutes to complete this task.*

| Goniometric Assessment: Iliofemoral Joint (Internal Rotation) | Course or Site / Assessor / Environment | | | | | |
|---|---|---|---|---|---|---|
| | | Test 1 | | Test 2 | | Test 3 |
| **Tester places patient and limb in appropriate position** | | **Y** | **N** | **Y** | **N** | **Y** | **N** |
| Seated with knees flexed to 90 degrees over the edge | | ○ | ○ | ○ | ○ | ○ | ○ |
| Hip in 90 degrees of flexion | | ○ | ○ | ○ | ○ | ○ | ○ |
| Towel placed under distal femur | | ○ | ○ | ○ | ○ | ○ | ○ |
| **Tester and goniometer placed in proper position** | | **Y** | **N** | **Y** | **N** | **Y** | **N** |
| Places fulcrum over the anterior aspect of the patella | | ○ | ○ | ○ | ○ | ○ | ○ |
| Fixed arm is lined up perpendicular to the floor | | ○ | ○ | ○ | ○ | ○ | ○ |
| Moving arm is placed in line with the anterior midline of the lower leg (tibial crest) | | ○ | ○ | ○ | ○ | ○ | ○ |
| **Tester performs test according to accepted guidelines** | | **Y** | **N** | **Y** | **N** | **Y** | **N** |
| The tester stabilizes the distal femur while other hand grasps the distal tibia to move the lower leg laterally | | ○ | ○ | ○ | ○ | ○ | ○ |
| The hand performing the motion also holds the lower leg in neutral position to prevent rotation at the knee joint | | ○ | ○ | ○ | ○ | ○ | ○ |
| Takes proper goniometric measurement | | ○ | ○ | ○ | ○ | ○ | ○ |
| Performs assessment bilaterally | | ○ | ○ | ○ | ○ | ○ | ○ |
| **Identifies implications** | | **Y** | **N** | **Y** | **N** | **Y** | **N** |
| Identifies normal ranges (internal rotation = 40 to 45 degrees) | | ○ | ○ | ○ | ○ | ○ | ○ |
| **Total** | | ___/11 | | ___/11 | | ___/11 | |
| **Must achieve >7 to pass this examination** | | Ⓟ | Ⓕ | Ⓟ | Ⓕ | Ⓟ | Ⓕ |

| Assessor: Date: | Test 1 Comments: |
|---|---|
| Assessor: Date: | Test 2 Comments: |
| Assessor: Date: | Test 3 Comments: |

**TEST ENVIRONMENTS**
**L:** Laboratory/Classroom
**C:** Clinical/Field Testing
**P:** Practicum
**A:** Assessment/Mock Exam

**TEST INFORMATION**
**Test Statistics:** N/A
**Reference(s):** Norkin & White (2009)

**MUSCULOSKELETAL SYSTEM—REGION 4: HIP AND PELVIS**
# OSTEOKINEMATIC JOINT MOTION

| NATA EC 5th | BOC RD6 | SKILL |
|---|---|---|
| CE-21d | D2-0203 | Goniometric Assessment:<br>Iliofemoral Joint (Internal Rotation) – Alternate |

**Supplies Needed:** Table, large goniometer

*This problem allows you the opportunity to demonstrate a* **goniometric assessment** *for the* **iliofemoral joint (internal rotation) – alternate**. *You have 2 minutes to complete this task.*

| Goniometric Assessment:<br>Iliofemoral Joint (Internal Rotation) –<br>Alternate | Course or Site _____  _____  _____<br>Assessor _____  _____  _____<br>Environment _____  _____  _____ | | | | | |
|---|---|---|---|---|---|---|
| | Test 1 | | Test 2 | | Test 3 | |
| | Y | N | Y | N | Y | N |
| **Tester places patient and limb in appropriate position** | Y | N | Y | N | Y | N |
| Prone with both legs extended | O | O | O | O | O | O |
| Knee flexed to 90 degrees on the side being tested | O | O | O | O | O | O |
| Strap placed across the pelvis for stabilization | O | O | O | O | O | O |
| **Tester and goniometer placed in proper position** | Y | N | Y | N | Y | N |
| Places fulcrum over the anterior aspect of the patella | O | O | O | O | O | O |
| Fixed arm is lined up perpendicular to the floor | O | O | O | O | O | O |
| Moving arm is placed in line with the anterior midline of the lower leg (tibial crest) | O | O | O | O | O | O |
| **Tester performs test according to accepted guidelines** | Y | N | Y | N | Y | N |
| The tester holds fixed arm while the other hand grasps the distal tibia to move the lower leg and moving arm laterally | O | O | O | O | O | O |
| The hand performing the motion also holds the lower leg in neutral position to prevent rotation at the knee joint | O | O | O | O | O | O |
| Takes proper goniometric measurement | O | O | O | O | O | O |
| Performs assessment bilaterally | O | O | O | O | O | O |
| **Identifies implications** | Y | N | Y | N | Y | N |
| Identifies normal ranges (internal rotation = 40 to 45 degrees) | O | O | O | O | O | O |
| Total | ____/11 | | ____/11 | | ____/11 | |
| Must achieve >7 to pass this examination | Ⓟ | Ⓕ | Ⓟ | Ⓕ | Ⓟ | Ⓕ |
| Assessor:<br>Date: | Test 1 Comments: | | | | | |
| Assessor:<br>Date: | Test 2 Comments: | | | | | |
| Assessor:<br>Date: | Test 3 Comments: | | | | | |

**TEST ENVIRONMENTS**
**L:** Laboratory/Classroom
**C:** Clinical/Field Testing
**P:** Practicum
**A:** Assessment/Mock Exam

**TEST INFORMATION**
**Test Statistics:** N/A
**Reference(s):** Norkin & White (2009)

MUSCULOSKELETAL SYSTEM—REGION 4: HIP AND PELVIS
# OSTEOKINEMATIC JOINT MOTION

| NATA EC 5th | BOC RD6 | SKILL |
|---|---|---|
| CE-21d | D2-0203 | Goniometric Assessment: Iliofemoral Joint (External Rotation) |

**Supplies Needed:** Table, towel, large goniometer

*This problem allows you the opportunity to demonstrate a* **goniometric assessment** *for the* **iliofemoral joint (external rotation)**. *You have 2 minutes to complete this task.*

| Goniometric Assessment: Iliofemoral Joint (External Rotation) | Course or Site _____ _____ _____ Assessor _____ _____ _____ Environment _____ _____ _____ | | | | | |
|---|---|---|---|---|---|---|
| | Test 1 | | Test 2 | | Test 3 | |
| **Tester places patient and limb in appropriate position** | Y | N | Y | N | Y | N |
| Seated with knees flexed to 90 degrees over the edge | ○ | ○ | ○ | ○ | ○ | ○ |
| Hip in 90 degrees of flexion | ○ | ○ | ○ | ○ | ○ | ○ |
| Towel placed under distal femur | ○ | ○ | ○ | ○ | ○ | ○ |
| Contralateral knee flexed past 90 degrees to allow full range of motion | ○ | ○ | ○ | ○ | ○ | ○ |
| **Tester and goniometer placed in proper position** | Y | N | Y | N | Y | N |
| Places fulcrum over the anterior aspect of the patella | ○ | ○ | ○ | ○ | ○ | ○ |
| Fixed arm is lined up perpendicular to the floor | ○ | ○ | ○ | ○ | ○ | ○ |
| Moving arm is placed in line with the anterior midline of the lower leg (tibial crest) | ○ | ○ | ○ | ○ | ○ | ○ |
| **Tester performs test according to accepted guidelines** | Y | N | Y | N | Y | N |
| The tester stabilizes the distal femur while other hand grasps the distal tibia to move the lower leg medially | ○ | ○ | ○ | ○ | ○ | ○ |
| The hand performing the motion also holds the lower leg in neutral position to prevent rotation at the knee joint | ○ | ○ | ○ | ○ | ○ | ○ |
| Takes proper goniometric measurement | ○ | ○ | ○ | ○ | ○ | ○ |
| Performs assessment bilaterally | ○ | ○ | ○ | ○ | ○ | ○ |
| **Identifies implications** | Y | N | Y | N | Y | N |
| Identifies normal ranges (external rotation = 45 to 50 degrees) | ○ | ○ | ○ | ○ | ○ | ○ |
| **Total** | ___/12 | | ___/12 | | ___/12 | |
| **Must achieve >8 to pass this examination** | Ⓟ | Ⓕ | Ⓟ | Ⓕ | Ⓟ | Ⓕ |

| Assessor: Date: | Test 1 Comments: |
|---|---|
| Assessor: Date: | Test 2 Comments: |
| Assessor: Date: | Test 3 Comments: |

**TEST ENVIRONMENTS**
**L:** Laboratory/Classroom
**C:** Clinical/Field Testing
**P:** Practicum
**A:** Assessment/Mock Exam

**TEST INFORMATION**
**Test Statistics:** N/A
**Reference(s):** Norkin & White (2009)

MUSCULOSKELETAL SYSTEM—REGION 4: HIP AND PELVIS
# OSTEOKINEMATIC JOINT MOTION

| NATA EC 5th | BOC RD6 | SKILL |
|---|---|---|
| CE-21d | D2-0203 | Goniometric Assessment: Iliofemoral Joint (External Rotation) – Alternate |

**Supplies Needed:** Table, large goniometer

*This problem allows you the opportunity to demonstrate a* **goniometric assessment** *for the* **iliofemoral joint (external rotation) – alternate**. *You have 2 minutes to complete this task.*

| Goniometric Assessment: Iliofemoral Joint (External Rotation) – Alternate | Course or Site Assessor Environment | | Test 1 | | Test 2 | | Test 3 |
|---|---|---|---|---|---|---|---|
| | | Y | N | Y | N | Y | N |
| **Tester places patient and limb in appropriate position** | | Y | N | Y | N | Y | N |
| Prone with both legs extended | | O | O | O | O | O | O |
| Knee flexed to 90 degrees on the side being tested | | O | O | O | O | O | O |
| Strap placed across the pelvis for stabilization | | O | O | O | O | O | O |
| **Tester and goniometer placed in proper position** | | Y | N | Y | N | Y | N |
| Places fulcrum over the anterior aspect of the patella | | O | O | O | O | O | O |
| Fixed arm is lined up perpendicular to the floor | | O | O | O | O | O | O |
| Moving arm is placed in line with the anterior midline of the lower leg (tibial crest) | | O | O | O | O | O | O |
| **Tester performs test according to accepted guidelines** | | Y | N | Y | N | Y | N |
| The tester stabilizes the distal femur while other hand grasps the distal tibia to move the lower leg medially | | O | O | O | O | O | O |
| The hand performing the motion also holds the lower leg in neutral position to prevent rotation at the knee joint | | O | O | O | O | O | O |
| Takes proper goniometric measurement | | O | O | O | O | O | O |
| Performs assessment bilaterally | | O | O | O | O | O | O |
| **Identifies implications** | | Y | N | Y | N | Y | N |
| Identifies normal ranges (external rotation = 45 to 50 degrees) | | O | O | O | O | O | O |
| **Total** | | __/11 | | __/11 | | __/11 | |
| **Must achieve >7 to pass this examination** | | (P) | (F) | (P) | (F) | (P) | (F) |

| Assessor: Date: | Test 1 Comments: |
|---|---|
| Assessor: Date: | Test 2 Comments: |
| Assessor: Date: | Test 3 Comments: |

**TEST ENVIRONMENTS**
**L:** Laboratory/Classroom
**C:** Clinical/Field Testing
**P:** Practicum
**A:** Assessment/Mock Exam

**TEST INFORMATION**
**Test Statistics:** N/A
**Reference(s):** Norkin & White (2009)

**MUSCULOSKELETAL SYSTEM—REGION 4: HIP AND PELVIS**
# OSTEOKINEMATIC JOINT MOTION

| NATA EC 5th | BOC RD6 | SKILL |
|---|---|---|
| CE-21d | D2-0203 | Goniometric Assessment: Iliofemoral Joint (Extension) |

**Supplies Needed:** Table, large goniometer

*This problem allows you the opportunity to demonstrate a* **goniometric assessment** *for the* **iliofemoral joint (extension)**. *You have 2 minutes to complete this task.*

| Goniometric Assessment: Iliofemoral Joint (Extension) | Course or Site Assessor Environment | | | | | |
|---|---|---|---|---|---|---|
| | | Test 1 | | Test 2 | | Test 3 |
| | | Y | N | Y | N | Y | N |
| Tester places patient and limb in appropriate position | | Y | N | Y | N | Y | N |
| Prone, with both knees extended | | O | O | O | O | O | O |
| Hip to be tested in neutral position | | O | O | O | O | O | O |
| Tester and goniometer placed in proper position | | Y | N | Y | N | Y | N |
| Places fulcrum over the greater trochanter | | O | O | O | O | O | O |
| Fixed arm is lined up with the lateral midline of the pelvis | | O | O | O | O | O | O |
| Moving arm is placed in line with the lateral midline of the femur, using lateral epicondyle for reference | | O | O | O | O | O | O |
| Tester performs test according to accepted guidelines | | Y | N | Y | N | Y | N |
| Extends the hip by raising the lower extremity from the table | | O | O | O | O | O | O |
| Maintains knee extension throughout the whole movement | | O | O | O | O | O | O |
| Takes proper goniometric measurement | | O | O | O | O | O | O |
| Performs assessment bilaterally | | O | O | O | O | O | O |
| Identifies implications | | Y | N | Y | N | Y | N |
| Identifies normal ranges (extension = 20 to 30 degrees) | | O | O | O | O | O | O |
| Total | | ___/10 | | ___/10 | | ___/10 |
| Must achieve >6 to pass this examination | | P | F | P | F | P | F |

| Assessor: Date: | Test 1 Comments: |
|---|---|
| Assessor: Date: | Test 2 Comments: |
| Assessor: Date: | Test 3 Comments: |

**TEST ENVIRONMENTS**
**L:** Laboratory/Classroom
**C:** Clinical/Field Testing
**P:** Practicum
**A:** Assessment/Mock Exam

**TEST INFORMATION**
**Test Statistics:** N/A
**Reference(s):** Norkin & White (2009)

# OSTEOKINEMATIC JOINT MOTION

| NATA EC 5th | BOC RD6 | SKILL |
|---|---|---|
| CE-21d | D2-0203 | Goniometric Assessment: Iliofemoral Joint (Flexion) |

**Supplies Needed:** Table, large goniometer

*This problem allows you the opportunity to demonstrate a* **goniometric assessment** *for the* **iliofemoral joint (flexion)**. *You have 2 minutes to complete this task.*

| Goniometric Assessment: Iliofemoral Joint (Flexion) | Course or Site<br>Assessor<br>Environment | | | | | |
|---|---|---|---|---|---|---|
| | **Test 1** | | **Test 2** | | **Test 3** | |
| **Tester places patient and limb in appropriate position** | **Y** | **N** | **Y** | **N** | **Y** | **N** |
| Supine with knees extended | O | O | O | O | O | O |
| Hips in neutral position | O | O | O | O | O | O |
| **Tester and goniometer placed in proper position** | **Y** | **N** | **Y** | **N** | **Y** | **N** |
| Places fulcrum on the lateral aspect of the hip over the greater trochanter | O | O | O | O | O | O |
| Fixed arm is lined up with the lateral midline of the trunk | O | O | O | O | O | O |
| Moving arm is placed in line with the lateral midline of the femur, using lateral epicondyle for reference | O | O | O | O | O | O |
| **Tester performs test according to accepted guidelines** | **Y** | **N** | **Y** | **N** | **Y** | **N** |
| Flexes the hip by lifting the lower extremity off the table | O | O | O | O | O | O |
| Maintains the extremity in neutral position | O | O | O | O | O | O |
| Stops the motion when resistance is felt or posterior tilting of the pelvis is observed | O | O | O | O | O | O |
| Takes proper goniometric measurement | O | O | O | O | O | O |
| Performs assessment bilaterally | O | O | O | O | O | O |
| **Identifies implications** | **Y** | **N** | **Y** | **N** | **Y** | **N** |
| Identifies normal ranges (flexion = 100 to 120 degrees) | O | O | O | O | O | O |
| **Total** | ___/11 | | ___/11 | | ___/11 | |
| **Must achieve >7 to pass this examination** | Ⓟ | Ⓕ | Ⓟ | Ⓕ | Ⓟ | Ⓕ |

| Assessor:<br>Date: | Test 1 Comments: |
|---|---|
| Assessor:<br>Date: | Test 2 Comments: |
| Assessor:<br>Date: | Test 3 Comments: |

**TEST ENVIRONMENTS**
**L:** Laboratory/Classroom
**C:** Clinical/Field Testing
**P:** Practicum
**A:** Assessment/Mock Exam

**TEST INFORMATION**
**Test Statistics:** N/A
**Reference(s):** Norkin & White (2009)

MUSCULOSKELETAL SYSTEM—REGION 4: HIP AND PELVIS
# CAPSULAR AND LIGAMENTOUS STRESS TESTING

| NATA EC 5th | BOC RD6 | SKILL |
|---|---|---|
| CE-21e | D2-0203 | Sacroiliac Compression Test |

**Supplies Needed:** Table

*This problem allows you the opportunity to demonstrate an* **orthopedic test** *known as the* **sacroiliac compression test** *for* **sacroiliac joint dysfunction**. *You have 2 minutes to complete this task.*

| Sacroiliac Compression Test | Course or Site<br>Assessor<br>Environment | | Test 1 | | Test 2 | | Test 3 | |
|---|---|---|---|---|---|---|---|---|
| **Tester places patient and limb in appropriate position** | | **Y** | **N** | **Y** | **N** | **Y** | **N** | |
| Side lying on opposite side of pain | | O | O | O | O | O | O | |
| **Tester placed in proper position** | | **Y** | **N** | **Y** | **N** | **Y** | **N** | |
| Stands to the side that will be tested | | O | O | O | O | O | O | |
| Places one hand on the iliac crest | | O | O | O | O | O | O | |
| **Tester performs test according to accepted guidelines** | | **Y** | **N** | **Y** | **N** | **Y** | **N** | |
| Applies a downward force through the ilium and holds for 30 seconds | | O | O | O | O | O | O | |
| Performs assessment bilaterally | | O | O | O | O | O | O | |
| **Identifies positive findings and implications** | | **Y** | **N** | **Y** | **N** | **Y** | **N** | |
| Reproduction of pain in the SI joint | | O | O | O | O | O | O | |
| **Total** | | __/6 | | __/6 | | __/6 | | |
| **Must achieve >4 to pass this examination** | | Ⓟ | Ⓕ | Ⓟ | Ⓕ | Ⓟ | Ⓕ | |

| Assessor:<br>Date: | Test 1 Comments: |
|---|---|
| Assessor:<br>Date: | Test 2 Comments: |
| Assessor:<br>Date: | Test 3 Comments: |

## TEST ENVIRONMENTS
**L:** Laboratory/Classroom
**C:** Clinical/Field Testing
**P:** Practicum
**A:** Assessment/Mock Exam

## TEST INFORMATION
**Test Statistics:** Sensitivity .07–.69
Specificity .63–1.00
(+) LR .70–3.95
(-) LR .40–1.03
**Reference(s):** Cook & Hegedus (2013)

# CAPSULAR AND LIGAMENTOUS STRESS TESTING

| NATA EC 5th | BOC RD6 | SKILL |
|---|---|---|
| CE-21e | D2-0203 | Sacroiliac Distraction Test |

**Supplies Needed:** Table

*This problem allows you the opportunity to demonstrate an* **orthopedic test** *known as the* **sacroiliac distraction test** *to rule out* **sacroiliac joint dysfunction**. *You have 2 minutes to complete this task.*

| Sacroiliac Distraction Test | Course or Site Assessor Environment | | Test 1 | | Test 2 | | Test 3 | |
|---|---|---|---|---|---|---|---|---|
| **Tester places patient and limb in appropriate position** | | | Y | N | Y | N | Y | N |
| Supine | | | O | O | O | O | O | O |
| **Tester placed in proper position** | | | Y | N | Y | N | Y | N |
| Stands on the side being tested | | | O | O | O | O | O | O |
| Palpates medial aspect of both ASIS | | | O | O | O | O | O | O |
| Crosses arms and places hands over ASIS | | | O | O | O | O | O | O |
| **Tester performs test according to accepted guidelines** | | | Y | N | Y | N | Y | N |
| Applies force in posterolateral direction to ASIS and holds for 30 seconds | | | O | O | O | O | O | O |
| **Identifies positive findings and implications** | | | Y | N | Y | N | Y | N |
| Reproduction of pain in the SI joint | | | O | O | O | O | O | O |
| **Total** | | | /6 | | /6 | | /6 | |
| **Must achieve >4 to pass this examination** | | | Ⓟ | Ⓕ | Ⓟ | Ⓕ | Ⓟ | Ⓕ |

| Assessor: Date: | Test 1 Comments: |
|---|---|
| Assessor: Date: | Test 2 Comments: |
| Assessor: Date: | Test 3 Comments: |

**TEST ENVIRONMENTS**
**L:** Laboratory/Classroom
**C:** Clinical/Field Testing
**P:** Practicum
**A:** Assessment/Mock Exam

**TEST INFORMATION**
**Test Statistics:** Sensitivity .04–.60
Specificity .74–1.00
(+) LR 1.10–3.20
(-) LR .50–.98
**Reference(s):** Cook & Hegedus (2013)

## MUSCULOSKELETAL SYSTEM—REGION 4: HIP AND PELVIS
# SPECIAL TESTS

| NATA EC 5th | BOC RD6 | SKILL |
|---|---|---|
| CE-21g, CE-20e | D2-0203 | Ely's Test |

**Supplies Needed:** Table

*This problem allows you the opportunity to demonstrate an* **orthopedic test** *known as* **Ely's test** *to rule out* **tightness of the rectus femoris***. You have 2 minutes to complete this task.*

| Ely's Test | Course or Site<br>Assessor<br>Environment<br>———— | Test 1 | | Test 2 | | Test 3 | |
|---|---|---|---|---|---|---|---|
| **Tester places patient and limb in appropriate position** | | Y | N | Y | N | Y | N |
| Prone | | O | O | O | O | O | O |
| **Tester placed in proper position** | | Y | N | Y | N | Y | N |
| Stands on the side being tested | | O | O | O | O | O | O |
| Grasps the lower leg around the malleoli with the caudal hand | | O | O | O | O | O | O |
| **Tester performs test according to accepted guidelines** | | Y | N | Y | N | Y | N |
| Passively flexes the patient's knee toward the buttocks | | O | O | O | O | O | O |
| **Identifies positive findings and implications** | | Y | N | Y | N | Y | N |
| The ipsilateral hip flexes, causing it to rise from the table | | O | O | O | O | O | O |
| Tightness of the rectus femoris | | O | O | O | O | O | O |
| **Total** | | ___/6 | | ___/6 | | ___/6 | |
| **Must achieve >4 to pass this examination** | | (P) | (F) | (P) | (F) | (P) | (F) |

| Assessor:<br>Date: | Test 1 Comments: |
|---|---|
| Assessor:<br>Date: | Test 2 Comments: |
| Assessor:<br>Date: | Test 3 Comments: |

**TEST ENVIRONMENTS**
**L:** Laboratory/Classroom
**C:** Clinical/Field Testing
**P:** Practicum
**A:** Assessment/Mock Exam

**TEST INFORMATION**
**Test Statistics:** No data available
**Reference(s):** Starkey & Brown (2015)

# SPECIAL TESTS

| NATA EC 5th | BOC RD6 | SKILL |
|---|---|---|
| CE-21g, CE-20e | D2-0203 | Flexion-Abduction-External Rotation (FABER) Test (Patrick's Test) |

**Supplies Needed:** Table

*This problem allows you the opportunity to demonstrate an* **orthopedic test** *known as the* **flexion-abduction-external rotation (FABER) test (Patrick's test)** *for* **sacroiliac joint dysfunction**. *You have 2 minutes to complete this task.*

| Flexion-Abduction-External Rotation (FABER) Test (Patrick's Test) | Course or Site / Assessor / Environment | | | | | |
|---|---|---|---|---|---|---|
| | Test 1 | | Test 2 | | Test 3 | |
| **Tester places patient and limb in appropriate position** | Y | N | Y | N | Y | N |
| Supine | O | O | O | O | O | O |
| Places foot of involved side crossed over the opposite thigh | O | O | O | O | O | O |
| **Tester placed in proper position** | Y | N | Y | N | Y | N |
| Stands to the side that will be tested | O | O | O | O | O | O |
| Places one hand on the cephalic hand on the opposite ASIS | O | O | O | O | O | O |
| Places the caudal hand on the medial aspect of the affected knee | O | O | O | O | O | O |
| **Tester performs test according to accepted guidelines** | Y | N | Y | N | Y | N |
| The extremity is allowed to rest into full external rotation | O | O | O | O | O | O |
| Applies gentle over pressure at the ASIS and medial knee | O | O | O | O | O | O |
| Performs assessment bilaterally | O | O | O | O | O | O |
| **Identifies positive findings and implications** | Y | N | Y | N | Y | N |
| Pain in the inguinal area anterior to the hip or pain in the SI area | O | O | O | O | O | O |
| Pain in the hip indicates hip pathology; pain in the SI area indicates SI joint pathology | O | O | O | O | O | O |
| **Total** | /10 | | /10 | | /10 | |
| **Must achieve >6 to pass this examination** | P | F | P | F | P | F |

| Assessor: Date: | Test 1 Comments: |
|---|---|
| Assessor: Date: | Test 2 Comments: |
| Assessor: Date: | Test 3 Comments: |

**TEST ENVIRONMENTS**
L: Laboratory/Classroom
C: Clinical/Field Testing
P: Practicum
A: Assessment/Mock Exam

**TEST INFORMATION**
**Test Statistics:** Sensitivity .42–.81
Specificity .18–.25
(+) LR .7–1.70
(-) LR .72–2.20
**Reference(s):** Reiman et al. (2015)
Starkey & Brown (2015)

## MUSCULOSKELETAL SYSTEM—REGION 4: HIP AND PELVIS
# SPECIAL TESTS

| NATA EC 5th | BOC RD6 | SKILL |
|---|---|---|
| CE-21g, CE-20e | D2-0203 | Flexion-Adduction-Internal Rotation (FADDIR) Test |

**Supplies Needed:** Table

*This problem allows you the opportunity to demonstrate an* **orthopedic test** *known as the* **flexion-adduction-internal rotation (FADDIR) test** *for* **hip labral pathology**. *You have 2 minutes to complete this task.*

| Flexion-Adduction-Internal Rotation (FADDIR) Test | Course or Site Assessor Environment | | Test 1 | | Test 2 | | Test 3 | |
|---|---|---|---|---|---|---|---|---|
| | | | Y | N | Y | N | Y | N |
| Tester places patient and limb in appropriate position | | | Y | N | Y | N | Y | N |
| Supine | | | ○ | ○ | ○ | ○ | ○ | ○ |
| Tester placed in proper position | | | Y | N | Y | N | Y | N |
| Places one hand on lateral aspect of knee | | | ○ | ○ | ○ | ○ | ○ | ○ |
| Places other hand around the ipsilateral ankle | | | ○ | ○ | ○ | ○ | ○ | ○ |
| Tester performs test according to accepted guidelines | | | Y | N | Y | N | Y | N |
| Passively flexes the hip and knee to 90 degrees | | | ○ | ○ | ○ | ○ | ○ | ○ |
| Passively and sequentially adducts and internally rotates the hip joint to its end range | | | ○ | ○ | ○ | ○ | ○ | ○ |
| Identifies positive findings and implications | | | Y | N | Y | N | Y | N |
| Reproduction of the patient's groin pain | | | ○ | ○ | ○ | ○ | ○ | ○ |
| Hip labral pathology | | | ○ | ○ | ○ | ○ | ○ | ○ |
| Total | | | ___/7 | | ___/7 | | ___/7 | |
| Must achieve >4 to pass this examination | | | Ⓟ | Ⓕ | Ⓟ | Ⓕ | Ⓟ | Ⓕ |

| Assessor: Date: | Test 1 Comments: |
|---|---|
| Assessor: Date: | Test 2 Comments: |
| Assessor: Date: | Test 3 Comments: |

**TEST ENVIRONMENTS**
**L:** Laboratory/Classroom
**C:** Clinical/Field Testing
**P:** Practicum
**A:** Assessment/Mock Exam

**TEST INFORMATION**
**Test Statistics:** Sensitivity .84–.90
Specificity .54–.74
(+) LR .73–1.70
(-) LR .72–2.20
**Reference(s):** Reiman et al. (2015)
Starkey & Brown (2015)

## MUSCULOSKELETAL SYSTEM—REGION 4: HIP AND PELVIS
# SPECIAL TESTS

| NATA EC 5th | BOC RD6 | SKILL |
|---|---|---|
| CE-21g, CE-20e | D2-0203 | Flexion-Adduction-Internal Rotation (FAIR) Test |

**Supplies Needed:** Table

*This problem allows you the opportunity to demonstrate an* **orthopedic test** *known as the* **flexion-adduction-internal rotation (FAIR) test** *for* **piriformis syndrome**. *You have 2 minutes to complete this task.*

| Flexion-Adduction-Internal Rotation (FAIR) Test | Course or Site Assessor Environment | Test 1 | | Test 2 | | Test 3 | |
|---|---|---|---|---|---|---|---|
| **Tester places patient and limb in appropriate position** | | Y | N | Y | N | Y | N |
| Side lying on side opposite being tested | | O | O | O | O | O | O |
| **Tester placed in proper position** | | Y | N | Y | N | Y | N |
| Passively brings the lower extremity to be tested into the combined motions of 90 degrees of hip flexion, maximal adduction, and 90 degrees of knee flexion | | O | O | O | O | O | O |
| Ensures that the pelvis remains level | | O | O | O | O | O | O |
| **Tester performs test according to accepted guidelines** | | Y | N | Y | N | Y | N |
| Applies upward and lateral pressure to the shin of the lower extremity to be tested, passively internally rotating the thigh to 45 degrees | | O | O | O | O | O | O |
| **Identifies positive findings and implications** | | Y | N | Y | N | Y | N |
| Pain elicited at the intersection of the sciatic nerve and piriformis | | O | O | O | O | O | O |
| Impinging of the sciatic nerve at the piriformis | | O | O | O | O | O | O |
| Total | | __/6 | | __/6 | | __/6 | |
| **Must achieve >4 to pass this examination** | | P | F | P | F | P | F |
| Assessor: Date: | Test 1 Comments: | | | | | | |
| Assessor: Date: | Test 2 Comments: | | | | | | |
| Assessor: Date: | Test 3 Comments: | | | | | | |

**TEST ENVIRONMENTS**
**L:** Laboratory/Classroom
**C:** Clinical/Field Testing
**P:** Practicum
**A:** Assessment/Mock Exam

**TEST INFORMATION**
**Test Statistics:** No data available
**Reference(s):** Cook & Hegedus (2013)

## MUSCULOSKELETAL SYSTEM—REGION 4: HIP AND PELVIS
# SPECIAL TESTS

| NATA EC 5th | BOC RD6 | SKILL |
|---|---|---|
| CE-21g, CE-20e | D2-0203 | Gaenslen's Test |

**Supplies Needed:** Table

*This problem allows you the opportunity to demonstrate an* **orthopedic test** *known as* **Gaenslen's test** *for* **sacroiliac pain**. *You have 2 minutes to complete this task.*

| Gaenslen's Test | Course or Site<br>Assessor<br>Environment | | | | | |
|---|---|---|---|---|---|---|
| | Test 1 | | Test 2 | | Test 3 | |
| | Y | N | Y | N | Y | N |
| **Tester places patient and limb in appropriate position** | **Y** | **N** | **Y** | **N** | **Y** | **N** |
| Supine | ○ | ○ | ○ | ○ | ○ | ○ |
| Painful leg resting very near the end of the treatment table | ○ | ○ | ○ | ○ | ○ | ○ |
| **Tester placed in proper position** | **Y** | **N** | **Y** | **N** | **Y** | **N** |
| Stands next to the patient's feet | ○ | ○ | ○ | ○ | ○ | ○ |
| **Tester performs test according to accepted guidelines** | **Y** | **N** | **Y** | **N** | **Y** | **N** |
| Passively flexes the nonpainful side of the hip (with knee bent) up to 90 degrees | ○ | ○ | ○ | ○ | ○ | ○ |
| Applies a downward force to the painful side while a counterforce is applied to the nonpainful side toward flexion | ○ | ○ | ○ | ○ | ○ | ○ |
| **Identifies positive findings and implications** | **Y** | **N** | **Y** | **N** | **Y** | **N** |
| The torque reproduces pain | ○ | ○ | ○ | ○ | ○ | ○ |
| SI pain or dysfunction | ○ | ○ | ○ | ○ | ○ | ○ |
| Total | ___/7 | | ___/7 | | ___/7 | |
| **Must achieve >4 to pass this examination** | Ⓟ | Ⓕ | Ⓟ | Ⓕ | Ⓟ | Ⓕ |

| Assessor:<br>Date: | Test 1 Comments: |
|---|---|
| Assessor:<br>Date: | Test 2 Comments: |
| Assessor:<br>Date: | Test 3 Comments: |

**TEST ENVIRONMENTS**
**L:** Laboratory/Classroom
**C:** Clinical/Field Testing
**P:** Practicum
**A:** Assessment/Mock Exam

**TEST INFORMATION**
**Test Statistics:** Sensitivity .36–.71
Specificity .26–.80
(+) LR 1.02–2.29
(-) LR .65–1.11
**Reference(s):** Cook & Hegedus (2013)

# SPECIAL TESTS

| NATA EC 5th | BOC RD6 | SKILL |
|---|---|---|
| CE-21g, CE-20e | D2-0203 | Hip Scouring |

**Supplies Needed:** Table

*This problem allows you the opportunity to demonstrate an* **orthopedic test** *known as* **hip scouring** *to rule out a possible* **defect of the articular surface** *or* **labral tear**. *You have 2 minutes to complete this task.*

| Hip Scouring | Course or Site Assessor Environment | | | | | |
|---|---|---|---|---|---|---|
| | | Test 1 | | Test 2 | | Test 3 |
| **Tester places patient and limb in appropriate position** | | Y | N | Y | N | Y | N |
| Supine | | ○ | ○ | ○ | ○ | ○ | ○ |
| Knee flexed to 90 degrees | | ○ | ○ | ○ | ○ | ○ | ○ |
| Hip flexed to 90 degrees | | ○ | ○ | ○ | ○ | ○ | ○ |
| **Tester placed in proper position** | | Y | N | Y | N | Y | N |
| Stands lateral to the involved side | | ○ | ○ | ○ | ○ | ○ | ○ |
| Stabilizes the medial portion of the tibia with dominant hand | | ○ | ○ | ○ | ○ | ○ | ○ |
| Stabilizes the anterior portion of the ankle mortise with nondominant hand | | ○ | ○ | ○ | ○ | ○ | ○ |
| **Tester performs test according to accepted guidelines** | | Y | N | Y | N | Y | N |
| Applies pressure downward along the shaft of the femur to compress joint surfaces | | ○ | ○ | ○ | ○ | ○ | ○ |
| Internally and externally rotates the femur with multiple angles of hip flexion | | ○ | ○ | ○ | ○ | ○ | ○ |
| **Identifies positive findings and implications** | | Y | N | Y | N | Y | N |
| Pain experienced during internal and external maneuvers | | ○ | ○ | ○ | ○ | ○ | ○ |
| **Total** | | __/9 | | __/9 | | __/9 |
| **Must achieve >6 to pass this examination** | | Ⓟ | Ⓕ | Ⓟ | Ⓕ | Ⓟ | Ⓕ |

| Assessor: Date: | Test 1 Comments: |
|---|---|
| Assessor: Date: | Test 2 Comments: |
| Assessor: Date: | Test 3 Comments: |

**TEST ENVIRONMENTS**
**L:** Laboratory/Classroom
**C:** Clinical/Field Testing
**P:** Practicum
**A:** Assessment/Mock Exam

**TEST INFORMATION**
**Test Statistics:** No data available
**Reference(s):** Starkey & Brown (2015)

## MUSCULOSKELETAL SYSTEM—REGION 4: HIP AND PELVIS
# SPECIAL TESTS

| NATA EC 5th | BOC RD6 | SKILL |
|---|---|---|
| CE-21g, CE-20e | D2-0203 | Ober's Test |

**Supplies Needed:** Table

*This problem allows you the opportunity to demonstrate an* **orthopedic test** *known as* **Ober's test** *for* **iliotibial band tightness**. *You have 2 minutes to complete this task.*

| Ober's Test | Course or Site<br>Assessor<br>Environment | | | | | |
|---|---|---|---|---|---|---|
| | | Test 1 | | Test 2 | | Test 3 |
| **Tester places patient and limb in appropriate position** | | Y | N | Y | N | Y | N |
| Lying on the side opposite that being tested | | ○ | ○ | ○ | ○ | ○ | ○ |
| The opposite hip is flexed 45 degrees and the knee flexed to 90 degrees to stabilize the torso and pelvis | | ○ | ○ | ○ | ○ | ○ | ○ |
| **Tester placed in proper position** | | Y | N | Y | N | Y | N |
| Stands behind the patient | | ○ | ○ | ○ | ○ | ○ | ○ |
| Stabilizes the patient's pelvis with one hand | | ○ | ○ | ○ | ○ | ○ | ○ |
| Supports the leg being tested along the medial aspect of the distal tibia with the opposite hand | | ○ | ○ | ○ | ○ | ○ | ○ |
| **Tester performs test according to accepted guidelines** | | Y | N | Y | N | Y | N |
| Passively abducts and extends the patient's hip to allow the tensor fasciae latae to clear the greater trochanter | | ○ | ○ | ○ | ○ | ○ | ○ |
| **Identifies positive findings and implications** | | Y | N | Y | N | Y | N |
| Minimal tightness: The femur adducts to horizontal | | ○ | ○ | ○ | ○ | ○ | ○ |
| Significant tightness: The femur is unable to adduct to horizontal | | ○ | ○ | ○ | ○ | ○ | ○ |
| Total | | ___/8 | | ___/8 | | ___/8 | |
| Must achieve >5 to pass this examination | | ⓟ | Ⓕ | ⓟ | Ⓕ | ⓟ | Ⓕ |

| Assessor:<br>Date: | Test 1 Comments: |
|---|---|
| Assessor:<br>Date: | Test 2 Comments: |
| Assessor:<br>Date: | Test 3 Comments: |

**TEST ENVIRONMENTS**
**L:** Laboratory/Classroom
**C:** Clinical/Field Testing
**P:** Practicum
**A:** Assessment/Mock Exam

**TEST INFORMATION**
**Test Statistics:** No data available
**Reference(s):** Starkey & Brown (2015)

## MUSCULOSKELETAL SYSTEM—REGION 4: HIP AND PELVIS
# SPECIAL TESTS

| NATA EC 5th | BOC RD6 | SKILL |
|---|---|---|
| CE-21g, CE-20e | D2-0203 | Thomas Test |

**Supplies Needed:** Table

*This problem allows you the opportunity to demonstrate an* **orthopedic test** *known as the* **Thomas test** *for* **hip flexor tightness**. *You have 2 minutes to complete this task.*

| Thomas Test | Course or Site Assessor Environment | | Test 1 | | Test 2 | | Test 3 | |
|---|---|---|---|---|---|---|---|---|
| **Tester places patient and limb in appropriate position** | | Y | N | Y | N | Y | N | |
| Supine at the edge of table | | O | O | O | O | O | O | |
| **Tester placed in proper position** | | Y | N | Y | N | Y | N | |
| Stands at the side of the patient | | O | O | O | O | O | O | |
| **Tester performs test according to accepted guidelines** | | Y | N | Y | N | Y | N | |
| Instructs the patient to lie back and pull both knees to chest | | O | O | O | O | O | O | |
| Holds symptomatic knee to chest and the other is slowly lowered into extension of the hip | | O | O | O | O | O | O | |
| **Identifies positive findings and implications** | | Y | N | Y | N | Y | N | |
| Inability of involved hip to fall to neutral | | O | O | O | O | O | O | |
| Involved knee begins to extend | | O | O | O | O | O | O | |
| Hip involvement indicates psoas tightness; knee involvement indicates rectus femoris tightness | | O | O | O | O | O | O | |
| **Total** | | ___/7 | | ___/7 | | ___/7 | | |
| **Must achieve >4 to pass this examination** | | P | F | P | F | P | F | |

| Assessor:<br>Date: | Test 1 Comments: |
|---|---|
| Assessor:<br>Date: | Test 2 Comments: |
| Assessor:<br>Date: | Test 3 Comments: |

**TEST ENVIRONMENTS**
**L:** Laboratory/Classroom
**C:** Clinical/Field Testing
**P:** Practicum
**A:** Assessment/Mock Exam

**TEST INFORMATION**
**Test Statistics:** No data available
**Reference(s):** Cook & Hegedus (2013)

## MUSCULOSKELETAL SYSTEM—REGION 4: HIP AND PELVIS
# SPECIAL TESTS

| NATA EC 5th | BOC RD6 | SKILL |
|---|---|---|
| CE-21g, CE-20e | D2-0203 | Trendelenburg's Sign |

**Supplies Needed:** Table

*This problem allows you the opportunity to demonstrate an* **orthopedic test** *known as* **Trendelenburg's sign** *for* **gluteal medius weakness**. *You have 2 minutes to complete this task.*

| Trendelenburg's Sign | Course or Site Assessor Environment | | Test 1 | | Test 2 | | Test 3 | |
|---|---|---|---|---|---|---|---|---|
| **Tester places patient and limb in appropriate position** | | | Y | N | Y | N | Y | N |
| Stands in front of the tester | | | O | O | O | O | O | O |
| **Tester placed in proper position** | | | Y | N | Y | N | Y | N |
| Stands behind the patient | | | O | O | O | O | O | O |
| Instructs the patient to stand on one leg | | | O | O | O | O | O | O |
| **Tester performs test according to accepted guidelines** | | | Y | N | Y | N | Y | N |
| Evaluates the degree of drop of the contralateral pelvis once the leg is lifted | | | O | O | O | O | O | O |
| Confirmation of abnormal pelvic drop is required during gait | | | O | O | O | O | O | O |
| **Identifies positive findings and implications** | | | Y | N | Y | N | Y | N |
| Asymmetric drop of one hip compared to the other during single stance | | | O | O | O | O | O | O |
| **Total** | | | __/6 | | __/6 | | __/6 | |
| **Must achieve >4 to pass this examination** | | | Ⓟ | Ⓕ | Ⓟ | Ⓕ | Ⓟ | Ⓕ |

| Assessor: Date: | Test 1 Comments: |
|---|---|
| Assessor: Date: | Test 2 Comments: |
| Assessor: Date: | Test 3 Comments: |

**TEST ENVIRONMENTS**
**L:** Laboratory/Classroom
**C:** Clinical/Field Testing
**P:** Practicum
**A:** Assessment/Mock Exam

**TEST INFORMATION**
**Test Statistics:** Sensitivity .38–.73
Specificity .77
(+) LR 3.15
(-) LR .35
**Reference(s):** Cook & Hegedus (2013)

## MUSCULOSKELETAL SYSTEM—REGION 4: HIP AND PELVIS
# SPECIAL TESTS

| NATA EC 5th | BOC RD6 | SKILL |
|---|---|---|
| CE-21g, CE-20e | D2-0203 | Leg Length Assessment (True) |

**Supplies Needed:** Table, tape measure

*This problem allows you the opportunity to demonstrate an* **orthopedic assessment** *for* **leg length assessment (true)**. *You have 2 minutes to complete this task.*

| Leg Length Assessment (True) | Course or Site Assessor Environment | | | | | |
|---|---|---|---|---|---|---|
| | | Test 1 | | Test 2 | | Test 3 |
| **Tester places patient and limb in appropriate position** | | Y | N | Y | N | Y | N |
| Supine with trunk, pelvis, and legs in straight alignment | | O | O | O | O | O | O |
| Hips in neutral position and legs close together | | O | O | O | O | O | O |
| **Tester performs test according to accepted guidelines** | | Y | N | Y | N | Y | N |
| Measures from the ipsilateral ASIS to the medial malleolus | | O | O | O | O | O | O |
| Takes proper length measurement | | O | O | O | O | O | O |
| Performs assessment bilaterally | | O | O | O | O | O | O |
| **Identifies implications** | | Y | N | Y | N | Y | N |
| Identifies significant differences (10 to 20 mm) | | O | O | O | O | O | O |
| **Total** | | ___/6 | | ___/6 | | ___/6 |
| **Must achieve >4 to pass this examination** | | Ⓟ | Ⓕ | Ⓟ | Ⓕ | Ⓟ | Ⓕ |

| Assessor: Date: | Test 1 Comments: |
|---|---|
| Assessor: Date: | Test 2 Comments: |
| Assessor: Date: | Test 3 Comments: |

**TEST ENVIRONMENTS**
L: Laboratory/Classroom
C: Clinical/Field Testing
P: Practicum
A: Assessment/Mock Exam

**TEST INFORMATION**
**Test Statistics:** N/A
**Reference(s):** Kendall et al. (2005)

MUSCULOSKELETAL SYSTEM—REGION 4: HIP AND PELVIS
# SPECIAL TESTS

| NATA EC 5th | BOC RD6 | SKILL |
|---|---|---|
| CE-21g, CE-20e | D2-0203 | Leg Length Assessment (Apparent) |

**Supplies Needed:** Table, tape measure

*This problem allows you the opportunity to demonstrate an* **orthopedic assessment** *for* **leg length assessment (apparent)**. *You have 2 minutes to complete this task.*

| Leg Length Assessment (Apparent) | Course or Site Assessor Environment | | | | | |
|---|---|---|---|---|---|---|
| | | Test 1 | | Test 2 | | Test 3 | |
| **Tester places patient and limb in appropriate position** | | Y | N | Y | N | Y | N |
| Supine with trunk, pelvis, and legs in straight alignment | | O | O | O | O | O | O |
| Hips in neutral position and legs close together | | O | O | O | O | O | O |
| **Tester performs test according to accepted guidelines** | | Y | N | Y | N | Y | N |
| Measures from umbilicus to the medial malleolus | | O | O | O | O | O | O |
| Takes proper length measurement | | O | O | O | O | O | O |
| Performs assessment bilaterally | | O | O | O | O | O | O |
| **Identifies implications** | | Y | N | Y | N | Y | N |
| Identifies significant differences  (10 to 20 mm) | | O | O | O | O | O | O |
| Total | | ___/6 | | ___/6 | | ___/6 | |
| **Must achieve >4 to pass this examination** | | P | F | P | F | P | F |

| Assessor: Date: | Test 1 Comments: |
|---|---|
| Assessor: Date: | Test 2 Comments: |
| Assessor: Date: | Test 3 Comments: |

**TEST ENVIRONMENTS**
**L:** Laboratory/Classroom
**C:** Clinical/Field Testing
**P:** Practicum
**A:** Assessment/Mock Exam

**TEST INFORMATION**
**Test Statistics:** N/A
**Reference(s):**  Kendall et al. (2005)
                   Starkey & Brown (2015)

# MUSCULOSKELETAL SYSTEM—REGION 4: HIP AND PELVIS
## SPECIAL TESTS

| NATA EC 5th | BOC RD6 | SKILL |
|---|---|---|
| CE-21g, CE-20e | D2-0203 | Girth Measurement (Thigh) |

**Supplies Needed:** Table, tape measure

*This problem allows you the opportunity to demonstrate an* **orthopedic assessment** *for* **girth measurement (thigh)**. *You have 2 minutes to complete this task.*

| Girth Measurement (Thigh) | Course or Site / Assessor / Environment | | Test 1 | | Test 2 | | Test 3 |
|---|---|---|---|---|---|---|---|
| **Tester, patient, and limb placed in appropriate position** | | Y | N | Y | N | Y | N |
| The patient is supine or standing | | ○ | ○ | ○ | ○ | ○ | ○ |
| The tester stands lateral to the patient | | ○ | ○ | ○ | ○ | ○ | ○ |
| **Tester performs test according to accepted guidelines** | | Y | N | Y | N | Y | N |
| Joint line is identified and measured at the 0-cm mark | | ○ | ○ | ○ | ○ | ○ | ○ |
| Measurements are taken at 5-, 10-, and 15-cm intervals above the joint line | | ○ | ○ | ○ | ○ | ○ | ○ |
| Takes proper girth measurement | | ○ | ○ | ○ | ○ | ○ | ○ |
| Performs assessment bilaterally | | ○ | ○ | ○ | ○ | ○ | ○ |
| **Identifies implications** | | Y | N | Y | N | Y | N |
| Identifies significant differences (±1 cm) | | ○ | ○ | ○ | ○ | ○ | ○ |
| **Total** | | ___/7 | | ___/7 | | ___/7 | |
| **Must achieve >4 to pass this examination** | | Ⓟ | Ⓕ | Ⓟ | Ⓕ | Ⓟ | Ⓕ |

| Assessor: Date: | Test 1 Comments: |
|---|---|
| Assessor: Date: | Test 2 Comments: |
| Assessor: Date: | Test 3 Comments: |

**TEST ENVIRONMENTS**
**L:** Laboratory/Classroom
**C:** Clinical/Field Testing
**P:** Practicum
**A:** Assessment/Mock Exam

**TEST INFORMATION**
**Test Statistics:** N/A
**Reference(s):** Starkey & Brown (2015)

## MUSCULOSKELETAL SYSTEM—REGION 4: HIP AND PELVIS
# SPECIAL TESTS

| NATA EC 5th | BOC RD6 | SKILL |
|---|---|---|
| CE-21g, CE-20e | D2-0203 | Postural Measurement (Q-Angle) |

**Supplies Needed:** Table, goniometer

*This problem allows you the opportunity to demonstrate an* **orthopedic assessment** *for* **postural measurement (Q-angle)**. *You have 2 minutes to complete this task.*

| Postural Measurement (Q-Angle) | Course or Site Assessor Environment | | Test 1 | | Test 2 | | Test 3 | |
|---|---|---|---|---|---|---|---|---|
| **Tester, patient, and limb placed in appropriate position** | | | **Y** | **N** | **Y** | **N** | **Y** | **N** |
| The patient is supine with knee fully extended with toes pointing up, or standing | | | ○ | ○ | ○ | ○ | ○ | ○ |
| The tester stands lateral to the side being tested | | | ○ | ○ | ○ | ○ | ○ | ○ |
| **Tester performs test according to accepted guidelines** | | | **Y** | **N** | **Y** | **N** | **Y** | **N** |
| Identifies and marks the ASIS, the midpoint of the patella, and the tibial tuberosity | | | ○ | ○ | ○ | ○ | ○ | ○ |
| Places fulcrum over the patellar midpoint, fixed arm in line with ASIS, moving arm in line with tibial tuberosity | | | ○ | ○ | ○ | ○ | ○ | ○ |
| Takes proper measurement | | | ○ | ○ | ○ | ○ | ○ | ○ |
| Performs assessment bilaterally | | | ○ | ○ | ○ | ○ | ○ | ○ |
| **Identifies implications** | | | **Y** | **N** | **Y** | **N** | **Y** | **N** |
| Identifies significant ranges (>13 degrees in men, >18 degrees in women) | | | ○ | ○ | ○ | ○ | ○ | ○ |
| | | Total | ___/7 | | ___/7 | | ___/7 | |
| | | Must achieve >4 to pass this examination | Ⓟ | Ⓕ | Ⓟ | Ⓕ | Ⓟ | Ⓕ |

| Assessor: Date: | Test 1 Comments: |
|---|---|
| Assessor: Date: | Test 2 Comments: |
| Assessor: Date: | Test 3 Comments: |

**TEST ENVIRONMENTS**
**L:** Laboratory/Classroom
**C:** Clinical/Field Testing
**P:** Practicum
**A:** Assessment/Mock Exam

**TEST INFORMATION**
**Test Statistics:** N/A
**Reference(s):** Starkey & Brown (2015)

# 8

# Musculoskeletal System— Region 5: Lumbar and Thoracic Spine

Hauth, J. M., Gloyeske, B. M., & Amato, H. K.
*Clinical Skills Documentation Guide for Athletic Training, Third Edition* (pp. 191-241).
© 2016 SLACK Incorporated.

## MUSCULOSKELETAL SYSTEM—REGION 5: LUMBAR AND THORACIC SPINE
# KNOWLEDGE AND SKILLS

| Musculoskeletal System—Region 5: Lumbar and Thoracic Spine | | | | Skill: Acquisition, Reinforcement, Proficiency | | |
|---|---|---|---|---|---|---|
| **NATA EC 5th** | **BOC RD6** | **Palpation** | **Page #** | | | |
| CE-21b, CE-20c | D2-0202 | Palpation: Lumbar and Thoracic Spine – 01 | 194 | | | |
| CE-21b, CE-20c | D2-0202 | Palpation: Lumbar and Thoracic Spine – 02 | 195 | | | |
| CE-21b, CE-20c | D2-0202 | Palpation: Lumbar and Thoracic Spine – 03 | 196 | | | |
| **NATA EC 5th** | **BOC RD6** | **Manual Muscle Testing** | **Page #** | | | |
| CE-21c | D2-0203 | MMT: Left Trunk Lateral Flexion (Left Internal Oblique/Left External Oblique/Left Quadratus Lumborum) | 197 | | | |
| CE-21c | D2-0203 | MMT: Left Trunk Rotation (Right Internal Oblique/Left External Oblique) | 198 | | | |
| CE-21c | D2-0203 | MMT: Right Trunk Lateral Flexion (Right External Oblique/Right Internal Oblique/Quadratus Lumborum) | 199 | | | |
| CE-21c | D2-0203 | MMT: Trunk Extension (Paraspinals) | 200 | | | |
| CE-21c | D2-0203 | MMT: Trunk Flexion (Rectus Abdominis) | 201 | | | |
| CE-21c | D2-0203 | MMT: Right Trunk Rotation (Left Internal Oblique/Right External Oblique) | 202 | | | |
| **NATA EC 5th** | **BOC RD6** | **Osteokinematic Joint Motion** | **Page #** | | | |
| CE-21d | D2-0203 | Goniometric Assessment: Trunk (Extension) | 203 | | | |
| CE-21d | D2-0203 | Goniometric Assessment: Trunk (Flexion) | 204 | | | |
| CE-21d | D2-0203 | Goniometric Assessment: Trunk (Lateral Flexion Left) | 205 | | | |
| CE-21d | D2-0203 | Goniometric Assessment: Trunk (Lateral Flexion Right) | 206 | | | |
| CE-21d | D2-0203 | Goniometric Assessment: Trunk (Rotation Left) | 207 | | | |
| CE-21d | D2-0203 | Goniometric Assessment: Trunk (Rotation Right) | 208 | | | |
| **NATA EC 5th** | **BOC RD6** | **Joint Play (Arthrokinematics)** | **Page #** | | | |
| CE-21f | D2-0203 | Spring Test | 209 | | | |
| **NATA EC 5th** | **BOC RD6** | **Special Tests** | **Page #** | | | |
| CE-21g, CE-20e | D2-0203 | Adam's Side Bending Test | 210 | | | |
| CE-21g, CE-20e | D2-0203 | Beevor's Sign | 211 | | | |
| CE-21g, CE-20e | D2-0203 | Bowstring Test (Cram Test/Popliteal Pressure Sign) | 212 | | | |
| CE-21g, CE-20e | D2-0203 | Extension Quadrant Test | 213 | | | |
| CE-21g, CE-20e | D2-0203 | Femoral Nerve Traction Test | 214 | | | |
| CE-21g, CE-20e | D2-0203 | Flexion Quadrant Test | 215 | | | |
| CE-21g, CE-20e | D2-0203 | Hoover's Sign | 216 | | | |
| CE-21g, CE-20e | D2-0203 | Kernig/Brudzinski Sign | 217 | | | |
| CE-21g, CE-20e | D2-0203 | Milgram's Test | 218 | | | |
| CE-21g, CE-20e | D2-0203 | Slump Test | 219 | | | |
| CE-21g, CE-20e | D2-0203 | Stork Stance Test | 220 | | | |
| CE-21g, CE-20e | D2-0203 | Straight Leg Raise (Unilateral Straight Leg Raise/Lasegue Test) | 221 | | | |
| CE-21g, CE-20e | D2-0203 | Tension Sign | 222 | | | |
| CE-21g, CE-20e | D2-0203 | Valsalva Test | 223 | | | |
| CE-21g, CE-20e | D2-0203 | Well Straight Leg Raise Test | 224 | | | |

*(continued on the next page)*

**MUSCULOSKELETAL SYSTEM—REGION 5: LUMBAR AND THORACIC SPINE**
# KNOWLEDGE AND SKILLS

| NATA EC 5th | BOC RD6 | Dermatome Testing | Page # | | | |
|---|---|---|---|---|---|---|
| CE-21h, CE-20f | D2-0203 | Dermatome: L1 | 225 | | | |
| CE-21h, CE-20f | D2-0203 | Dermatome: L2 | 226 | | | |
| CE-21h, CE-20f | D2-0203 | Dermatome: L3 | 227 | | | |
| CE-21h, CE-20f | D2-0203 | Dermatome: L4 | 228 | | | |
| CE-21h, CE-20f | D2-0203 | Dermatome: L5 | 229 | | | |
| CE-21h, CE-20f | D2-0203 | Dermatome: S1 | 230 | | | |
| CE-21h, CE-20f | D2-0203 | Dermatome: S2 | 231 | | | |
| NATA EC 5th | BOC RD6 | Myotome Testing | Page # | | | |
| CE-21h, CE-20f | D2-0203 | Myotome: L1/L2 | 232 | | | |
| CE-21h, CE-20f | D2-0203 | Myotome: L3 | 233 | | | |
| CE-21h, CE-20f | D2-0203 | Myotome: L4 | 234 | | | |
| CE-21h, CE-20f | D2-0203 | Myotome: L5 | 235 | | | |
| CE-21h, CE-20f | D2-0203 | Myotome: S1 | 236 | | | |
| CE-21h, CE-20f | D2-0203 | Myotome: S2 | 237 | | | |
| NATA EC 5th | BOC RD6 | Reflex Testing | Page # | | | |
| CE-21h, CE-20f | D2-0203 | Reflex Testing: L2/L3/L4 | 238 | | | |
| CE-21h, CE-20f | D2-0203 | Reflex Testing: L5 | 239 | | | |
| CE-21h, CE-20f | D2-0203 | Reflex Testing: S1 | 240 | | | |
| CE-21h, CE-20f | D2-0203 | Reflex Testing: S2 | 241 | | | |

## MUSCULOSKELETAL SYSTEM—REGION 5: LUMBAR AND THORACIC SPINE
# PALPATION

| NATA EC 5th | BOC RD6 | SKILL |
|---|---|---|
| CE-21b, CE-20c | D2-0202 | Palpation: Lumbar and Thoracic Spine – 01 |

**Supplies Needed:** Table

*This problem allows you the opportunity to demonstrate your ability to **palpate** the **lumbar and thoracic spine**. You have 2 minutes to complete this task.*

| Palpation: Lumbar and Thoracic Spine – 01 | Course or Site Assessor Environment _____ _____ _____ | Test 1 | | Test 2 | | Test 3 | |
|---|---|---|---|---|---|---|---|
| | | Y | N | Y | N | Y | N |
| Ribs 11-12 | | O | O | O | O | O | O |
| Quadratus lumborum muscle | | O | O | O | O | O | O |
| Spinous processes of L4-L5 | | O | O | O | O | O | O |
| Paraspinal muscles | | O | O | O | O | O | O |
| Thoracolumbar fascia | | O | O | O | O | O | O |
| Transverse processes of T1-T4 | | O | O | O | O | O | O |
| Supraspinous ligament | | O | O | O | O | O | O |
| Total | | ____/7 | | ____/7 | | ____/7 | |
| Must achieve >4 to pass this examination | | P | F | P | F | P | F |
| Assessor: Date: | Test 1 Comments: | | | | | | |
| Assessor: Date: | Test 2 Comments: | | | | | | |
| Assessor: Date: | Test 3 Comments: | | | | | | |

**TEST ENVIRONMENTS**
**L:** Laboratory/Classroom
**C:** Clinical/Field Testing
**P:** Practicum
**A:** Assessment/Mock Exam

**TEST INFORMATION**
**Test Statistics:** N/A
**Reference(s):** Starkey & Brown (2015)

## MUSCULOSKELETAL SYSTEM—REGION 5: LUMBAR AND THORACIC SPINE
# PALPATION

| NATA EC 5th | BOC RD6 | SKILL |
|---|---|---|
| CE-21b, CE-20c | D2-0202 | Palpation: Lumbar and Thoracic Spine – 02 |

**Supplies Needed:** Table

*This problem allows you the opportunity to demonstrate your ability to* **palpate** *the* **lumbar and thoracic spine**. *You have 2 minutes to complete this task.*

| Palpation: Lumbar and Thoracic Spine – 02 | Course or Site Assessor Environment | | Test 1 | | Test 2 | | Test 3 |
|---|---|---|---|---|---|---|---|
| | | Y | N | Y | N | Y | N |
| Supraspinous ligament | | ○ | ○ | ○ | ○ | ○ | ○ |
| Ribs 5-8 | | ○ | ○ | ○ | ○ | ○ | ○ |
| Spinous processes of T1-4 | | ○ | ○ | ○ | ○ | ○ | ○ |
| Paraspinal muscles | | ○ | ○ | ○ | ○ | ○ | ○ |
| Thoracolumbar fascia | | ○ | ○ | ○ | ○ | ○ | ○ |
| Costovertebral junction | | ○ | ○ | ○ | ○ | ○ | ○ |
| Transverse processes of L4-S1 | | ○ | ○ | ○ | ○ | ○ | ○ |
| **Total** | | __/7 | | __/7 | | __/7 | |
| **Must achieve >4 to pass this examination** | | Ⓟ | Ⓕ | Ⓟ | Ⓕ | Ⓟ | Ⓕ |

| Assessor: Date: | Test 1 Comments: |
|---|---|
| Assessor: Date: | Test 2 Comments: |
| Assessor: Date: | Test 3 Comments: |

**TEST ENVIRONMENTS**
**L:** Laboratory/Classroom
**C:** Clinical/Field Testing
**P:** Practicum
**A:** Assessment/Mock Exam

**TEST INFORMATION**
**Test Statistics:** N/A
**Reference(s):** Starkey & Brown (2015)

## MUSCULOSKELETAL SYSTEM—REGION 5: LUMBAR AND THORACIC SPINE
# PALPATION

| NATA EC 5th | BOC RD6 | SKILL |
|---|---|---|
| CE-21b, CE-20c | D2-0202 | Palpation: Lumbar and Thoracic Spine – 03 |

**Supplies Needed:** Table

*This problem allows you the opportunity to demonstrate your ability to* **palpate** *the* **lumbar and thoracic spine**. *You have 2 minutes to complete this task.*

| Palpation: Lumbar and Thoracic Spine – 03 | Course or Site / Assessor / Environment | Test 1 | | Test 2 | | Test 3 | |
|---|---|---|---|---|---|---|---|
| | | Y | N | Y | N | Y | N |
| Supraspinous ligament | | ○ | ○ | ○ | ○ | ○ | ○ |
| Ribs 8-10 | | ○ | ○ | ○ | ○ | ○ | ○ |
| Spinous processes of L1-L3 | | ○ | ○ | ○ | ○ | ○ | ○ |
| Paraspinal muscles | | ○ | ○ | ○ | ○ | ○ | ○ |
| Thoracolumbar fascia | | ○ | ○ | ○ | ○ | ○ | ○ |
| Interspinalis muscle | | ○ | ○ | ○ | ○ | ○ | ○ |
| Transverse processes of T5-T9 | | ○ | ○ | ○ | ○ | ○ | ○ |
| Total | | ___/7 | | ___/7 | | ___/7 | |
| Must achieve >4 to pass this examination | | Ⓟ | Ⓕ | Ⓟ | Ⓕ | Ⓟ | Ⓕ |

Assessor: Date: — Test 1 Comments:

Assessor: Date: — Test 2 Comments:

Assessor: Date: — Test 3 Comments:

**TEST ENVIRONMENTS**
L: Laboratory/Classroom
C: Clinical/Field Testing
P: Practicum
A: Assessment/Mock Exam

**TEST INFORMATION**
**Test Statistics:** N/A
**Reference(s):** Starkey & Brown (2015)

## MUSCULOSKELETAL SYSTEM—REGION 5: LUMBAR AND THORACIC SPINE
# MANUAL MUSCLE TESTING

| NATA EC 5th | BOC RD6 | SKILL |
|---|---|---|
| CE-21c | D2-0203 | MMT: Left Trunk Lateral Flexion (Left Internal Oblique/Left External Oblique/ Left Quadratus Lumborum) |

**Supplies Needed:** Table, pillow

*This problem allows you the opportunity to demonstrate a* **manual muscle test** *for* **left trunk lateral flexion.** *You have 2 minutes to complete this task.*

| MMT: Left Trunk Lateral Flexion (Left Internal Oblique/Left External Oblique/Left Quadratus Lumborum) | Course or Site Assessor Environment | Test 1 | | Test 2 | | Test 3 | |
|---|---|---|---|---|---|---|---|
| **Tester places patient and limbs in appropriate position** | | **Y** | **N** | **Y** | **N** | **Y** | **N** |
| Side lying on right hip with a pillow between thighs | | ○ | ○ | ○ | ○ | ○ | ○ |
| Pelvis and spine in neutral position, legs straight | | ○ | ○ | ○ | ○ | ○ | ○ |
| **Tester placed in proper position** | | **Y** | **N** | **Y** | **N** | **Y** | **N** |
| Fixes pelvis to thigh but allows pelvis to tilt downward | | ○ | ○ | ○ | ○ | ○ | ○ |
| **Tester performs test according to accepted guidelines** | | **Y** | **N** | **Y** | **N** | **Y** | **N** |
| Instructs the patient to raise trunk directly sideways | | ○ | ○ | ○ | ○ | ○ | ○ |
| Ensures no trunk rotation occurs | | ○ | ○ | ○ | ○ | ○ | ○ |
| Resistance is held for 5 seconds | | ○ | ○ | ○ | ○ | ○ | ○ |
| Performs assessment bilaterally | | ○ | ○ | ○ | ○ | ○ | ○ |
| **Identifies implications** | | **Y** | **N** | **Y** | **N** | **Y** | **N** |
| Correctly grades the MMT | | ○ | ○ | ○ | ○ | ○ | ○ |
| | Total | __/8 | | __/8 | | __/8 | |
| | Must achieve >5 to pass this examination | Ⓟ | Ⓕ | Ⓟ | Ⓕ | Ⓟ | Ⓕ |

| Assessor: Date: | Test 1 Comments: |
|---|---|
| Assessor: Date: | Test 2 Comments: |
| Assessor: Date: | Test 3 Comments: |

**TEST ENVIRONMENTS**
**L:** Laboratory/Classroom
**C:** Clinical/Field Testing
**P:** Practicum
**A:** Assessment/Mock Exam

**TEST INFORMATION**
**Test Statistics:** N/A
**Reference(s):** Kendall et al. (2005)

MUSCULOSKELETAL SYSTEM—REGION 5: LUMBAR AND THORACIC SPINE
# MANUAL MUSCLE TESTING

| NATA EC 5th | BOC RD6 | SKILL |
|---|---|---|
| CE-21c | D2-0203 | MMT: Left Trunk Rotation (Right Internal Oblique/Left External Oblique) |

**Supplies Needed:** Table

*This problem allows you the opportunity to demonstrate a* **manual muscle test** *for* **left trunk rotation**. *You have 2 minutes to complete this task.*

| MMT: Left Trunk Rotation (Right Internal Oblique/ Left External Oblique) | Course or Site Assessor Environment | | Test 1 | | Test 2 | | Test 3 | |
|---|---|---|---|---|---|---|---|---|
| Tester places patient and limbs in appropriate position | | Y | N | Y | N | Y | N | |
| Supine with hands clasped behind head | | ○ | ○ | ○ | ○ | ○ | ○ | |
| Tester placed in proper position | | Y | N | Y | N | Y | N | |
| Stands lateral at the patient's waist level | | ○ | ○ | ○ | ○ | ○ | ○ | |
| Tester performs test according to accepted guidelines | | Y | N | Y | N | Y | N | |
| Instructs the patient to bring right elbow to left knee | | ○ | ○ | ○ | ○ | ○ | ○ | |
| Observes motion to ensure scapular clearance | | ○ | ○ | ○ | ○ | ○ | ○ | |
| Performs assessment bilaterally | | ○ | ○ | ○ | ○ | ○ | ○ | |
| Identifies implications | | Y | N | Y | N | Y | N | |
| Correctly grades the MMT | | ○ | ○ | ○ | ○ | ○ | ○ | |
| Total | | ___/6 | | ___/6 | | ___/6 | | |
| Must achieve >4 to pass this examination | | Ⓟ | Ⓕ | Ⓟ | Ⓕ | Ⓟ | Ⓕ | |

| Assessor: Date: | Test 1 Comments: |
|---|---|
| Assessor: Date: | Test 2 Comments: |
| Assessor: Date: | Test 3 Comments: |

**TEST ENVIRONMENTS**
**L:** Laboratory/Classroom
**C:** Clinical/Field Testing
**P:** Practicum
**A:** Assessment/Mock Exam

**TEST INFORMATION**
**Test Statistics:** N/A
**Reference(s):**   Hislop & Montgomery (2007)

# MANUAL MUSCLE TESTING

| NATA EC 5th | BOC RD6 | SKILL |
|---|---|---|
| CE-21c | D2-0203 | MMT: Right Trunk Lateral Flexion (Right External Oblique/Right Internal Oblique/ Quadratus Lumborum) |

**Supplies Needed:** Table, pillow

*This problem allows you the opportunity to demonstrate a* **manual muscle test** *for* **right trunk lateral flexion***. You have 2 minutes to complete this task.*

| MMT: Right Trunk Lateral Flexion (Right External Oblique/Right Internal Oblique/Quadratus Lumborum) | Course or Site Assessor Environment | | Test 1 | | Test 2 | | Test 3 |
|---|---|---|---|---|---|---|---|
| **Tester places patient and limbs in appropriate position** | | Y | N | Y | N | Y | N |
| Side lying on left hip with a pillow between thighs | | O | O | O | O | O | O |
| Pelvis and spine in neutral position, legs straight | | O | O | O | O | O | O |
| **Tester placed in proper position** | | Y | N | Y | N | Y | N |
| Fixes pelvis to thigh but allows pelvis to tilt downward | | O | O | O | O | O | O |
| **Tester performs test according to accepted guidelines** | | Y | N | Y | N | Y | N |
| Instructs the patient to raise trunk directly sideways | | O | O | O | O | O | O |
| Ensures no trunk rotation occurs | | O | O | O | O | O | O |
| Resistance is held for 5 seconds | | O | O | O | O | O | O |
| Performs assessment bilaterally | | O | O | O | O | O | O |
| **Identifies implications** | | Y | N | Y | N | Y | N |
| Correctly grades the MMT | | O | O | O | O | O | O |
| Total | | /8 | | /8 | | /8 | |
| Must achieve >5 to pass this examination | | P | F | P | F | P | F |

| Assessor: Date: | Test 1 Comments: |
|---|---|
| Assessor: Date: | Test 2 Comments: |
| Assessor: Date: | Test 3 Comments: |

**TEST ENVIRONMENTS**
**L:** Laboratory/Classroom
**C:** Clinical/Field Testing
**P:** Practicum
**A:** Assessment/Mock Exam

**TEST INFORMATION**
**Test Statistics:** N/A
**Reference(s):** Kendall et al. (2005)

# MANUAL MUSCLE TESTING

| NATA EC 5th | BOC RD6 | SKILL |
|---|---|---|
| CE-21c | D2-0203 | MMT: Trunk Extension (Paraspinals) |

**Supplies Needed:** Table

*This problem allows you the opportunity to demonstrate a* **manual muscle test** *for* **trunk extension (paraspinals)**. *You have 2 minutes to complete this task.*

| MMT: Trunk Extension (Paraspinals) | Course or Site Assessor Environment | | Test 1 | | Test 2 | | Test 3 | |
|---|---|---|---|---|---|---|---|---|
| | | | Y | N | Y | N | Y | N |
| **Tester places patient and limbs in appropriate position** | | | Y | N | Y | N | Y | N |
| Prone with hands clasped behind head | | | O | O | O | O | O | O |
| **Tester placed in proper position** | | | Y | N | Y | N | Y | N |
| Stands next to the patient's lower extremities | | | O | O | O | O | O | O |
| **Tester performs test according to accepted guidelines** | | | Y | N | Y | N | Y | N |
| Instructs the patient to extend trunk to full range of motion | | | O | O | O | O | O | O |
| Holds lower extremity to stabilize through the motion | | | O | O | O | O | O | O |
| Resistance is held for 5 seconds | | | O | O | O | O | O | O |
| Performs assessment bilaterally | | | O | O | O | O | O | O |
| **Identifies implications** | | | Y | N | Y | N | Y | N |
| Correctly grades the MMT | | | O | O | O | O | O | O |
| **Total** | | | __/7 | | __/7 | | __/7 | |
| **Must achieve >4 to pass this examination** | | | Ⓟ | Ⓕ | Ⓟ | Ⓕ | Ⓟ | Ⓕ |

| Assessor:<br>Date: | Test 1 Comments: |
|---|---|
| Assessor:<br>Date: | Test 2 Comments: |
| Assessor:<br>Date: | Test 3 Comments: |

**TEST ENVIRONMENTS**
**L:** Laboratory/Classroom
**C:** Clinical/Field Testing
**P:** Practicum
**A:** Assessment/Mock Exam

**TEST INFORMATION**
**Test Statistics:** N/A
**Reference(s):** Kendall et al. (2005)

MUSCULOSKELETAL SYSTEM—REGION 5: LUMBAR AND THORACIC SPINE
# MANUAL MUSCLE TESTING

| NATA EC 5th | BOC RD6 | SKILL |
|---|---|---|
| CE-21c | D2-0203 | MMT: Trunk Flexion (Rectus Abdominis) |

**Supplies Needed:** Table

*This problem allows you the opportunity to demonstrate a* **manual muscle test** *for* **trunk flexion (rectus abdominis)**. *You have 2 minutes to complete this task.*

| MMT: Trunk Flexion (Rectus Abdominis) | Course or Site Assessor Environment | | Test 1 | | Test 2 | | Test 3 | |
|---|---|---|---|---|---|---|---|---|
| | | Y | N | Y | N | Y | N | |
| **Tester places patient and limbs in appropriate position** | | Y | N | Y | N | Y | N |
| Supine with arms crossed behind head | | O | O | O | O | O | O |
| **Tester placed in proper position** | | Y | N | Y | N | Y | N |
| Stands lateral to the patient | | O | O | O | O | O | O |
| **Tester performs test according to accepted guidelines** | | Y | N | Y | N | Y | N |
| Instructs the patient to curl up, bringing head, shoulders, and arms off the table | | O | O | O | O | O | O |
| Stabilizes the pelvis through the motion | | O | O | O | O | O | O |
| Resistance is held for 5 seconds | | O | O | O | O | O | O |
| **Identifies implications** | | Y | N | Y | N | Y | N |
| Correctly grades the MMT | | O | O | O | O | O | O |
| Total | | __/6 | | __/6 | | __/6 | |
| Must achieve >4 to pass this examination | | Ⓟ | Ⓕ | Ⓟ | Ⓕ | Ⓟ | Ⓕ |

| Assessor: Date: | Test 1 Comments: |
|---|---|
| Assessor: Date: | Test 2 Comments: |
| Assessor: Date: | Test 3 Comments: |

**TEST ENVIRONMENTS**
**L:** Laboratory/Classroom
**C:** Clinical/Field Testing
**P:** Practicum
**A:** Assessment/Mock Exam

**TEST INFORMATION**
**Test Statistics:** N/A
**Reference(s):** Hislop & Montgomery (2007)

## MUSCULOSKELETAL SYSTEM—REGION 5: LUMBAR AND THORACIC SPINE
# MANUAL MUSCLE TESTING

| NATA EC 5th | BOC RD6 | SKILL |
|---|---|---|
| CE-21c | D2-0203 | MMT: Right Trunk Rotation (Left Internal Oblique/Right External Oblique) |

**Supplies Needed:** Table

*This problem allows you the opportunity to demonstrate a* **manual muscle test** *for* **right trunk rotation**. *You have 2 minutes to complete this task.*

| MMT: Right Trunk Rotation (Left Internal Oblique/ Right External Oblique) | Course or Site Assessor Environment | | Test 1 | | Test 2 | | Test 3 | |
|---|---|---|---|---|---|---|---|---|
| **Tester places patient and limbs in appropriate position** | | | Y | N | Y | N | Y | N |
| Supine with hands clasped behind head | | | ○ | ○ | ○ | ○ | ○ | ○ |
| **Tester placed in proper position** | | | Y | N | Y | N | Y | N |
| Stands lateral at the patient's waist level | | | ○ | ○ | ○ | ○ | ○ | ○ |
| **Tester performs test according to accepted guidelines** | | | Y | N | Y | N | Y | N |
| Instructs the patient to bring left elbow to right knee | | | ○ | ○ | ○ | ○ | ○ | ○ |
| Observes motion to ensure scapular clearance | | | ○ | ○ | ○ | ○ | ○ | ○ |
| Performs assessment bilaterally | | | ○ | ○ | ○ | ○ | ○ | ○ |
| **Identifies implications** | | | Y | N | Y | N | Y | N |
| Correctly grades the MMT | | | ○ | ○ | ○ | ○ | ○ | ○ |
| Total | | | __/6 | | __/6 | | __/6 | |
| Must achieve >4 to pass this examination | | | Ⓟ | Ⓕ | Ⓟ | Ⓕ | Ⓟ | Ⓕ |
| **Assessor:** **Date:** | Test 1 Comments: | | | | | | | |
| **Assessor:** **Date:** | Test 2 Comments: | | | | | | | |
| **Assessor:** **Date:** | Test 3 Comments: | | | | | | | |

**TEST ENVIRONMENTS**
**L:** Laboratory/Classroom
**C:** Clinical/Field Testing
**P:** Practicum
**A:** Assessment/Mock Exam

**TEST INFORMATION**
**Test Statistics:** N/A
**Reference(s):** Hislop & Montgomery (2007)

## MUSCULOSKELETAL SYSTEM—REGION 5: LUMBAR AND THORACIC SPINE
# OSTEOKINEMATIC JOINT MOTION

| NATA EC 5th | BOC RD6 | SKILL |
|:---:|:---:|:---:|
| CE-21d | D2-0203 | Goniometric Assessment: Trunk (Extension) |

**Supplies Needed:** Table, two inclinometers

*This problem allows you the opportunity to demonstrate a* **goniometric assessment** *for the* **trunk (extension)**. *You have 2 minutes to complete this task.*

| Goniometric Assessment: Trunk (Extension) | Course or Site Assessor Environment | | | | | |
|---|---|---|---|---|---|---|
| | Test 1 | | Test 2 | | Test 3 | |
| **Tester places patient in appropriate position** | Y | N | Y | N | Y | N |
| Stands with feet shoulder width apart | O | O | O | O | O | O |
| Cervical, thoracic, and lumbar spine in neutral position | O | O | O | O | O | O |
| **Tester and goniometer placed in proper position** | Y | N | Y | N | Y | N |
| Stands behind the patient | O | O | O | O | O | O |
| T12 and S1 vertebrae are marked in the correct location | O | O | O | O | O | O |
| One inclinometer is placed over T12 and one is placed over S1 | O | O | O | O | O | O |
| Both inclinometers are zeroed prior to measuring | O | O | O | O | O | O |
| **Tester performs test according to accepted guidelines** | Y | N | Y | N | Y | N |
| Instructs the patient to extend the spine as far as possible, keeping trunk erect and feet flat on the floor | O | O | O | O | O | O |
| Stops the motion when the patient's pelvis begins to tilt posteriorly | O | O | O | O | O | O |
| Takes proper goniometric measurement | O | O | O | O | O | O |
| **Identifies implications** | Y | N | Y | N | Y | N |
| Identifies normal ranges (trunk extension = 25 degrees) | O | O | O | O | O | O |
| **Total** | ___/10 | | ___/10 | | ___/10 | |
| **Must achieve >6 to pass this examination** | Ⓟ | Ⓕ | Ⓟ | Ⓕ | Ⓟ | Ⓕ |

| Assessor: Date: | Test 1 Comments: |
|---|---|
| Assessor: Date: | Test 2 Comments: |
| Assessor: Date: | Test 3 Comments: |

**TEST ENVIRONMENTS**
**L:** Laboratory/Classroom
**C:** Clinical/Field Testing
**P:** Practicum
**A:** Assessment/Mock Exam

**TEST INFORMATION**
**Test Statistics:** N/A
**Reference(s):** Norkin & White (2009)

## MUSCULOSKELETAL SYSTEM—REGION 5: LUMBAR AND THORACIC SPINE
# OSTEOKINEMATIC JOINT MOTION

| NATA EC 5th | BOC RD6 | SKILL |
|---|---|---|
| CE-21d | D2-0203 | Goniometric Assessment: Trunk (Flexion) |

**Supplies Needed:** Table, two inclinometers

*This problem allows you the opportunity to demonstrate a* **goniometric assessment** *for the* **trunk (flexion)**.
*You have 2 minutes to complete this task.*

| Goniometric Assessment: Trunk (Flexion) | Course or Site Assessor Environment | | | | | |
|---|---|---|---|---|---|---|
| | | Test 1 | | Test 2 | | Test 3 |
| **Tester places patient in appropriate position** | | **Y** | **N** | **Y** | **N** | **Y** | **N** |
| Stands with feet shoulder width apart | | O | O | O | O | O | O |
| Cervical, thoracic, and lumbar spine in neutral position | | O | O | O | O | O | O |
| **Tester and goniometer placed in proper position** | | **Y** | **N** | **Y** | **N** | **Y** | **N** |
| Stands behind the patient | | O | O | O | O | O | O |
| T12 and S1 vertebrae are marked in the correct location | | O | O | O | O | O | O |
| One inclinometer is placed over T12 and one is placed over S1 | | O | O | O | O | O | O |
| Both inclinometers are zeroed prior to measuring | | O | O | O | O | O | O |
| **Tester performs test according to accepted guidelines** | | **Y** | **N** | **Y** | **N** | **Y** | **N** |
| Instructs the patient to bend forward as far as possible, keeping arms relaxed | | O | O | O | O | O | O |
| Stops the motion when the patient's pelvis begins to tilt anteriorly | | O | O | O | O | O | O |
| Takes proper goniometric measurement by subtracting the degrees on the S1 inclinometer from the T12 inclinometer | | O | O | O | O | O | O |
| **Identifies implications** | | **Y** | **N** | **Y** | **N** | **Y** | **N** |
| Identifies normal ranges (trunk flexion = 60 degrees) | | O | O | O | O | O | O |
| | **Total** | __/10 | | __/10 | | __/10 | |
| | **Must achieve >6 to pass this examination** | Ⓟ | Ⓕ | Ⓟ | Ⓕ | Ⓟ | Ⓕ |

| Assessor: Date: | Test 1 Comments: |
|---|---|
| Assessor: Date: | Test 2 Comments: |
| Assessor: Date: | Test 3 Comments: |

**TEST ENVIRONMENTS**
**L:** Laboratory/Classroom
**C:** Clinical/Field Testing
**P:** Practicum
**A:** Assessment/Mock Exam

**TEST INFORMATION**
**Test Statistics:** N/A
**Reference(s):** Norkin & White (2009)

## MUSCULOSKELETAL SYSTEM—REGION 5: LUMBAR AND THORACIC SPINE
# OSTEOKINEMATIC JOINT MOTION

| NATA EC 5th | BOC RD6 | SKILL |
|---|---|---|
| CE-21d | D2-0203 | Goniometric Assessment: Trunk (Lateral Flexion Left) |

**Supplies Needed:** Table, two inclinometers

*This problem allows you the opportunity to demonstrate a* **goniometric assessment** *for the* **trunk (lateral flexion left)***. You have 2 minutes to complete this task.*

| Goniometric Assessment: Trunk (Lateral Flexion Left) | Course or Site / Assessor / Environment | | | | | |
|---|---|---|---|---|---|---|
| | | Test 1 | | Test 2 | | Test 3 |
| **Tester places patient in appropriate position** | | Y | N | Y | N | Y | N |
| Seated with feet on the floor | | O | O | O | O | O | O |
| Cervical, thoracic, and lumbar spine in neutral position | | O | O | O | O | O | O |
| **Tester and goniometer placed in proper position** | | Y | N | Y | N | Y | N |
| Stands behind the patient | | O | O | O | O | O | O |
| T12 and S1 vertebrae are marked in the correct location | | O | O | O | O | O | O |
| One inclinometer is placed over T12 and one is placed over S1 | | O | O | O | O | O | O |
| Both inclinometers are zeroed prior to measuring | | O | O | O | O | O | O |
| **Tester performs test according to accepted guidelines** | | Y | N | Y | N | Y | N |
| Instructs the patient to bend laterally to the left, while keeping both feet flat on the ground and knees straight | | O | O | O | O | O | O |
| Stops the motion when the patient's pelvis begins to tilt anteriorly | | O | O | O | O | O | O |
| Takes proper goniometric measurement by subtracting the degrees on the S1 inclinometer from the T12 inclinometer | | O | O | O | O | O | O |
| **Identifies implications** | | Y | N | Y | N | Y | N |
| Identifies normal ranges (trunk lateral flexion left = 25 degrees) | | O | O | O | O | O | O |
| **Total** | | ___/10 | | ___/10 | | ___/10 | |
| **Must achieve >6 to pass this examination** | | Ⓟ | Ⓕ | Ⓟ | Ⓕ | Ⓟ | Ⓕ |

| Assessor: Date: | Test 1 Comments: |
|---|---|
| Assessor: Date: | Test 2 Comments: |
| Assessor: Date: | Test 3 Comments: |

**TEST ENVIRONMENTS**
**L:** Laboratory/Classroom
**C:** Clinical/Field Testing
**P:** Practicum
**A:** Assessment/Mock Exam

**TEST INFORMATION**
**Test Statistics:** N/A
**Reference(s):** Norkin & White (2009)

MUSCULOSKELETAL SYSTEM—REGION 5: LUMBAR AND THORACIC SPINE
# OSTEOKINEMATIC JOINT MOTION

| NATA EC 5th | BOC RD6 | SKILL |
|---|---|---|
| CE-21d | D2-0203 | Goniometric Assessment: Trunk (Lateral Flexion Right) |

**Supplies Needed:** Table, two inclinometers

*This problem allows you the opportunity to demonstrate a* **goniometric assessment** *for the* **trunk (lateral flexion right)**. *You have 2 minutes to complete this task.*

| Goniometric Assessment: Trunk (Lateral Flexion Right) | Course or Site _____ _____ _____ Assessor _____ _____ _____ Environment _____ _____ _____ | | | | | |
|---|---|---|---|---|---|---|
| | | Test 1 | | Test 2 | | Test 3 | |
| **Tester places patient in appropriate position** | | Y | N | Y | N | Y | N |
| Seated with feet on the floor | | O | O | O | O | O | O |
| Cervical, thoracic, and lumbar spine in neutral position | | O | O | O | O | O | O |
| **Tester and goniometer placed in proper position** | | Y | N | Y | N | Y | N |
| Stands behind the patient | | O | O | O | O | O | O |
| T12 and S1 vertebrae are marked in the correct location | | O | O | O | O | O | O |
| One inclinometer is placed over T12 and one is placed over S1 | | O | O | O | O | O | O |
| Both inclinometers are zeroed prior to measuring | | O | O | O | O | O | O |
| **Tester performs test according to accepted guidelines** | | Y | N | Y | N | Y | N |
| Instructs the patient to bend laterally to the right, while keeping both feet flat on the ground and knees straight | | O | O | O | O | O | O |
| Stops the motion when the patient's pelvis begins to tilt anteriorly | | O | O | O | O | O | O |
| Takes proper goniometric measurement by subtracting the degrees on the S1 inclinometer from the T12 inclinometer | | O | O | O | O | O | O |
| **Identifies implications** | | Y | N | Y | N | Y | N |
| Identifies normal ranges (trunk lateral flexion right = 25 degrees) | | O | O | O | O | O | O |
| Total | | ___/10 | | ___/10 | | ___/10 | |
| Must achieve >6 to pass this examination | | Ⓟ | Ⓕ | Ⓟ | Ⓕ | Ⓟ | Ⓕ |

| Assessor: Date: | Test 1 Comments: |
|---|---|
| Assessor: Date: | Test 2 Comments: |
| Assessor: Date: | Test 3 Comments: |

**TEST ENVIRONMENTS**
**L:** Laboratory/Classroom
**C:** Clinical/Field Testing
**P:** Practicum
**A:** Assessment/Mock Exam

**TEST INFORMATION**
**Test Statistics:** N/A
**Reference(s):** Norkin & White (2009)

**MUSCULOSKELETAL SYSTEM—REGION 5: LUMBAR AND THORACIC SPINE**
# OSTEOKINEMATIC JOINT MOTION

| NATA EC 5th | BOC RD6 | SKILL |
|---|---|---|
| CE-21d | D2-0203 | Goniometric Assessment: Trunk (Rotation Left) |

**Supplies Needed:** Table, large goniometer

*This problem allows you the opportunity to demonstrate a* **goniometric assessment** *for the* **trunk (rotation left)**. *You have 2 minutes to complete this task.*

| Goniometric Assessment: Trunk (Rotation Left) | Course or Site Assessor Environment | | | | | |
|---|---|---|---|---|---|---|
| | | Test 1 | | Test 2 | | Test 3 |
| **Tester places patient in appropriate position** | | **Y** | **N** | **Y** | **N** | **Y** | **N** |
| Seated with feet on the floor | | O | O | O | O | O | O |
| Cervical, thoracic, and lumbar spine in neutral position | | O | O | O | O | O | O |
| **Tester and goniometer placed in proper position** | | **Y** | **N** | **Y** | **N** | **Y** | **N** |
| Stands behind the patient | | O | O | O | O | O | O |
| Places fulcrum over the center of the cranial aspect of the patient's head | | O | O | O | O | O | O |
| Fixed arm is lined up parallel with an imaginary line between the iliac crests | | O | O | O | O | O | O |
| Distal arm is lined up parallel with the two acromion processes | | O | O | O | O | O | O |
| **Tester performs test according to accepted guidelines** | | **Y** | **N** | **Y** | **N** | **Y** | **N** |
| Instructs the patient to turn to the left as far as possible, keeping trunk erect and feet flat on the floor | | O | O | O | O | O | O |
| Stops the motion when the patient's pelvis starts to rotate | | O | O | O | O | O | O |
| Takes proper goniometric measurement | | O | O | O | O | O | O |
| Performs assessment bilaterally | | O | O | O | O | O | O |
| **Identifies implications** | | **Y** | **N** | **Y** | **N** | **Y** | **N** |
| Identifies normal ranges (trunk rotation = 45 degrees) | | O | O | O | O | O | O |
| **Total** | | __/11 | | __/11 | | __/11 |
| **Must achieve >7 to pass this examination** | | Ⓟ | Ⓕ | Ⓟ | Ⓕ | Ⓟ | Ⓕ |

| Assessor: Date: | Test 1 Comments: |
|---|---|
| Assessor: Date: | Test 2 Comments: |
| Assessor: Date: | Test 3 Comments: |

**TEST ENVIRONMENTS**
**L:** Laboratory/Classroom
**C:** Clinical/Field Testing
**P:** Practicum
**A:** Assessment/Mock Exam

**TEST INFORMATION**
**Test Statistics:** N/A
**Reference(s):** Norkin & White (2009)

# MUSCULOSKELETAL SYSTEM—REGION 5: LUMBAR AND THORACIC SPINE
## OSTEOKINEMATIC JOINT MOTION

| NATA EC 5th | BOC RD6 | SKILL |
|---|---|---|
| CE-21d | D2-0203 | Goniometric Assessment: Trunk (Rotation Right) |

**Supplies Needed:** Table, large goniometer

*This problem allows you the opportunity to demonstrate a* **goniometric assessment** *for the* **trunk (rotation right)**. *You have 2 minutes to complete this task.*

| Goniometric Assessment: Trunk (Rotation Right) | Course or Site<br>Assessor<br>Environment | | | | | |
|---|---|---|---|---|---|---|
| | Test 1 | | Test 2 | | Test 3 | |
| **Tester places patient in appropriate position** | **Y** | **N** | **Y** | **N** | **Y** | **N** |
| Seated with feet on the floor | O | O | O | O | O | O |
| Cervical, thoracic, and lumbar spine in neutral position | O | O | O | O | O | O |
| **Tester and goniometer placed in proper position** | **Y** | **N** | **Y** | **N** | **Y** | **N** |
| Stands behind the patient | O | O | O | O | O | O |
| Places fulcrum over the center of the cranial aspect of the patient's head | O | O | O | O | O | O |
| Fixed arm is lined up parallel with an imaginary line between the iliac crests | O | O | O | O | O | O |
| Distal arm is lined up parallel with the two acromion processes | O | O | O | O | O | O |
| **Tester performs test according to accepted guidelines** | **Y** | **N** | **Y** | **N** | **Y** | **N** |
| Instructs the patient to turn to the right as far as possible, keeping trunk erect and feet flat on the floor | O | O | O | O | O | O |
| Stops the motion when the patient's pelvis starts to rotate | O | O | O | O | O | O |
| Takes proper goniometric measurement | O | O | O | O | O | O |
| Performs assessment bilaterally | O | O | O | O | O | O |
| **Identifies implications** | **Y** | **N** | **Y** | **N** | **Y** | **N** |
| Identifies normal ranges (trunk rotation = 45 degrees) | O | O | O | O | O | O |
| **Total** | __/11 | | __/11 | | __/11 | |
| **Must achieve >7 to pass this examination** | Ⓟ | Ⓕ | Ⓟ | Ⓕ | Ⓟ | Ⓕ |

| Assessor:<br>Date: | **Test 1 Comments:** |
|---|---|
| Assessor:<br>Date: | **Test 2 Comments:** |
| Assessor:<br>Date: | **Test 3 Comments:** |

**TEST ENVIRONMENTS**
**L:** Laboratory/Classroom
**C:** Clinical/Field Testing
**P:** Practicum
**A:** Assessment/Mock Exam

**TEST INFORMATION**
**Test Statistics:** N/A
**Reference(s):** Norkin & White (2009)

## MUSCULOSKELETAL SYSTEM—REGION 5: LUMBAR AND THORACIC SPINE
# JOINT PLAY (ARTHROKINEMATICS)

| NATA EC 5th | BOC RD6 | SKILL |
|---|---|---|
| CE-21f | D2-0203 | Spring Test |

**Supplies Needed:** Table

*This problem allows you the opportunity to demonstrate an* **orthopedic test** *known as the* **spring test** *to rule out* **facet joint mobility***. You have 2 minutes to complete this task.*

| Spring Test | Course or Site Assessor Environment | | Test 1 | | Test 2 | | Test 3 | |
|---|---|---|---|---|---|---|---|---|
| | | | Y | N | Y | N | Y | N |
| **Tester places patient and limb in appropriate position** | | | Y | N | Y | N | Y | N |
| Prone | | | ○ | ○ | ○ | ○ | ○ | ○ |
| **Tester placed in proper position** | | | Y | N | Y | N | Y | N |
| Stands over the patient with thumbs placed over the spinous process to be tested | | | ○ | ○ | ○ | ○ | ○ | ○ |
| **Tester performs test according to accepted guidelines** | | | Y | N | Y | N | Y | N |
| Carefully pushes the spinous process anteriorly, feeling for the springing of the vertebrae | | | ○ | ○ | ○ | ○ | ○ | ○ |
| **Identifies positive findings and implications** | | | Y | N | Y | N | Y | N |
| Vertebrae does not "spring" or move | | | ○ | ○ | ○ | ○ | ○ | ○ |
| Total | | | ___/4 | | ___/4 | | ___/4 | |
| **Must achieve >2 to pass this examination** | | | Ⓟ | Ⓕ | Ⓟ | Ⓕ | Ⓟ | Ⓕ |

| Assessor: Date: | Test 1 Comments: |
|---|---|
| Assessor: Date: | Test 2 Comments: |
| Assessor: Date: | Test 3 Comments: |

**TEST ENVIRONMENTS**
**L:** Laboratory/Classroom
**C:** Clinical/Field Testing
**P:** Practicum
**A:** Assessment/Mock Exam

**TEST INFORMATION**
**Test Statistics:** No data available
**Reference(s):** Starkey & Brown (2015)

## MUSCULOSKELETAL SYSTEM—REGION 5: LUMBAR AND THORACIC SPINE
# SPECIAL TESTS

| NATA EC 5th | BOC RD6 | SKILL |
|---|---|---|
| CE-21g, CE-20e | D2-0203 | Adam's Side Bending Test |

**Supplies Needed:** Table

*This problem allows you the opportunity to demonstrate an* **orthopedic test** *known as* **Adam's side bending test** *to rule out* **scoliosis***. You have 2 minutes to complete this task.*

| Adam's Side Bending Test | Course or Site Assessor Environment | | Test 1 | | Test 2 | | Test 3 | |
|---|---|---|---|---|---|---|---|---|
| **Tester places patient and limb in appropriate position** | | | Y | N | Y | N | Y | N |
| Stands | | | ○ | ○ | ○ | ○ | ○ | ○ |
| **Tester placed in proper position** | | | Y | N | Y | N | Y | N |
| Behind the patient | | | ○ | ○ | ○ | ○ | ○ | ○ |
| **Tester performs test according to accepted guidelines** | | | Y | N | Y | N | Y | N |
| The patient bends forward, sliding the hands down the front of each leg | | | ○ | ○ | ○ | ○ | ○ | ○ |
| **Identifies positive findings and implications** | | | Y | N | Y | N | Y | N |
| An asymmetrical hump is observed along the lateral aspect of the thoracolumbar spine and rib cage | | | ○ | ○ | ○ | ○ | ○ | ○ |
| | Total | | ___/4 | | ___/4 | | ___/4 | |
| | **Must achieve >2 to pass this examination** | | Ⓟ | Ⓕ | Ⓟ | Ⓕ | Ⓟ | Ⓕ |
| **Assessor:** **Date:** | Test 1 Comments: | | | | | | | |
| **Assessor:** **Date:** | Test 2 Comments: | | | | | | | |
| **Assessor:** **Date:** | Test 3 Comments: | | | | | | | |

**TEST ENVIRONMENTS**
**L:** Laboratory/Classroom
**C:** Clinical/Field Testing
**P:** Practicum
**A:** Assessment/Mock Exam

**TEST INFORMATION**
**Test Statistics**: No data available
**Reference(s):**    Starkey & Brown (2015)

## MUSCULOSKELETAL SYSTEM—REGION 5: LUMBAR AND THORACIC SPINE
# SPECIAL TESTS

| NATA EC 5th | BOC RD6 | SKILL |
|---|---|---|
| CE-21g, CE-20e | D2-0203 | Beevor's Sign |

**Supplies Needed:** Table

*This problem allows you the opportunity to demonstrate an* **orthopedic test** *known as* **Beevor's sign** *to rule out* **thoracic nerve inhibition**. *You have 2 minutes to complete this task.*

| Beevor's Sign | Course or Site / Assessor / Environment | | Test 1 | | Test 2 | | Test 3 | |
|---|---|---|---|---|---|---|---|---|
| **Tester places patient and limb in appropriate position** | | | Y | N | Y | N | Y | N |
| Hook lying | | | O | O | O | O | O | O |
| **Tester placed in proper position** | | | Y | N | Y | N | Y | N |
| At the side of the patient | | | O | O | O | O | O | O |
| **Tester performs test according to accepted guidelines** | | | Y | N | Y | N | Y | N |
| The patient performs an abdominal curl (partial sit-up) | | | O | O | O | O | O | O |
| **Identifies positive findings and implications** | | | Y | N | Y | N | Y | N |
| The umbilicus moves up, down, or to one side | | | O | O | O | O | O | O |
| | | Total | ___/4 | | ___/4 | | ___/4 | |
| | **Must achieve >2 to pass this examination** | | P | F | P | F | P | F |

| Assessor: Date: | **Test 1 Comments:** |
|---|---|
| Assessor: Date: | **Test 2 Comments:** |
| Assessor: Date: | **Test 3 Comments:** |

**TEST ENVIRONMENTS**
**L:** Laboratory/Classroom
**C:** Clinical/Field Testing
**P:** Practicum
**A:** Assessment/Mock Exam

**TEST INFORMATION**
**Test Statistics:** No data available
**Reference(s):** Starkey & Brown (2015)

## MUSCULOSKELETAL SYSTEM—REGION 5: LUMBAR AND THORACIC SPINE
# SPECIAL TESTS

| NATA EC 5th | BOC RD6 | SKILL |
|---|---|---|
| CE-21g, CE-20e | D2-0203 | Bowstring Test<br>(Cram Test/Popliteal Pressure Sign) |

**Supplies Needed:** Table

*This problem allows you the opportunity to demonstrate an* **orthopedic test** *known as the* **Bowstring test (cram test/popliteal pressure sign)** *to rule out* **sciatic nerve irritation***. You have 2 minutes to complete this task.*

| Bowstring Test (Cram Test/Popliteal Pressure Sign) | Course or Site Assessor Environment | | Test 1 | | Test 2 | | Test 3 |
|---|---|---|---|---|---|---|---|
| | | **Y** | **N** | **Y** | **N** | **Y** | **N** |
| **Tester places patient and limb in appropriate position** | | **Y** | **N** | **Y** | **N** | **Y** | **N** |
| Supine | | O | O | O | O | O | O |
| Hip flexed to 90 degrees | | O | O | O | O | O | O |
| Knee flexed to 90 degrees | | O | O | O | O | O | O |
| **Tester placed in proper position** | | **Y** | **N** | **Y** | **N** | **Y** | **N** |
| Stands to the side of the patient (may kneel on the table) | | O | O | O | O | O | O |
| Grasps posterior ankle at level of medial malleoli | | O | O | O | O | O | O |
| Places thumb at central popliteal fossa | | O | O | O | O | O | O |
| **Tester performs test according to accepted guidelines** | | **Y** | **N** | **Y** | **N** | **Y** | **N** |
| Performs passive knee extension until symptoms occur | | O | O | O | O | O | O |
| Slightly flexes knee until symptoms subside | | O | O | O | O | O | O |
| Applies force into popliteal space | | O | O | O | O | O | O |
| **Identifies positive findings and implications** | | **Y** | **N** | **Y** | **N** | **Y** | **N** |
| Pain reoccurs when thumb pressure is applied to popliteal space | | O | O | O | O | O | O |
| **Total** | | | /10 | | /10 | | /10 |
| **Must achieve >6 to pass this examination** | | Ⓟ | Ⓕ | Ⓟ | Ⓕ | Ⓟ | Ⓕ |

| Assessor:<br>Date: | Test 1 Comments: |
|---|---|
| Assessor:<br>Date: | Test 2 Comments: |
| Assessor:<br>Date: | Test 3 Comments: |

**TEST ENVIRONMENTS**
**L:** Laboratory/Classroom
**C:** Clinical/Field Testing
**P:** Practicum
**A:** Assessment/Mock Exam

**TEST INFORMATION**
**Test Statistics:** No data available
**Reference(s):** Konin et al. (2016)
Starkey & Brown (2015)

**MUSCULOSKELETAL SYSTEM—REGION 5: LUMBAR AND THORACIC SPINE**
# SPECIAL TESTS

| NATA EC 5th | BOC RD6 | SKILL |
|---|---|---|
| CE-21g, CE-20e | D2-0203 | Extension Quadrant Test |

**Supplies Needed:** Table

*This problem allows you the opportunity to demonstrate an* **orthopedic test** *known as the* **extension quadrant test** *to rule out a possible* **facet joint pathology**. *You have 2 minutes to complete this task.*

| Extension Quadrant Test | Course or Site Assessor Environment | | | | | |
|---|---|---|---|---|---|---|
| | | Test 1 | | Test 2 | | Test 3 |
| | | Y | N | Y | N | Y | N |
| **Tester places patient and limb in appropriate position** | | Y | N | Y | N | Y | N |
| Stands | | O | O | O | O | O | O |
| **Tester placed in proper position** | | Y | N | Y | N | Y | N |
| Stands behind the patient, grasping the patient's shoulders | | O | O | O | O | O | O |
| **Tester performs test according to accepted guidelines** | | Y | N | Y | N | Y | N |
| The patient extends spine as far as possible, then side bends and rotates to the involved side | | O | O | O | O | O | O |
| Examiner provides overpressure through the shoulders, supporting the patient as needed | | O | O | O | O | O | O |
| **Identifies positive findings and implications** | | Y | N | Y | N | Y | N |
| Reproduction of pain | | O | O | O | O | O | O |
| Total | | __/5 | | __/5 | | __/5 | |
| Must achieve >3 to pass this examination | | P | F | P | F | P | F |

| Assessor:<br>Date: | Test 1 Comments: |
|---|---|
| Assessor:<br>Date: | Test 2 Comments: |
| Assessor:<br>Date: | Test 3 Comments: |

**TEST ENVIRONMENTS**
**L:** Laboratory/Classroom
**C:** Clinical/Field Testing
**P:** Practicum
**A:** Assessment/Mock Exam

**TEST INFORMATION**
**Test Statistics:** Sensitivity .70
**Reference(s):** Cook & Hegedus (2013)
Starkey & Brown (2015)

## MUSCULOSKELETAL SYSTEM—REGION 5: LUMBAR AND THORACIC SPINE
## SPECIAL TESTS

| NATA EC 5th | BOC RD6 | SKILL |
|---|---|---|
| CE-21g, CE-20e | D2-0203 | Femoral Nerve Traction Test |

**Supplies Needed:** Table, pillow or small bolster

*This problem allows you the opportunity to demonstrate an* **orthopedic test** *known as the* **femoral nerve traction test** *for* **nerve root impingement (L2, L3, or L4)**. *You have 2 minutes to complete this task.*

| Femoral Nerve Traction Test | Course or Site / Assessor / Environment | Test 1 | | Test 2 | | Test 3 | |
|---|---|---|---|---|---|---|---|
| **Tester places patient and limb in appropriate position** | | Y | N | Y | N | Y | N |
| Prone with pillow under the abdomen | | ○ | ○ | ○ | ○ | ○ | ○ |
| **Tester placed in proper position** | | Y | N | Y | N | Y | N |
| Stands on the side not being tested | | ○ | ○ | ○ | ○ | ○ | ○ |
| Places caudal hand on the lateral aspect of the knee being tested | | ○ | ○ | ○ | ○ | ○ | ○ |
| Places cephalic hand on ipsilateral PSIS (to stabilize) | | ○ | ○ | ○ | ○ | ○ | ○ |
| **Tester performs test according to accepted guidelines** | | Y | N | Y | N | Y | N |
| Passively flexes the knee to 90 degrees | | ○ | ○ | ○ | ○ | ○ | ○ |
| Passively extends the hip to end range with caudal hand while stabilizing the PSIS with the cephalic hand | | ○ | ○ | ○ | ○ | ○ | ○ |
| **Identifies positive findings and implications** | | Y | N | Y | N | Y | N |
| Pain is elicited in the anterior and lateral thigh | | ○ | ○ | ○ | ○ | ○ | ○ |
| Nerve root impingement at the L2, L3, or L4 level | | ○ | ○ | ○ | ○ | ○ | ○ |
| **Total** | | __/8 | | __/8 | | __/8 | |
| **Must achieve >5 to pass this examination** | | Ⓟ | Ⓕ | Ⓟ | Ⓕ | Ⓟ | Ⓕ |

| Assessor: Date: | Test 1 Comments: |
|---|---|
| Assessor: Date: | Test 2 Comments: |
| Assessor: Date: | Test 3 Comments: |

**TEST ENVIRONMENTS**
**L:** Laboratory/Classroom
**C:** Clinical/Field Testing
**P:** Practicum
**A:** Assessment/Mock Exam

**TEST INFORMATION**
**Test Statistics:** Sensitivity .84
**Reference(s):** Cook & Hegedus (2013)
Starkey & Brown (2015)

## MUSCULOSKELETAL SYSTEM—REGION 5: LUMBAR AND THORACIC SPINE
# SPECIAL TESTS

| NATA EC 5th | BOC RD6 | SKILL |
|---|---|---|
| CE-21g, CE-20e | D2-0203 | Flexion Quadrant Test |

**Supplies Needed:** N/A

*This problem allows you the opportunity to demonstrate an* **orthopedic test** *known as the* **flexion quadrant test** *to identify* **lumbar flexion dysfunction**. *You have 2 minutes to complete this task.*

| Flexion Quadrant Test | Course or Site Assessor Environment | | Test 1 | | Test 2 | | Test 3 | |
|---|---|---|---|---|---|---|---|---|
| **Tester places patient and limb in appropriate position** | | Y | N | Y | N | Y | N |
| Stands | | ○ | ○ | ○ | ○ | ○ | ○ |
| **Tester placed in proper position** | | Y | N | Y | N | Y | N |
| Stands facing the patient | | ○ | ○ | ○ | ○ | ○ | ○ |
| **Tester performs test according to accepted guidelines** | | Y | N | Y | N | Y | N |
| The patient is instructed to reach forward and touch one foot with both hands, repeated on the opposite side | | ○ | ○ | ○ | ○ | ○ | ○ |
| **Identifies positive findings and implications** | | Y | N | Y | N | Y | N |
| Reproduction of pain | | ○ | ○ | ○ | ○ | ○ | ○ |
| Total | | ___/4 | | ___/4 | | ___/4 | |
| Must achieve >2 to pass this examination | | Ⓟ | Ⓕ | Ⓟ | Ⓕ | Ⓟ | Ⓕ |

| Assessor: Date: | Test 1 Comments: |
|---|---|
| Assessor: Date: | Test 2 Comments: |
| Assessor: Date: | Test 3 Comments: |

**TEST ENVIRONMENTS**
**L:** Laboratory/Classroom
**C:** Clinical/Field Testing
**P:** Practicum
**A:** Assessment/Mock Exam

**TEST INFORMATION**
**Test Statistics:** No data available
**Reference(s):** Cook & Hegedus (2013)

## MUSCULOSKELETAL SYSTEM—REGION 5: LUMBAR AND THORACIC SPINE
# SPECIAL TESTS

| NATA EC 5th | BOC RD6 | SKILL |
|---|---|---|
| CE-21g, CE-20e | D2-0203 | Hoover's Sign |

**Supplies Needed:** Table, bolster

*This problem allows you the opportunity to demonstrate an* **orthopedic test** *known as* **Hoover's sign** *to rule out* **malingering***. You have 2 minutes to complete this task.*

| Hoover's Sign | Course or Site Assessor Environment | Test 1 | | Test 2 | | Test 3 | |
|---|---|---|---|---|---|---|---|
| | | Y | N | Y | N | Y | N |
| **Tester places patient and limb in appropriate position** | | Y | N | Y | N | Y | N |
| Supine with the knee extended | | ○ | ○ | ○ | ○ | ○ | ○ |
| **Tester placed in proper position** | | Y | N | Y | N | Y | N |
| Stands at the feet of the patient | | ○ | ○ | ○ | ○ | ○ | ○ |
| Cups the heel of the patient | | ○ | ○ | ○ | ○ | ○ | ○ |
| **Tester performs test according to accepted guidelines** | | Y | N | Y | N | Y | N |
| Instructs the patient to lift the leg of the involved side | | ○ | ○ | ○ | ○ | ○ | ○ |
| **Identifies positive findings and implications** | | Y | N | Y | N | Y | N |
| The patient makes no attempt to lift the involved leg | | ○ | ○ | ○ | ○ | ○ | ○ |
| The tester does not sense any pressure in hand | | ○ | ○ | ○ | ○ | ○ | ○ |
| Total | | ___/6 | | ___/6 | | ___/6 | |
| Must achieve >4 to pass this examination | | Ⓟ | Ⓕ | Ⓟ | Ⓕ | Ⓟ | Ⓕ |
| Assessor: Date: | Test 1 Comments: | | | | | | |
| Assessor: Date: | Test 2 Comments: | | | | | | |
| Assessor: Date: | Test 3 Comments: | | | | | | |

**TEST ENVIRONMENTS**
**L:** Laboratory/Classroom
**C:** Clinical/Field Testing
**P:** Practicum
**A:** Assessment/Mock Exam

**TEST INFORMATION**
**Test Statistics:** No data available
**Reference(s):** Prentice (2014)

## MUSCULOSKELETAL SYSTEM—REGION 5: LUMBAR AND THORACIC SPINE
# SPECIAL TESTS

| NATA EC 5th | BOC RD6 | SKILL |
|---|---|---|
| CE-21g, CE-20e | D2-0203 | Kernig/Brudzinski Sign |

**Supplies Needed:** Table

*This problem allows you the opportunity to demonstrate an* **orthopedic test** *known as the* **Kernig/Brudzinski sign** *for* **nerve root impingement**. *You have 2 minutes to complete this task.*

| Kernig/Brudzinski Sign | Course or Site<br>Assessor<br>Environment | | Test 1 | | Test 2 | | Test 3 |
|---|---|---|---|---|---|---|---|
| **Tester places patient and limb in appropriate position** | | Y | N | Y | N | Y | N |
| Supine | | ○ | ○ | ○ | ○ | ○ | ○ |
| **Tester placed in proper position** | | Y | N | Y | N | Y | N |
| Stands lateral to the side being tested | | ○ | ○ | ○ | ○ | ○ | ○ |
| **Tester performs test according to accepted guidelines** | | Y | N | Y | N | Y | N |
| The patient performs a unilateral active straight leg raise with the knee extended until pain occurs | | ○ | ○ | ○ | ○ | ○ | ○ |
| After pain occurs, the patient flexes the knee | | ○ | ○ | ○ | ○ | ○ | ○ |
| **Identifies positive findings and implications** | | Y | N | Y | N | Y | N |
| Pain experienced in the spine and radiating into lower extremity | | ○ | ○ | ○ | ○ | ○ | ○ |
| Pain is relieved when the patient flexes the knee | | ○ | ○ | ○ | ○ | ○ | ○ |
| Total | | \_\_\_/6 | | \_\_\_/6 | | \_\_\_/6 | |
| **Must achieve >4 to pass this examination** | | Ⓟ | Ⓕ | Ⓟ | Ⓕ | Ⓟ | Ⓕ |
| Assessor:<br>Date: | Test 1 Comments: | | | | | | |
| Assessor:<br>Date: | Test 2 Comments: | | | | | | |
| Assessor:<br>Date: | Test 3 Comments: | | | | | | |

**TEST ENVIRONMENTS**
L: Laboratory/Classroom
C: Clinical/Field Testing
P: Practicum
A: Assessment/Mock Exam

**TEST INFORMATION**
**Test Statistics:** No data available
**Reference(s):** Starkey & Brown (2015)

## MUSCULOSKELETAL SYSTEM—REGION 5: LUMBAR AND THORACIC SPINE
## SPECIAL TESTS

| NATA EC 5th | BOC RD6 | SKILL |
|---|---|---|
| CE-21g, CE-20e | D2-0203 | Milgram's Test |

**Supplies Needed:** Table

*This problem allows you the opportunity to demonstrate an* **orthopedic test** *known as* **Milgram's test** *for a* **herniated disc**. *You have 2 minutes to complete this task.*

| Milgram's Test | Course or Site<br>Assessor<br>Environment | | | | | |
|---|---|---|---|---|---|---|
| | | \_\_\_\_ | | \_\_\_\_ | | \_\_\_\_ |
| | | \_\_\_\_ | | \_\_\_\_ | | \_\_\_\_ |
| | | **Test 1** | | **Test 2** | | **Test 3** |
| **Tester places patient and limb in appropriate position** | | Y | N | Y | N | Y | N |
| Supine on the table | | ○ | ○ | ○ | ○ | ○ | ○ |
| **Tester placed in proper position** | | Y | N | Y | N | Y | N |
| Stands at the feet of the patient | | ○ | ○ | ○ | ○ | ○ | ○ |
| **Tester performs test according to accepted guidelines** | | Y | N | Y | N | Y | N |
| The patient performs a bilateral straight leg raise to the height of 2 to 6 inches and is asked to hold the position for 30 seconds | | ○ | ○ | ○ | ○ | ○ | ○ |
| **Identifies positive findings and implications** | | Y | N | Y | N | Y | N |
| The patient is unable to hold the position or lift leg | | ○ | ○ | ○ | ○ | ○ | ○ |
| | **Total** | \_\_\_\_/4 | | \_\_\_\_/4 | | \_\_\_\_/4 |
| | **Must achieve >2 to pass this examination** | Ⓟ | Ⓕ | Ⓟ | Ⓕ | Ⓟ | Ⓕ |
| **Assessor:**<br>**Date:** | **Test 1 Comments:** | | | | | |
| **Assessor:**<br>**Date:** | **Test 2 Comments:** | | | | | |
| **Assessor:**<br>**Date:** | **Test 3 Comments:** | | | | | |

**TEST ENVIRONMENTS**
**L:** Laboratory/Classroom
**C:** Clinical/Field Testing
**P:** Practicum
**A:** Assessment/Mock Exam

**TEST INFORMATION**
**Test Statistics:** No data available
**Reference(s):** Starkey & Brown (2015)

## MUSCULOSKELETAL SYSTEM—REGION 5: LUMBAR AND THORACIC SPINE
# SPECIAL TESTS

| NATA EC 5th | BOC RD6 | SKILL |
|---|---|---|
| CE-21g, CE-20e | D2-0203 | Slump Test |

**Supplies Needed:** Table

*This problem allows you the opportunity to demonstrate an* **orthopedic test** *known as the* **slump test** *for* **dural lining impingement***. You have 2 minutes to complete this task.*

| Slump Test | Course or Site Assessor Environment | | | | | |
|---|---|---|---|---|---|---|
| | | Test 1 | | Test 2 | | Test 3 |
| **Tester places patient and limb in appropriate position** | | Y | N | Y | N | Y | N |
| Seated | | ○ | ○ | ○ | ○ | ○ | ○ |
| **Tester placed in proper position** | | Y | N | Y | N | Y | N |
| Stands at the side of the patient | | ○ | ○ | ○ | ○ | ○ | ○ |
| **Tester performs test according to accepted guidelines** | | Y | N | Y | N | Y | N |
| The patient slumps forward along the thoracolumbar spine, rounding shoulders while keeping the cervical spine in neutral, overpressure is applied | | ○ | ○ | ○ | ○ | ○ | ○ |
| The patient flexes the cervical spine by bringing the chin to chest; clinician holds the patient in this position | | ○ | ○ | ○ | ○ | ○ | ○ |
| Knee is actively extended | | ○ | ○ | ○ | ○ | ○ | ○ |
| The ankle is dorsiflexed | | ○ | ○ | ○ | ○ | ○ | ○ |
| Repeat all steps on opposite side | | ○ | ○ | ○ | ○ | ○ | ○ |
| **Identifies positive findings and implications** | | Y | N | Y | N | Y | N |
| Sciatic pain | | ○ | ○ | ○ | ○ | ○ | ○ |
| Reproduction of other neurologic issues | | ○ | ○ | ○ | ○ | ○ | ○ |
| | Total | __/9 | | __/9 | | __/9 |
| | Must achieve >6 to pass this examination | Ⓟ | Ⓕ | Ⓟ | Ⓕ | Ⓟ | Ⓕ |

| Assessor: Date: | Test 1 Comments: |
|---|---|
| Assessor: Date: | Test 2 Comments: |
| Assessor: Date: | Test 3 Comments: |

**TEST ENVIRONMENTS**
**L:** Laboratory/Classroom
**C:** Clinical/Field Testing
**P:** Practicum
**A:** Assessment/Mock Exam

**TEST INFORMATION**
**Test Statistics:** Sensitivity .41–.84
Specificity .55–.83
(+) LR 1.82–4.94
(-) LR .19–.32
**Reference(s):** Cook & Hegedus (2013)
Starkey & Brown (2015)

## MUSCULOSKELETAL SYSTEM—REGION 5: LUMBAR AND THORACIC SPINE
# SPECIAL TESTS

| NATA EC 5th | BOC RD6 | SKILL |
|---|---|---|
| CE-21g, CE-20e | D2-0203 | Stork Stance Test |

**Supplies Needed:** Table

*This problem allows you the opportunity to demonstrate an* **orthopedic test** *known as the* **stork stance test** *for* **radiographic instability** *of the spine. You have 2 minutes to complete this task.*

| Stork Stance Test | Course or Site Assessor Environment | | Test 1 | | Test 2 | | Test 3 | |
|---|---|---|---|---|---|---|---|---|
| **Tester places patient and limb in appropriate position** | | | Y | N | Y | N | Y | N |
| Stands with hands on hips | | | ◯ | ◯ | ◯ | ◯ | ◯ | ◯ |
| **Tester placed in proper position** | | | Y | N | Y | N | Y | N |
| Stands behind the patient ready to provide support if the patient becomes unstable | | | ◯ | ◯ | ◯ | ◯ | ◯ | ◯ |
| **Tester performs test according to accepted guidelines** | | | Y | N | Y | N | Y | N |
| Instructs the patient to extend backward | | | ◯ | ◯ | ◯ | ◯ | ◯ | ◯ |
| **Identifies positive findings and implications** | | | Y | N | Y | N | Y | N |
| Pain during extension | | | ◯ | ◯ | ◯ | ◯ | ◯ | ◯ |
| | | Total | ___/4 | | ___/4 | | ___/4 | |
| | Must achieve >2 to pass this examination | | ℗ | Ⓕ | ℗ | Ⓕ | ℗ | Ⓕ |
| **Assessor:** **Date:** | **Test 1 Comments:** | | | | | | | |
| **Assessor:** **Date:** | **Test 2 Comments:** | | | | | | | |
| **Assessor:** **Date:** | **Test 3 Comments:** | | | | | | | |

**TEST ENVIRONMENTS**
**L:** Laboratory/Classroom
**C:** Clinical/Field Testing
**P:** Practicum
**A:** Assessment/Mock Exam

**TEST INFORMATION**
**Test Statistics:** No data available
**Reference(s):** Cook & Hegedus (2013)

**MUSCULOSKELETAL SYSTEM—REGION 5: LUMBAR AND THORACIC SPINE**
# SPECIAL TESTS

| NATA EC 5th | BOC RD6 | SKILL |
|---|---|---|
| CE-21g, CE-20e | D2-0203 | Straight Leg Raise (Unilateral Straight Leg Raise/Lasegue Test) |

**Supplies Needed:** Table

*This problem allows you the opportunity to demonstrate an* **orthopedic test** *known as the* **straight leg raise (unilateral straight leg raise/Lasegue test)** *for* **sciatic nerve irritation/herniated disc**. *You have 2 minutes to complete this task.*

| Straight Leg Raise (Unilateral Straight Leg Raise/ Lasegue Test) | Course or Site Assessor Environment | | | | | | |
|---|---|---|---|---|---|---|---|
| | | _____ | | _____ | | _____ | |
| | | **Test 1** | | **Test 2** | | **Test 3** | |
| **Tester places patient and limb in appropriate position** | | Y | N | Y | N | Y | N |
| Supine | | ○ | ○ | ○ | ○ | ○ | ○ |
| **Tester placed in proper position** | | Y | N | Y | N | Y | N |
| Stands at the side being tested | | ○ | ○ | ○ | ○ | ○ | ○ |
| Places one hand under heel and one hand on anterior knee | | ○ | ○ | ○ | ○ | ○ | ○ |
| **Tester performs test according to accepted guidelines** | | Y | N | Y | N | Y | N |
| Passively flexes hip while keeping knee in full extension until discomfort or full range of motion | | ○ | ○ | ○ | ○ | ○ | ○ |
| **Identifies positive findings and implications** | | Y | N | Y | N | Y | N |
| The patient complains of pain before the end of normal range of motion (70 degrees) | | ○ | ○ | ○ | ○ | ○ | ○ |
| The patient complains of pain before or at 30 degrees of hip flexion | | ○ | ○ | ○ | ○ | ○ | ○ |
| **Total** | | \_\_\_\_/6 | | \_\_\_\_/6 | | \_\_\_\_/6 | |
| **Must achieve >4 to pass this examination** | | Ⓟ | Ⓕ | Ⓟ | Ⓕ | Ⓟ | Ⓕ |
| Assessor: Date: | Test 1 Comments: | | | | | | |
| Assessor: Date: | Test 2 Comments: | | | | | | |
| Assessor: Date: | Test 3 Comments: | | | | | | |

**TEST ENVIRONMENTS**
**L:** Laboratory/Classroom
**C:** Clinical/Field Testing
**P:** Practicum
**A:** Assessment/Mock Exam

**TEST INFORMATION**
**Test Statistics:** Sensitivity .16–.98
Specificity .10–.89
(+) LR 1.03–4.72
(-) LR .05–.90
**Reference(s):** Cook & Hegedus (2013)
Starkey & Brown (2015)

## MUSCULOSKELETAL SYSTEM—REGION 5: LUMBAR AND THORACIC SPINE
# SPECIAL TESTS

| NATA EC 5th | BOC RD6 | SKILL |
|---|---|---|
| CE-21g, CE-20e | D2-0203 | Tension Sign |

**Supplies Needed:** Table

*This problem allows you the opportunity to demonstrate an* **orthopedic test** *known as the* **tension sign** *to rule out a* **sciatic nerve irritation**. *You have 2 minutes to complete this task.*

| Tension Sign | Course or Site<br>Assessor<br>Environment | | Test 1 | | Test 2 | | Test 3 |
|---|---|---|---|---|---|---|---|
| **Tester places patient and limb in appropriate position** | | Y | N | Y | N | Y | N |
| Supine | | O | O | O | O | O | O |
| **Tester placed in proper position** | | Y | N | Y | N | Y | N |
| Stands to the side of limb being tested | | O | O | O | O | O | O |
| Places one hand under the heel | | O | O | O | O | O | O |
| Places other hand under the knee joint | | O | O | O | O | O | O |
| **Tester performs test according to accepted guidelines** | | Y | N | Y | N | Y | N |
| Passively flexes the hip to 90 degrees with the knee flexed to 90 degrees | | O | O | O | O | O | O |
| The knee is then extended as far as possible with the examiner palpating the tibial portion of the sciatic nerve | | O | O | O | O | O | O |
| **Identifies positive findings and implications** | | Y | N | Y | N | Y | N |
| Exquisite tenderness | | O | O | O | O | O | O |
| Duplication of sciatic nerve symptoms | | O | O | O | O | O | O |
| | Total | ___/8 | | ___/8 | | ___/8 | |
| | **Must achieve >5 to pass this examination** | P | F | P | F | P | F |

| Assessor:<br>Date: | Test 1 Comments: |
|---|---|
| Assessor:<br>Date: | Test 2 Comments: |
| Assessor:<br>Date: | Test 3 Comments: |

**TEST ENVIRONMENTS**
**L:** Laboratory/Classroom
**C:** Clinical/Field Testing
**P:** Practicum
**A:** Assessment/Mock Exam

**TEST INFORMATION**
**Test Statistics:** No data available
**Reference(s):** Starkey & Brown (2015)

## MUSCULOSKELETAL SYSTEM—REGION 5: LUMBAR AND THORACIC SPINE
# SPECIAL TESTS

| NATA EC 5th | BOC RD6 | SKILL |
|---|---|---|
| CE-21g, CE-20e | D2-0203 | Valsalva Test |

**Supplies Needed:** Table

*This problem allows you the opportunity to demonstrate an* **orthopedic test** *known as the* **Valsalva test** *to rule out a* **space-occupying lesion**. *You have 2 minutes to complete this task.*

| Valsalva Test | Course or Site Assessor Environment | | Test 1 | | Test 2 | | Test 3 | |
|---|---|---|---|---|---|---|---|---|
| **Tester places patient and limb in appropriate position** | | | Y | N | Y | N | Y | N |
| Seated | | | ○ | ○ | ○ | ○ | ○ | ○ |
| Knee is extended and quadriceps are relaxed | | | ○ | ○ | ○ | ○ | ○ | ○ |
| **Tester placed in proper position** | | | Y | N | Y | N | Y | N |
| Stands in front of the patient | | | ○ | ○ | ○ | ○ | ○ | ○ |
| **Tester performs test according to accepted guidelines** | | | Y | N | Y | N | Y | N |
| The patient is instructed to take a deep breath while bearing down | | | ○ | ○ | ○ | ○ | ○ | ○ |
| **Identifies positive findings and implications** | | | Y | N | Y | N | Y | N |
| Increased spinal or radicular pain | | | ○ | ○ | ○ | ○ | ○ | ○ |
| **Total** | | | ___/5 | | ___/5 | | ___/5 | |
| **Must achieve >3 to pass this examination** | | | Ⓟ | Ⓕ | Ⓟ | Ⓕ | Ⓟ | Ⓕ |

| Assessor: Date: | Test 1 Comments: |
|---|---|
| Assessor: Date: | Test 2 Comments: |
| Assessor: Date: | Test 3 Comments: |

**TEST ENVIRONMENTS**
**L:** Laboratory/Classroom
**C:** Clinical/Field Testing
**P:** Practicum
**A:** Assessment/Mock Exam

**TEST INFORMATION**
**Test Statistics:** No data available
**Reference(s):** Starkey & Brown (2015)

**MUSCULOSKELETAL SYSTEM—REGION 5: LUMBAR AND THORACIC SPINE**
# SPECIAL TESTS

| NATA EC 5th | BOC RD6 | SKILL |
|---|---|---|
| CE-21g, CE-20e | D2-0203 | Well Straight Leg Raise Test |

**Supplies Needed:** Table

*This problem allows you the opportunity to demonstrate an* **orthopedic test** *known as the* **well straight leg raise test** *to rule out a possible* **herniated intervertebral disc**. *You have 2 minutes to complete this task.*

| Well Straight Leg Raise Test | Course or Site Assessor Environment | Test 1 | | Test 2 | | Test 3 | |
|---|---|---|---|---|---|---|---|
| | | **Y** | **N** | **Y** | **N** | **Y** | **N** |
| **Tester places patient and limb in appropriate position** | | **Y** | **N** | **Y** | **N** | **Y** | **N** |
| Supine | | ○ | ○ | ○ | ○ | ○ | ○ |
| The patient's head, neck, shoulders, and hip in neutral | | ○ | ○ | ○ | ○ | ○ | ○ |
| **Tester placed in proper position** | | **Y** | **N** | **Y** | **N** | **Y** | **N** |
| Stands lateral to the noninvolved side | | ○ | ○ | ○ | ○ | ○ | ○ |
| Stabilizes the posterior aspect of the patient's ankle, maintaining knee extension and neutral dorsiflexion | | ○ | ○ | ○ | ○ | ○ | ○ |
| **Tester performs test according to accepted guidelines** | | **Y** | **N** | **Y** | **N** | **Y** | **N** |
| Raises the patient's leg into hip flexion until symptom reproduction | | ○ | ○ | ○ | ○ | ○ | ○ |
| **Identifies positive findings and implications** | | **Y** | **N** | **Y** | **N** | **Y** | **N** |
| Pain experienced during straight leg maneuver of opposite leg | | ○ | ○ | ○ | ○ | ○ | ○ |
| | Total | ___/6 | | ___/6 | | ___/6 | |
| | Must achieve >4 to pass this examination | Ⓟ | Ⓕ | Ⓟ | Ⓕ | Ⓟ | Ⓕ |
| **Assessor:** **Date:** | **Test 1 Comments:** | | | | | | |
| **Assessor:** **Date:** | **Test 2 Comments:** | | | | | | |
| **Assessor:** **Date:** | **Test 3 Comments:** | | | | | | |

**TEST ENVIRONMENTS**
**L:** Laboratory/Classroom
**C:** Clinical/Field Testing
**P:** Practicum
**A:** Assessment/Mock Exam

**TEST INFORMATION**
**Test Statistics:** Sensitivity .23–.43
Specificity .88–1.00
(+) LR 1.91–14.30
(-) LR .59–.86
**Reference(s):** Cook & Hegedus (2013)

## MUSCULOSKELETAL SYSTEM—REGION 5: LUMBAR AND THORACIC SPINE
# DERMATOME TESTING

| NATA EC 5th | BOC RD6 | SKILL |
|---|---|---|
| CE-21h, CE-20f | D2-0203 | Dermatome: L1 |

**Supplies Needed:** Table, neurological hammer, cotton-tipped applicator, toothpicks

*This problem allows you the opportunity to demonstrate a* **dermatome assessment** *for* **L1**. *You have 2 minutes to complete this task.*

| Dermatome: L1 | Course or Site Assessor Environment | | Test 1 | | Test 2 | | Test 3 | |
|---|---|---|---|---|---|---|---|---|
| **Tester places patient and limb in appropriate position** | | | Y | N | Y | N | Y | N |
| Seated, legs over the table | | | O | O | O | O | O | O |
| Upright position | | | O | O | O | O | O | O |
| **Tester placed in proper position** | | | Y | N | Y | N | Y | N |
| Stands in front of the patient | | | O | O | O | O | O | O |
| **Tester performs test according to accepted guidelines** | | | Y | N | Y | N | Y | N |
| Instructs the patient in the differences in sharp/dull | | | O | O | O | O | O | O |
| Instructs the patient to close eyes and look away | | | O | O | O | O | O | O |
| Applies sharp/dull sensation in randomized order over the adductor/groin region | | | O | O | O | O | O | O |
| Instructs the patient to identify sharp/dull | | | O | O | O | O | O | O |
| **Identifies implications** | | | Y | N | Y | N | Y | N |
| Unable to differentiate | | | O | O | O | O | O | O |
| | | Total | __/8 | | __/8 | | __/8 | |
| | Must achieve >5 to pass this examination | | Ⓟ | Ⓕ | Ⓟ | Ⓕ | Ⓟ | Ⓕ |

| Assessor: Date: | Test 1 Comments: |
|---|---|
| Assessor: Date: | Test 2 Comments: |
| Assessor: Date: | Test 3 Comments: |

**TEST ENVIRONMENTS**
**L:** Laboratory/Classroom
**C:** Clinical/Field Testing
**P:** Practicum
**A:** Assessment/Mock Exam

**TEST INFORMATION**
**Test Statistics:** N/A
**Reference(s):** Starkey & Brown (2015)

## MUSCULOSKELETAL SYSTEM—REGION 5: LUMBAR AND THORACIC SPINE
# DERMATOME TESTING

| NATA EC 5th | BOC RD6 | SKILL |
|---|---|---|
| CE-21h, CE-20f | D2-0203 | Dermatome: L2 |

**Supplies Needed:** Table, neurological hammer, cotton-tipped applicator, toothpicks

*This problem allows you the opportunity to demonstrate a* **dermatome assessment** *for* **L2**. *You have 2 minutes to complete this task.*

| Dermatome: L2 | Course or Site Assessor Environment | | Test 1 | | Test 2 | | Test 3 |
|---|---|---|---|---|---|---|---|
| **Tester places patient and limb in appropriate position** | | Y | N | Y | N | Y | N |
| Seated, legs over the table | | ○ | ○ | ○ | ○ | ○ | ○ |
| Upright position | | ○ | ○ | ○ | ○ | ○ | ○ |
| **Tester placed in proper position** | | Y | N | Y | N | Y | N |
| Stands in front of the patient | | ○ | ○ | ○ | ○ | ○ | ○ |
| **Tester performs test according to accepted guidelines** | | Y | N | Y | N | Y | N |
| Instructs the patient in the differences in sharp/dull | | ○ | ○ | ○ | ○ | ○ | ○ |
| Instructs the patient to close eyes and look away | | ○ | ○ | ○ | ○ | ○ | ○ |
| Applies sharp/dull sensation in randomized order over the adductor/groin region | | ○ | ○ | ○ | ○ | ○ | ○ |
| Instructs the patient to identify sharp/dull | | ○ | ○ | ○ | ○ | ○ | ○ |
| **Identifies implications** | | Y | N | Y | N | Y | N |
| Unable to differentiate | | ○ | ○ | ○ | ○ | ○ | ○ |
| Total | | /8 | | /8 | | /8 | |
| Must achieve >5 to pass this examination | | Ⓟ | Ⓕ | Ⓟ | Ⓕ | Ⓟ | Ⓕ |

| Assessor:<br>Date: | Test 1 Comments: |
|---|---|
| Assessor:<br>Date: | Test 2 Comments: |
| Assessor:<br>Date: | Test 3 Comments: |

**TEST ENVIRONMENTS**
**L:** Laboratory/Classroom
**C:** Clinical/Field Testing
**P:** Practicum
**A:** Assessment/Mock Exam

**TEST INFORMATION**
**Test Statistics:** N/A
**Reference(s):** Starkey & Brown (2015)

## MUSCULOSKELETAL SYSTEM—REGION 5: LUMBAR AND THORACIC SPINE
# DERMATOME TESTING

| NATA EC 5th | BOC RD6 | SKILL |
|---|---|---|
| CE-21h, CE-20f | D2-0203 | Dermatome: L3 |

**Supplies Needed:** Table, neurological hammer, cotton-tipped applicator, toothpicks

*This problem allows you the opportunity to demonstrate a* **dermatome assessment** *for* **L3.** *You have 2 minutes to complete this task.*

| Dermatome: L3 | Course or Site<br>Assessor<br>Environment | | | | | | |
|---|---|---|---|---|---|---|---|
| | | Test 1 | | Test 2 | | Test 3 | |
| **Tester places patient and limb in appropriate position** | | Y | N | Y | N | Y | N |
| Seated, legs over the table | | O | O | O | O | O | O |
| Upright position | | O | O | O | O | O | O |
| **Tester placed in proper position** | | Y | N | Y | N | Y | N |
| Stands in front of the patient | | O | O | O | O | O | O |
| **Tester performs test according to accepted guidelines** | | Y | N | Y | N | Y | N |
| Instructs the patient in the differences in sharp/dull | | O | O | O | O | O | O |
| Instructs the patient to close eyes and look away | | O | O | O | O | O | O |
| Applies sharp/dull sensation in randomized order over the mid-thigh region | | O | O | O | O | O | O |
| Instructs the patient to identify sharp/dull | | O | O | O | O | O | O |
| **Identifies implications** | | Y | N | Y | N | Y | N |
| Unable to differentiate | | O | O | O | O | O | O |
| Total | | __/8 | | __/8 | | __/8 | |
| Must achieve >5 to pass this examination | | Ⓟ | Ⓕ | Ⓟ | Ⓕ | Ⓟ | Ⓕ |

| Assessor:<br>Date: | Test 1 Comments: |
|---|---|
| Assessor:<br>Date: | Test 2 Comments: |
| Assessor:<br>Date: | Test 3 Comments: |

**TEST ENVIRONMENTS**
**L:** Laboratory/Classroom
**C:** Clinical/Field Testing
**P:** Practicum
**A:** Assessment/Mock Exam

**TEST INFORMATION**
**Test Statistics:** N/A
**Reference(s):** Starkey & Brown (2015)

MUSCULOSKELETAL SYSTEM—REGION 5: LUMBAR AND THORACIC SPINE
# DERMATOME TESTING

| NATA EC 5th | BOC RD6 | SKILL |
|---|---|---|
| CE-21h, CE-20f | D2-0203 | Dermatome: L4 |

**Supplies Needed:** Table, neurological hammer, cotton-tipped applicator, toothpicks

*This problem allows you the opportunity to demonstrate a **dermatome assessment** for **L4**. You have 2 minutes to complete this task.*

| Dermatome: L4 | Course or Site Assessor Environment | | Test 1 | | Test 2 | | Test 3 | |
|---|---|---|---|---|---|---|---|---|
| | | | **Y** | **N** | **Y** | **N** | **Y** | **N** |
| **Tester places patient and limb in appropriate position** | | | Y | N | Y | N | Y | N |
| Seated, legs over the table | | | O | O | O | O | O | O |
| Upright position | | | O | O | O | O | O | O |
| **Tester placed in proper position** | | | Y | N | Y | N | Y | N |
| Stands in front of the patient | | | O | O | O | O | O | O |
| **Tester performs test according to accepted guidelines** | | | Y | N | Y | N | Y | N |
| Instructs the patient in the differences in sharp/dull | | | O | O | O | O | O | O |
| Instructs the patient to close eyes and look away | | | O | O | O | O | O | O |
| Applies sharp/dull sensation in randomized order over the mid-thigh to medial lower leg | | | O | O | O | O | O | O |
| Instructs the patient to identify sharp/dull | | | O | O | O | O | O | O |
| **Identifies implications** | | | Y | N | Y | N | Y | N |
| Unable to differentiate | | | O | O | O | O | O | O |
| Total | | | ___/8 | | ___/8 | | ___/8 | |
| Must achieve >5 to pass this examination | | | Ⓟ | Ⓕ | Ⓟ | Ⓕ | Ⓟ | Ⓕ |
| Assessor: Date: | Test 1 Comments: | | | | | | | |
| Assessor: Date: | Test 2 Comments: | | | | | | | |
| Assessor: Date: | Test 3 Comments: | | | | | | | |

**TEST ENVIRONMENTS**
**L:** Laboratory/Classroom
**C:** Clinical/Field Testing
**P:** Practicum
**A:** Assessment/Mock Exam

**TEST INFORMATION**
**Test Statistics:** N/A
**Reference(s):** Starkey & Brown (2015)

## MUSCULOSKELETAL SYSTEM—REGION 5: LUMBAR AND THORACIC SPINE
# DERMATOME TESTING

| NATA EC 5th | BOC RD6 | SKILL |
|---|---|---|
| CE-21h, CE-20f | D2-0203 | Dermatome: L5 |

**Supplies Needed:** Table, neurological hammer, cotton-tipped applicator, toothpicks

*This problem allows you the opportunity to demonstrate a* **dermatome assessment** *for* **L5**. *You have 2 minutes to complete this task.*

| Dermatome: L5 | Course or Site Assessor Environment | | Test 1 | | Test 2 | | Test 3 |
|---|---|---|---|---|---|---|---|
| **Tester places patient and limb in appropriate position** | | Y | N | Y | N | Y | N |
| Seated, legs over the table | | ○ | ○ | ○ | ○ | ○ | ○ |
| Upright position | | ○ | ○ | ○ | ○ | ○ | ○ |
| **Tester placed in proper position** | | Y | N | Y | N | Y | N |
| Stands in front of the patient | | ○ | ○ | ○ | ○ | ○ | ○ |
| **Tester performs test according to accepted guidelines** | | Y | N | Y | N | Y | N |
| Instructs the patient in the differences in sharp/dull | | ○ | ○ | ○ | ○ | ○ | ○ |
| Instructs the patient to close eyes and look away | | ○ | ○ | ○ | ○ | ○ | ○ |
| Applies sharp/dull sensation in randomized order over the superolateral lower leg to great toe | | ○ | ○ | ○ | ○ | ○ | ○ |
| Instructs the patient to identify sharp/dull | | ○ | ○ | ○ | ○ | ○ | ○ |
| **Identifies implications** | | Y | N | Y | N | Y | N |
| Unable to differentiate | | ○ | ○ | ○ | ○ | ○ | ○ |
| Total | | \_\_\_/8 | | \_\_\_/8 | | \_\_\_/8 | |
| Must achieve >5 to pass this examination | | Ⓟ | Ⓕ | Ⓟ | Ⓕ | Ⓟ | Ⓕ |

| Assessor:<br>Date: | Test 1 Comments: |
|---|---|
| Assessor:<br>Date: | Test 2 Comments: |
| Assessor:<br>Date: | Test 3 Comments: |

**TEST ENVIRONMENTS**
**L:** Laboratory/Classroom
**C:** Clinical/Field Testing
**P:** Practicum
**A:** Assessment/Mock Exam

**TEST INFORMATION**
**Test Statistics:** N/A
**Reference(s):** Starkey & Brown (2015)

## MUSCULOSKELETAL SYSTEM—REGION 5: LUMBAR AND THORACIC SPINE
# DERMATOME TESTING

| NATA EC 5th | BOC RD6 | SKILL |
|---|---|---|
| CE-21h, CE-20f | D2-0203 | Dermatome: S1 |

**Supplies Needed:** Table, neurological hammer, cotton-tipped applicator, toothpicks

*This problem allows you the opportunity to demonstrate a* **dermatome assessment** *for* **S1**. *You have 2 minutes to complete this task.*

| Dermatome: S1 | Course or Site / Assessor / Environment | | Test 1 | | Test 2 | | Test 3 | |
|---|---|---|---|---|---|---|---|---|
| **Tester places patient and limb in appropriate position** | | | Y | N | Y | N | Y | N |
| Seated, legs over the table | | | ○ | ○ | ○ | ○ | ○ | ○ |
| Upright position | | | ○ | ○ | ○ | ○ | ○ | ○ |
| **Tester placed in proper position** | | | Y | N | Y | N | Y | N |
| Stands in front of the patient | | | ○ | ○ | ○ | ○ | ○ | ○ |
| **Tester performs test according to accepted guidelines** | | | Y | N | Y | N | Y | N |
| Instructs the patient in the differences in sharp/dull | | | ○ | ○ | ○ | ○ | ○ | ○ |
| Instructs the patient to close eyes and look away | | | ○ | ○ | ○ | ○ | ○ | ○ |
| Applies sharp/dull sensation in randomized order over the lateral aspect of lower leg and lateral aspect of the hamstring muscles | | | ○ | ○ | ○ | ○ | ○ | ○ |
| Instructs the patient to identify sharp/dull | | | ○ | ○ | ○ | ○ | ○ | ○ |
| **Identifies implications** | | | Y | N | Y | N | Y | N |
| Unable to differentiate | | | ○ | ○ | ○ | ○ | ○ | ○ |
| **Total** | | | ____/8 | | ____/8 | | ____/8 | |
| **Must achieve >5 to pass this examination** | | | Ⓟ | Ⓕ | Ⓟ | Ⓕ | Ⓟ | Ⓕ |
| **Assessor:** **Date:** | **Test 1 Comments:** | | | | | | | |
| **Assessor:** **Date:** | **Test 2 Comments:** | | | | | | | |
| **Assessor:** **Date:** | **Test 3 Comments:** | | | | | | | |

**TEST ENVIRONMENTS**
**L:** Laboratory/Classroom
**C:** Clinical/Field Testing
**P:** Practicum
**A:** Assessment/Mock Exam

**TEST INFORMATION**
**Test Statistics:** N/A
**Reference(s):** Starkey & Brown (2015)

## MUSCULOSKELETAL SYSTEM—REGION 5: LUMBAR AND THORACIC SPINE
# DERMATOME TESTING

| NATA EC 5th | BOC RD6 | SKILL |
|---|---|---|
| CE-21h, CE-20f | D2-0203 | Dermatome: S2 |

**Supplies Needed:** Table, neurological hammer, cotton-tipped applicator, toothpicks

*This problem allows you the opportunity to demonstrate a* **dermatome assessment** *for* **S2**. *You have 2 minutes to complete this task.*

| Dermatome: S2 | Course or Site Assessor Environment | | Test 1 | | Test 2 | | Test 3 | |
|---|---|---|---|---|---|---|---|---|
| | | | Y | N | Y | N | Y | N |
| **Tester places patient and limb in appropriate position** | | | Y | N | Y | N | Y | N |
| Seated, legs over the table | | | O | O | O | O | O | O |
| Upright position | | | O | O | O | O | O | O |
| **Tester placed in proper position** | | | Y | N | Y | N | Y | N |
| Stands in front of the patient | | | O | O | O | O | O | O |
| **Tester performs test according to accepted guidelines** | | | Y | N | Y | N | Y | N |
| Instructs the patient in the differences in sharp/dull | | | O | O | O | O | O | O |
| Instructs the patient to close eyes and look away | | | O | O | O | O | O | O |
| Applies sharp/dull sensation in randomized order over the middle of the hamstring muscles | | | O | O | O | O | O | O |
| Instructs the patient to identify sharp/dull | | | O | O | O | O | O | O |
| **Identifies implications** | | | Y | N | Y | N | Y | N |
| Unable to differentiate | | | O | O | O | O | O | O |
| Total | | | __/8 | | __/8 | | __/8 | |
| **Must achieve >5 to pass this examination** | | | Ⓟ | Ⓕ | Ⓟ | Ⓕ | Ⓟ | Ⓕ |

| Assessor: Date: | Test 1 Comments: |
|---|---|
| Assessor: Date: | Test 2 Comments: |
| Assessor: Date: | Test 3 Comments: |

**TEST ENVIRONMENTS**
**L:** Laboratory/Classroom
**C:** Clinical/Field Testing
**P:** Practicum
**A:** Assessment/Mock Exam

**TEST INFORMATION**
**Test Statistics:** N/A
**Reference(s):** Starkey & Brown (2015)

## MUSCULOSKELETAL SYSTEM—REGION 5: LUMBAR AND THORACIC SPINE
# MYOTOME TESTING

| NATA EC 5th | BOC RD6 | SKILL |
|---|---|---|
| CE-21h, CE-20f | D2-0203 | Myotome: L1/L2 |

**Supplies Needed:** Table

*This problem allows you the opportunity to demonstrate a* **myotome assessment** *for* **L1/L2**.
*You have 2 minutes to complete this task.*

| Myotome: L1/L2 / Course or Site / Assessor / Environment | Test 1 | | Test 2 | | Test 3 | |
|---|---|---|---|---|---|---|
| | Y | N | Y | N | Y | N |
| **Tester places patient and limb in appropriate position** | **Y** | **N** | **Y** | **N** | **Y** | **N** |
| Seated, legs over the table | ○ | ○ | ○ | ○ | ○ | ○ |
| Upright position | ○ | ○ | ○ | ○ | ○ | ○ |
| **Tester placed in proper position** | **Y** | **N** | **Y** | **N** | **Y** | **N** |
| Stands at the side being tested | ○ | ○ | ○ | ○ | ○ | ○ |
| **Tester performs test according to accepted guidelines** | **Y** | **N** | **Y** | **N** | **Y** | **N** |
| Applies manual resistance against hip flexion | ○ | ○ | ○ | ○ | ○ | ○ |
| Stabilizes appropriately | ○ | ○ | ○ | ○ | ○ | ○ |
| Performs bilaterally | ○ | ○ | ○ | ○ | ○ | ○ |
| **Identifies implications** | **Y** | **N** | **Y** | **N** | **Y** | **N** |
| Inability to maintain position | ○ | ○ | ○ | ○ | ○ | ○ |
| Total | ___/7 | | ___/7 | | ___/7 | |
| **Must achieve >4 to pass this examination** | Ⓟ | Ⓕ | Ⓟ | Ⓕ | Ⓟ | Ⓕ |

| Assessor:<br>Date: | Test 1 Comments: |
|---|---|
| Assessor:<br>Date: | Test 2 Comments: |
| Assessor:<br>Date: | Test 3 Comments: |

**TEST ENVIRONMENTS**
**L:** Laboratory/Classroom
**C:** Clinical/Field Testing
**P:** Practicum
**A:** Assessment/Mock Exam

**TEST INFORMATION**
**Test Statistics:** N/A
**Reference(s):**    Starkey & Brown (2015)

## MUSCULOSKELETAL SYSTEM—REGION 5: LUMBAR AND THORACIC SPINE
# MYOTOME TESTING

| NATA EC 5th | BOC RD6 | SKILL |
|---|---|---|
| CE-21h, CE-20f | D2-0203 | Myotome: L3 |

**Supplies Needed:** Table

*This problem allows you the opportunity to demonstrate a* **myotome assessment** *for* **L3**. *You have 2 minutes to complete this task.*

| Myotome: L3 | Course or Site Assessor Environment | | Test 1 | | Test 2 | | Test 3 | |
|---|---|---|---|---|---|---|---|---|
| **Tester places patient and limb in appropriate position** | | Y | N | Y | N | Y | N |
| Seated, legs over the table | | O | O | O | O | O | O |
| Upright position | | O | O | O | O | O | O |
| **Tester placed in proper position** | | Y | N | Y | N | Y | N |
| Stands at the side being tested | | O | O | O | O | O | O |
| **Tester performs test according to accepted guidelines** | | Y | N | Y | N | Y | N |
| Applies manual resistance against knee extension | | O | O | O | O | O | O |
| Stabilizes appropriately | | O | O | O | O | O | O |
| Performs bilaterally | | O | O | O | O | O | O |
| **Identifies implications** | | Y | N | Y | N | Y | N |
| Inability to maintain position | | O | O | O | O | O | O |
| **Total** | | __/7 | | __/7 | | __/7 | |
| **Must achieve >4 to pass this examination** | | Ⓟ | Ⓕ | Ⓟ | Ⓕ | Ⓟ | Ⓕ |

| Assessor:<br>Date: | Test 1 Comments: |
|---|---|
| Assessor:<br>Date: | Test 2 Comments: |
| Assessor:<br>Date: | Test 3 Comments: |

**TEST ENVIRONMENTS**
**L:** Laboratory/Classroom
**C:** Clinical/Field Testing
**P:** Practicum
**A:** Assessment/Mock Exam

**TEST INFORMATION**
**Test Statistics:** N/A
**Reference(s):** Starkey & Brown (2015)

MUSCULOSKELETAL SYSTEM—REGION 5: LUMBAR AND THORACIC SPINE
# MYOTOME TESTING

| NATA EC 5th | BOC RD6 | SKILL |
|---|---|---|
| CE-21h, CE-20f | D2-0203 | Myotome: L4 |

**Supplies Needed:** Table

*This problem allows you the opportunity to demonstrate a* **myotome assessment** *for* **L4**. *You have 2 minutes to complete this task.*

| Myotome: L4 / Course or Site Assessor Environment | Test 1 | | Test 2 | | Test 3 | |
|---|---|---|---|---|---|---|
| | Y | N | Y | N | Y | N |
| **Tester places patient and limb in appropriate position** | Y | N | Y | N | Y | N |
| Seated on the edge of the table | ○ | ○ | ○ | ○ | ○ | ○ |
| Upright position | ○ | ○ | ○ | ○ | ○ | ○ |
| **Tester placed in proper position** | Y | N | Y | N | Y | N |
| Stands at the side being tested | ○ | ○ | ○ | ○ | ○ | ○ |
| **Tester performs test according to accepted guidelines** | Y | N | Y | N | Y | N |
| Applies manual resistance against ankle dorsiflexion | ○ | ○ | ○ | ○ | ○ | ○ |
| Stabilizes appropriately | ○ | ○ | ○ | ○ | ○ | ○ |
| Performs bilaterally | ○ | ○ | ○ | ○ | ○ | ○ |
| **Identifies implications** | Y | N | Y | N | Y | N |
| Inability to maintain position | ○ | ○ | ○ | ○ | ○ | ○ |
| Total | __/7 | | __/7 | | __/7 | |
| **Must achieve >4 to pass this examination** | Ⓟ | Ⓕ | Ⓟ | Ⓕ | Ⓟ | Ⓕ |

| Assessor: Date: | Test 1 Comments: |
|---|---|
| Assessor: Date: | Test 2 Comments: |
| Assessor: Date: | Test 3 Comments: |

**TEST ENVIRONMENTS**
**L:** Laboratory/Classroom
**C:** Clinical/Field Testing
**P:** Practicum
**A:** Assessment/Mock Exam

**TEST INFORMATION**
**Test Statistics:** N/A
**Reference(s):** Starkey & Brown (2015)

## MUSCULOSKELETAL SYSTEM—REGION 5: LUMBAR AND THORACIC SPINE
# MYOTOME TESTING

| NATA EC 5th | BOC RD6 | SKILL |
|---|---|---|
| CE-21h, CE-20f | D2-0203 | Myotome: L5 |

**Supplies Needed:** Table

*This problem allows you the opportunity to demonstrate a **myotome assessment** for **L5**. You have 2 minutes to complete this task.*

| Myotome: L5 | Course or Site Assessor Environment | | | | | | |
|---|---|---|---|---|---|---|---|
| | | Test 1 | | Test 2 | | Test 3 | |
| **Tester places patient and limb in appropriate position** | | Y | N | Y | N | Y | N |
| Seated, legs over the table | | ○ | ○ | ○ | ○ | ○ | ○ |
| Upright position | | ○ | ○ | ○ | ○ | ○ | ○ |
| **Tester placed in proper position** | | Y | N | Y | N | Y | N |
| Stands at the side being tested | | ○ | ○ | ○ | ○ | ○ | ○ |
| **Tester performs test according to accepted guidelines** | | Y | N | Y | N | Y | N |
| Applies manual resistance against great toe extension | | ○ | ○ | ○ | ○ | ○ | ○ |
| Stabilizes appropriately | | ○ | ○ | ○ | ○ | ○ | ○ |
| Performs bilaterally | | ○ | ○ | ○ | ○ | ○ | ○ |
| **Identifies implications** | | Y | N | Y | N | Y | N |
| Inability to maintain position | | ○ | ○ | ○ | ○ | ○ | ○ |
| Total | | ___/7 | | ___/7 | | ___/7 | |
| **Must achieve >4 to pass this examination** | | Ⓟ | Ⓕ | Ⓟ | Ⓕ | Ⓟ | Ⓕ |
| **Assessor:** **Date:** | Test 1 Comments: | | | | | | |
| **Assessor:** **Date:** | Test 2 Comments: | | | | | | |
| **Assessor:** **Date:** | Test 3 Comments: | | | | | | |

**TEST ENVIRONMENTS**
**L:** Laboratory/Classroom
**C:** Clinical/Field Testing
**P:** Practicum
**A:** Assessment/Mock Exam

**TEST INFORMATION**
**Test Statistics:** N/A
**Reference(s):** Starkey & Brown (2015)

MUSCULOSKELETAL SYSTEM—REGION 5: LUMBAR AND THORACIC SPINE
# MYOTOME TESTING

| NATA EC 5th | BOC RD6 | SKILL |
|---|---|---|
| CE-21h, CE-20f | D2-0203 | Myotome: S1 |

**Supplies Needed:** Table

*This problem allows you the opportunity to demonstrate a* **myotome assessment** *for* **S1**. *You have 2 minutes to complete this task.*

| Myotome: S1 — Course or Site / Assessor / Environment | Test 1 Y | Test 1 N | Test 2 Y | Test 2 N | Test 3 Y | Test 3 N |
|---|---|---|---|---|---|---|
| **Tester places patient and limb in appropriate position** | **Y** | **N** | **Y** | **N** | **Y** | **N** |
| Seated, legs over the table | ○ | ○ | ○ | ○ | ○ | ○ |
| Upright position | ○ | ○ | ○ | ○ | ○ | ○ |
| **Tester placed in proper position** | **Y** | **N** | **Y** | **N** | **Y** | **N** |
| Stands at the side being tested | ○ | ○ | ○ | ○ | ○ | ○ |
| **Tester performs test according to accepted guidelines** | **Y** | **N** | **Y** | **N** | **Y** | **N** |
| Applies manual resistance against ankle eversion | ○ | ○ | ○ | ○ | ○ | ○ |
| Stabilizes appropriately | ○ | ○ | ○ | ○ | ○ | ○ |
| Performs bilaterally | ○ | ○ | ○ | ○ | ○ | ○ |
| **Identifies implications** | **Y** | **N** | **Y** | **N** | **Y** | **N** |
| Inability to maintain position | ○ | ○ | ○ | ○ | ○ | ○ |
| Total | /7 | | /7 | | /7 | |
| Must achieve >4 to pass this examination | Ⓟ | Ⓕ | Ⓟ | Ⓕ | Ⓟ | Ⓕ |

| Assessor: Date: | **Test 1 Comments:** |
|---|---|
| Assessor: Date: | **Test 2 Comments:** |
| Assessor: Date: | **Test 3 Comments:** |

**TEST ENVIRONMENTS**
**L:** Laboratory/Classroom
**C:** Clinical/Field Testing
**P:** Practicum
**A:** Assessment/Mock Exam

**TEST INFORMATION**
**Test Statistics:** N/A
**Reference(s):** Starkey & Brown (2015)

## MUSCULOSKELETAL SYSTEM—REGION 5: LUMBAR AND THORACIC SPINE
# MYOTOME TESTING

| NATA EC 5th | BOC RD6 | SKILL |
|---|---|---|
| CE-21h, CE-20f | D2-0203 | Myotome: S2 |

**Supplies Needed:** Table

*This problem allows you the opportunity to demonstrate a* **myotome assessment** *for* **S2.** *You have 2 minutes to complete this task.*

| Myotome: S2 / Course or Site / Assessor / Environment | Test 1 | | Test 2 | | Test 3 | |
|---|---|---|---|---|---|---|
| | Y | N | Y | N | Y | N |
| **Tester places patient and limb in appropriate position** | Y | N | Y | N | Y | N |
| Seated, legs over the table | ○ | ○ | ○ | ○ | ○ | ○ |
| Upright position | ○ | ○ | ○ | ○ | ○ | ○ |
| **Tester placed in proper position** | Y | N | Y | N | Y | N |
| Stands at the side being tested | ○ | ○ | ○ | ○ | ○ | ○ |
| **Tester performs test according to accepted guidelines** | Y | N | Y | N | Y | N |
| Applies manual resistance against knee flexion | ○ | ○ | ○ | ○ | ○ | ○ |
| Stabilizes appropriately | ○ | ○ | ○ | ○ | ○ | ○ |
| Performs bilaterally | ○ | ○ | ○ | ○ | ○ | ○ |
| **Identifies implications** | Y | N | Y | N | Y | N |
| Inability to maintain position | ○ | ○ | ○ | ○ | ○ | ○ |
| **Total** | ___/7 | | ___/7 | | ___/7 | |
| **Must achieve >4 to pass this examination** | Ⓟ | Ⓕ | Ⓟ | Ⓕ | Ⓟ | Ⓕ |

| Assessor: Date: | **Test 1 Comments:** |
|---|---|
| Assessor: Date: | **Test 2 Comments:** |
| Assessor: Date: | **Test 3 Comments:** |

**TEST ENVIRONMENTS**
**L:** Laboratory/Classroom
**C:** Clinical/Field Testing
**P:** Practicum
**A:** Assessment/Mock Exam

**TEST INFORMATION**
**Test Statistics:** N/A
**Reference(s):** Starkey & Brown (2015)

## MUSCULOSKELETAL SYSTEM—REGION 5: LUMBAR AND THORACIC SPINE
# REFLEX TESTING

| NATA EC 5th | BOC RD6 | SKILL |
|---|---|---|
| CE-21h, CE-20f | D2-0203 | Reflex Testing: L2/L3/L4 |

**Supplies Needed:** Table, reflex hammer

*This problem allows you the opportunity to demonstrate a **reflex test** for **L2/L3/L4**. You have 2 minutes to complete this task.*

| Reflex Testing: L2/L3/L4 | Course or Site / Assessor / Environment | | Test 1 | | Test 2 | | Test 3 | |
|---|---|---|---|---|---|---|---|---|
| **Tester places patient and limb in appropriate position** | | | Y | N | Y | N | Y | N |
| Seated, legs over the table | | | ○ | ○ | ○ | ○ | ○ | ○ |
| Looking away from the tester | | | ○ | ○ | ○ | ○ | ○ | ○ |
| **Tester placed in proper position** | | | Y | N | Y | N | Y | N |
| Stands at the side being tested | | | ○ | ○ | ○ | ○ | ○ | ○ |
| **Tester performs test according to accepted guidelines** | | | Y | N | Y | N | Y | N |
| Uses reflex hammer to tap patellar tendon | | | ○ | ○ | ○ | ○ | ○ | ○ |
| Performs bilaterally | | | ○ | ○ | ○ | ○ | ○ | ○ |
| **Identifies implications** | | | Y | N | Y | N | Y | N |
| No reflex | | | ○ | ○ | ○ | ○ | ○ | ○ |
| Total | | | ___/6 | | ___/6 | | ___/6 | |
| Must achieve >3 to pass this examination | | | Ⓟ | Ⓕ | Ⓟ | Ⓕ | Ⓟ | Ⓕ |

| Assessor: Date: | Test 1 Comments: |
|---|---|
| Assessor: Date: | Test 2 Comments: |
| Assessor: Date: | Test 3 Comments: |

**TEST ENVIRONMENTS**
**L:** Laboratory/Classroom
**C:** Clinical/Field Testing
**P:** Practicum
**A:** Assessment/Mock Exam

**TEST INFORMATION**
**Test Statistics:** N/A
**Reference(s):** Starkey & Brown (2015)

## MUSCULOSKELETAL SYSTEM—REGION 5: LUMBAR AND THORACIC SPINE
# REFLEX TESTING

| NATA EC 5th | BOC RD6 | SKILL |
|---|---|---|
| CE-21h, CE-20f | D2-0203 | Reflex Testing: L5 |

**Supplies Needed:** Table, reflex hammer

*This problem allows you the opportunity to demonstrate a* **reflex test** *for* **L5**. *You have 2 minutes to complete this task.*

| Reflex Testing: L5 | Course or Site / Assessor / Environment | | Test 1 | | Test 2 | | Test 3 | |
|---|---|---|---|---|---|---|---|---|
| **Tester places patient and limb in appropriate position** | | | Y | N | Y | N | Y | N |
| Supine, ankle off the table | | | ○ | ○ | ○ | ○ | ○ | ○ |
| Looking away from the tester | | | ○ | ○ | ○ | ○ | ○ | ○ |
| **Tester placed in proper position** | | | Y | N | Y | N | Y | N |
| Stands at the side being tested | | | ○ | ○ | ○ | ○ | ○ | ○ |
| **Tester performs test according to accepted guidelines** | | | Y | N | Y | N | Y | N |
| Uses reflex hammer to tap tibialis posterior tendon | | | ○ | ○ | ○ | ○ | ○ | ○ |
| Performs bilaterally | | | ○ | ○ | ○ | ○ | ○ | ○ |
| **Identifies implications** | | | Y | N | Y | N | Y | N |
| No reflex | | | ○ | ○ | ○ | ○ | ○ | ○ |
| Total | | | ___/6 | | ___/6 | | ___/6 | |
| Must achieve >3 to pass this examination | | | Ⓟ | Ⓕ | Ⓟ | Ⓕ | Ⓟ | Ⓕ |

| Assessor: Date: | Test 1 Comments: |
|---|---|
| Assessor: Date: | Test 2 Comments: |
| Assessor: Date: | Test 3 Comments: |

**TEST ENVIRONMENTS**
L: Laboratory/Classroom
C: Clinical/Field Testing
P: Practicum
A: Assessment/Mock Exam

**TEST INFORMATION**
**Test Statistics:** N/A
**Reference(s):** Starkey & Brown (2015)

## MUSCULOSKELETAL SYSTEM—REGION 5: LUMBAR AND THORACIC SPINE
# REFLEX TESTING

| NATA EC 5th | BOC RD6 | SKILL |
|---|---|---|
| CE-21h, CE-20f | D2-0203 | Reflex Testing: S1 |

**Supplies Needed:** Table, reflex hammer

*This problem allows you the opportunity to demonstrate a* **reflex test** *for* **S1**. *You have 2 minutes to complete this task.*

| Reflex Testing: S1 | Course or Site / Assessor / Environment | | Test 1 | | Test 2 | | Test 3 | |
|---|---|---|---|---|---|---|---|---|
| **Tester places patient and limb in appropriate position** | | | Y | N | Y | N | Y | N |
| Prone, legs over the table | | | ○ | ○ | ○ | ○ | ○ | ○ |
| **Tester placed in proper position** | | | Y | N | Y | N | Y | N |
| Stands at the side being tested | | | ○ | ○ | ○ | ○ | ○ | ○ |
| Supports the patient's ankle | | | ○ | ○ | ○ | ○ | ○ | ○ |
| **Tester performs test according to accepted guidelines** | | | Y | N | Y | N | Y | N |
| Uses reflex hammer to tap Achilles tendon | | | ○ | ○ | ○ | ○ | ○ | ○ |
| Performs bilaterally | | | ○ | ○ | ○ | ○ | ○ | ○ |
| **Identifies implications** | | | Y | N | Y | N | Y | N |
| No reflex | | | ○ | ○ | ○ | ○ | ○ | ○ |
| Total | | | ___/6 | | ___/6 | | ___/6 | |
| Must achieve >3 to pass this examination | | | Ⓟ | Ⓕ | Ⓟ | Ⓕ | Ⓟ | Ⓕ |

| Assessor: Date: | Test 1 Comments: |
|---|---|
| Assessor: Date: | Test 2 Comments: |
| Assessor: Date: | Test 3 Comments: |

**TEST ENVIRONMENTS**
**L:** Laboratory/Classroom
**C:** Clinical/Field Testing
**P:** Practicum
**A:** Assessment/Mock Exam

**TEST INFORMATION**
**Test Statistics:** N/A
**Reference(s):** Starkey & Brown (2015)

## MUSCULOSKELETAL SYSTEM—REGION 5: LUMBAR AND THORACIC SPINE
# REFLEX TESTING

| NATA EC 5th | BOC RD6 | SKILL |
|---|---|---|
| CE-21h, CE-20f | D2-0203 | Reflex Testing: S2 |

**Supplies Needed:** Table, reflex hammer

*This problem allows you the opportunity to demonstrate a* **reflex test** *for* **S2**. *You have 2 minutes to complete this task.*

| Reflex Testing: S2 | Course or Site Assessor Environment | | | | | |
|---|---|---|---|---|---|---|
| | | Test 1 | | Test 2 | | Test 3 |
| **Tester places patient and limb in appropriate position** | | Y | N | Y | N | Y | N |
| Prone | | O | O | O | O | O | O |
| Lower leg in 90 degrees flexion | | O | O | O | O | O | O |
| **Tester placed in proper position** | | Y | N | Y | N | Y | N |
| Stands at the side being tested | | O | O | O | O | O | O |
| Supports the patient's lower leg | | O | O | O | O | O | O |
| **Tester performs test according to accepted guidelines** | | Y | N | Y | N | Y | N |
| Uses reflex hammer to tap biceps femoris tendon | | O | O | O | O | O | O |
| Performs bilaterally | | O | O | O | O | O | O |
| **Identifies implications** | | Y | N | Y | N | Y | N |
| No reflex | | O | O | O | O | O | O |
| **Total** | | ___/7 | | ___/7 | | ___/7 |
| **Must achieve >4 to pass this examination** | | Ⓟ | Ⓕ | Ⓟ | Ⓕ | Ⓟ | Ⓕ |

| Assessor: Date: | Test 1 Comments: |
|---|---|
| Assessor: Date: | Test 2 Comments: |
| Assessor: Date: | Test 3 Comments: |

**TEST ENVIRONMENTS**
**L:** Laboratory/Classroom
**C:** Clinical/Field Testing
**P:** Practicum
**A:** Assessment/Mock Exam

**TEST INFORMATION**
**Test Statistics:** N/A
**Reference(s):** Starkey & Brown (2015)

# 9

# MUSCULOSKELETAL SYSTEM—
# REGION 6: CERVICAL SPINE

Hauth, J. M., Gloyeske, B. M., & Amato, H. K.
*Clinical Skills Documentation Guide for Athletic Training, Third Edition* (pp. 242-289).
© 2016 SLACK Incorporated.

## MUSCULOSKELETAL SYSTEM—REGION 6: CERVICAL SPINE
# KNOWLEDGE AND SKILLS

| *Musculoskeletal System—Region 6: Cervical Spine* | | | | *Skill: Acquisition, Reinforcement, Proficiency* | | |
|---|---|---|---|---|---|---|
| **NATA EC 5th** | **BOC RD6** | **Palpation** | **Page #** | | | |
| CE-21b, CE-20c | D2-0202 | Palpation: Cervical Spine – 01 | 245 | | | |
| CE-21b, CE-20c | D2-0202 | Palpation: Cervical Spine – 02 | 246 | | | |
| CE-21b, CE-20c | D2-0202 | Palpation: Cervical Spine – 03 | 247 | | | |
| **NATA EC 5th** | **BOC RD6** | **Manual Muscle Testing** | **Page #** | | | |
| CE-21c | D2-0203 | MMT: Cervical Extension (Sternocleidomastoid/ Upper Trapezius) | 248 | | | |
| CE-21c | D2-0203 | MMT: Cervical Flexion (Sternocleidomastoid/ Scalenus Anterior) | 249 | | | |
| CE-21c | D2-0203 | MMT: Cervical Lateral Flexion (Sternocleidomastoid/ Scalenus Anterior/Scalenus Medius/Scalenus Posterior/Upper Trapezius) | 250 | | | |
| CE-21c | D2-0203 | MMT: Cervical Rotation (Sternocleidomastoid/ Scalenus Anterior/Scalenus Medius/ Scalenus Posterior/Upper Trapezius) | 251 | | | |
| **NATA EC 5th** | **BOC RD6** | **Osteokinematic Joint Motion** | **Page #** | | | |
| CE-21d | D2-0203 | Goniometric Assessment: Cervical Spine (Extension) | 252 | | | |
| CE-21d | D2-0203 | Goniometric Assessment: Cervical Spine (Flexion) | 253 | | | |
| CE-21d | D2-0203 | Goniometric Assessment: Cervical Spine (Lateral Flexion Left) | 254 | | | |
| CE-21d | D2-0203 | Goniometric Assessment: Cervical Spine (Lateral Flexion Right) | 255 | | | |
| CE-21d | D2-0203 | Goniometric Assessment: Cervical Spine (Rotation Left) | 256 | | | |
| CE-21d | D2-0203 | Goniometric Assessment: Cervical Spine (Rotation Right) | 257 | | | |
| **NATA EC 5th** | **BOC RD6** | **Special Tests** | **Page #** | | | |
| CE-21g, CE-20e | D2-0203 | Adson's Test | 258 | | | |
| CE-21g, CE-20e | D2-0203 | Allen's Test | 259 | | | |
| CE-21g, CE-20e | D2-0203 | Brachial Plexus Traction Test | 260 | | | |
| CE-21g, CE-20e | D2-0203 | Cervical Compression Test | 261 | | | |
| CE-21g, CE-20e | D2-0203 | Cervical Distraction Test | 262 | | | |
| CE-21g, CE-20e | D2-0203 | Cervical-Flexion Rotation Test | 263 | | | |
| CE-21g, CE-20e | D2-0203 | Military Brace Test | 264 | | | |
| CE-21g, CE-20e | D2-0203 | Roos' Test (Elevated Arm Stress Test) | 265 | | | |
| CE-21g, CE-20e | D2-0203 | Shoulder Abduction Test | 266 | | | |
| CE-21g, CE-20e | D2-0203 | Spurling's Test | 267 | | | |
| CE-21g, CE-20e | D2-0203 | Upper Limb Tension Test | 268 | | | |
| CE-21g, CE-20e | D2-0203 | Vertebral Basilar Insufficiency Test (Vertebral Artery Test) | 269 | | | |

*(continued on the next page)*

## MUSCULOSKELETAL SYSTEM—REGION 6: CERVICAL SPINE
# KNOWLEDGE AND SKILLS

| NATA EC 5th | BOC RD6 | Dermatome Testing | Page # | | | |
|---|---|---|---|---|---|---|
| CE-21h, CE-20f | D2-0203 | Dermatome: C1 | 270 | | | |
| CE-21h, CE-20f | D2-0203 | Dermatome: C2 | 271 | | | |
| CE-21h, CE-20f | D2-0203 | Dermatome: C3 | 272 | | | |
| CE-21h, CE-20f | D2-0203 | Dermatome: C4 | 273 | | | |
| CE-21h, CE-20f | D2-0203 | Dermatome: C5 | 274 | | | |
| CE-21h, CE-20f | D2-0203 | Dermatome: C6 | 275 | | | |
| CE-21h, CE-20f | D2-0203 | Dermatome: C7 | 276 | | | |
| CE-21h, CE-20f | D2-0203 | Dermatome: C8 | 277 | | | |
| CE-21h, CE-20f | D2-0203 | Dermatome: T1 | 278 | | | |
| NATA EC 5th | BOC RD6 | Myotome Testing | Page # | | | |
| CE-21h, CE-20f | D2-0203 | Myotome: C2 | 279 | | | |
| CE-21h, CE-20f | D2-0203 | Myotome: C3 | 280 | | | |
| CE-21h, CE-20f | D2-0203 | Myotome: C4 | 281 | | | |
| CE-21h, CE-20f | D2-0203 | Myotome: C5 | 282 | | | |
| CE-21h, CE-20f | D2-0203 | Myotome: C6 | 283 | | | |
| CE-21h, CE-20f | D2-0203 | Myotome: C7 | 284 | | | |
| CE-21h, CE-20f | D2-0203 | Myotome: C8 | 285 | | | |
| CE-21h, CE-20f | D2-0203 | Myotome: T1 | 286 | | | |
| NATA EC 5th | BOC RD6 | Reflex Testing | Page # | | | |
| CE-21h, CE-20f | D2-0203 | Reflex Testing: C5 | 287 | | | |
| CE-21h, CE-20f | D2-0203 | Reflex Testing: C6 | 288 | | | |
| CE-21h, CE-20f | D2-0203 | Reflex Testing: C7 | 289 | | | |

## MUSCULOSKELETAL SYSTEM—REGION 6: CERVICAL SPINE
## PALPATION

| NATA EC 5th | BOC RD6 | SKILL |
|---|---|---|
| CE-21b, CE-20c | D2-0202 | Palpation: Cervical Spine – 01 |

**Supplies Needed:** Table

*This problem allows you the opportunity to demonstrate your ability to* **palpate** *the* **cervical spine**. *You have 2 minutes to complete this task.*

| Palpation: Cervical Spine – 01 | Course or Site<br>Assessor<br>Environment | | | | | |
|---|---|---|---|---|---|---|
| | | Test 1 | | Test 2 | | Test 3 |
| | | Y | N | Y | N | Y | N |
| Spinous processes of C3-C4 | | ○ | ○ | ○ | ○ | ○ | ○ |
| Middle scalene muscles | | ○ | ○ | ○ | ○ | ○ | ○ |
| Ligamentum nuchae | | ○ | ○ | ○ | ○ | ○ | ○ |
| Origin of upper trapezius muscle | | ○ | ○ | ○ | ○ | ○ | ○ |
| Interspinalis | | ○ | ○ | ○ | ○ | ◉ | ○ |
| Transverse processes of C6-C7 | | ○ | ○ | ○ | ○ | ○ | ○ |
| Supraspinous ligament of C4-C5 | | ○ | ○ | ○ | ○ | ○ | ○ |
| **Total** | | __/7 | | __/7 | | __/7 |
| **Must achieve >4 to pass this examination** | | ⓟ | Ⓕ | ⓟ | Ⓕ | ⓟ | Ⓕ |

| Assessor:<br>Date: | Test 1 Comments: |
|---|---|
| Assessor:<br>Date: | Test 2 Comments: |
| Assessor:<br>Date: | Test 3 Comments: |

**TEST ENVIRONMENTS**
**L:** Laboratory/Classroom
**C:** Clinical/Field Testing
**P:** Practicum
**A:** Assessment/Mock Exam

**TEST INFORMATION**
**Test Statistics:** N/A
**Reference(s):** Starkey & Brown (2015)

## MUSCULOSKELETAL SYSTEM—REGION 6: CERVICAL SPINE
# PALPATION

| NATA EC 5th | BOC RD6 | SKILL |
|---|---|---|
| CE-21b, CE-20c | D2-0202 | Palpation: Cervical Spine – 02 |

**Supplies Needed:** Table

*This problem allows you the opportunity to demonstrate your ability to* **palpate** *the* **cervical spine**. *You have 2 minutes to complete this task.*

| Palpation: Cervical Spine – 02 | Course or Site<br>Assessor<br>Environment | | | | | |
|---|---|---|---|---|---|---|
| | | Test 1 | | Test 2 | | Test 3 |
| | | Y | N | Y | N | Y | N |
| Insertion of upper trapezius muscle | | O | O | O | O | O | O |
| Spinous processes of atlas | | O | O | O | O | O | O |
| Intertransversarii muscle | | O | O | O | O | O | O |
| Supraspinous ligament of C6-C7 | | O | O | O | O | O | O |
| Transverse processes of C3-C4 | | O | O | O | O | O | O |
| Anterior scalene muscles | | O | O | O | O | O | O |
| Rotator muscles | | O | O | O | O | O | O |
| **Total** | | __/7 | | __/7 | | __/7 | |
| **Must achieve >4 to pass this examination** | | (P) | (F) | (P) | (F) | (P) | (F) |
| Assessor:<br>Date: | Test 1 Comments: | | | | | | |
| Assessor:<br>Date: | Test 2 Comments: | | | | | | |
| Assessor:<br>Date: | Test 3 Comments: | | | | | | |

**TEST ENVIRONMENTS**
L: Laboratory/Classroom
C: Clinical/Field Testing
P: Practicum
A: Assessment/Mock Exam

**TEST INFORMATION**
**Test Statistics:** N/A
**Reference(s):** Starkey & Brown (2015)

## MUSCULOSKELETAL SYSTEM—REGION 6: CERVICAL SPINE
# PALPATION

| NATA EC 5th | BOC RD6 | SKILL |
|---|---|---|
| CE-21b, CE-20c | D2-0202 | Palpation: Cervical Spine – 03 |

**Supplies Needed:** Table

*This problem allows you the opportunity to demonstrate your ability to **palpate** the **cervical spine**. You have 2 minutes to complete this task.*

| Palpation: Cervical Spine – 03 | Course or Site Assessor Environment | Test 1 | | Test 2 | | Test 3 | |
|---|---|---|---|---|---|---|---|
| | | Y | N | Y | N | Y | N |
| Multifidi muscles | | ○ | ○ | ○ | ○ | ○ | ○ |
| Spinous processes of C6-C7 | | ○ | ○ | ○ | ○ | ○ | ○ |
| Origin of lower trapezius | | ○ | ○ | ○ | ○ | ○ | ○ |
| Transverse processes of C2-C3 | | ○ | ○ | ○ | ○ | ○ | ○ |
| Insertion of splenius cervicis muscle | | ○ | ○ | ○ | ○ | ○ | ○ |
| Oblique capitis inferior muscle | | ○ | ○ | ○ | ○ | ○ | ○ |
| Supraspinous ligament of C4-C5 | | ○ | ○ | ○ | ○ | ○ | ○ |
| | Total | ___/7 | | ___/7 | | ___/7 | |
| Must achieve >4 to pass this examination | | Ⓟ | Ⓕ | Ⓟ | Ⓕ | Ⓟ | Ⓕ |
| **Assessor:** **Date:** | **Test 1 Comments:** | | | | | | |
| **Assessor:** **Date:** | **Test 2 Comments:** | | | | | | |
| **Assessor:** **Date:** | **Test 3 Comments:** | | | | | | |

**TEST ENVIRONMENTS**
**L:** Laboratory/Classroom
**C:** Clinical/Field Testing
**P:** Practicum
**A:** Assessment/Mock Exam

**TEST INFORMATION**
**Test Statistics:** N/A
**Reference(s):** Starkey & Brown (2015)

## MUSCULOSKELETAL SYSTEM—REGION 6: CERVICAL SPINE
# MANUAL MUSCLE TESTING

| NATA EC 5th | BOC RD6 | SKILL |
|---|---|---|
| CE-21c | D2-0203 | MMT: Cervical Extension (Sternocleidomastoid/Upper Trapezius) |

**Supplies Needed:** Table

*This problem allows you the opportunity to demonstrate a* **manual muscle test** *for* **cervical extension**. *You have 2 minutes to complete this task.*

| MMT: Cervical Extension (Sternocleidomastoid/Upper Trapezius) | Course or Site _____ Assessor _____ Environment _____ | | | | | |
|---|---|---|---|---|---|---|
| | | Test 1 | | Test 2 | | Test 3 |
| **Tester places patient and limbs in appropriate position** | | Y | N | Y | N | Y | N |
| Prone, shoulders abducted to 90 degrees, elbows flexed to 90 degrees | | ○ | ○ | ○ | ○ | ○ | ○ |
| Cervical spine and head in neutral position | | ○ | ○ | ○ | ○ | ○ | ○ |
| **Tester placed in proper position** | | Y | N | Y | N | Y | N |
| Stands on side of the patient with hand on the back of the head | | ○ | ○ | ○ | ○ | ○ | ○ |
| **Tester performs test according to accepted guidelines** | | Y | N | Y | N | Y | N |
| Instructs the patient to extend head against pressure | | ○ | ○ | ○ | ○ | ○ | ○ |
| Resistance is applied anteriorly | | ○ | ○ | ○ | ○ | ○ | ○ |
| Resistance is held for 5 seconds | | ○ | ○ | ○ | ○ | ○ | ○ |
| **Identifies implications** | | Y | N | Y | N | Y | N |
| Correctly grades the MMT | | ○ | ○ | ○ | ○ | ○ | ○ |
| Total | | ___/7 | | ___/7 | | ___/7 | |
| Must achieve >4 to pass this examination | | Ⓟ | Ⓕ | Ⓟ | Ⓕ | Ⓟ | Ⓕ |

| Assessor: Date: | Test 1 Comments: |
|---|---|
| Assessor: Date: | Test 2 Comments: |
| Assessor: Date: | Test 3 Comments: |

**TEST ENVIRONMENTS**
**L:** Laboratory/Classroom
**C:** Clinical/Field Testing
**P:** Practicum
**A:** Assessment/Mock Exam

**TEST INFORMATION**
**Test Statistics:** N/A
**Reference(s):** Kendall et al. (2005)
Starkey & Brown (2015)

MUSCULOSKELETAL SYSTEM—REGION 6: CERVICAL SPINE
# MANUAL MUSCLE TESTING

| NATA EC 5th | BOC RD6 | SKILL |
|---|---|---|
| CE-21c | D2-0203 | MMT: Cervical Flexion (Sternocleidomastoid/Scalenus Anterior) |

**Supplies Needed:** Table

*This problem allows you the opportunity to demonstrate a* **manual muscle test** *for* **cervical flexion**. *You have 2 minutes to complete this task.*

| MMT: Cervical Flexion (Sternocleidomastoid/Scalenus Anterior) | Course or Site Assessor Environment | Test 1 | | Test 2 | | Test 3 | |
|---|---|---|---|---|---|---|---|
| **Tester places patient and limbs in appropriate position** | | **Y** | **N** | **Y** | **N** | **Y** | **N** |
| Supine with shoulders abducted to 90 degrees and elbows flexed to 90 degrees | | ○ | ○ | ○ | ○ | ○ | ○ |
| Cervical spine and head in neutral position | | ○ | ○ | ○ | ○ | ○ | ○ |
| **Tester placed in proper position** | | **Y** | **N** | **Y** | **N** | **Y** | **N** |
| Stands to the side of the patient with one hand on the forehead and one hand on the chest | | ○ | ○ | ○ | ○ | ○ | ○ |
| **Tester performs test according to accepted guidelines** | | **Y** | **N** | **Y** | **N** | **Y** | **N** |
| Instructs the patient to tuck chin and completely flex neck | | ○ | ○ | ○ | ○ | ○ | ○ |
| Applies resistance to forehead | | ○ | ○ | ○ | ○ | ○ | ○ |
| Resistance is held for 5 seconds | | ○ | ○ | ○ | ○ | ○ | ○ |
| **Identifies implications** | | **Y** | **N** | **Y** | **N** | **Y** | **N** |
| Correctly grades the MMT | | ○ | ○ | ○ | ○ | ○ | ○ |
| | Total | ___/7 | | ___/7 | | ___/7 | |
| | Must achieve >4 to pass this examination | Ⓟ | Ⓕ | Ⓟ | Ⓕ | Ⓟ | Ⓕ |

| Assessor: Date: | Test 1 Comments: |
|---|---|
| Assessor: Date: | Test 2 Comments: |
| Assessor: Date: | Test 3 Comments: |

**TEST ENVIRONMENTS**
**L:** Laboratory/Classroom
**C:** Clinical/Field Testing
**P:** Practicum
**A:** Assessment/Mock Exam

**TEST INFORMATION**
**Test Statistics:** N/A
**Reference(s):** Kendall et al. (2005)
Starkey & Brown (2015)

## MUSCULOSKELETAL SYSTEM—REGION 6: CERVICAL SPINE
# MANUAL MUSCLE TESTING

| NATA EC 5th | BOC RD6 | SKILL |
|---|---|---|
| CE-21c | D2-0203 | MMT: Cervical Lateral Flexion (Sternocleidomastoid/Scalenus Anterior/Scalenus Medius/Scalenus Posterior/Upper Trapezius) |

**Supplies Needed:** Table

*This problem allows you the opportunity to demonstrate a* **manual muscle test** *for* **cervical lateral flexion.** *You have 2 minutes to complete this task.*

| MMT: Cervical Lateral Flexion (Sternocleidomastoid/Scalenus Anterior/Scalenus Medius/Scalenus Posterior/Upper Trapezius) | Course or Site Assessor Environment | | Test 1 | | Test 2 | | Test 3 | |
|---|---|---|---|---|---|---|---|---|
| **Tester places patient and limbs in appropriate position** | | **Y** | **N** | **Y** | **N** | **Y** | **N** | |
| Seated on table, legs over side of table | | ○ | ○ | ○ | ○ | ○ | ○ | |
| Cervical spine and head in neutral position | | ○ | ○ | ○ | ○ | ○ | ○ | |
| **Tester placed in proper position** | | **Y** | **N** | **Y** | **N** | **Y** | **N** | |
| Stands behind or next to the patient | | ○ | ○ | ○ | ○ | ○ | ○ | |
| Places one hand on the side of the head being tested and one hand on the same side shoulder | | ○ | ○ | ○ | ○ | ○ | ○ | |
| **Tester performs test according to accepted guidelines** | | **Y** | **N** | **Y** | **N** | **Y** | **N** | |
| Instructs the patient to bring ear to shoulder | | ○ | ○ | ○ | ○ | ○ | ○ | |
| Applies resistance over temporal and parietal bones | | ○ | ○ | ○ | ○ | ○ | ○ | |
| Resistance is held for 5 seconds | | ○ | ○ | ○ | ○ | ○ | ○ | |
| Performs assessment bilaterally | | ○ | ○ | ○ | ○ | ○ | ○ | |
| **Identifies implications** | | **Y** | **N** | **Y** | **N** | **Y** | **N** | |
| Correctly grades the MMT | | ○ | ○ | ○ | ○ | ○ | ○ | |
| **Total** | | _____/9 | | _____/9 | | _____/9 | | |
| **Must achieve >6 to pass this examination** | | Ⓟ | Ⓕ | Ⓟ | Ⓕ | Ⓟ | Ⓕ | |

| **Assessor:** **Date:** | **Test 1 Comments:** |
|---|---|
| **Assessor:** **Date:** | **Test 2 Comments:** |
| **Assessor:** **Date:** | **Test 3 Comments:** |

**TEST ENVIRONMENTS**
**L:** Laboratory/Classroom
**C:** Clinical/Field Testing
**P:** Practicum
**A:** Assessment/Mock Exam

**TEST INFORMATION**
**Test Statistics:** N/A
**Reference(s):** Kendall et al. (2005)
Starkey & Brown (2015)

## MUSCULOSKELETAL SYSTEM—REGION 6: CERVICAL SPINE
# MANUAL MUSCLE TESTING

| NATA EC 5th | BOC RD6 | SKILL |
|---|---|---|
| CE-21c | D2-0203 | MMT: Cervical Rotation (Sternocleidomastoid/ Scalenus Anterior/Scalenus Medius/ Scalenus Posterior/Upper Trapezius) |

**Supplies Needed:** Table

*This problem allows you the opportunity to demonstrate a* **manual muscle test** *for* **cervical rotation**. *You have 2 minutes to complete this task.*

| MMT: Cervical Rotation (Sternocleidomastoid/Scalenus Anterior/Scalenus Medius/ Scalenus Posterior/Upper Trapezius) | Course or Site Assessor Environment | | | | | | |
|---|---|---|---|---|---|---|---|
| | | Test 1 | | Test 2 | | Test 3 | |
| **Tester places patient and limbs in appropriate position** | | **Y** | **N** | **Y** | **N** | **Y** | **N** |
| Supine with shoulders abducted to 90 degrees and elbows flexed to 90 degrees | | ○ | ○ | ○ | ○ | ○ | ○ |
| The patient starts with head rotated to side opposite being tested | | ○ | ○ | ○ | ○ | ○ | ○ |
| **Tester placed in proper position** | | **Y** | **N** | **Y** | **N** | **Y** | **N** |
| Stands next to the patient | | ○ | ○ | ○ | ○ | ○ | ○ |
| Places one hand over the sternum and one hand over the temporal bone | | ○ | ○ | ○ | ○ | ○ | ○ |
| **Tester performs test according to accepted guidelines** | | **Y** | **N** | **Y** | **N** | **Y** | **N** |
| Instructs the patient to rotate head back toward midline, against resistance | | ○ | ○ | ○ | ○ | ○ | ○ |
| Applies resistance over temporal bone | | ○ | ○ | ○ | ○ | ○ | ○ |
| Resistance is held for 5 seconds | | ○ | ○ | ○ | ○ | ○ | ○ |
| Performs assessment bilaterally | | ○ | ○ | ○ | ○ | ○ | ○ |
| **Identifies implications** | | **Y** | **N** | **Y** | **N** | **Y** | **N** |
| Correctly grades the MMT | | ○ | ○ | ○ | ○ | ○ | ○ |
| Total | | ___/9 | | ___/9 | | ___/9 | |
| Must achieve >6 to pass this examination | | Ⓟ | Ⓕ | Ⓟ | Ⓕ | Ⓟ | Ⓕ |
| Assessor: Date: | Test 1 Comments: | | | | | | |
| Assessor: Date: | Test 2 Comments: | | | | | | |
| Assessor: Date: | Test 3 Comments: | | | | | | |

**TEST ENVIRONMENTS**
**L:** Laboratory/Classroom
**C:** Clinical/Field Testing
**P:** Practicum
**A:** Assessment/Mock Exam

**TEST INFORMATION**
**Test Statistics:** N/A
**Reference(s):** Kendall et al. (2005)
Starkey & Brown (2015)

MUSCULOSKELETAL SYSTEM—REGION 6: CERVICAL SPINE
# OSTEOKINEMATIC JOINT MOTION

| NATA EC 5th | BOC RD6 | SKILL |
|---|---|---|
| CE-21d | D2-0203 | Goniometric Assessment: Cervical Spine (Extension) |

**Supplies Needed:** Chair, two inclinometers

*This problem allows you the opportunity to demonstrate a* **goniometric assessment** *for the* **cervical spine (extension)**. *You have 2 minutes to complete this task.*

| Goniometric Assessment: Cervical Spine (Extension) | Course or Site Assessor Environment _____ _____ _____ | | | | | |
|---|---|---|---|---|---|---|
| | | Test 1 | | Test 2 | | Test 3 |
| **Tester places patient in appropriate position** | | Y | N | Y | N | Y | N |
| Seated with back well supported by back of chair | | ○ | ○ | ○ | ○ | ○ | ○ |
| Cervical spine in 0 degrees of rotation and lateral flexion | | ○ | ○ | ○ | ○ | ○ | ○ |
| **Tester and goniometer placed in proper position** | | Y | N | Y | N | Y | N |
| Places one hand on the back of the patient's head | | ○ | ○ | ○ | ○ | ○ | ○ |
| Places center of fulcrum over the external auditory meatus | | ○ | ○ | ○ | ○ | ○ | ○ |
| Stationary arm perpendicular or parallel to the ground | | ○ | ○ | ○ | ○ | ○ | ○ |
| Align moving arm with base of nose | | ○ | ○ | ○ | ○ | ○ | ○ |
| **Tester performs test according to accepted guidelines** | | Y | N | Y | N | Y | N |
| Instructs the patient to extend the head as far as possible | | ○ | ○ | ○ | ○ | ○ | ○ |
| Once the patient reaches end range, the tester takes proper goniometric measurement | | ○ | ○ | ○ | ○ | ○ | ○ |
| **Identifies implications** | | Y | N | Y | N | Y | N |
| Identifies normal ranges (cervical extension = 50 degrees) | | ○ | ○ | ○ | ○ | ○ | ○ |
| Total | | ___/9 | | ___/9 | | ___/9 | |
| **Must achieve >6 to pass this examination** | | Ⓟ | Ⓕ | Ⓟ | Ⓕ | Ⓟ | Ⓕ |

| Assessor: Date: | Test 1 Comments: |
|---|---|
| Assessor: Date: | Test 2 Comments: |
| Assessor: Date: | Test 3 Comments: |

**TEST ENVIRONMENTS**
**L:** Laboratory/Classroom
**C:** Clinical/Field Testing
**P:** Practicum
**A:** Assessment/Mock Exam

**TEST INFORMATION**
**Test Statistics:** N/A
**Reference(s):** Norkin & White (2009)

# OSTEOKINEMATIC JOINT MOTION

| NATA EC 5th | BOC RD6 | SKILL |
|---|---|---|
| CE-21d | D2-0203 | Goniometric Assessment: Cervical Spine (Flexion) |

**Supplies Needed:** Chair, two inclinometers

*This problem allows you the opportunity to demonstrate a* **goniometric assessment** *for the* **cervical spine (flexion)**. *You have 2 minutes to complete this task.*

| Goniometric Assessment: Cervical Spine (Flexion) | Course or Site Assessor Environment ___ ___ ___ | | Test 1 | | Test 2 | | Test 3 | |
|---|---|---|---|---|---|---|---|---|
| **Tester places patient in appropriate position** | | | **Y** | **N** | **Y** | **N** | **Y** | **N** |
| Seated with back well supported by back of chair | | | ○ | ○ | ○ | ○ | ○ | ○ |
| Cervical spine in 0 degrees of rotation and lateral flexion | | | ○ | ○ | ○ | ○ | ○ | ○ |
| **Tester and goniometer placed in proper position** | | | **Y** | **N** | **Y** | **N** | **Y** | **N** |
| Stands on the side of the patient | | | ○ | ○ | ○ | ○ | ○ | ○ |
| Places center of fulcrum over the external auditory meatus | | | ○ | ○ | ○ | ○ | ○ | ○ |
| Stationary arm perpendicular or parallel to the ground | | | ○ | ○ | ○ | ○ | ○ | ○ |
| Align moving arm with base of nose | | | ○ | ○ | ○ | ○ | ○ | ○ |
| **Tester performs test according to accepted guidelines** | | | **Y** | **N** | **Y** | **N** | **Y** | **N** |
| Instructs the patient to bend the head forward as far as possible, chin to chest | | | ○ | ○ | ○ | ○ | ○ | ○ |
| Once the patient reaches end range, the tester takes proper goniometric measurement | | | ○ | ○ | ○ | ○ | ○ | ○ |
| **Identifies implications** | | | **Y** | **N** | **Y** | **N** | **Y** | **N** |
| Identifies normal ranges (cervical flexion = 40 degrees) | | | ○ | ○ | ○ | ○ | ○ | ○ |
| Total | | | ___/9 | | ___/9 | | ___/9 | |
| Must achieve >6 to pass this examination | | | Ⓟ | Ⓕ | Ⓟ | Ⓕ | Ⓟ | Ⓕ |

| Assessor: Date: | Test 1 Comments: |
|---|---|
| Assessor: Date: | Test 2 Comments: |
| Assessor: Date: | Test 3 Comments: |

**TEST ENVIRONMENTS**
**L:** Laboratory/Classroom
**C:** Clinical/Field Testing
**P:** Practicum
**A:** Assessment/Mock Exam

**TEST INFORMATION**
**Test Statistics:** N/A
**Reference(s):** Norkin & White (2009)

MUSCULOSKELETAL SYSTEM—REGION 6: CERVICAL SPINE
# OSTEOKINEMATIC JOINT MOTION

| NATA EC 5th | BOC RD6 | SKILL |
|---|---|---|
| CE-21d | D2-0203 | Goniometric Assessment: Cervical Spine (Lateral Flexion Left) |

**Supplies Needed:** Table, two inclinometers

*This problem allows you the opportunity to demonstrate a* **goniometric assessment** *for the* **cervical spine (lateral flexion left)**. *You have 2 minutes to complete this task*

| Goniometric Assessment: Cervical Spine (Lateral Flexion Left) | Course or Site Assessor Environment | | Test 1 | | Test 2 | | Test 3 | |
|---|---|---|---|---|---|---|---|---|
| | | | Y | N | Y | N | Y | N |
| **Tester places patient in appropriate position** | | | Y | N | Y | N | Y | N |
| Seated upright | | | O | O | O | O | O | O |
| Cervical spine in 0 degrees on flexion, extension, and rotation | | | O | O | O | O | O | O |
| **Tester and goniometer placed in proper position** | | | Y | N | Y | N | Y | N |
| Tester stands behind the patient | | | O | O | O | O | O | O |
| Places center of fulcrum over the spinous process of C7 | | | O | O | O | O | O | O |
| Stationary arm perpendicular to the ground | | | O | O | O | O | O | O |
| Align moving arm with dorsal midline of the head | | | O | O | O | O | O | O |
| **Tester performs test according to accepted guidelines** | | | Y | N | Y | N | Y | N |
| Instructs the patient to laterally bend the head to the left, ear to shoulder | | | O | O | O | O | O | O |
| Once the patient reaches end range, the tester takes proper goniometric measurement | | | O | O | O | O | O | O |
| **Identifies implications** | | | Y | N | Y | N | Y | N |
| Identifies normal ranges (cervical lateral flexion left = 22 degrees) | | | O | O | O | O | O | O |
| Total | | | ___/9 | | ___/9 | | ___/9 | |
| Must achieve >6 to pass this examination | | | Ⓟ | Ⓕ | Ⓟ | Ⓕ | Ⓟ | Ⓕ |

| Assessor: Date: | Test 1 Comments: |
|---|---|
| Assessor: Date: | Test 2 Comments: |
| Assessor: Date: | Test 3 Comments: |

**TEST ENVIRONMENTS**
**L:** Laboratory/Classroom
**C:** Clinical/Field Testing
**P:** Practicum
**A:** Assessment/Mock Exam

**TEST INFORMATION**
**Test Statistics:** N/A
**Reference(s):** Norkin & White (2009)

## MUSCULOSKELETAL SYSTEM—REGION 6: CERVICAL SPINE
# OSTEOKINEMATIC JOINT MOTION

| NATA EC 5th | BOC RD6 | SKILL |
|---|---|---|
| CE-21d | D2-0203 | Goniometric Assessment: Cervical Spine (Lateral Flexion Right) |

**Supplies Needed:** Table, two inclinometers

*This problem allows you the opportunity to demonstrate a* **goniometric assessment** *for the* **cervical spine (lateral flexion right)**. *You have 2 minutes to complete this task.*

| Goniometric Assessment: Cervical Spine (Lateral Flexion Right) | Course or Site Assessor Environment | | Test 1 | | Test 2 | | Test 3 | |
|---|---|---|---|---|---|---|---|---|
| **Tester places patient in appropriate position** | | **Y** | **N** | **Y** | **N** | **Y** | **N** | |
| Seated upright, feet on the floor | | O | O | O | O | O | O | |
| Cervical spine in 0 degrees on flexion, extension, and rotation | | O | O | O | O | O | O | |
| **Tester and goniometer placed in proper position** | | **Y** | **N** | **Y** | **N** | **Y** | **N** | |
| Stands behind the patient | | O | O | O | O | O | O | |
| Places the center of fulcrum over the spinous process of C7 | | O | O | O | O | O | O | |
| Stationary arm perpendicular to the ground | | O | O | O | O | O | O | |
| Align moving arm with dorsal midline of the head | | O | O | O | O | O | O | |
| **Tester performs test according to accepted guidelines** | | **Y** | **N** | **Y** | **N** | **Y** | **N** | |
| Instructs the patient to laterally bend the head to the right, ear to shoulder | | O | O | O | O | O | O | |
| Once the patient reaches end range, the tester takes proper goniometric measurement | | O | O | O | O | O | O | |
| **Identifies implications** | | **Y** | **N** | **Y** | **N** | **Y** | **N** | |
| Identifies normal ranges (cervical lateral flexion right = 22 degrees) | | O | O | O | O | O | O | |
| **Total** | | ___/9 | | ___/9 | | ___/9 | | |
| **Must achieve >6 to pass this examination** | | Ⓟ | Ⓕ | Ⓟ | Ⓕ | Ⓟ | Ⓕ | |

| Assessor: Date: | Test 1 Comments: |
|---|---|
| Assessor: Date: | Test 2 Comments: |
| Assessor: Date: | Test 3 Comments: |

**TEST ENVIRONMENTS**
**L:** Laboratory/Classroom
**C:** Clinical/Field Testing
**P:** Practicum
**A:** Assessment/Mock Exam

**TEST INFORMATION**
**Test Statistics:** N/A
**Reference(s):** Norkin & White (2009)

MUSCULOSKELETAL SYSTEM—REGION 6: CERVICAL SPINE
# OSTEOKINEMATIC JOINT MOTION

| NATA EC 5th | BOC RD6 | SKILL |
|---|---|---|
| CE-21d | D2-0203 | Goniometric Assessment: Cervical Spine (Rotation Left) |

**Supplies Needed:** Chair, large goniometer

*This problem allows you the opportunity to demonstrate a* **goniometric assessment** *for the* **cervical spine (rotation left)**. *You have 2 minutes to complete this task.*

| Goniometric Assessment: Cervical Spine (Rotation Left) | Course or Site Assessor Environment | Test 1 | | Test 2 | | Test 3 | |
|---|---|---|---|---|---|---|---|
| **Tester places patient in appropriate position** | | **Y** | **N** | **Y** | **N** | **Y** | **N** |
| Seated with back well supported by back of chair | | O | O | O | O | O | O |
| Cervical spine in 0 degrees of flexion, extension, and lateral flexion | | O | O | O | O | O | O |
| **Tester and goniometer placed in proper position** | | **Y** | **N** | **Y** | **N** | **Y** | **N** |
| Stands behind the patient | | O | O | O | O | O | O |
| Places center of fulcrum over the center of cranial aspect of head | | O | O | O | O | O | O |
| Stationary arm parallel to an imaginary line between the two acromial processes | | O | O | O | O | O | O |
| Align moving arm with tip of the nose | | O | O | O | O | O | O |
| **Tester performs test according to accepted guidelines** | | **Y** | **N** | **Y** | **N** | **Y** | **N** |
| Instructs the patient to turn head to the left as far as possible, look over left shoulder | | O | O | O | O | O | O |
| Once the patient reaches end range, the tester takes proper goniometric measurement | | O | O | O | O | O | O |
| **Identifies implications** | | **Y** | **N** | **Y** | **N** | **Y** | **N** |
| Identifies normal ranges (cervical rotation left = 49 degrees) | | O | O | O | O | O | O |
| **Total** | | ___/9 | | ___/9 | | ___/9 | |
| **Must achieve >6 to pass this examination** | | Ⓟ | Ⓕ | Ⓟ | Ⓕ | Ⓟ | Ⓕ |

| Assessor: Date: | Test 1 Comments: |
|---|---|
| Assessor: Date: | Test 2 Comments: |
| Assessor: Date: | Test 3 Comments: |

**TEST ENVIRONMENTS**
**L:** Laboratory/Classroom
**C:** Clinical/Field Testing
**P:** Practicum
**A:** Assessment/Mock Exam

**TEST INFORMATION**
**Test Statistics:** N/A
**Reference(s):** Norkin & White (2009)

## MUSCULOSKELETAL SYSTEM—REGION 6: CERVICAL SPINE
# OSTEOKINEMATIC JOINT MOTION

| NATA EC 5th | BOC RD6 | SKILL |
|:---:|:---:|:---:|
| CE-21d | D2-0203 | Goniometric Assessment: Cervical Spine (Rotation Right) |

**Supplies Needed:** Chair, large goniometer

*This problem allows you the opportunity to demonstrate a* **goniometric assessment** *for the* **cervical spine (rotation right)**. *You have 2 minutes to complete this task.*

| Goniometric Assessment: Cervical Spine (Rotation Right) | Course or Site Assessor Environment | | Test 1 | | Test 2 | | Test 3 | |
|---|---|---|:---:|:---:|:---:|:---:|:---:|:---:|
| | | | **Y** | **N** | **Y** | **N** | **Y** | **N** |
| **Tester places patient in appropriate position** | | | **Y** | **N** | **Y** | **N** | **Y** | **N** |
| Seated with back well supported by back of chair | | | O | O | O | O | O | O |
| Cervical spine in 0 degrees of flexion, extension, and lateral flexion | | | O | O | O | O | O | O |
| **Tester and goniometer placed in proper position** | | | **Y** | **N** | **Y** | **N** | **Y** | **N** |
| Stands behind the patient | | | O | O | O | O | O | O |
| Places center of fulcrum over the center of cranial aspect of head | | | O | O | O | O | O | O |
| Stationary arm parallel to an imaginary line between the two acromial processes | | | O | O | O | O | O | O |
| Align moving arm with tip of the nose | | | O | O | O | O | O | O |
| **Tester performs test according to accepted guidelines** | | | **Y** | **N** | **Y** | **N** | **Y** | **N** |
| Instructs the patient to turn head to the right as far as possible, look over right shoulder | | | O | O | O | O | O | O |
| Once the patient reaches end range, the tester takes proper goniometric measurement | | | O | O | O | O | O | O |
| **Identifies implications** | | | **Y** | **N** | **Y** | **N** | **Y** | **N** |
| Identifies normal ranges (cervical rotation right = 51 degrees) | | | O | O | O | O | O | O |
| Total | | | ___/9 | | ___/9 | | ___/9 | |
| Must achieve >6 to pass this examination | | | Ⓟ | Ⓕ | Ⓟ | Ⓕ | Ⓟ | Ⓕ |

| Assessor: Date: | Test 1 Comments: |
|---|---|
| Assessor: Date: | Test 2 Comments: |
| Assessor: Date: | Test 3 Comments: |

**TEST ENVIRONMENTS**
**L:** Laboratory/Classroom
**C:** Clinical/Field Testing
**P:** Practicum
**A:** Assessment/Mock Exam

**TEST INFORMATION**
**Test Statistics:** N/A
**Reference(s):** Norkin & White (2009)

MUSCULOSKELETAL SYSTEM—REGION 6: CERVICAL SPINE
# SPECIAL TESTS

| NATA EC 5th | BOC RD6 | SKILL |
|---|---|---|
| CE-21g, CE-20e | D2-0203 | Adson's Test |

**Supplies Needed:** Table

*This problem allows you the opportunity to demonstrate an* **orthopedic test** *known as* **Adson's test** *to rule out* **thoracic outlet syndrome***. You have 2 minutes to complete this task.*

| Adson's Test | Course or Site Assessor Environment | | | | | |
|---|---|---|---|---|---|---|
| | Test 1 | | Test 2 | | Test 3 | |
| **Tester places patient and limb in appropriate position** | Y | N | Y | N | Y | N |
| Seated with knees off the table | O | O | O | O | O | O |
| Humerus external rotation, shoulder abducted to 30 degrees, elbow extended with thumb pointing upward | O | O | O | O | O | O |
| **Tester placed in proper position** | Y | N | Y | N | Y | N |
| Behind the patient | O | O | O | O | O | O |
| Palpating the radial pulse on the testing side | O | O | O | O | O | O |
| **Tester performs test according to accepted guidelines** | Y | N | Y | N | Y | N |
| While maintaining a feel for the radial pulse, the tester externally rotates and extends the patient's shoulder | O | O | O | O | O | O |
| The patient is instructed to turn (rotate his/her face) to the same side and inhale deeply and hold the breath | O | O | O | O | O | O |
| **Identifies positive findings and implications** | Y | N | Y | N | Y | N |
| The radial pulse disappears or markedly diminishes as compared to the opposite side | O | O | O | O | O | O |
| Subclavian artery is being occluded between the anterior and middle scalene muscles and the pectoralis minor | O | O | O | O | O | O |
| Total | __/8 | | __/8 | | __/8 | |
| **Must achieve >5 to pass this examination** | Ⓟ | Ⓕ | Ⓟ | Ⓕ | Ⓟ | Ⓕ |

| Assessor: Date: | Test 1 Comments: |
|---|---|
| Assessor: Date: | Test 2 Comments: |
| Assessor: Date: | Test 3 Comments: |

**TEST ENVIRONMENTS**
**L:** Laboratory/Classroom
**C:** Clinical/Field Testing
**P:** Practicum
**A:** Assessment/Mock Exam

**TEST INFORMATION**
**Test Statistics:** Sensitivity .94
Specificity .18–.87
(+) LR 3.2
(-) LR .28
**Reference(s):** Malanga, Landes, et al. (2003)
Starkey & Brown (2015)

## MUSCULOSKELETAL SYSTEM—REGION 6: CERVICAL SPINE
## SPECIAL TESTS

| NATA EC 5th | BOC RD6 | SKILL |
|---|---|---|
| CE-21g, CE-20e | D2-0203 | Allen's Test |

**Supplies Needed:** Table or chair

*This problem allows you the opportunity to demonstrate an* **orthopedic test** *known as* **Allen's test** *to rule out* **thoracic outlet syndrome***. You have 2 minutes to complete this task.*

| Allen's Test | Course or Site Assessor Environment | | Test 1 | | Test 2 | | Test 3 | |
|---|---|---|---|---|---|---|---|---|
| **Tester places patient and limb in appropriate position** | | **Y** | **N** | **Y** | **N** | **Y** | **N** | |
| Seated, head facing forward | | ○ | ○ | ○ | ○ | ○ | ○ | |
| **Tester placed in proper position** | | **Y** | **N** | **Y** | **N** | **Y** | **N** | |
| Stands behind the patient | | ○ | ○ | ○ | ○ | ○ | ○ | |
| One hand positioned so that the radial pulse is felt | | ○ | ○ | ○ | ○ | ○ | ○ | |
| **Tester performs test according to accepted guidelines** | | **Y** | **N** | **Y** | **N** | **Y** | **N** | |
| Elbow is passively flexed to 90 degrees and shoulder is abducted to 90 degrees | | ○ | ○ | ○ | ○ | ○ | ○ | |
| Shoulder is passively horizontally abducted and placed into external rotation | | ○ | ○ | ○ | ○ | ○ | ○ | |
| The patient then rotates the head toward the opposite shoulder | | ○ | ○ | ○ | ○ | ○ | ○ | |
| **Identifies positive findings and implications** | | **Y** | **N** | **Y** | **N** | **Y** | **N** | |
| The radial pulse disappears or reproduction of neurologic symptoms | | ○ | ○ | ○ | ○ | ○ | ○ | |
| The pectoralis minor is compressing the neurovascular bundle | | ○ | ○ | ○ | ○ | ○ | ○ | |
| **Total** | | __/8 | | __/8 | | __/8 | | |
| **Must achieve >5 to pass this examination** | | Ⓟ | Ⓕ | Ⓟ | Ⓕ | Ⓟ | Ⓕ | |

| Assessor:<br>Date: | Test 1 Comments: |
|---|---|
| Assessor:<br>Date: | Test 2 Comments: |
| Assessor:<br>Date: | Test 3 Comments: |

**TEST ENVIRONMENTS**
**L:** Laboratory/Classroom
**C:** Clinical/Field Testing
**P:** Practicum
**A:** Assessment/Mock Exam

**TEST INFORMATION**
**Test Statistics:** No data available
**Reference(s):** Starkey & Brown (2015)

## MUSCULOSKELETAL SYSTEM—REGION 6: CERVICAL SPINE
# SPECIAL TESTS

| NATA EC 5th | BOC RD6 | SKILL |
|---|---|---|
| CE-21g, CE-20e | D2-0203 | Brachial Plexus Traction Test |

**Supplies Needed:** Table or chair

*This problem allows you the opportunity to demonstrate an* **orthopedic test** *known as the* **brachial plexus traction test** *to rule out* **brachial plexus neuropraxia**. *You have 2 minutes to complete this task.*

| Brachial Plexus Traction Test | Course or Site Assessor Environment | | Test 1 | | Test 2 | | Test 3 | |
|---|---|---|---|---|---|---|---|---|
| **Tester places patient and limb in appropriate position** | | | **Y** | **N** | **Y** | **N** | **Y** | **N** |
| Seated (if the patient is taller than the tester) or standing | | | O | O | O | O | O | O |
| **Tester placed in proper position** | | | **Y** | **N** | **Y** | **N** | **Y** | **N** |
| Stands behind the patient | | | O | O | O | O | O | O |
| **Tester performs test according to accepted guidelines** | | | **Y** | **N** | **Y** | **N** | **Y** | **N** |
| One hand is placed on the side of the patient's head | | | O | O | O | O | O | O |
| One hand is placed over the AC joint on the side being tested | | | O | O | O | O | O | O |
| The cervical spine is laterally bent away from the implicated side | | | O | O | O | O | O | O |
| The shoulder is depressed | | | O | O | O | O | O | O |
| **Identifies positive findings and implications** | | | **Y** | **N** | **Y** | **N** | **Y** | **N** |
| Reproduction of pain and/or paresthesia symptoms throughout the involved upper extremity | | | O | O | O | O | O | O |
| Brachial plexus neuropraxia | | | O | O | O | O | O | O |
| Total | | | ___/8 | | ___/8 | | ___/8 | |
| Must achieve >5 to pass this examination | | | (P) | (F) | (P) | (F) | (P) | (F) |

| Assessor:<br>Date: | Test 1 Comments: |
|---|---|
| Assessor:<br>Date: | Test 2 Comments: |
| Assessor:<br>Date: | Test 3 Comments: |

**TEST ENVIRONMENTS**
**L:** Laboratory/Classroom
**C:** Clinical/Field Testing
**P:** Practicum
**A:** Assessment/Mock Exam

**TEST INFORMATION**
**Test Statistics:** No data available
**Reference(s):** Starkey & Brown (2015)

## MUSCULOSKELETAL SYSTEM—REGION 6: CERVICAL SPINE
# SPECIAL TESTS

| NATA EC 5th | BOC RD6 | SKILL |
|---|---|---|
| CE-21g, CE-20e | D2-0203 | Cervical Compression Test |

**Supplies Needed:** Table or chair

*This problem allows you the opportunity to demonstrate an* **orthopedic test** *known as the* **cervical compression test** *to rule out a possible* **intervertebral foramen pathology.** *You have 2 minutes to complete this task.*

| Cervical Compression Test | Course or Site / Assessor / Environment | | Test 1 | | Test 2 | | Test 3 | |
|---|---|---|---|---|---|---|---|---|
| **Tester places patient and limb in appropriate position** | | | Y | N | Y | N | Y | N |
| Seated | | | O | O | O | O | O | O |
| **Tester placed in proper position** | | | Y | N | Y | N | Y | N |
| Stands behind the patient, with hands clasped over the top (crown) of the patient's head | | | O | O | O | O | O | O |
| **Tester performs test according to accepted guidelines** | | | Y | N | Y | N | Y | N |
| Presses down on the crown of the patient's head, creating an axial force | | | O | O | O | O | O | O |
| **Identifies positive findings and implications** | | | Y | N | Y | N | Y | N |
| Reproduction of symptoms in the upper cervical spine, upper extremity, or both | | | O | O | O | O | O | O |
| Compression of the facet joints and narrowing of the intervertebral foramen | | | O | O | O | O | O | O |
| Total | | | ___/5 | | ___/5 | | ___/5 | |
| **Must achieve >3 to pass this examination** | | | Ⓟ | Ⓕ | Ⓟ | Ⓕ | Ⓟ | Ⓕ |

| Assessor: Date: | Test 1 Comments: |
|---|---|
| Assessor: Date: | Test 2 Comments: |
| Assessor: Date: | Test 3 Comments: |

**TEST ENVIRONMENTS**
**L:** Laboratory/Classroom
**C:** Clinical/Field Testing
**P:** Practicum
**A:** Assessment/Mock Exam

**TEST INFORMATION**
**Test Statistics:** No data available
**Reference(s):** Starkey & Brown (2015)

**MUSCULOSKELETAL SYSTEM—REGION 6: CERVICAL SPINE**
# SPECIAL TESTS

| NATA EC 5th | BOC RD6 | SKILL |
|---|---|---|
| CE-21g, CE-20e | D2-0203 | Cervical Distraction Test |

**Supplies Needed:** Table, small bolster (placed under the patient's knees)

*This problem allows you the opportunity to demonstrate an* **orthopedic test** *known as the* **cervical distraction test** *for* **intervertebral foramen** *or* **neural foramina pathology**. *You have 2 minutes to complete this task.*

| Cervical Distraction Test | Course or Site Assessor Environment | | Test 1 | | Test 2 | | Test 3 | |
|---|---|---|---|---|---|---|---|---|
| **Tester places patient and limb in appropriate position** | | **Y** | **N** | **Y** | **N** | **Y** | **N** | |
| Supine to relax the cervical spine postural muscles | | ○ | ○ | ○ | ○ | ○ | ○ | |
| **Tester placed in proper position** | | **Y** | **N** | **Y** | **N** | **Y** | **N** | |
| Stands at the patient's head | | ○ | ○ | ○ | ○ | ○ | ○ | |
| One hand beneath the head of the patient grasping the occiput, the other hand placed palm down on top of the patient's forehead | | ○ | ○ | ○ | ○ | ○ | ○ | |
| **Tester performs test according to accepted guidelines** | | **Y** | **N** | **Y** | **N** | **Y** | **N** | |
| The tester slightly flexes the patient's neck and applies a traction force to the skull | | ○ | ○ | ○ | ○ | ○ | ○ | |
| **Identifies positive findings and implications** | | **Y** | **N** | **Y** | **N** | **Y** | **N** | |
| The patient's symptoms are relieved or reduced | | ○ | ○ | ○ | ○ | ○ | ○ | |
| The patient experiences compression of the cervical facet joints and/or stenosis of the neural foramina | | ○ | ○ | ○ | ○ | ○ | ○ | |
| **Total** | | ____ /6 | | ____ /6 | | ____ /6 | | |
| **Must achieve >4 to pass this examination** | | Ⓟ | Ⓕ | Ⓟ | Ⓕ | Ⓟ | Ⓕ | |

| Assessor:<br>Date: | Test 1 Comments: |
|---|---|
| Assessor:<br>Date: | Test 2 Comments: |
| Assessor:<br>Date: | Test 3 Comments: |

**TEST ENVIRONMENTS**
**L:** Laboratory/Classroom
**C:** Clinical/Field Testing
**P:** Practicum
**A:** Assessment/Mock Exam

**TEST INFORMATION**
**Test Statistics:** No data available
**Reference(s):** Starkey & Brown (2015)

## MUSCULOSKELETAL SYSTEM—REGION 6: CERVICAL SPINE
# SPECIAL TESTS

| NATA EC 5th | BOC RD6 | SKILL |
|---|---|---|
| CE-21g, CE-20e | D2-0203 | Cervical-Flexion Rotation Test |

**Supplies Needed:** Table, bolster (placed under the patient's knees)

*This problem allows you the opportunity to demonstrate an* **orthopedic test** *known as the* **cervical-flexion rotation test** *to identify* **cervicogenic headache***. You have 2 minutes to complete this task.*

| Cervical-Flexion Rotation Test | Course or Site Assessor Environment | | Test 1 | | Test 2 | | Test 3 | |
|---|---|---|---|---|---|---|---|---|
| **Tester places patient and limb in appropriate position** | | **Y** | **N** | **Y** | **N** | **Y** | **N** | |
| Supine on the table | | ○ | ○ | ○ | ○ | ○ | ○ | |
| **Tester placed in proper position** | | **Y** | **N** | **Y** | **N** | **Y** | **N** | |
| Stands at the head of the patient | | ○ | ○ | ○ | ○ | ○ | ○ | |
| Resting symptoms are assessed | | ○ | ○ | ○ | ○ | ○ | ○ | |
| **Tester performs test according to accepted guidelines** | | **Y** | **N** | **Y** | **N** | **Y** | **N** | |
| The patient actively moves his/her neck into maximum flexion | | ○ | ○ | ○ | ○ | ○ | ○ | |
| Examiner applies a full rotation force to both sides | | ○ | ○ | ○ | ○ | ○ | ○ | |
| **Identifies positive findings and implications** | | **Y** | **N** | **Y** | **N** | **Y** | **N** | |
| Reproduction of pain | | ○ | ○ | ○ | ○ | ○ | ○ | |
| Cervicogenic headache is indicated | | ○ | ○ | ○ | ○ | ○ | ○ | |
| Total | | ___ /7 | | ___ /7 | | ___ /7 | | |
| **Must achieve >4 to pass this examination** | | Ⓟ | Ⓕ | Ⓟ | Ⓕ | Ⓟ | Ⓕ | |

| Assessor: Date: | Test 1 Comments: |
|---|---|
| Assessor: Date: | Test 2 Comments: |
| Assessor: Date: | Test 3 Comments: |

**TEST ENVIRONMENTS**
**L:** Laboratory/Classroom
**C:** Clinical/Field Testing
**P:** Practicum
**A:** Assessment/Mock Exam

**TEST INFORMATION**
**Test Statistics:** No data available
**Reference(s):** Cook & Hegedus (2013)

## MUSCULOSKELETAL SYSTEM—REGION 6: CERVICAL SPINE
# SPECIAL TESTS

| NATA EC 5th | BOC RD6 | SKILL |
|---|---|---|
| CE-21g, CE-20e | D2-0203 | Military Brace Test |

**Supplies Needed:** N/A

*This problem allows you the opportunity to demonstrate an* **orthopedic test** *known as the* **military brace test** *to rule out* **thoracic outlet syndrome**. *You have 2 minutes to complete this task.*

| Military Brace Test | Course or Site Assessor Environment | | Test 1 | | Test 2 | | Test 3 | |
|---|---|---|---|---|---|---|---|---|
| **Tester places patient and limb in appropriate position** | | | Y | N | Y | N | Y | N |
| Stands | | | ○ | ○ | ○ | ○ | ○ | ○ |
| Shoulders should be relaxed, the patient looking forward | | | ○ | ○ | ○ | ○ | ○ | ○ |
| **Tester placed in proper position** | | | Y | N | Y | N | Y | N |
| Stands behind the patient | | | ○ | ○ | ○ | ○ | ○ | ○ |
| One hand palpates the radial pulse on the involved extremity | | | ○ | ○ | ○ | ○ | ○ | ○ |
| **Tester performs test according to accepted guidelines** | | | Y | N | Y | N | Y | N |
| The patient retracts and depresses the shoulders as if coming to military attention | | | ○ | ○ | ○ | ○ | ○ | ○ |
| The humerus is extended and abducted to 30 degrees | | | ○ | ○ | ○ | ○ | ○ | ○ |
| The neck and head are hyperextended | | | ○ | ○ | ○ | ○ | ○ | ○ |
| **Identifies positive findings and implications** | | | Y | N | Y | N | Y | N |
| The radial pulse disappears | | | ○ | ○ | ○ | ○ | ○ | ○ |
| The subclavian artery is being blocked by the costoclavicular structures of the shoulder | | | ○ | ○ | ○ | ○ | ○ | ○ |
| **Total** | | | __/9 | | __/9 | | __/9 | |
| **Must achieve >6 to pass this examination** | | | Ⓟ | Ⓕ | Ⓟ | Ⓕ | Ⓟ | Ⓕ |

| Assessor: Date: | Test 1 Comments: |
|---|---|
| Assessor: Date: | Test 2 Comments: |
| Assessor: Date: | Test 3 Comments: |

**TEST ENVIRONMENTS**
L: Laboratory/Classroom
C: Clinical/Field Testing
P: Practicum
A: Assessment/Mock Exam

**TEST INFORMATION**
**Test Statistics:** No data available
**Reference(s):** Starkey & Brown (2015)

## MUSCULOSKELETAL SYSTEM—REGION 6: CERVICAL SPINE
# SPECIAL TESTS

| NATA EC 5th | BOC RD6 | SKILL |
|---|---|---|
| CE-21g, CE-20e | D2-0203 | Roos' Test (Elevated Arm Stress Test) |

**Supplies Needed:** Table

*This problem allows you the opportunity to demonstrate an* **orthopedic test** *known as* **Roos' test (elevated arm stress test)** *for* **thoracic outlet syndrome**. *You have 2 minutes to complete this task.*

| Roos' Test (Elevated Arm Stress Test) | Course or Site Assessor Environment | Test 1 | | Test 2 | | Test 3 | |
|---|---|---|---|---|---|---|---|
| **Tester places patient and limb in appropriate position** | | **Y** | **N** | **Y** | **N** | **Y** | **N** |
| Seated or standing | | O | O | O | O | O | O |
| The shoulders are abducted to 90 degrees, the elbows are flexed to 90 degrees, and the humerus is externally rotated | | O | O | O | O | O | O |
| **Tester placed in proper position** | | **Y** | **N** | **Y** | **N** | **Y** | **N** |
| Stands in front of the patient | | O | O | O | O | O | O |
| **Tester performs test according to accepted guidelines** | | **Y** | **N** | **Y** | **N** | **Y** | **N** |
| The patient rapidly opens and closes both hands for 3 minutes | | O | O | O | O | O | O |
| **Identifies positive findings and implications** | | **Y** | **N** | **Y** | **N** | **Y** | **N** |
| The patient is unable to maintain the testing position or replication of sensory and/or motor symptoms in the upper extremity | | O | O | O | O | O | O |
| Thoracic outlet syndrome of neurologic origin | | O | O | O | O | O | O |
| **Total** | | ___/6 | | ___/6 | | ___/6 | |
| **Must achieve >4 to pass this examination** | | Ⓟ | Ⓕ | Ⓟ | Ⓕ | Ⓟ | Ⓕ |
| **Assessor:** **Date:** | **Test 1 Comments:** | | | | | | |
| **Assessor:** **Date:** | **Test 2 Comments:** | | | | | | |
| **Assessor:** **Date:** | **Test 3 Comments:** | | | | | | |

**TEST ENVIRONMENTS**
**L:** Laboratory/Classroom
**C:** Clinical/Field Testing
**P:** Practicum
**A:** Assessment/Mock Exam

**TEST INFORMATION**
**Test Statistics:** (+) LR 1.2
(-) LR .52
**Reference(s):** Starkey & Brown (2015)

## MUSCULOSKELETAL SYSTEM—REGION 6: CERVICAL SPINE
# SPECIAL TESTS

| NATA EC 5th | BOC RD6 | SKILL |
|---|---|---|
| CE-21g, CE-20e | D2-0203 | Shoulder Abduction Test |

**Supplies Needed:** Table or chair

*This problem allows you the opportunity to demonstrate an* **orthopedic test** *known as the* **shoulder abduction test** *for* **cervical radiculopathy**. *You have 2 minutes to complete this task.*

| Shoulder Abduction Test | Course or Site Assessor Environment | | Test 1 | | Test 2 | | Test 3 | |
|---|---|---|---|---|---|---|---|---|
| | | | Y | N | Y | N | Y | N |
| **Tester places patient and limb in appropriate position** | | | Y | N | Y | N | Y | N |
| Seated or standing | | | O | O | O | O | O | O |
| **Tester placed in proper position** | | | Y | N | Y | N | Y | N |
| Stands in front of the patient | | | O | O | O | O | O | O |
| **Tester performs test according to accepted guidelines** | | | Y | N | Y | N | Y | N |
| The patient actively abducts the arm so that the hand is resting on top of the head and maintains this position for 30 seconds | | | O | O | O | O | O | O |
| **Identifies positive findings and implications** | | | Y | N | Y | N | Y | N |
| Decrease in the patient's symptoms secondary to decreased tension on the involved nerve root | | | O | O | O | O | O | O |
| Herniated disk or nerve root compression | | | O | O | O | O | O | O |
| Total | | | ___/5 | | ___/5 | | ___/5 | |
| Must achieve >3 to pass this examination | | | Ⓟ | Ⓕ | Ⓟ | Ⓕ | Ⓟ | Ⓕ |

| Assessor: Date: | Test 1 Comments: |
|---|---|
| Assessor: Date: | Test 2 Comments: |
| Assessor: Date: | Test 3 Comments: |

**TEST ENVIRONMENTS**
**L:** Laboratory/Classroom
**C:** Clinical/Field Testing
**P:** Practicum
**A:** Assessment/Mock Exam

**TEST INFORMATION**
**Test Statistics:** No data available
**Reference(s):** Starkey & Brown (2015)

**MUSCULOSKELETAL SYSTEM—REGION 6: CERVICAL SPINE**
# SPECIAL TESTS

| NATA EC 5th | BOC RD6 | SKILL |
|---|---|---|
| CE-21g, CE-20e | D2-0203 | Spurling's Test |

**Supplies Needed:** Table or chair

*This problem allows you the opportunity to demonstrate an* **orthopedic test** *known as* **Spurling's test** *for* **cervical radiculopathy**. *You have 2 minutes to complete this task.*

| Spurling's Test | Course or Site Assessor Environment | | Test 1 | | Test 2 | | Test 3 |
|---|---|---|---|---|---|---|---|
| | | Y | N | Y | N | Y | N |
| **Tester places patient and limb in appropriate position** | | Y | N | Y | N | Y | N |
| Seated | | ○ | ○ | ○ | ○ | ○ | ○ |
| **Tester placed in proper position** | | Y | N | Y | N | Y | N |
| Stands behind the patient with the hands interlocked over the crown of the patient's head | | ○ | ○ | ○ | ○ | ○ | ○ |
| **Tester performs test according to accepted guidelines** | | Y | N | Y | N | Y | N |
| The patient laterally flexes the cervical spine | | ○ | ○ | ○ | ○ | ○ | ○ |
| A compressive (axial) force is then placed along the cervical spine | | ○ | ○ | ○ | ○ | ○ | ○ |
| **Identifies positive findings and implications** | | Y | N | Y | N | Y | N |
| Pain/reproduction of symptoms radiating down the patient's arm | | ○ | ○ | ○ | ○ | ○ | ○ |
| Nerve root impingement by narrowing of the neural foramina | | ○ | ○ | ○ | ○ | ○ | ○ |
| **Total** | | ___/6 | | ___/6 | | ___/6 | |
| **Must achieve >4 to pass this examination** | | Ⓟ | Ⓕ | Ⓟ | Ⓕ | Ⓟ | Ⓕ |

| Assessor: Date: | Test 1 Comments: |
|---|---|
| Assessor: Date: | Test 2 Comments: |
| Assessor: Date: | Test 3 Comments: |

**TEST ENVIRONMENTS**
**L:** Laboratory/Classroom
**C:** Clinical/Field Testing
**P:** Practicum
**A:** Assessment/Mock Exam

**TEST INFORMATION**
**Test Statistics:** Sensitivity .3–.93
Specificity .5–1
(+) LR 1.92–18.6
(-) LR .07–.75
**Reference(s):** Starkey & Brown (2015)
Wainner et al. (2003)

## MUSCULOSKELETAL SYSTEM—REGION 6: CERVICAL SPINE
# SPECIAL TESTS

| NATA EC 5th | BOC RD6 | SKILL |
|---|---|---|
| CE-21g, CE-20e | D2-0203 | Upper Limb Tension Test |

**Supplies Needed:** Table, bolster (placed under the patient's knees)

*This problem allows you the opportunity to demonstrate an* **orthopedic test** *known as the* **upper limb tension test** *for* **cervical radiculopathy**. *You have 2 minutes to complete this task.*

| Upper Limb Tension Test | Course or Site / Assessor / Environment | Test 1 | | Test 2 | | Test 3 | |
|---|---|---|---|---|---|---|---|
| **Tester places patient and limb in appropriate position** | | **Y** | **N** | **Y** | **N** | **Y** | **N** |
| Supine on table with bolster under the knees | | ○ | ○ | ○ | ○ | ○ | ○ |
| **Tester placed in proper position** | | **Y** | **N** | **Y** | **N** | **Y** | **N** |
| Stands to the side of the patient | | ○ | ○ | ○ | ○ | ○ | ○ |
| The tester will maintain each of the following movements for the duration of the test | | ○ | ○ | ○ | ○ | ○ | ○ |
| **Tester performs test according to accepted guidelines** | | **Y** | **N** | **Y** | **N** | **Y** | **N** |
| Depresses the shoulder girdle | | ○ | ○ | ○ | ○ | ○ | ○ |
| Passively abducts the GH joint to 110 degrees | | ○ | ○ | ○ | ○ | ○ | ○ |
| Supinates the forearm and extends the wrist and fingers | | ○ | ○ | ○ | ○ | ○ | ○ |
| Passively extends the elbow | | ○ | ○ | ○ | ○ | ○ | ○ |
| The patient laterally flexes the neck to the contralateral side | | ○ | ○ | ○ | ○ | ○ | ○ |
| The tester should discontinue assessment if symptoms are elicited | | ○ | ○ | ○ | ○ | ○ | ○ |
| **Identifies positive findings and implications** | | **Y** | **N** | **Y** | **N** | **Y** | **N** |
| Reproduction of neurological symptoms | | ○ | ○ | ○ | ○ | ○ | ○ |
| Cervical radiculopathy or ulnar neuropathy | | ○ | ○ | ○ | ○ | ○ | ○ |
| **Total** | | ___/11 | | ___/11 | | ___/11 | |
| **Must achieve >7 to pass this examination** | | Ⓟ | Ⓕ | Ⓟ | Ⓕ | Ⓟ | Ⓕ |

| Assessor: Date: | Test 1 Comments: |
|---|---|
| Assessor: Date: | Test 2 Comments: |
| Assessor: Date: | Test 3 Comments: |

**TEST ENVIRONMENTS**
**L:** Laboratory/Classroom
**C:** Clinical/Field Testing
**P:** Practicum
**A:** Assessment/Mock Exam

**TEST INFORMATION**
**Test Statistics:** No data available
**Reference(s):** Cook & Hegedus (2013)

## MUSCULOSKELETAL SYSTEM—REGION 6: CERVICAL SPINE
# SPECIAL TESTS

| NATA EC 5th | BOC RD6 | SKILL |
|---|---|---|
| CE-21g, CE-20e | D2-0203 | Vertebral Basilar Insufficiency Test (Vertebral Artery Test) |

**Supplies Needed:** Table, bolster (placed under the patient's knees)

*This problem allows you the opportunity to demonstrate an* **orthopedic test** *known as the* **vertebral basilar insufficiency test (vertebral artery test)** *for* **vertebral artery dysfunction**. *You have 2 minutes to complete this task.*

| Vertebral Basilar Insufficiency Test (Vertebral Artery Test) | Course or Site Assessor Environment | | Test 1 | | Test 2 | | Test 3 | |
|---|---|---|---|---|---|---|---|---|
| **Tester places patient and limb in appropriate position** | | Y | N | Y | N | Y | N | |
| Supine | | O | O | O | O | O | O | |
| **Tester placed in proper position** | | Y | N | Y | N | Y | N | |
| Seated at the head of the patient, cupping the patient's head | | O | O | O | O | O | O | |
| **Tester performs test according to accepted guidelines** | | Y | N | Y | N | Y | N | |
| Passively extends, laterally flexes, and rotates the head | | O | O | O | O | O | O | |
| Maintains this position for 10 seconds | | O | O | O | O | O | O | |
| Repeats test to opposite side | | O | O | O | O | O | O | |
| **Identifies positive findings and implications** | | Y | N | Y | N | Y | N | |
| The patient displays dizziness, diplopia, dysphasia, dysarthria, nausea, and nystagmus | | O | O | O | O | O | O | |
| Vertebral artery insufficiency is indicated | | O | O | O | O | O | O | |
| Total | | ___/7 | | ___/7 | | ___/7 | | |
| **Must achieve >4 to pass this examination** | | Ⓟ | Ⓕ | Ⓟ | Ⓕ | Ⓟ | Ⓕ | |

| Assessor: Date: | Test 1 Comments: |
|---|---|
| Assessor: Date: | Test 2 Comments: |
| Assessor: Date: | Test 3 Comments: |

**TEST ENVIRONMENTS**
**L:** Laboratory/Classroom
**C:** Clinical/Field Testing
**P:** Practicum
**A:** Assessment/Mock Exam

**TEST INFORMATION**
**Test Statistics:** No data available
**Reference(s):** Cook & Hegedus (2013)

MUSCULOSKELETAL SYSTEM—REGION 6: CERVICAL SPINE
# DERMATOME TESTING

| NATA EC 5th | BOC RD6 | SKILL |
|---|---|---|
| CE-21h, CE-20f | D2-0203 | Dermatome: C1 |

**Supplies Needed:** Table, neurological hammer, cotton-tipped applicator, toothpicks

*This problem allows you the opportunity to demonstrate a* **dermatome assessment** *for* **C1**. *You have 2 minutes to complete this task.*

| Dermatome: C1 | Course or Site / Assessor / Environment | | Test 1 | | Test 2 | | Test 3 | |
|---|---|---|---|---|---|---|---|---|
| **Tester places patient and limb in appropriate position** | | | Y | N | Y | N | Y | N |
| Seated, legs over the table | | | O | O | O | O | O | O |
| Upright position | | | O | O | O | O | O | O |
| **Tester placed in proper position** | | | Y | N | Y | N | Y | N |
| Stands in front of the patient | | | O | O | O | O | O | O |
| **Tester performs test according to accepted guidelines** | | | Y | N | Y | N | Y | N |
| Instructs the patient in the differences in sharp/dull | | | O | O | O | O | O | O |
| Instructs the patient to close eyes and look away | | | O | O | O | O | O | O |
| Applies sharp/dull sensation in randomized order over the superior head | | | O | O | O | O | O | O |
| Instructs the patient to identify sharp/dull | | | O | O | O | O | O | O |
| **Identifies implications** | | | Y | N | Y | N | Y | N |
| Unable to differentiate | | | O | O | O | O | O | O |
| | Total | | /8 | | /8 | | /8 | |
| | Must achieve >5 to pass this examination | | P | F | P | F | P | F |
| Assessor: Date: | Test 1 Comments: | | | | | | | |
| Assessor: Date: | Test 2 Comments: | | | | | | | |
| Assessor: Date: | Test 3 Comments: | | | | | | | |

**TEST ENVIRONMENTS**
**L:** Laboratory/Classroom
**C:** Clinical/Field Testing
**P:** Practicum
**A:** Assessment/Mock Exam

**TEST INFORMATION**
**Test Statistics:** N/A
**Reference(s):** Starkey & Brown (2015)

## MUSCULOSKELETAL SYSTEM—REGION 6: CERVICAL SPINE
# DERMATOME TESTING

| NATA EC 5th | BOC RD6 | SKILL |
|---|---|---|
| CE-21h, CE-20f | D2-0203 | Dermatome: C2 |

**Supplies Needed:** Table, neurological hammer, cotton-tipped applicator, toothpicks

*This problem allows you the opportunity to demonstrate a* **dermatome assessment** *for* **C2**. *You have 2 minutes to complete this task.*

| Dermatome: C2 | Course or Site / Assessor / Environment | Test 1 | | Test 2 | | Test 3 | |
|---|---|---|---|---|---|---|---|
| | | Y | N | Y | N | Y | N |
| **Tester places patient and limb in appropriate position** | | Y | N | Y | N | Y | N |
| Seated, legs over the table | | O | O | O | O | O | O |
| Upright position | | O | O | O | O | O | O |
| **Tester placed in proper position** | | Y | N | Y | N | Y | N |
| Stands in front of the patient | | O | O | O | O | O | O |
| **Tester performs test according to accepted guidelines** | | Y | N | Y | N | Y | N |
| Instructs the patient in the differences in sharp/dull | | O | O | O | O | O | O |
| Instructs the patient to close eyes and look away | | O | O | O | O | O | O |
| Applies sharp/dull sensation in randomized order over the back of head to ear | | O | O | O | O | O | O |
| Instructs the patient to identify sharp/dull | | O | O | O | O | O | O |
| **Identifies implications** | | Y | N | Y | N | Y | N |
| Unable to differentiate | | O | O | O | O | O | O |
| Total | | ___/8 | | ___/8 | | ___/8 | |
| **Must achieve >5 to pass this examination** | | Ⓟ | Ⓕ | Ⓟ | Ⓕ | Ⓟ | Ⓕ |
| Assessor: Date: | **Test 1 Comments:** | | | | | | |
| Assessor: Date: | **Test 2 Comments:** | | | | | | |
| Assessor: Date: | **Test 3 Comments:** | | | | | | |

**TEST ENVIRONMENTS**
**L:** Laboratory/Classroom
**C:** Clinical/Field Testing
**P:** Practicum
**A:** Assessment/Mock Exam

**TEST INFORMATION**
**Test Statistics:** N/A
**Reference(s):** Starkey & Brown (2015)

MUSCULOSKELETAL SYSTEM—REGION 6: CERVICAL SPINE
# DERMATOME TESTING

| NATA EC 5th | BOC RD6 | SKILL |
|---|---|---|
| CE-21h, CE-20f | D2-0203 | Dermatome: C3 |

**Supplies Needed:** Table, neurological hammer, cotton-tipped applicator, toothpicks

*This problem allows you the opportunity to demonstrate a* **dermatome assessment** *for* **C3**. *You have 2 minutes to complete this task.*

| Dermatome: C3 | Course or Site Assessor Environment | | Test 1 | | Test 2 | | Test 3 | |
|---|---|---|---|---|---|---|---|---|
| **Tester places patient and limb in appropriate position** | | | Y | N | Y | N | Y | N |
| Seated, legs over the table | | | ○ | ○ | ○ | ○ | ○ | ○ |
| Upright position | | | ○ | ○ | ○ | ○ | ○ | ○ |
| **Tester placed in proper position** | | | Y | N | Y | N | Y | N |
| Stands in front of the patient | | | ○ | ○ | ○ | ○ | ○ | ○ |
| **Tester performs test according to accepted guidelines** | | | Y | N | Y | N | Y | N |
| Instructs the patient in the differences in sharp/dull | | | ○ | ○ | ○ | ○ | ○ | ○ |
| Instructs the patient to close eyes and look away | | | ○ | ○ | ○ | ○ | ○ | ○ |
| Applies sharp/dull sensation in randomized order over the middle to lateral neck | | | ○ | ○ | ○ | ○ | ○ | ○ |
| Instructs the patient to identify sharp/dull | | | ○ | ○ | ○ | ○ | ○ | ○ |
| **Identifies implications** | | | Y | N | Y | N | Y | N |
| Unable to differentiate | | | ○ | ○ | ○ | ○ | ○ | ○ |
| Total | | | ___/8 | | ___/8 | | ___/8 | |
| Must achieve >5 to pass this examination | | | Ⓟ | Ⓕ | Ⓟ | Ⓕ | Ⓟ | Ⓕ |
| Assessor: Date: | Test 1 Comments: | | | | | | | |
| Assessor: Date: | Test 2 Comments: | | | | | | | |
| Assessor: Date: | Test 3 Comments: | | | | | | | |

**TEST ENVIRONMENTS**
**L:** Laboratory/Classroom
**C:** Clinical/Field Testing
**P:** Practicum
**A:** Assessment/Mock Exam

**TEST INFORMATION**
**Test Statistics:** N/A
**Reference(s):** Starkey & Brown (2015)

## MUSCULOSKELETAL SYSTEM—REGION 6: CERVICAL SPINE
# DERMATOME TESTING

| NATA EC 5th | BOC RD6 | SKILL |
|---|---|---|
| CE-21h, CE-20f | D2-0203 | Dermatome: C4 |

**Supplies Needed:** Table, neurological hammer, cotton-tipped applicator, toothpicks

*This problem allows you the opportunity to demonstrate a* **dermatome assessment** *for* **C4.** *You have 2 minutes to complete this task.*

| Dermatome: C4 | Course or Site Assessor Environment | Test 1 | | Test 2 | | Test 3 | |
|---|---|---|---|---|---|---|---|
| | | Y | N | Y | N | Y | N |
| **Tester places patient and limb in appropriate position** | | **Y** | **N** | **Y** | **N** | **Y** | **N** |
| Seated, legs over the table | | O | O | O | O | O | O |
| Upright position | | O | O | O | O | O | O |
| **Tester placed in proper position** | | **Y** | **N** | **Y** | **N** | **Y** | **N** |
| Stands in front of the patient | | O | O | O | O | O | O |
| **Tester performs test according to accepted guidelines** | | **Y** | **N** | **Y** | **N** | **Y** | **N** |
| Instructs the patient in the differences in sharp/dull | | O | O | O | O | O | O |
| Instructs the patient to close eyes and look away | | O | O | O | O | O | O |
| Applies sharp/dull sensation in randomized order over the suprascapular area and traps | | O | O | O | O | O | O |
| Instructs the patient to identify sharp/dull | | O | O | O | O | O | O |
| **Identifies implications** | | **Y** | **N** | **Y** | **N** | **Y** | **N** |
| Unable to differentiate | | O | O | O | O | O | O |
| | Total | ___/8 | | ___/8 | | ___/8 | |
| | **Must achieve >5 to pass this examination** | Ⓟ | Ⓕ | Ⓟ | Ⓕ | Ⓟ | Ⓕ |

| Assessor: Date: | Test 1 Comments: |
|---|---|
| Assessor: Date: | Test 2 Comments: |
| Assessor: Date: | Test 3 Comments: |

**TEST ENVIRONMENTS**
**L:** Laboratory/Classroom
**C:** Clinical/Field Testing
**P:** Practicum
**A:** Assessment/Mock Exam

**TEST INFORMATION**
**Test Statistics:** N/A
**Reference(s):** Starkey & Brown (2015)

## MUSCULOSKELETAL SYSTEM—REGION 6: CERVICAL SPINE
# DERMATOME TESTING

| NATA EC 5th | BOC RD6 | SKILL |
|---|---|---|
| CE-21h, CE-20f | D2-0203 | Dermatome: C5 |

**Supplies Needed:** Table, neurological hammer, cotton-tipped applicator, toothpicks

*This problem allows you the opportunity to demonstrate a* **dermatome assessment** *for* **C5**. *You have 2 minutes to complete this task.*

| Dermatome: C5 / Course or Site / Assessor / Environment | Test 1 | | Test 2 | | Test 3 | |
|---|---|---|---|---|---|---|
| | Y | N | Y | N | Y | N |
| **Tester places patient and limb in appropriate position** | Y | N | Y | N | Y | N |
| Seated, legs over the table | O | O | O | O | O | O |
| Upright position | O | O | O | O | O | O |
| **Tester placed in proper position** | Y | N | Y | N | Y | N |
| Stands in front of the patient | O | O | O | O | O | O |
| **Tester performs test according to accepted guidelines** | Y | N | Y | N | Y | N |
| Instructs the patient in the differences in sharp/dull | O | O | O | O | O | O |
| Instructs the patient to close eyes and look away | O | O | O | O | O | O |
| Applies sharp/dull sensation in randomized order over the deltoid patch | O | O | O | O | O | O |
| Instructs the patient to identify sharp/dull | O | O | O | O | O | O |
| **Identifies implications** | Y | N | Y | N | Y | N |
| Unable to differentiate | O | O | O | O | O | O |
| Total | ___/8 | | ___/8 | | ___/8 | |
| **Must achieve >5 to pass this examination** | Ⓟ | Ⓕ | Ⓟ | Ⓕ | Ⓟ | Ⓕ |

| Assessor: Date: | Test 1 Comments: |
|---|---|
| Assessor: Date: | Test 2 Comments: |
| Assessor: Date: | Test 3 Comments: |

**TEST ENVIRONMENTS**
**L:** Laboratory/Classroom
**C:** Clinical/Field Testing
**P:** Practicum
**A:** Assessment/Mock Exam

**TEST INFORMATION**
**Test Statistics:** N/A
**Reference(s):** Starkey & Brown (2015)

## MUSCULOSKELETAL SYSTEM—REGION 6: CERVICAL SPINE
# DERMATOME TESTING

| NATA EC 5th | BOC RD6 | SKILL |
|---|---|---|
| CE-21h, CE-20f | D2-0203 | Dermatome: C6 |

**Supplies Needed:** Table, neurological hammer, cotton-tipped applicator, toothpicks

*This problem allows you the opportunity to demonstrate a* **dermatome assessment** *for* **C6**. *You have 2 minutes to complete this task.*

| Dermatome: C6 | Course or Site Assessor Environment | | | | | | |
|---|---|---|---|---|---|---|---|
| | | Test 1 | | Test 2 | | Test 3 | |
| **Tester places patient and limb in appropriate position** | | Y | N | Y | N | Y | N |
| Seated, legs over the table | | ○ | ○ | ○ | ○ | ○ | ○ |
| Upright position | | ○ | ○ | ○ | ○ | ○ | ○ |
| **Tester placed in proper position** | | Y | N | Y | N | Y | N |
| Stands in front of the patient | | ○ | ○ | ○ | ○ | ○ | ○ |
| **Tester performs test according to accepted guidelines** | | Y | N | Y | N | Y | N |
| Instructs the patient in the differences in sharp/dull | | ○ | ○ | ○ | ○ | ○ | ○ |
| Instructs the patient to close eyes and look away | | ○ | ○ | ○ | ○ | ○ | ○ |
| Applies sharp/dull sensation in randomized order over the lateral forearm | | ○ | ○ | ○ | ○ | ○ | ○ |
| Instructs the patient to identify sharp/dull | | ○ | ○ | ○ | ○ | ○ | ○ |
| **Identifies implications** | | Y | N | Y | N | Y | N |
| Unable to differentiate | | ○ | ○ | ○ | ○ | ○ | ○ |
| Total | | ___/8 | | ___/8 | | ___/8 | |
| **Must achieve >5 to pass this examination** | | Ⓟ | Ⓕ | Ⓟ | Ⓕ | Ⓟ | Ⓕ |

| Assessor: Date: | Test 1 Comments: |
|---|---|
| Assessor: Date: | Test 2 Comments: |
| Assessor: Date: | Test 3 Comments: |

**TEST ENVIRONMENTS**
**L:** Laboratory/Classroom
**C:** Clinical/Field Testing
**P:** Practicum
**A:** Assessment/Mock Exam

**TEST INFORMATION**
**Test Statistics:** N/A
**Reference(s):** Starkey & Brown (2015)

## MUSCULOSKELETAL SYSTEM—REGION 6: CERVICAL SPINE
# DERMATOME TESTING

| NATA EC 5th | BOC RD6 | SKILL |
|---|---|---|
| CE-21h, CE-20f | D2-0203 | Dermatome: C7 |

**Supplies Needed:** Table, neurological hammer, cotton-tipped applicator, toothpicks

*This problem allows you the opportunity to demonstrate a* **dermatome assessment** *for* **C7**. *You have 2 minutes to complete this task.*

| Dermatome: C7 | Course or Site Assessor Environment | Test 1 | | Test 2 | | Test 3 | |
|---|---|---|---|---|---|---|---|
| | | Y | N | Y | N | Y | N |
| **Tester places patient and limb in appropriate position** | | Y | N | Y | N | Y | N |
| Seated, legs over the table | | ○ | ○ | ○ | ○ | ○ | ○ |
| Upright position | | ○ | ○ | ○ | ○ | ○ | ○ |
| **Tester placed in proper position** | | Y | N | Y | N | Y | N |
| Stands in front of the patient | | ○ | ○ | ○ | ○ | ○ | ○ |
| **Tester performs test according to accepted guidelines** | | Y | N | Y | N | Y | N |
| Instructs the patient in the differences in sharp/dull | | ○ | ○ | ○ | ○ | ○ | ○ |
| Instructs the patient to close eyes and look away | | ○ | ○ | ○ | ○ | ○ | ○ |
| Applies sharp/dull sensation in randomized order over the tip of the middle finger | | ○ | ○ | ○ | ○ | ○ | ○ |
| Instructs the patient to identify sharp/dull | | ○ | ○ | ○ | ○ | ○ | ○ |
| **Identifies implications** | | Y | N | Y | N | Y | N |
| Unable to differentiate | | ○ | ○ | ○ | ○ | ○ | ○ |
| | Total | __/8 | | __/8 | | __/8 | |
| | Must achieve >5 to pass this examination | Ⓟ | Ⓕ | Ⓟ | Ⓕ | Ⓟ | Ⓕ |

| Assessor: Date: | Test 1 Comments: |
|---|---|
| Assessor: Date: | Test 2 Comments: |
| Assessor: Date: | Test 3 Comments: |

**TEST ENVIRONMENTS**
**L:** Laboratory/Classroom
**C:** Clinical/Field Testing
**P:** Practicum
**A:** Assessment/Mock Exam

**TEST INFORMATION**
**Test Statistics:** N/A
**Reference(s):** Starkey & Brown (2015)

**MUSCULOSKELETAL SYSTEM—REGION 6: CERVICAL SPINE**
# DERMATOME TESTING

| NATA EC 5th | BOC RD6 | SKILL |
|---|---|---|
| CE-21h, CE-20f | D2-0203 | Dermatome: C8 |

**Supplies Needed:** Table, neurological hammer, cotton-tipped applicator, toothpicks

*This problem allows you the opportunity to demonstrate a* **dermatome assessment** *for* **C8**. *You have 2 minutes to complete this task.*

| Dermatome: C8 | Course or Site Assessor Environment | | Test 1 | | Test 2 | | Test 3 |
|---|---|---|---|---|---|---|---|
| | | **Y** | **N** | **Y** | **N** | **Y** | **N** |
| **Tester places patient and limb in appropriate position** | | **Y** | **N** | **Y** | **N** | **Y** | **N** |
| Seated, legs over the table | | O | O | O | O | O | O |
| Upright position | | O | O | O | O | O | O |
| **Tester placed in proper position** | | **Y** | **N** | **Y** | **N** | **Y** | **N** |
| Stands in front of the patient | | O | O | O | O | O | O |
| **Tester performs test according to accepted guidelines** | | **Y** | **N** | **Y** | **N** | **Y** | **N** |
| Instructs the patient in the differences in sharp/dull | | O | O | O | O | O | O |
| Instructs the patient to close eyes and look away | | O | O | O | O | O | O |
| Applies sharp/dull sensation in randomized order over the middle forearm and the ring and little finger | | O | O | O | O | O | O |
| Instructs the patient to identify sharp/dull | | O | O | O | O | O | O |
| **Identifies implications** | | **Y** | **N** | **Y** | **N** | **Y** | **N** |
| Unable to differentiate | | O | O | O | O | O | O |
| **Total** | | __/8 | | __/8 | | __/8 | |
| **Must achieve >5 to pass this examination** | | Ⓟ | Ⓕ | Ⓟ | Ⓕ | Ⓟ | Ⓕ |

| Assessor: Date: | Test 1 Comments: |
|---|---|
| Assessor: Date: | Test 2 Comments: |
| Assessor: Date: | Test 3 Comments: |

**TEST ENVIRONMENTS**
**L:** Laboratory/Classroom
**C:** Clinical/Field Testing
**P:** Practicum
**A:** Assessment/Mock Exam

**TEST INFORMATION**
**Test Statistics:** N/A
**Reference(s):** Starkey & Brown (2015)

## MUSCULOSKELETAL SYSTEM—REGION 6: CERVICAL SPINE
# DERMATOME TESTING

| NATA EC 5th | BOC RD6 | SKILL |
|---|---|---|
| CE-21h, CE-20f | D2-0203 | Dermatome: T1 |

**Supplies Needed:** Table, neurological hammer, cotton-tipped applicator, toothpicks

*This problem allows you the opportunity to demonstrate a* **dermatome assessment** *for* **T1**. *You have 2 minutes to complete this task.*

| Dermatome: T1 | Course or Site Assessor Environment | | | | | |
|---|---|---|---|---|---|---|
| | | Test 1 | | Test 2 | | Test 3 |
| **Tester places patient and limb in appropriate position** | | Y | N | Y | N | Y | N |
| Seated, legs over the table | | O | O | O | O | O | O |
| Upright position | | O | O | O | O | O | O |
| **Tester placed in proper position** | | Y | N | Y | N | Y | N |
| Stands in front of the patient | | O | O | O | O | O | O |
| **Tester performs test according to accepted guidelines** | | Y | N | Y | N | Y | N |
| Instructs the patient in the differences in sharp/dull | | O | O | O | O | O | O |
| Instructs the patient to close eyes and look away | | O | O | O | O | O | O |
| Applies sharp/dull sensation in randomized order over the medial elbow | | O | O | O | O | O | O |
| Instructs the patient to identify sharp/dull | | O | O | O | O | O | O |
| **Identifies implications** | | Y | N | Y | N | Y | N |
| Unable to differentiate | | O | O | O | O | O | O |
| Total | | __/8 | | __/8 | | __/8 |
| Must achieve >5 to pass this examination | | (P) | (F) | (P) | (F) | (P) | (F) |

| Assessor: Date: | Test 1 Comments: |
|---|---|
| Assessor: Date: | Test 2 Comments: |
| Assessor: Date: | Test 3 Comments: |

**TEST ENVIRONMENTS**
**L:** Laboratory/Classroom
**C:** Clinical/Field Testing
**P:** Practicum
**A:** Assessment/Mock Exam

**TEST INFORMATION**
**Test Statistics:** N/A
**Reference(s):** Starkey & Brown (2015)

**MUSCULOSKELETAL SYSTEM—REGION 6: CERVICAL SPINE**
# MYOTOME TESTING

| NATA EC 5th | BOC RD6 | SKILL |
|---|---|---|
| CE-21h, CE-20f | D2-0203 | Myotome: C2 |

**Supplies Needed:** Table

*This problem allows you the opportunity to demonstrate a* **myotome assessment** *for* **C2***. You have 2 minutes to complete this task.*

| Myotome: C2 | Course or Site / Assessor / Environment | | Test 1 | | Test 2 | | Test 3 | |
|---|---|---|---|---|---|---|---|---|
| **Tester places patient and limb in appropriate position** | | **Y** | **N** | **Y** | **N** | **Y** | **N** | |
| Seated, legs over the table | | ○ | ○ | ○ | ○ | ○ | ○ | |
| Upright position | | ○ | ○ | ○ | ○ | ○ | ○ | |
| **Tester placed in proper position** | | **Y** | **N** | **Y** | **N** | **Y** | **N** | |
| Stands at the side being tested | | ○ | ○ | ○ | ○ | ○ | ○ | |
| **Tester performs test according to accepted guidelines** | | **Y** | **N** | **Y** | **N** | **Y** | **N** | |
| Applies manual resistance against cervical rotation | | ○ | ○ | ○ | ○ | ○ | ○ | |
| Applies manual resistance against cervical flexion | | ○ | ○ | ○ | ○ | ○ | ○ | |
| Stabilizes appropriately | | ○ | ○ | ○ | ○ | ○ | ○ | |
| Performs bilaterally | | ○ | ○ | ○ | ○ | ○ | ○ | |
| **Identifies implications** | | **Y** | **N** | **Y** | **N** | **Y** | **N** | |
| Inability to maintain position | | ○ | ○ | ○ | ○ | ○ | ○ | |
| **Total** | | ___/8 | | ___/8 | | ___/8 | | |
| **Must achieve >5 to pass this examination** | | Ⓟ | Ⓕ | Ⓟ | Ⓕ | Ⓟ | Ⓕ | |

| Assessor: Date: | Test 1 Comments: |
|---|---|
| Assessor: Date: | Test 2 Comments: |
| Assessor: Date: | Test 3 Comments: |

**TEST ENVIRONMENTS**
**L:** Laboratory/Classroom
**C:** Clinical/Field Testing
**P:** Practicum
**A:** Assessment/Mock Exam

**TEST INFORMATION**
**Test Statistics:** N/A
**Reference(s):** Starkey & Brown (2015)

## MUSCULOSKELETAL SYSTEM—REGION 6: CERVICAL SPINE
# MYOTOME TESTING

| NATA EC 5th | BOC RD6 | SKILL |
|---|---|---|
| CE-21h, CE-20f | D2-0203 | Myotome: C3 |

**Supplies Needed:** Table

*This problem allows you the opportunity to demonstrate a* **myotome assessment** *for* **C3**. *You have 2 minutes to complete this task.*

| Myotome: C3 | Course or Site Assessor Environment | | | | | |
|---|---|---|---|---|---|---|
| | | Test 1 | | Test 2 | | Test 3 |
| **Tester places patient and limb in appropriate position** | | Y | N | Y | N | Y | N |
| Seated, legs over the table | | ○ | ○ | ○ | ○ | ○ | ○ |
| Upright position | | ○ | ○ | ○ | ○ | ○ | ○ |
| **Tester placed in proper position** | | Y | N | Y | N | Y | N |
| Stands at the side being tested | | ○ | ○ | ○ | ○ | ○ | ○ |
| **Tester performs test according to accepted guidelines** | | Y | N | Y | N | Y | N |
| Applies manual resistance against cervical lateral rotation | | ○ | ○ | ○ | ○ | ○ | ○ |
| Stabilizes appropriately | | ○ | ○ | ○ | ○ | ○ | ○ |
| Performs bilaterally | | ○ | ○ | ○ | ○ | ○ | ○ |
| **Identifies implications** | | Y | N | Y | N | Y | N |
| Inability to maintain position | | ○ | ○ | ○ | ○ | ○ | ○ |
| | Total | ___/7 | | ___/7 | | ___/7 |
| | Must achieve >4 to pass this examination | Ⓟ | Ⓕ | Ⓟ | Ⓕ | Ⓟ | Ⓕ |

| Assessor: Date: | Test 1 Comments: |
|---|---|
| Assessor: Date: | Test 2 Comments: |
| Assessor: Date: | Test 3 Comments: |

**TEST ENVIRONMENTS**
**L:** Laboratory/Classroom
**C:** Clinical/Field Testing
**P:** Practicum
**A:** Assessment/Mock Exam

**TEST INFORMATION**
**Test Statistics:** N/A
**Reference(s):** Starkey & Brown (2015)

## MUSCULOSKELETAL SYSTEM—REGION 6: CERVICAL SPINE
# MYOTOME TESTING

| NATA EC 5th | BOC RD6 | SKILL |
|---|---|---|
| CE-21h, CE-20f | D2-0203 | Myotome: C4 |

**Supplies Needed:** Table

*This problem allows you the opportunity to demonstrate a* **myotome assessment** *for* **C4**. *You have 2 minutes to complete this task.*

| Myotome: C4 | Course or Site / Assessor / Environment | | Test 1 | | Test 2 | | Test 3 | |
|---|---|---|---|---|---|---|---|---|
| | | | **Y** | **N** | **Y** | **N** | **Y** | **N** |
| **Tester places patient and limb in appropriate position** | | | Y | N | Y | N | Y | N |
| Seated, legs over the table | | | O | O | O | O | O | O |
| Upright position | | | O | O | O | O | O | O |
| **Tester placed in proper position** | | | Y | N | Y | N | Y | N |
| Stands at the side being tested | | | O | O | O | O | O | O |
| **Tester performs test according to accepted guidelines** | | | Y | N | Y | N | Y | N |
| Applies manual resistance against shoulder elevation | | | O | O | O | O | O | O |
| Stabilizes appropriately | | | O | O | O | O | O | O |
| Performs bilaterally | | | O | O | O | O | O | O |
| **Identifies implications** | | | Y | N | Y | N | Y | N |
| Inability to maintain position | | | O | O | O | O | O | O |
| Total | | | ___/7 | | ___/7 | | ___/7 | |
| Must achieve >4 to pass this examination | | | P | F | P | F | P | F |

| Assessor: Date: | Test 1 Comments: |
|---|---|
| Assessor: Date: | Test 2 Comments: |
| Assessor: Date: | Test 3 Comments: |

**TEST ENVIRONMENTS**
**L:** Laboratory/Classroom
**C:** Clinical/Field Testing
**P:** Practicum
**A:** Assessment/Mock Exam

**TEST INFORMATION**
**Test Statistics:** N/A
**Reference(s):** Starkey & Brown (2015)

## MUSCULOSKELETAL SYSTEM—REGION 6: CERVICAL SPINE
# MYOTOME TESTING

| NATA EC 5th | BOC RD6 | SKILL |
|---|---|---|
| CE-21h, CE-20f | D2-0203 | Myotome: C5 |

**Supplies Needed:** Table

*This problem allows you the opportunity to demonstrate a* **myotome assessment** *for* **C5**. *You have 2 minutes to complete this task.*

| Myotome: C5 | Course or Site / Assessor / Environment | | Test 1 | | Test 2 | | Test 3 | |
|---|---|---|---|---|---|---|---|---|
| | | | Y | N | Y | N | Y | N |
| **Tester places patient and limb in appropriate position** | | | Y | N | Y | N | Y | N |
| Seated, legs over the table | | | O | O | O | O | O | O |
| Upright position | | | O | O | O | O | O | O |
| **Tester placed in proper position** | | | Y | N | Y | N | Y | N |
| Stands at the side being tested | | | O | O | O | O | O | O |
| **Tester performs test according to accepted guidelines** | | | Y | N | Y | N | Y | N |
| Applies manual resistance against elbow flexion | | | O | O | O | O | O | O |
| Applies manual resistance against shoulder abduction | | | O | O | O | O | O | O |
| Stabilizes appropriately | | | O | O | O | O | O | O |
| Performs bilaterally | | | O | O | O | O | O | O |
| **Identifies implications** | | | Y | N | Y | N | Y | N |
| Inability to maintain position | | | O | O | O | O | O | O |
| **Total** | | | __/8 | | __/8 | | __/8 | |
| **Must achieve >5 to pass this examination** | | | Ⓟ | Ⓕ | Ⓟ | Ⓕ | Ⓟ | Ⓕ |

| Assessor:<br>Date: | Test 1 Comments: |
|---|---|
| Assessor:<br>Date: | Test 2 Comments: |
| Assessor:<br>Date: | Test 3 Comments: |

**TEST ENVIRONMENTS**
**L:** Laboratory/Classroom
**C:** Clinical/Field Testing
**P:** Practicum
**A:** Assessment/Mock Exam

**TEST INFORMATION**
**Test Statistics:** N/A
**Reference(s):**   Starkey & Brown (2015)

# MYOTOME TESTING

| NATA EC 5th | BOC RD6 | SKILL |
|---|---|---|
| CE-21h, CE-20f | D2-0203 | Myotome: C6 |

**Supplies Needed:** Table

*This problem allows you the opportunity to demonstrate a* **myotome assessment** *for* **C6**. *You have 2 minutes to complete this task.*

| Myotome: C6 | Course or Site Assessor Environment | | Test 1 | | Test 2 | | Test 3 | |
|---|---|---|---|---|---|---|---|---|
| **Tester places patient and limb in appropriate position** | | **Y** | **N** | **Y** | **N** | **Y** | **N** | |
| Seated, legs over the table | | O | O | O | O | O | O | |
| Upright position | | O | O | O | O | O | O | |
| **Tester placed in proper position** | | **Y** | **N** | **Y** | **N** | **Y** | **N** | |
| Stands at the side being tested | | O | O | O | O | O | O | |
| **Tester performs test according to accepted guidelines** | | **Y** | **N** | **Y** | **N** | **Y** | **N** | |
| Applies manual resistance against wrist extension | | O | O | O | O | O | O | |
| Stabilizes appropriately | | O | O | O | O | O | O | |
| Performs bilaterally | | O | O | O | O | O | O | |
| **Identifies implications** | | **Y** | **N** | **Y** | **N** | **Y** | **N** | |
| Inability to maintain position | | O | O | O | O | O | O | |
| Total | | ___/7 | | ___/7 | | ___/7 | | |
| **Must achieve >4 to pass this examination** | | Ⓟ | Ⓕ | Ⓟ | Ⓕ | Ⓟ | Ⓕ | |

| Assessor: Date: | Test 1 Comments: |
|---|---|
| Assessor: Date: | Test 2 Comments: |
| Assessor: Date: | Test 3 Comments: |

**TEST ENVIRONMENTS**
**L:** Laboratory/Classroom
**C:** Clinical/Field Testing
**P:** Practicum
**A:** Assessment/Mock Exam

**TEST INFORMATION**
**Test Statistics:** N/A
**Reference(s):** Starkey & Brown (2015)

MUSCULOSKELETAL SYSTEM—REGION 6: CERVICAL SPINE
# MYOTOME TESTING

| NATA EC 5th | BOC RD6 | SKILL |
|---|---|---|
| CE-21h, CE-20f | D2-0203 | Myotome: C7 |

**Supplies Needed:** Table

*This problem allows you the opportunity to demonstrate a* **myotome assessment** *for* **C7**. *You have 2 minutes to complete this task.*

| Myotome: C7 | Course or Site<br>Assessor<br>Environment | | | | | |
|---|---|---|---|---|---|---|
| | | Test 1 | | Test 2 | | Test 3 | |
| **Tester places patient and limb in appropriate position** | | Y | N | Y | N | Y | N |
| Seated, legs over the table | | O | O | O | O | O | O |
| Upright position | | O | O | O | O | O | O |
| **Tester placed in proper position** | | Y | N | Y | N | Y | N |
| Stands at the side being tested | | O | O | O | O | O | O |
| **Tester performs test according to accepted guidelines** | | Y | N | Y | N | Y | N |
| Applies manual resistance against wrist flexion | | O | O | O | O | O | O |
| Applies manual resistance against finger extension | | O | O | O | O | O | O |
| Applies manual resistance against elbow extension | | O | O | O | O | O | O |
| Stabilizes appropriately | | O | O | O | O | O | O |
| Performs bilaterally | | O | O | O | O | O | O |
| **Identifies implications** | | Y | N | Y | N | Y | N |
| Inability to maintain position | | O | O | O | O | O | O |
| **Total** | | /9 | | /9 | | /9 | |
| **Must achieve >6 to pass this examination** | | Ⓟ | Ⓕ | Ⓟ | Ⓕ | Ⓟ | Ⓕ |

| Assessor:<br>Date: | Test 1 Comments: |
|---|---|
| Assessor:<br>Date: | Test 2 Comments: |
| Assessor:<br>Date: | Test 3 Comments: |

**TEST ENVIRONMENTS**
**L:** Laboratory/Classroom
**C:** Clinical/Field Testing
**P:** Practicum
**A:** Assessment/Mock Exam

**TEST INFORMATION**
**Test Statistics:** N/A
**Reference(s):** Starkey & Brown (2015)

**MUSCULOSKELETAL SYSTEM—REGION 6: CERVICAL SPINE**
# MYOTOME TESTING

| NATA EC 5th | BOC RD6 | SKILL |
|---|---|---|
| CE-21h, CE-20f | D2-0203 | Myotome: C8 |

**Supplies Needed:** Table

*This problem allows you the opportunity to demonstrate a* **myotome assessment** *for* **C8**. *You have 2 minutes to complete this task.*

| Myotome: C8 | Course or Site Assessor Environment | | Test 1 | | Test 2 | | Test 3 |
|---|---|---|---|---|---|---|---|
| | | Y | N | Y | N | Y | N |
| **Tester places patient and limb in appropriate position** | | Y | N | Y | N | Y | N |
| Seated, legs over the table | | O | O | O | O | O | O |
| Upright position | | O | O | O | O | O | O |
| **Tester placed in proper position** | | Y | N | Y | N | Y | N |
| Stands at the side being tested | | O | O | O | O | O | O |
| **Tester performs test according to accepted guidelines** | | Y | N | Y | N | Y | N |
| Applies manual resistance against finger flexion | | O | O | O | O | O | O |
| Applies manual resistance against thumb extension | | O | O | O | O | O | O |
| Stabilizes appropriately | | O | O | O | O | O | O |
| Performs bilaterally | | O | O | O | O | O | O |
| **Identifies implications** | | Y | N | Y | N | Y | N |
| Inability to maintain position | | O | O | O | O | O | O |
| Total | | /8 | | /8 | | /8 | |
| Must achieve >5 to pass this examination | | P | F | P | F | P | F |

| Assessor: Date: | Test 1 Comments: |
|---|---|
| Assessor: Date: | Test 2 Comments: |
| Assessor: Date: | Test 3 Comments: |

**TEST ENVIRONMENTS**
L: Laboratory/Classroom
C: Clinical/Field Testing
P: Practicum
A: Assessment/Mock Exam

**TEST INFORMATION**
**Test Statistics:** N/A
**Reference(s):** Starkey & Brown (2015)

## MUSCULOSKELETAL SYSTEM—REGION 6: CERVICAL SPINE
# MYOTOME TESTING

| NATA EC 5th | BOC RD6 | SKILL |
|---|---|---|
| CE-21h, CE-20f | D2-0203 | Myotome: T1 |

**Supplies Needed:** Table

*This problem allows you the opportunity to demonstrate a* **myotome assessment** *for* **T1.** *You have 2 minutes to complete this task.*

| Myotome: T1 | Course or Site / Assessor / Environment | | | | | |
|---|---|---|---|---|---|---|
| | | Test 1 | | Test 2 | | Test 3 |
| | | Y | N | Y | N | Y | N |
| **Tester places patient and limb in appropriate position** | | Y | N | Y | N | Y | N |
| Seated, legs over the table | | ○ | ○ | ○ | ○ | ○ | ○ |
| Upright position | | ○ | ○ | ○ | ○ | ○ | ○ |
| **Tester placed in proper position** | | Y | N | Y | N | Y | N |
| Stands at the side being tested | | ○ | ○ | ○ | ○ | ○ | ○ |
| **Tester performs test according to accepted guidelines** | | Y | N | Y | N | Y | N |
| Applies manual resistance against finger abduction | | ○ | ○ | ○ | ○ | ○ | ○ |
| Applies manual resistance against finger adduction | | ○ | ○ | ○ | ○ | ○ | ○ |
| Stabilizes appropriately | | ○ | ○ | ○ | ○ | ○ | ○ |
| Performs bilaterally | | ○ | ○ | ○ | ○ | ○ | ○ |
| **Identifies implications** | | Y | N | Y | N | Y | N |
| Inability to maintain position | | ○ | ○ | ○ | ○ | ○ | ○ |
| **Total** | | __/8 | | __/8 | | __/8 | |
| **Must achieve >5 to pass this examination** | | Ⓟ | Ⓕ | Ⓟ | Ⓕ | Ⓟ | Ⓕ |

| Assessor:<br>Date: | Test 1 Comments: |
|---|---|
| Assessor:<br>Date: | Test 2 Comments: |
| Assessor:<br>Date: | Test 3 Comments: |

**TEST ENVIRONMENTS**
**L:** Laboratory/Classroom
**C:** Clinical/Field Testing
**P:** Practicum
**A:** Assessment/Mock Exam

**TEST INFORMATION**
**Test Statistics:** N/A
**Reference(s):** Starkey & Brown (2015)

## MUSCULOSKELETAL SYSTEM—REGION 6: CERVICAL SPINE
# REFLEX TESTING

| NATA EC 5th | BOC RD6 | SKILL |
|---|---|---|
| CE-21h, CE-20f | D2-0203 | Reflex Testing: C5 |

**Supplies Needed:** Table, reflex hammer

*This problem allows you the opportunity to demonstrate a* **reflex test** *for* **C5**. *You have 2 minutes to complete this task.*

| Reflex Testing: C5 | Course or Site Assessor Environment | | Test 1 | | Test 2 | | Test 3 |
|---|---|---|---|---|---|---|---|
| **Tester places patient and limb in appropriate position** | | Y | N | Y | N | Y | N |
| Seated, legs over the table | | ○ | ○ | ○ | ○ | ○ | ○ |
| Looking away from the tester | | ○ | ○ | ○ | ○ | ○ | ○ |
| **Tester placed in proper position** | | Y | N | Y | N | Y | N |
| Stands at the side being tested | | ○ | ○ | ○ | ○ | ○ | ○ |
| Thumb is placed over biceps tendon | | ○ | ○ | ○ | ○ | ○ | ○ |
| **Tester performs test according to accepted guidelines** | | Y | N | Y | N | Y | N |
| Uses reflex hammer to tap thumb | | ○ | ○ | ○ | ○ | ○ | ○ |
| Performs bilaterally | | ○ | ○ | ○ | ○ | ○ | ○ |
| **Identifies implications** | | Y | N | Y | N | Y | N |
| No reflex | | ○ | ○ | ○ | ○ | ○ | ○ |
| Total | | ___/7 | | ___/7 | | ___/7 | |
| **Must achieve >4 to pass this examination** | | Ⓟ | Ⓕ | Ⓟ | Ⓕ | Ⓟ | Ⓕ |

| Assessor:<br>Date: | Test 1 Comments: |
|---|---|
| Assessor:<br>Date: | Test 2 Comments: |
| Assessor:<br>Date: | Test 3 Comments: |

**TEST ENVIRONMENTS**
**L:** Laboratory/Classroom
**C:** Clinical/Field Testing
**P:** Practicum
**A:** Assessment/Mock Exam

**TEST INFORMATION**
**Test Statistics:** N/A
**Reference(s):** Starkey & Brown (2015)

## MUSCULOSKELETAL SYSTEM—REGION 6: CERVICAL SPINE
# REFLEX TESTING

| NATA EC 5th | BOC RD6 | SKILL |
|---|---|---|
| CE-21h, CE-20f | D2-0203 | Reflex Testing: C6 |

**Supplies Needed:** Table, reflex hammer

*This problem allows you the opportunity to demonstrate a **reflex test** for **C6**. You have 2 minutes to complete this task.*

| Reflex Testing: C6 | Course or Site Assessor Environment | | Test 1 | | Test 2 | | Test 3 | |
|---|---|---|---|---|---|---|---|---|
| | | | | | | | | |
| **Tester places patient and limb in appropriate position** | | | Y | N | Y | N | Y | N |
| Seated, legs over the table | | | ○ | ○ | ○ | ○ | ○ | ○ |
| Looking away from the tester | | | ○ | ○ | ○ | ○ | ○ | ○ |
| Elbow is passively flexed to 60 degrees | | | ○ | ○ | ○ | ○ | ○ | ○ |
| **Tester placed in proper position** | | | Y | N | Y | N | Y | N |
| Stands at the side being tested | | | ○ | ○ | ○ | ○ | ○ | ○ |
| Cradles the patient's arm | | | ○ | ○ | ○ | ○ | ○ | ○ |
| **Tester performs test according to accepted guidelines** | | | Y | N | Y | N | Y | N |
| Uses reflex hammer to tap distal portion of the brachioradialis tendon | | | ○ | ○ | ○ | ○ | ○ | ○ |
| Performs bilaterally | | | ○ | ○ | ○ | ○ | ○ | ○ |
| **Identifies implications** | | | Y | N | Y | N | Y | N |
| No reflex | | | ○ | ○ | ○ | ○ | ○ | ○ |
| | | **Total** | __/8 | | __/8 | | __/8 | |
| | **Must achieve >5 to pass this examination** | | Ⓟ | Ⓕ | Ⓟ | Ⓕ | Ⓟ | Ⓕ |
| **Assessor:** **Date:** | **Test 1 Comments:** | | | | | | | |
| **Assessor:** **Date:** | **Test 2 Comments:** | | | | | | | |
| **Assessor:** **Date:** | **Test 3 Comments:** | | | | | | | |

**TEST ENVIRONMENTS**
**L:** Laboratory/Classroom
**C:** Clinical/Field Testing
**P:** Practicum
**A:** Assessment/Mock Exam

**TEST INFORMATION**
**Test Statistics:** N/A
**Reference(s):** Starkey & Brown (2015)

## MUSCULOSKELETAL SYSTEM—REGION 6: CERVICAL SPINE
# REFLEX TESTING

| NATA EC 5th | BOC RD6 | SKILL |
|---|---|---|
| CE-21h, CE-20f | D2-0203 | Reflex Testing: C7 |

**Supplies Needed:** Table, reflex hammer

*This problem allows you the opportunity to demonstrate a **reflex test** for **C7**. You have 2 minutes to complete this task.*

| Reflex Testing: C7 | Course or Site / Assessor / Environment | Test 1 Y | Test 1 N | Test 2 Y | Test 2 N | Test 3 Y | Test 3 N |
|---|---|---|---|---|---|---|---|
| **Tester places patient and limb in appropriate position** | | Y | N | Y | N | Y | N |
| Seated, legs over the table | | O | O | O | O | O | O |
| Looking away from the tester | | O | O | O | O | O | O |
| Shoulder is passively abducted to 90 degrees | | O | O | O | O | O | O |
| Elbow is passively flexed to 90 degrees | | O | O | O | O | O | O |
| **Tester placed in proper position** | | Y | N | Y | N | Y | N |
| Stands at the side being tested | | O | O | O | O | O | O |
| Supports the patient's arm | | O | O | O | O | O | O |
| **Tester performs test according to accepted guidelines** | | Y | N | Y | N | Y | N |
| Uses reflex hammer to tap the distal triceps brachii tendon | | O | O | O | O | O | O |
| Performs bilaterally | | O | O | O | O | O | O |
| **Identifies implications** | | Y | N | Y | N | Y | N |
| No reflex | | O | O | O | O | O | O |
| Total | | __/9 | | __/9 | | __/9 | |
| **Must achieve >6 to pass this examination** | | Ⓟ | Ⓕ | Ⓟ | Ⓕ | Ⓟ | Ⓕ |

| Assessor: Date: | Test 1 Comments: |
|---|---|
| Assessor: Date: | Test 2 Comments: |
| Assessor: Date: | Test 3 Comments: |

**TEST ENVIRONMENTS**
**L:** Laboratory/Classroom
**C:** Clinical/Field Testing
**P:** Practicum
**A:** Assessment/Mock Exam

**TEST INFORMATION**
**Test Statistics:** N/A
**Reference(s):** Starkey & Brown (2015)

# 10

# MUSCULOSKELETAL SYSTEM— REGION 7: SHOULDER

Hauth, J. M., Gloyeske, B. M., & Amato, H. K.
*Clinical Skills Documentation Guide for Athletic Training, Third Edition* (pp. 290-343).
© 2016 SLACK Incorporated.

## Musculoskeletal System—Region 7: Shoulder
# Knowledge and Skills

| Musculoskeletal System—Region 7: Shoulder | | | | Skill: Acquisition, Reinforcement, Proficiency | | |
|---|---|---|---|---|---|---|
| **NATA EC 5th** | **BOC RD6** | **Palpation** | **Page #** | | | |
| CE-21b, CE-20c | D2-0202 | Palpation: Shoulder – 01 | 293 | | | |
| CE-21b, CE-20c | D2-0202 | Palpation: Shoulder – 02 | 294 | | | |
| CE-21b, CE-20c | D2-0202 | Palpation: Shoulder – 03 | 295 | | | |
| **NATA EC 5th** | **BOC RD6** | **Manual Muscle Testing** | **Page #** | | | |
| CE-21c | D2-0203 | MMT: Coracobrachialis | 296 | | | |
| CE-21c | D2-0203 | MMT: Deltoid (Anterior) | 297 | | | |
| CE-21c | D2-0203 | MMT: Deltoid (Middle) | 298 | | | |
| CE-21c | D2-0203 | MMT: Deltoid (Posterior) | 299 | | | |
| CE-21c | D2-0203 | MMT: Infraspinatus | 300 | | | |
| CE-21c | D2-0203 | MMT: Latissimus Dorsi | 301 | | | |
| CE-21c | D2-0203 | MMT: Pectoralis Major (Upper Portion) | 302 | | | |
| CE-21c | D2-0203 | MMT: Pectoralis Major (Lower Portion) | 303 | | | |
| CE-21c | D2-0203 | MMT: Pectoralis Minor | 304 | | | |
| CE-21c | D2-0203 | MMT: Rhomboid Alternate Test | 305 | | | |
| CE-21c | D2-0203 | MMT: Rhomboid/Levator | 306 | | | |
| CE-21c | D2-0203 | MMT: Serratus Anterior | 307 | | | |
| CE-21c | D2-0203 | MMT: Serratus Anterior (Preferred Test) | 308 | | | |
| CE-21c | D2-0203 | MMT: Subscapularis | 309 | | | |
| CE-21c | D2-0203 | MMT: Supraspinatus | 310 | | | |
| CE-21c | D2-0203 | MMT: Teres Major | 311 | | | |
| CE-21c | D2-0203 | MMT: Teres Minor | 312 | | | |
| CE-21c | D2-0203 | MMT: Trapezius (Lower) | 313 | | | |
| CE-21c | D2-0203 | MMT: Trapezius (Middle) | 314 | | | |
| CE-21c | D2-0203 | MMT: Trapezius (Upper) | 315 | | | |
| **NATA EC 5th** | **BOC RD6** | **Osteokinematic Joint Motion** | **Page #** | | | |
| CE-21d | D2-0203 | Goniometric Assessment: Glenohumeral Joint (Flexion) | 316 | | | |
| CE-21d | D2-0203 | Goniometric Assessment: Glenohumeral Joint (Extension) | 317 | | | |
| CE-21d | D2-0203 | Goniometric Assessment: Glenohumeral Joint (Internal/External Rotation) | 318 | | | |
| CE-21d | D2-0203 | Goniometric Assessment: Glenohumeral Joint (Abduction) | 319 | | | |
| **NATA EC 5th** | **BOC RD6** | **Capsular and Ligamentous Stress Testing** | **Page #** | | | |
| CE-21e | D2-0203 | Acromioclavicular Joint Compression Test (Shear Test) | 320 | | | |
| CE-21e | D2-0203 | Acromioclavicular Joint Distraction Test | 321 | | | |
| CE-21e | D2-0203 | Anterior Drawer Test for the Shoulder | 322 | | | |
| CE-21e | D2-0203 | Apprehension Test (Crank Test) | 323 | | | |
| CE-21e | D2-0203 | Feagin Test | 324 | | | |
| CE-21e | D2-0203 | Jerk Test (Clunk Test) | 325 | | | |
| CE-21e | D2-0203 | Posterior Apprehension (Stress) Test | 326 | | | |
| CE-21e | D2-0203 | Posterior Drawer Test for the Shoulder | 327 | | | |
| CE-21e | D2-0203 | Relocation Test (Jobe's Test) | 328 | | | |
| CE-21e | D2-0203 | Sternoclavicular Joint Stress Test | 329 | | | |
| CE-21e | D2-0203 | Sulcus Sign | 330 | | | |
| CE-21e | D2-0203 | Surprise Test (Anterior Release Test) | 331 | | | |

*(continued on the next page)*

## Musculoskeletal System—Region 7: Shoulder
# Knowledge and Skills

| NATA EC 5th | BOC RD6 | Joint Play (Arthrokinematics) | Page # | | | |
|---|---|---|---|---|---|---|
| CE-21f | D2-0203 | Acromioclavicular Joint Play | 332 | | | |
| CE-21f | D2-0203 | Glenohumeral Joint Play | 333 | | | |
| CE-21f | D2-0203 | Sternoclavicular Joint Play | 334 | | | |
| NATA EC 5th | BOC RD6 | Special Tests | Page # | | | |
| CE-21g, CE-20e | D2-0203 | Active Compression Test (O'Brien Test) | 335 | | | |
| CE-21g, CE-20e | D2-0203 | Apley's Scratch Test | 336 | | | |
| CE-21g, CE-20e | D2-0203 | Drop Arm Test (Codman's Test) | 337 | | | |
| CE-21g, CE-20e | D2-0203 | Empty Can Test (Supraspinatus Test) | 338 | | | |
| CE-21g, CE-20e | D2-0203 | Hawkins-Kennedy Test | 339 | | | |
| CE-21g, CE-20e | D2-0203 | Neer Impingement Test | 340 | | | |
| CE-21g, CE-20e | D2-0203 | Pectoralis Major Contracture Test | 341 | | | |
| CE-21g, CE-20e | D2-0203 | Speed's Test (Straight Arm Test) | 342 | | | |
| CE-21g, CE-20e | D2-0203 | Yergason's Test | 343 | | | |

## MUSCULOSKELETAL SYSTEM—REGION 7: SHOULDER
## PALPATION

| NATA EC 5th | BOC RD6 | SKILL |
|---|---|---|
| CE-21b, CE-20c | D2-0202 | Palpation: Shoulder – 01 |

**Supplies Needed:** Table

*This problem allows you the opportunity to demonstrate your ability to* **palpate** *the* **shoulder**.
*You have 2 minutes to complete this task.*

| Palpation: Shoulder – 01 | Course or Site Assessor Environment | Test 1 | | Test 2 | | Test 3 | |
|---|---|---|---|---|---|---|---|
| | | Y | N | Y | N | Y | N |
| Acromion process | | O | O | O | O | O | O |
| Long head of the biceps brachii | | O | O | O | O | O | O |
| Manubrium of sternum | | O | O | O | O | O | O |
| Inferior angle of the scapula | | O | O | O | O | O | O |
| Deltoid tuberosity | | O | O | O | O | O | O |
| Upper trapezius muscle | | O | O | O | O | O | O |
| Coracobrachialis muscle | | O | O | O | O | O | O |
| Total | | ___/7 | | ___/7 | | ___/7 | |
| Must achieve >4 to pass this examination | | Ⓟ | Ⓕ | Ⓟ | Ⓕ | Ⓟ | Ⓕ |

| Assessor: Date: | Test 1 Comments: |
|---|---|
| Assessor: Date: | Test 2 Comments: |
| Assessor: Date: | Test 3 Comments: |

**TEST ENVIRONMENTS**
**L:** Laboratory/Classroom
**C:** Clinical/Field Testing
**P:** Practicum
**A:** Assessment/Mock Exam

**TEST INFORMATION**
**Test Statistics:** N/A
**Reference(s):**  Starkey & Brown (2015)

## MUSCULOSKELETAL SYSTEM—REGION 7: SHOULDER
# PALPATION

| NATA EC 5th | BOC RD6 | SKILL |
|---|---|---|
| CE-21b, CE-20c | D2-0202 | Palpation: Shoulder – 02 |

**Supplies Needed:** Table

*This problem allows you the opportunity to demonstrate your ability to* **palpate** *the* **shoulder**.
*You have 2 minutes to complete this task.*

| Palpation: Shoulder – 02 | Course or Site Assessor Environment | | | | | |
|---|---|---|---|---|---|---|
| | | Test 1 | | Test 2 | | Test 3 |
| | | Y | N | Y | N | Y | N |
| Coracoid process | | ○ | ○ | ○ | ○ | ○ | ○ |
| Bicipital groove | | ○ | ○ | ○ | ○ | ○ | ○ |
| Pectoralis major muscle | | ○ | ○ | ○ | ○ | ○ | ○ |
| Sternoclavicular joint | | ○ | ○ | ○ | ○ | ○ | ○ |
| Teres minor muscle | | ○ | ○ | ○ | ○ | ○ | ○ |
| Spine of the scapula | | ○ | ○ | ○ | ○ | ○ | ○ |
| Triceps brachii muscle | | ○ | ○ | ○ | ○ | ○ | ○ |
| **Total** | | __/7 | | __/7 | | __/7 | |
| **Must achieve >4 to pass this examination** | | Ⓟ | Ⓕ | Ⓟ | Ⓕ | Ⓟ | Ⓕ |

| Assessor: Date: | Test 1 Comments: |
|---|---|
| Assessor: Date: | Test 2 Comments: |
| Assessor: Date: | Test 3 Comments: |

**TEST ENVIRONMENTS**
**L:** Laboratory/Classroom
**C:** Clinical/Field Testing
**P:** Practicum
**A:** Assessment/Mock Exam

**TEST INFORMATION**
**Test Statistics:** N/A
**Reference(s):** Starkey & Brown (2015)

## MUSCULOSKELETAL SYSTEM—REGION 7: SHOULDER
## PALPATION

| NATA EC 5th | BOC RD6 | SKILL |
|---|---|---|
| CE-21b, CE-20c | D2-0202 | Palpation: Shoulder – 03 |

**Supplies Needed:** Table

*This problem allows you the opportunity to demonstrate your ability to* **palpate** *the* **shoulder**.
*You have 2 minutes to complete this task.*

| Palpation: Shoulder – 03 | Course or Site Assessor Environment | Test 1 | | Test 2 | | Test 3 | |
|---|---|---|---|---|---|---|---|
| | | Y | N | Y | N | Y | N |
| Acromioclavicular joint | | O | O | O | O | O | O |
| Superior angle of the scapula | | O | O | O | O | O | O |
| Lesser tuberosity | | O | O | O | O | O | O |
| Xiphoid process | | O | O | O | O | O | O |
| Pectoralis minor muscle | | O | O | O | O | O | O |
| Supraspinatus muscle | | O | O | O | O | O | O |
| Rhomboids muscle | | O | O | O | O | O | O |
| **Total** | | __/7 | | __/7 | | __/7 | |
| **Must achieve >4 to pass this examination** | | ℗ | Ⓕ | ℗ | Ⓕ | ℗ | Ⓕ |

| Assessor:<br>Date: | Test 1 Comments: |
|---|---|
| Assessor:<br>Date: | Test 2 Comments: |
| Assessor:<br>Date: | Test 3 Comments: |

**TEST ENVIRONMENTS**
**L:** Laboratory/Classroom
**C:** Clinical/Field Testing
**P:** Practicum
**A:** Assessment/Mock Exam

**TEST INFORMATION**
**Test Statistics:** N/A
**Reference(s):** Starkey & Brown (2015)

## MUSCULOSKELETAL SYSTEM—REGION 7: SHOULDER
# MANUAL MUSCLE TESTING

| NATA EC 5th | BOC RD6 | SKILL |
|---|---|---|
| CE-21c | D2-0203 | MMT: Coracobrachialis |

**Supplies Needed:** Table

*This problem allows you the opportunity to demonstrate a* **manual muscle test** *for the* **coracobrachialis**.
*You have 2 minutes to complete this task.*

| MMT: Coracobrachialis | Course or Site Assessor Environment | Test 1 | | Test 2 | | Test 3 | |
|---|---|---|---|---|---|---|---|
| | | Y | N | Y | N | Y | N |
| **Tester places patient and limb in appropriate position** | | Y | N | Y | N | Y | N |
| Seated or supine (trunk fixated) | | ○ | ○ | ○ | ○ | ○ | ○ |
| Shoulder flexed to approximately 75 degrees | | ○ | ○ | ○ | ○ | ○ | ○ |
| Shoulder placed in lateral rotation | | ○ | ○ | ○ | ○ | ○ | ○ |
| Elbow flexed to 90 degrees and forearm supinated | | ○ | ○ | ○ | ○ | ○ | ○ |
| **Tester placed in proper position** | | Y | N | Y | N | Y | N |
| Stands to the side of the patient | | ○ | ○ | ○ | ○ | ○ | ○ |
| Places one hand on anteromedial surface of distal one third humerus | | ○ | ○ | ○ | ○ | ○ | ○ |
| **Tester performs test according to accepted guidelines** | | Y | N | Y | N | Y | N |
| Instructs the patient to hold the position | | ○ | ○ | ○ | ○ | ○ | ○ |
| Applies resistance downward in the direction of extension and light abduction | | ○ | ○ | ○ | ○ | ○ | ○ |
| Holds resistance for 5 seconds | | ○ | ○ | ○ | ○ | ○ | ○ |
| Performs assessment bilaterally | | ○ | ○ | ○ | ○ | ○ | ○ |
| **Identifies implications** | | Y | N | Y | N | Y | N |
| Correctly grades the MMT | | ○ | ○ | ○ | ○ | ○ | ○ |
| | **Total** | ___/11 | | ___/11 | | ___/11 | |
| | **Must achieve >7 to pass this examination** | Ⓟ | Ⓕ | Ⓟ | Ⓕ | Ⓟ | Ⓕ |

| Assessor: Date: | Test 1 Comments: |
|---|---|
| Assessor: Date: | Test 2 Comments: |
| Assessor: Date: | Test 3 Comments: |

**TEST ENVIRONMENTS**
**L:** Laboratory/Classroom
**C:** Clinical/Field Testing
**P:** Practicum
**A:** Assessment/Mock Exam

**TEST INFORMATION**
**Test Statistics:** N/A
**Reference(s):** Kendall et al. (2005)

## MUSCULOSKELETAL SYSTEM—REGION 7: SHOULDER
# MANUAL MUSCLE TESTING

| NATA EC 5th | BOC RD6 | SKILL |
|---|---|---|
| CE-21c | D2-0203 | MMT: Deltoid (Anterior) |

**Supplies Needed:** Table or chair

*This problem allows you the opportunity to demonstrate a* **manual muscle test** *for the* **anterior deltoid muscle.** *You have 2 minutes to complete this task.*

| MMT: Deltoid (Anterior) | Course or Site Assessor Environment | | Test 1 | | Test 2 | | Test 3 | |
|---|---|---|---|---|---|---|---|---|
| **Tester places patient and limb in appropriate position** | | | **Y** | **N** | **Y** | **N** | **Y** | **N** |
| Seated or supine | | | O | O | O | O | O | O |
| Shoulder abducted to 90 degrees in slight flexion | | | O | O | O | O | O | O |
| Shoulder placed in slight external rotation | | | O | O | O | O | O | O |
| Elbow flexed to 90 degrees (palmar surface facing downward) | | | O | O | O | O | O | O |
| **Tester placed in proper position** | | | **Y** | **N** | **Y** | **N** | **Y** | **N** |
| Stands facing the patient | | | O | O | O | O | O | O |
| Places one hand around the distal humerus | | | O | O | O | O | O | O |
| Places other hand posteriorly on shoulder girdle and applies counterpressure | | | O | O | O | O | O | O |
| **Tester performs test according to accepted guidelines** | | | **Y** | **N** | **Y** | **N** | **Y** | **N** |
| Instructs the patient to hold this position | | | O | O | O | O | O | O |
| Applies resistance anteromedial side of the arm in the direction of adduction and slight extension | | | O | O | O | O | O | O |
| Holds resistance for 5 seconds | | | O | O | O | O | O | O |
| Performs assessment bilaterally | | | O | O | O | O | O | O |
| **Identifies implications** | | | **Y** | **N** | **Y** | **N** | **Y** | **N** |
| Correctly grades the MMT | | | O | O | O | O | O | O |
| | | Total | ___/12 | | ___/12 | | ___/12 | |
| | Must achieve >8 to pass this examination | | Ⓟ | Ⓕ | Ⓟ | Ⓕ | Ⓟ | Ⓕ |

| Assessor: Date: | Test 1 Comments: |
|---|---|
| Assessor: Date: | Test 2 Comments: |
| Assessor: Date: | Test 3 Comments: |

**TEST ENVIRONMENTS**
**L:** Laboratory/Classroom
**C:** Clinical/Field Testing
**P:** Practicum
**A:** Assessment/Mock Exam

**TEST INFORMATION**
**Test Statistics:** N/A
**Reference(s):** Kendall et al. (2005)

## MUSCULOSKELETAL SYSTEM—REGION 7: SHOULDER
## MANUAL MUSCLE TESTING

| NATA EC 5th | BOC RD6 | SKILL |
|---|---|---|
| CE-21c | D2-0203 | MMT: Deltoid (Middle) |

**Supplies Needed:** Table or chair

*This problem allows you the opportunity to demonstrate a* **manual muscle test** *for the* **middle deltoid muscle***. You have 2 minutes to complete this task.*

| MMT: Deltoid (Middle) | Course or Site Assessor Environment | Test 1 | | Test 2 | | Test 3 | |
|---|---|---|---|---|---|---|---|
| | | Y | N | Y | N | Y | N |
| **Tester places patient and limb in appropriate position** | | Y | N | Y | N | Y | N |
| Seated | | O | O | O | O | O | O |
| Shoulder abducted to 90 degrees | | O | O | O | O | O | O |
| Elbow flexed to 90 degrees (palmar surface facing downward | | O | O | O | O | O | O |
| **Tester placed in proper position** | | Y | N | Y | N | Y | N |
| Stands behind or to the side of the patient | | O | O | O | O | O | O |
| Places one hand around the distal end of the humerus | | O | O | O | O | O | O |
| **Tester performs test according to accepted guidelines** | | Y | N | Y | N | Y | N |
| Instructs the patient to hold the position | | O | O | O | O | O | O |
| Applies resistance downward in direction of adduction | | O | O | O | O | O | O |
| Holds resistance for 5 seconds | | O | O | O | O | O | O |
| Performs assessment bilaterally | | O | O | O | O | O | O |
| **Identifies implications** | | Y | N | Y | N | Y | N |
| Correctly grades the MMT | | O | O | O | O | O | O |
| | Total | __/10 | | __/10 | | __/10 | |
| | Must achieve >6 to pass this examination | (P) | (F) | (P) | (F) | (P) | (F) |
| **Assessor:** **Date:** | **Test 1 Comments:** | | | | | | |
| **Assessor:** **Date:** | **Test 2 Comments:** | | | | | | |
| **Assessor:** **Date:** | **Test 3 Comments:** | | | | | | |

**TEST ENVIRONMENTS**
**L:** Laboratory/Classroom
**C:** Clinical/Field Testing
**P:** Practicum
**A:** Assessment/Mock Exam

**TEST INFORMATION**
**Test Statistics:** N/A
**Reference(s):** Kendall et al. (2005)

MUSCULOSKELETAL SYSTEM—REGION 7: SHOULDER
# MANUAL MUSCLE TESTING

| NATA EC 5th | BOC RD6 | SKILL |
|---|---|---|
| CE-21c | D2-0203 | MMT: Deltoid (Posterior) |

**Supplies Needed:** Table or chair

*This problem allows you the opportunity to demonstrate a* **manual muscle test** *for the* **posterior deltoid muscle.** *You have 2 minutes to complete this task.*

| MMT: Deltoid (Posterior) | Course or Site Assessor Environment | | Test 1 | | Test 2 | | Test 3 | |
|---|---|---|---|---|---|---|---|---|
| **Tester places patient and limb in appropriate position** | | | Y | N | Y | N | Y | N |
| Seated or prone | | | O | O | O | O | O | O |
| Shoulder abducted to 90 degrees (slight extension) | | | O | O | O | O | O | O |
| Shoulder placed in slight medial rotation | | | O | O | O | O | O | O |
| Elbow flexed to 90 degrees (palmar surface facing downward) | | | O | O | O | O | O | O |
| **Tester placed in proper position** | | | Y | N | Y | N | Y | N |
| Stands behind the patient | | | O | O | O | O | O | O |
| Places one hand on posterolateral surface of distal humerus | | | O | O | O | O | O | O |
| Applies counterpressure anteriorly to the shoulder girdle with other hand | | | O | O | O | O | O | O |
| **Tester performs test according to accepted guidelines** | | | Y | N | Y | N | Y | N |
| Instructs the patient to hold the position | | | O | O | O | O | O | O |
| Applies resistance downward in direction of adduction and slight flexion | | | O | O | O | O | O | O |
| Holds resistance for 5 seconds | | | O | O | O | O | O | O |
| Performs assessment bilaterally | | | O | O | O | O | O | O |
| **Identifies implications** | | | Y | N | Y | N | Y | N |
| Correctly grades the MMT | | | O | O | O | O | O | O |
| **Total** | | | __/12 | | __/12 | | __/12 | |
| **Must achieve >8 to pass this examination** | | | Ⓟ | Ⓕ | Ⓟ | Ⓕ | Ⓟ | Ⓕ |

| Assessor: Date: | Test 1 Comments: |
|---|---|
| Assessor: Date: | Test 2 Comments: |
| Assessor: Date: | Test 3 Comments: |

**TEST ENVIRONMENTS**
**L:** Laboratory/Classroom
**C:** Clinical/Field Testing
**P:** Practicum
**A:** Assessment/Mock Exam

**TEST INFORMATION**
**Test Statistics:** N/A
**Reference(s):** Kendall et al. (2005)

## MUSCULOSKELETAL SYSTEM—REGION 7: SHOULDER
# MANUAL MUSCLE TESTING

| NATA EC 5th | BOC RD6 | SKILL |
|---|---|---|
| CE-21c | D2-0203 | MMT: Infraspinatus |

**Supplies Needed:** Table

*This problem allows you the opportunity to demonstrate a* **manual muscle test** *for the* **infraspinatus muscle.** *You have 2 minutes to complete this task.*

| MMT: Infraspinatus | Course or Site / Assessor / Environment | | Test 1 | | Test 2 | | Test 3 | |
|---|---|---|---|---|---|---|---|---|
| **Tester places patient and limb in appropriate position** | | | Y | N | Y | N | Y | N |
| Prone (head turned away from the test arm) | | | ○ | ○ | ○ | ○ | ○ | ○ |
| Shoulder flexed to 90 degrees and externally rotated to approximately 90 degrees | | | ○ | ○ | ○ | ○ | ○ | ○ |
| Elbow flexed to 90 degrees (elbow off table edge) | | | ○ | ○ | ○ | ○ | ○ | ○ |
| **Tester placed in proper position** | | | Y | N | Y | N | Y | N |
| Stands on the side of the patient's test arm | | | ○ | ○ | ○ | ○ | ○ | ○ |
| Places one hand under the arm near the elbow; stabilizes humerus | | | ○ | ○ | ○ | ○ | ○ | ○ |
| Places the other hand on the distal forearm | | | ○ | ○ | ○ | ○ | ○ | ○ |
| **Tester performs test according to accepted guidelines** | | | Y | N | Y | N | Y | N |
| Instructs the patient to hold this position | | | ○ | ○ | ○ | ○ | ○ | ○ |
| Applies resistance downward in the direction of medial rotation | | | ○ | ○ | ○ | ○ | ○ | ○ |
| Holds resistance for 5 seconds | | | ○ | ○ | ○ | ○ | ○ | ○ |
| Performs assessment bilaterally | | | ○ | ○ | ○ | ○ | ○ | ○ |
| **Identifies implications** | | | Y | N | Y | N | Y | N |
| Correctly grades the MMT | | | ○ | ○ | ○ | ○ | ○ | ○ |
| Total | | | __/11 | | __/11 | | __/11 | |
| Must achieve >7 to pass this examination | | | Ⓟ | Ⓕ | Ⓟ | Ⓕ | Ⓟ | Ⓕ |

| Assessor: Date: | Test 1 Comments: |
|---|---|
| Assessor: Date: | Test 2 Comments: |
| Assessor: Date: | Test 3 Comments: |

**TEST ENVIRONMENTS**
**L:** Laboratory/Classroom
**C:** Clinical/Field Testing
**P:** Practicum
**A:** Assessment/Mock Exam

**TEST INFORMATION**
**Test Statistics:** N/A
**Reference(s):** Kendall et al. (2005)

# MANUAL MUSCLE TESTING

| NATA EC 5th | BOC RD6 | SKILL |
|---|---|---|
| CE-21c | D2-0203 | MMT: Latissimus Dorsi |

**Supplies Needed:** Table

*This problem allows you the opportunity to demonstrate a* **manual muscle test** *for the* **latissimus dorsi muscle**. *You have 2 minutes to complete this task.*

| MMT: Latissimus Dorsi | Course or Site / Assessor / Environment | | | | | |
|---|---|---|---|---|---|---|
| | Test 1 | | Test 2 | | Test 3 | |
| **Tester places patient and limb in appropriate position** | Y | N | Y | N | Y | N |
| Prone | ○ | ○ | ○ | ○ | ○ | ○ |
| Shoulder placed in slight extension and adduction | ○ | ○ | ○ | ○ | ○ | ○ |
| Shoulder internally rotated, forearm facing body | ○ | ○ | ○ | ○ | ○ | ○ |
| **Tester placed in proper position** | Y | N | Y | N | Y | N |
| Stands at side of the patient | ○ | ○ | ○ | ○ | ○ | ○ |
| Places one hand on the medial forearm | ○ | ○ | ○ | ○ | ○ | ○ |
| **Tester performs test according to accepted guidelines** | Y | N | Y | N | Y | N |
| Instructs the patient to hold this position | ○ | ○ | ○ | ○ | ○ | ○ |
| Applies resistance in the direction of extension and adduction | ○ | ○ | ○ | ○ | ○ | ○ |
| Holds resistance for 5 seconds | ○ | ○ | ○ | ○ | ○ | ○ |
| Performs assessment bilaterally | ○ | ○ | ○ | ○ | ○ | ○ |
| **Identifies implications** | Y | N | Y | N | Y | N |
| Correctly grades the MMT | ○ | ○ | ○ | ○ | ○ | ○ |
| **Total** | __/10 | | __/10 | | __/10 | |
| **Must achieve >6 to pass this examination** | Ⓟ | Ⓕ | Ⓟ | Ⓕ | Ⓟ | Ⓕ |

| Assessor: Date: | Test 1 Comments: |
|---|---|
| Assessor: Date: | Test 2 Comments: |
| Assessor: Date: | Test 3 Comments: |

**TEST ENVIRONMENTS**
**L:** Laboratory/Classroom
**C:** Clinical/Field Testing
**P:** Practicum
**A:** Assessment/Mock Exam

**TEST INFORMATION**
**Test Statistics:** N/A
**Reference(s):** Hislop & Montgomery (2007)
Kendall et al. (2005)

## MUSCULOSKELETAL SYSTEM—REGION 7: SHOULDER
## MANUAL MUSCLE TESTING

| NATA EC 5th | BOC RD6 | SKILL |
|:---:|:---:|:---:|
| CE-21c | D2-0203 | MMT: Pectoralis Major (Upper Portion) |

**Supplies Needed:** Table

*This problem allows you the opportunity to demonstrate a* **manual muscle test** *for the* **pectoralis major (upper portion) muscle**. *You have 2 minutes to complete this task.*

| MMT: Pectoralis Major (Upper Portion) | Course or Site _____ _____ _____<br>Assessor _____ _____ _____<br>Environment _____ _____ _____ | | | | | |
|---|---|:---:|:---:|:---:|:---:|:---:|:---:|
| | | Test 1 | | Test 2 | | Test 3 | |
| **Tester places patient and limb in appropriate position** | | **Y** | **N** | **Y** | **N** | **Y** | **N** |
| Supine | | ○ | ○ | ○ | ○ | ○ | ○ |
| Shoulder placed in 90 degrees flexion and slight medial rotation | | ○ | ○ | ○ | ○ | ○ | ○ |
| Elbow placed in full extension | | ○ | ○ | ○ | ○ | ○ | ○ |
| **Tester placed in proper position** | | **Y** | **N** | **Y** | **N** | **Y** | **N** |
| Stands at side of the patient, above the patient's head | | ○ | ○ | ○ | ○ | ○ | ○ |
| Places one hand on the medial forearm | | ○ | ○ | ○ | ○ | ○ | ○ |
| Places other hand on the patient's opposite shoulder (stabilizing body) | | ○ | ○ | ○ | ○ | ○ | ○ |
| **Tester performs test according to accepted guidelines** | | **Y** | **N** | **Y** | **N** | **Y** | **N** |
| Instructs the patient to hold this position | | ○ | ○ | ○ | ○ | ○ | ○ |
| Applies resistance in the direction of horizontal adduction (horizontal extension) | | ○ | ○ | ○ | ○ | ○ | ○ |
| Holds resistance for 5 seconds | | ○ | ○ | ○ | ○ | ○ | ○ |
| Performs assessment bilaterally | | ○ | ○ | ○ | ○ | ○ | ○ |
| **Identifies implications** | | **Y** | **N** | **Y** | **N** | **Y** | **N** |
| Correctly grades the MMT | | ○ | ○ | ○ | ○ | ○ | ○ |
| **Total** | | ____/11 | | ____/11 | | ____/11 | |
| **Must achieve >7 to pass this examination** | | Ⓟ | Ⓕ | Ⓟ | Ⓕ | Ⓟ | Ⓕ |

| Assessor:<br>Date: | Test 1 Comments: |
|---|---|
| Assessor:<br>Date: | Test 2 Comments: |
| Assessor:<br>Date: | Test 3 Comments: |

**TEST ENVIRONMENTS**
**L:** Laboratory/Classroom
**C:** Clinical/Field Testing
**P:** Practicum
**A:** Assessment/Mock Exam

**TEST INFORMATION**
**Test Statistics:** N/A
**Reference(s):**  Hislop & Montgomery (2007)
Kendall et al. (2005)

## MUSCULOSKELETAL SYSTEM—REGION 7: SHOULDER
## MANUAL MUSCLE TESTING

| NATA EC 5th | BOC RD6 | SKILL |
|---|---|---|
| CE-21c | D2-0203 | MMT: Pectoralis Major (Lower Portion) |

**Supplies Needed:** Table

*This problem allows you the opportunity to demonstrate a* **manual muscle test** *for the* **pectoralis major (lower portion) muscle***. You have 2 minutes to complete this task.*

| MMT: Pectoralis Major (Lower Portion) | Course or Site Assessor Environment | | Test 1 | | Test 2 | | Test 3 | |
|---|---|---|---|---|---|---|---|---|
| **Tester places patient and limb in appropriate position** | | Y | N | Y | N | Y | N | |
| Supine | | ○ | ○ | ○ | ○ | ○ | ○ | |
| Shoulder placed in 90 degrees flexion and slight medial rotation | | ○ | ○ | ○ | ○ | ○ | ○ | |
| Arm obliquely adducted toward opposite iliac crest | | ○ | ○ | ○ | ○ | ○ | ○ | |
| Elbow placed in full extension | | ○ | ○ | ○ | ○ | ○ | ○ | |
| **Tester placed in proper position** | | Y | N | Y | N | Y | N | |
| Stands at side of the patient, above the patient's head | | ○ | ○ | ○ | ○ | ○ | ○ | |
| Places one hand on the medial forearm | | ○ | ○ | ○ | ○ | ○ | ○ | |
| Places other hand on the patient's opposite iliac crest (stabilizing body) | | ○ | ○ | ○ | ○ | ○ | ○ | |
| **Tester performs test according to accepted guidelines** | | Y | N | Y | N | Y | N | |
| Instructs the patient to hold this position | | ○ | ○ | ○ | ○ | ○ | ○ | |
| Applies resistance obliquely in the direction of horizontal abduction (horizontal extension) | | ○ | ○ | ○ | ○ | ○ | ○ | |
| Holds resistance for 5 seconds | | ○ | ○ | ○ | ○ | ○ | ○ | |
| Performs assessment bilaterally | | ○ | ○ | ○ | ○ | ○ | ○ | |
| **Identifies implications** | | Y | N | Y | N | Y | N | |
| Correctly grades the MMT | | ○ | ○ | ○ | ○ | ○ | ○ | |
| **Total** | | /12 | | /12 | | /12 | | |
| **Must achieve >8 to pass this examination** | | Ⓟ | Ⓕ | Ⓟ | Ⓕ | Ⓟ | Ⓕ | |

| Assessor: Date: | Test 1 Comments: |
|---|---|
| Assessor: Date: | Test 2 Comments: |
| Assessor: Date: | Test 3 Comments: |

**TEST ENVIRONMENTS**
**L:** Laboratory/Classroom
**C:** Clinical/Field Testing
**P:** Practicum
**A:** Assessment/Mock Exam

**TEST INFORMATION**
**Test Statistics:** N/A
**Reference(s):** Hislop & Montgomery (2007)
Kendall et al. (2005)

## MUSCULOSKELETAL SYSTEM—REGION 7: SHOULDER
# MANUAL MUSCLE TESTING

| NATA EC 5th | BOC RD6 | SKILL |
|---|---|---|
| CE-21c | D2-0203 | MMT: Pectoralis Minor |

**Supplies Needed:** Table

*This problem allows you the opportunity to demonstrate a* **manual muscle test** *for the* **pectoralis minor muscle**. *You have 2 minutes to complete this task.*

| MMT: Pectoralis Minor | Course or Site Assessor Environment | | Test 1 | | Test 2 | | Test 3 | |
|---|---|---|---|---|---|---|---|---|
| **Tester places patient and limb in appropriate position** | | | Y | N | Y | N | Y | N |
| Supine (head at end of table) | | | ○ | ○ | ○ | ○ | ○ | ○ |
| Arm at the patient's side | | | ○ | ○ | ○ | ○ | ○ | ○ |
| **Tester placed in proper position** | | | Y | N | Y | N | Y | N |
| Stands at side of the patient, facing the patient | | | ○ | ○ | ○ | ○ | ○ | ○ |
| Places one hand on the anterior aspect of the shoulder | | | ○ | ○ | ○ | ○ | ○ | ○ |
| **Tester performs test according to accepted guidelines** | | | Y | N | Y | N | Y | N |
| Instructs the patient to actively thrust shoulder forward (lift off table) | | | ○ | ○ | ○ | ○ | ○ | ○ |
| Applies downward resistance against anterior shoulder (toward table) | | | ○ | ○ | ○ | ○ | ○ | ○ |
| Holds resistance for 5 seconds | | | ○ | ○ | ○ | ○ | ○ | ○ |
| Performs assessment bilaterally | | | ○ | ○ | ○ | ○ | ○ | ○ |
| **Identifies implications** | | | Y | N | Y | N | Y | N |
| Correctly grades the MMT | | | ○ | ○ | ○ | ○ | ○ | ○ |
| Total | | | __/9 | | __/9 | | __/9 | |
| Must achieve >6 to pass this examination | | | Ⓟ | Ⓕ | Ⓟ | Ⓕ | Ⓟ | Ⓕ |

| Assessor: Date: | Test 1 Comments: |
|---|---|
| Assessor: Date: | Test 2 Comments: |
| Assessor: Date: | Test 3 Comments: |

**TEST ENVIRONMENTS**
**L:** Laboratory/Classroom
**C:** Clinical/Field Testing
**P:** Practicum
**A:** Assessment/Mock Exam

**TEST INFORMATION**
**Test Statistics:** N/A
**Reference(s):** Hislop & Montgomery (2007)
Kendall et al. (2005)

| NATA EC 5th | BOC RD6 | SKILL |
|---|---|---|
| CE-21c | D2-0203 | MMT: Rhomboid Alternate Test |

**Supplies Needed:** Table

*This problem allows you the opportunity to demonstrate the* **rhomboid alternate test**. *You have 2 minutes to complete this task.*

| MMT: Rhomboid Alternate Test | Course or Site Assessor Environment | | | | | |
|---|---|---|---|---|---|---|
| | | Test 1 | | Test 2 | | Test 3 |
| **Tester places patient and limb in appropriate position** | | Y | N | Y | N | Y | N |
| Prone | | ○ | ○ | ○ | ○ | ○ | ○ |
| Shoulder abducted to 90 degrees | | ○ | ○ | ○ | ○ | ○ | ○ |
| Shoulder medially rotated with thumb pointing downward | | ○ | ○ | ○ | ○ | ○ | ○ |
| **Tester placed in proper position** | | Y | N | Y | N | Y | N |
| Stands at side of the patient, facing the patient | | ○ | ○ | ○ | ○ | ○ | ○ |
| Places one hand on the opposite scapula | | ○ | ○ | ○ | ○ | ○ | ○ |
| Places other hand against distal forearm (radius/ulna) | | ○ | ○ | ○ | ○ | ○ | ○ |
| **Tester performs test according to accepted guidelines** | | Y | N | Y | N | Y | N |
| Instructs the patient to actively horizontally extend the shoulder | | ○ | ○ | ○ | ○ | ○ | ○ |
| Applies resistance against arm in direction of horizontal flexion (downward direction toward the table) | | ○ | ○ | ○ | ○ | ○ | ○ |
| Holds resistance for 5 seconds | | ○ | ○ | ○ | ○ | ○ | ○ |
| Performs assessment bilaterally | | ○ | ○ | ○ | ○ | ○ | ○ |
| **Identifies implications** | | Y | N | Y | N | Y | N |
| Correctly grades the MMT | | ○ | ○ | ○ | ○ | ○ | ○ |
| Total | | __/11 | | __/11 | | __/11 |
| Must achieve >7 to pass this examination | | Ⓟ | Ⓕ | Ⓟ | Ⓕ | Ⓟ | Ⓕ |

| Assessor: Date: | Test 1 Comments: |
|---|---|
| Assessor: Date: | Test 2 Comments: |
| Assessor: Date: | Test 3 Comments: |

**TEST ENVIRONMENTS**
**L:** Laboratory/Classroom
**C:** Clinical/Field Testing
**P:** Practicum
**A:** Assessment/Mock Exam

**TEST INFORMATION**
**Test Statistics:** N/A
**Reference(s):** Hislop & Montgomery (2007)
Kendall et al. (2005)

## MUSCULOSKELETAL SYSTEM—REGION 7: SHOULDER
# MANUAL MUSCLE TESTING

| NATA EC 5th | BOC RD6 | SKILL |
|---|---|---|
| CE-21c | D2-0203 | MMT: Rhomboid/Levator |

**Supplies Needed:** Table

*This problem allows you the opportunity to demonstrate a* **manual muscle test** *for the* **rhomboid/levator muscle.** *You have 2 minutes to complete this task.*

| MMT: Rhomboid/Levator | Course or Site / Assessor / Environment | | | | | |
|---|---|---|---|---|---|---|
| | Test 1 | | Test 2 | | Test 3 | |
| **Tester places patient and limb in appropriate position** | Y | N | Y | N | Y | N |
| Prone (shoulder at edge of table) | ○ | ○ | ○ | ○ | ○ | ○ |
| Shoulder extended (hyperextended)/slight lateral rotation and full adduction | ○ | ○ | ○ | ○ | ○ | ○ |
| Elbow flexed to 90 degrees | ○ | ○ | ○ | ○ | ○ | ○ |
| **Tester placed in proper position** | Y | N | Y | N | Y | N |
| Stands at side of the patient, facing the patient | ○ | ○ | ○ | ○ | ○ | ○ |
| Places one hand on the shoulder/scapula | ○ | ○ | ○ | ○ | ○ | ○ |
| Places other hand against medial aspect of the elbow | ○ | ○ | ○ | ○ | ○ | ○ |
| **Tester performs test according to accepted guidelines** | Y | N | Y | N | Y | N |
| Instructs the patient to actively attain the position | ○ | ○ | ○ | ○ | ○ | ○ |
| Applies resistance against arm in direction of abduction/ lateral rotation of the inferior angle of the scapula | ○ | ○ | ○ | ○ | ○ | ○ |
| Applies depressive force to the shoulder with the other hand | ○ | ○ | ○ | ○ | ○ | ○ |
| Holds resistance for 5 seconds | ○ | ○ | ○ | ○ | ○ | ○ |
| Performs assessment bilaterally | ○ | ○ | ○ | ○ | ○ | ○ |
| **Identifies implications** | Y | N | Y | N | Y | N |
| Correctly grades the MMT | ○ | ○ | ○ | ○ | ○ | ○ |
| Total | __/12 | | __/12 | | __/12 | |
| Must achieve >8 to pass this examination | Ⓟ | Ⓕ | Ⓟ | Ⓕ | Ⓟ | Ⓕ |

| Assessor: Date: | Test 1 Comments: |
|---|---|
| Assessor: Date: | Test 2 Comments: |
| Assessor: Date: | Test 3 Comments: |

**TEST ENVIRONMENTS**
**L:** Laboratory/Classroom
**C:** Clinical/Field Testing
**P:** Practicum
**A:** Assessment/Mock Exam

**TEST INFORMATION**
**Test Statistics:** N/A
**Reference(s):** Hislop & Montgomery (2007)
Kendall et al. (2005)

## MUSCULOSKELETAL SYSTEM—REGION 7: SHOULDER
# MANUAL MUSCLE TESTING

| NATA EC 5th | BOC RD6 | SKILL |
|---|---|---|
| CE-21c | D2-0203 | MMT: Serratus Anterior |

**Supplies Needed:** Table

*This problem allows you the opportunity to demonstrate a* **manual muscle test** *for the* **serratus anterior muscle**. *You have 2 minutes to complete this task.*

| MMT: Serratus Anterior | Course or Site / Assessor / Environment | | Test 1 | | Test 2 | | Test 3 | |
|---|---|---|---|---|---|---|---|---|
| **Tester places patient and limb in appropriate position** | | **Y** | **N** | **Y** | **N** | **Y** | **N** | |
| Supine | | ○ | ○ | ○ | ○ | ○ | ○ | |
| Shoulder flexed to 90 degrees | | ○ | ○ | ○ | ○ | ○ | ○ | |
| Shoulder elevated off the table (abduction of the scapula/punching movement) | | ○ | ○ | ○ | ○ | ○ | ○ | |
| Fingers clenched in a fist | | ○ | ○ | ○ | ○ | ○ | ○ | |
| **Tester placed in proper position** | | **Y** | **N** | **Y** | **N** | **Y** | **N** | |
| Stands at side of the patient, facing the patient (the tester may need to stand on a stool) | | ○ | ○ | ○ | ○ | ○ | ○ | |
| Places one (or both) hand(s) over the elevated fist | | ○ | ○ | ○ | ○ | ○ | ○ | |
| **Tester performs test according to accepted guidelines** | | **Y** | **N** | **Y** | **N** | **Y** | **N** | |
| Instructs the patient to maintain the elevated position | | ○ | ○ | ○ | ○ | ○ | ○ | |
| Applies downward resistance against the clenched fist (axial pressure pushing shoulder back down to the table) | | ○ | ○ | ○ | ○ | ○ | ○ | |
| Holds resistance for 5 seconds | | ○ | ○ | ○ | ○ | ○ | ○ | |
| Performs assessment bilaterally | | ○ | ○ | ○ | ○ | ○ | ○ | |
| **Identifies implications** | | **Y** | **N** | **Y** | **N** | **Y** | **N** | |
| Correctly grades the MMT | | ○ | ○ | ○ | ○ | ○ | ○ | |
| | Total | ___/11 | | ___/11 | | ___/11 | | |
| | Must achieve >7 to pass this examination | Ⓟ | Ⓕ | Ⓟ | Ⓕ | Ⓟ | Ⓕ | |

| Assessor: Date: | Test 1 Comments: |
|---|---|
| Assessor: Date: | Test 2 Comments: |
| Assessor: Date: | Test 3 Comments: |

**TEST ENVIRONMENTS**
**L:** Laboratory/Classroom
**C:** Clinical/Field Testing
**P:** Practicum
**A:** Assessment/Mock Exam

**TEST INFORMATION**
**Test Statistics:** N/A
**Reference(s):** Kendall et al. (2005)

MUSCULOSKELETAL SYSTEM—REGION 7: SHOULDER
# MANUAL MUSCLE TESTING

| NATA EC 5th | BOC RD6 | SKILL |
|---|---|---|
| CE-21c | D2-0203 | MMT: Serratus Anterior (Preferred Test) |

**Supplies Needed:** Table

*This problem allows you the opportunity to demonstrate a* **manual muscle test** *for the* **serratus anterior muscle (preferred test)**. *You have 2 minutes to complete this task.*

| MMT: Serratus Anterior (Preferred Test) | Course or Site Assessor Environment | | | | | |
|---|---|---|---|---|---|---|
| | Test 1 | | Test 2 | | Test 3 | |
| **Tester places patient and limb in appropriate position** | Y | N | Y | N | Y | N |
| Seated | ○ | ○ | ○ | ○ | ○ | ○ |
| Shoulder flexed to 120 to 130 degrees | ○ | ○ | ○ | ○ | ○ | ○ |
| Instructs the patient to hold on to table with opposite hand | ○ | ○ | ○ | ○ | ○ | ○ |
| **Tester placed in proper position** | Y | N | Y | N | Y | N |
| Stands on side to be tested | ○ | ○ | ○ | ○ | ○ | ○ |
| Grasps dorsal surface of arm between shoulder and elbow | ○ | ○ | ○ | ○ | ○ | ○ |
| Places other hand along inferior angle with thumb against lateral border | ○ | ○ | ○ | ○ | ○ | ○ |
| **Tester performs test according to accepted guidelines** | Y | N | Y | N | Y | N |
| Instructs the patient to maintain this position | ○ | ○ | ○ | ○ | ○ | ○ |
| Applies downward resistance into shoulder extension | ○ | ○ | ○ | ○ | ○ | ○ |
| Applies slight pressure against lateral border with opposite hand | ○ | ○ | ○ | ○ | ○ | ○ |
| Holds resistance for 5 seconds | ○ | ○ | ○ | ○ | ○ | ○ |
| Performs assessment bilaterally | ○ | ○ | ○ | ○ | ○ | ○ |
| **Identifies implications** | Y | N | Y | N | Y | N |
| Correctly grades the MMT | ○ | ○ | ○ | ○ | ○ | ○ |
| **Total** | __/12 | | __/12 | | __/12 | |
| **Must achieve >8 to pass this examination** | Ⓟ | Ⓕ | Ⓟ | Ⓕ | Ⓟ | Ⓕ |

| Assessor: Date: | Test 1 Comments: |
|---|---|
| Assessor: Date: | Test 2 Comments: |
| Assessor: Date: | Test 3 Comments: |

**TEST ENVIRONMENTS**
**L:** Laboratory/Classroom
**C:** Clinical/Field Testing
**P:** Practicum
**A:** Assessment/Mock Exam

**TEST INFORMATION**
**Test Statistics:** N/A
**Reference(s):** Kendall et al. (2005)

## MUSCULOSKELETAL SYSTEM—REGION 7: SHOULDER
# MANUAL MUSCLE TESTING

| NATA EC 5th | BOC RD6 | SKILL |
|---|---|---|
| CE-21c | D2-0203 | MMT: Subscapularis |

**Supplies Needed:** Table, towel or bolster

*This problem allows you the opportunity to demonstrate a* **manual muscle test** *for the* **subscapularis muscle**. *You have 2 minutes to complete this task.*

| MMT: Subscapularis | Course or Site Assessor Environment | | | | | |
|---|---|---|---|---|---|---|
| | | Test 1 | | Test 2 | | Test 3 |
| **Tester places patient and limb in appropriate position** | | Y | N | Y | N | Y | N |
| Prone (head turned toward test side) | | O | O | O | O | O | O |
| Shoulder abducted 90 degrees and internally rotated ~45 degrees | | O | O | O | O | O | O |
| Elbow flexed to 90 degrees with forearm hanging over side of table | | O | O | O | O | O | O |
| Distal arm at elbow supported by folded towel or bolster | | O | O | O | O | O | O |
| **Tester placed in proper position** | | Y | N | Y | N | Y | N |
| Stands on the test side of the patient | | O | O | O | O | O | O |
| Places one hand under arm at elbow to stabilize humerus | | O | O | O | O | O | O |
| Places other hand on volar aspect of distal forearm | | O | O | O | O | O | O |
| **Tester performs test according to accepted guidelines** | | Y | N | Y | N | Y | N |
| Instructs the patient to hold this position | | O | O | O | O | O | O |
| Applies resistance downward in direction of lateral rotation | | O | O | O | O | O | O |
| Holds resistance for 5 seconds | | O | O | O | O | O | O |
| Performs assessment bilaterally | | O | O | O | O | O | O |
| **Identifies implications** | | Y | N | Y | N | Y | N |
| Correctly grades the MMT | | O | O | O | O | O | O |
| **Total** | | ___/12 | | ___/12 | | ___/12 | |
| **Must achieve >8 to pass this examination** | | Ⓟ | Ⓕ | Ⓟ | Ⓕ | Ⓟ | Ⓕ |

| Assessor: Date: | Test 1 Comments: |
|---|---|
| Assessor: Date: | Test 2 Comments: |
| Assessor: Date: | Test 3 Comments: |

**TEST ENVIRONMENTS**
**L:** Laboratory/Classroom
**C:** Clinical/Field Testing
**P:** Practicum
**A:** Assessment/Mock Exam

**TEST INFORMATION**
**Test Statistics:** N/A
**Reference(s):** Hislop & Montgomery (2007)
Kendall et al. (2005)

### MUSCULOSKELETAL SYSTEM—REGION 7: SHOULDER
# MANUAL MUSCLE TESTING

| NATA EC 5th | BOC RD6 | SKILL |
|---|---|---|
| CE-21c | D2-0203 | MMT: Supraspinatus |

**Supplies Needed:** Table or chair

*This problem allows you the opportunity to demonstrate a* **manual muscle test** *for the* **supraspinatus muscle**. *You have 2 minutes to complete this task.*

| MMT: Supraspinatus | Course or Site / Assessor / Environment | | Test 1 | | Test 2 | | Test 3 |
|---|---|---|---|---|---|---|---|
| **Tester places patient and limb in appropriate position** | | Y | N | Y | N | Y | N |
| Seated or standing | | ○ | ○ | ○ | ○ | ○ | ○ |
| Arm placed at side of the patient (palm flat against the side) | | ○ | ○ | ○ | ○ | ○ | ○ |
| Head and neck extended and laterally flexed toward test side | | ○ | ○ | ○ | ○ | ○ | ○ |
| Head and neck are laterally rotated to opposite side | | ○ | ○ | ○ | ○ | ○ | ○ |
| **Tester placed in proper position** | | Y | N | Y | N | Y | N |
| Stands facing the patient | | ○ | ○ | ○ | ○ | ○ | ○ |
| Stabilizes the opposite shoulder with one hand | | ○ | ○ | ○ | ○ | ○ | ○ |
| Places other hand at distal forearm | | ○ | ○ | ○ | ○ | ○ | ○ |
| **Tester performs test according to accepted guidelines** | | Y | N | Y | N | Y | N |
| Instructs the patient to initiate abduction of the shoulder | | ○ | ○ | ○ | ○ | ○ | ○ |
| Applies resistance in direction of adduction | | ○ | ○ | ○ | ○ | ○ | ○ |
| Holds resistance for 5 seconds | | ○ | ○ | ○ | ○ | ○ | ○ |
| Performs assessment bilaterally | | ○ | ○ | ○ | ○ | ○ | ○ |
| **Identifies implications** | | Y | N | Y | N | Y | N |
| Correctly grades the MMT | | ○ | ○ | ○ | ○ | ○ | ○ |
| **Total** | | ___/12 | | ___/12 | | ___/12 | |
| **Must achieve >8 to pass this examination** | | P | F | P | F | P | F |

| Assessor: Date: | Test 1 Comments: |
|---|---|
| Assessor: Date: | Test 2 Comments: |
| Assessor: Date: | Test 3 Comments: |

**TEST ENVIRONMENTS**
**L:** Laboratory/Classroom
**C:** Clinical/Field Testing
**P:** Practicum
**A:** Assessment/Mock Exam

**TEST INFORMATION**
**Test Statistics:** N/A
**Reference(s):** Hislop & Montgomery (2007)
Kendall et al. (2005)

## MUSCULOSKELETAL SYSTEM—REGION 7: SHOULDER
# MANUAL MUSCLE TESTING

| NATA EC 5th | BOC RD6 | SKILL |
|---|---|---|
| CE-21c | D2-0203 | MMT: Teres Major |

**Supplies Needed:** Table

*This problem allows you the opportunity to demonstrate a* **manual muscle test** *for the* **teres major muscle.** *You have 2 minutes to complete this task.*

| MMT: Teres Major | Course or Site / Assessor / Environment | Test 1 | | Test 2 | | Test 3 | |
|---|---|---|---|---|---|---|---|
| | | Y | N | Y | N | Y | N |
| **Tester places patient and limb in appropriate position** | | Y | N | Y | N | Y | N |
| Prone (head facing test arm) | | ○ | ○ | ○ | ○ | ○ | ○ |
| Shoulder extended, adducted, and medially rotated | | ○ | ○ | ○ | ○ | ○ | ○ |
| Palmar surface of hand facing upward | | ○ | ○ | ○ | ○ | ○ | ○ |
| **Tester placed in proper position** | | Y | N | Y | N | Y | N |
| Stands on the test arm side of the patient | | ○ | ○ | ○ | ○ | ○ | ○ |
| Places one hand on the distal humerus just proximal to elbow | | ○ | ○ | ○ | ○ | ○ | ○ |
| **Tester performs test according to accepted guidelines** | | Y | N | Y | N | Y | N |
| Instructs the patient to hold the position | | ○ | ○ | ○ | ○ | ○ | ○ |
| Applies resistance downward in direction of abduction and flexion | | ○ | ○ | ○ | ○ | ○ | ○ |
| Holds resistance for 5 seconds | | ○ | ○ | ○ | ○ | ○ | ○ |
| Performs assessment bilaterally | | ○ | ○ | ○ | ○ | ○ | ○ |
| **Identifies implications** | | Y | N | Y | N | Y | N |
| Correctly grades the MMT | | ○ | ○ | ○ | ○ | ○ | ○ |
| Total | | ___/10 | | ___/10 | | ___/10 | |
| Must achieve >7 to pass this examination | | Ⓟ | Ⓕ | Ⓟ | Ⓕ | Ⓟ | Ⓕ |

| Assessor: Date: | Test 1 Comments: |
|---|---|
| Assessor: Date: | Test 2 Comments: |
| Assessor: Date: | Test 3 Comments: |

**TEST ENVIRONMENTS**
**L:** Laboratory/Classroom
**C:** Clinical/Field Testing
**P:** Practicum
**A:** Assessment/Mock Exam

**TEST INFORMATION**
**Test Statistics:** N/A
**Reference(s):** Kendall et al. (2005)

MUSCULOSKELETAL SYSTEM—REGION 7: SHOULDER
# MANUAL MUSCLE TESTING

| NATA EC 5th | BOC RD6 | SKILL |
|---|---|---|
| CE-21c | D2-0203 | MMT: Teres Minor |

**Supplies Needed:** Table

*This problem allows you the opportunity to demonstrate a* **manual muscle test** *for the* **teres minor muscle**. *You have 2 minutes to complete this task.*

| MMT: Teres Minor | Course or Site Assessor Environment | | | | | |
|---|---|---|---|---|---|---|
| | | Test 1 | | Test 2 | | Test 3 |
| **Tester places patient and limb in appropriate position** | | **Y** | **N** | **Y** | **N** | **Y** | **N** |
| Prone (head facing away from test arm) | | ○ | ○ | ○ | ○ | ○ | ○ |
| Shoulder flexed to 90 degrees and externally rotated to ~90 degrees | | ○ | ○ | ○ | ○ | ○ | ○ |
| Elbow flexed to 90 degrees (elbow off edge of the table) | | ○ | ○ | ○ | ○ | ○ | ○ |
| **Tester placed in proper position** | | **Y** | **N** | **Y** | **N** | **Y** | **N** |
| Stands on the side of the patient at test arm | | ○ | ○ | ○ | ○ | ○ | ○ |
| Places one hand under arm near the elbow to stabilize the humerus | | ○ | ○ | ○ | ○ | ○ | ○ |
| Places other hand on the distal forearm | | ○ | ○ | ○ | ○ | ○ | ○ |
| **Tester performs test according to accepted guidelines** | | **Y** | **N** | **Y** | **N** | **Y** | **N** |
| Instructs the patient to hold the position | | ○ | ○ | ○ | ○ | ○ | ○ |
| Applies resistance downward in direction of medial rotation | | ○ | ○ | ○ | ○ | ○ | ○ |
| Holds resistance for 5 seconds | | ○ | ○ | ○ | ○ | ○ | ○ |
| Performs assessment bilaterally | | ○ | ○ | ○ | ○ | ○ | ○ |
| **Identifies implications** | | **Y** | **N** | **Y** | **N** | **Y** | **N** |
| Correctly grades the MMT | | ○ | ○ | ○ | ○ | ○ | ○ |
| **Total** | | ___/11 | | ___/11 | | ___/11 | |
| **Must achieve >7 to pass this examination** | | Ⓟ | Ⓕ | Ⓟ | Ⓕ | Ⓟ | Ⓕ |

| Assessor: Date: | Test 1 Comments: |
|---|---|
| Assessor: Date: | Test 2 Comments: |
| Assessor: Date: | Test 3 Comments: |

**TEST ENVIRONMENTS**
**L:** Laboratory/Classroom
**C:** Clinical/Field Testing
**P:** Practicum
**A:** Assessment/Mock Exam

**TEST INFORMATION**
**Test Statistics:** N/A
**Reference(s):** Kendall et al. (2005)

## MUSCULOSKELETAL SYSTEM—REGION 7: SHOULDER
# MANUAL MUSCLE TESTING

| NATA EC 5th | BOC RD6 | SKILL |
|---|---|---|
| CE-21c | D2-0203 | MMT: Trapezius (Lower) |

**Supplies Needed:** Table

*This problem allows you the opportunity to demonstrate a* **manual muscle test** *for the* **trapezius (lower) muscle**. *You have 2 minutes to complete this task.*

| MMT: Trapezius (Lower) | Course or Site Assessor Environment _____ _____ _____ | | Test 1 | | Test 2 | | Test 3 |
|---|---|---|---|---|---|---|---|
| | | **Y** | **N** | **Y** | **N** | **Y** | **N** |
| **Tester places patient and limb in appropriate position** | | **Y** | **N** | **Y** | **N** | **Y** | **N** |
| Prone (shoulder at edge of table) | | O | O | O | O | O | O |
| Shoulder abducted to approximately 130 to 145 degrees | | O | O | O | O | O | O |
| Shoulder laterally rotated with thumb pointing upward | | O | O | O | O | O | O |
| **Tester placed in proper position** | | **Y** | **N** | **Y** | **N** | **Y** | **N** |
| Stands at side of the patient, facing the patient | | O | O | O | O | O | O |
| Places one hand over the distal humerus or forearm | | O | O | O | O | O | O |
| Places other hand (fingertips) below scapular spine on same side | | O | O | O | O | O | O |
| **Tester performs test according to accepted guidelines** | | **Y** | **N** | **Y** | **N** | **Y** | **N** |
| Instructs the patient to actively horizontally extend the shoulder | | O | O | O | O | O | O |
| Applies downward resistance in the direction of horizontal flexion | | O | O | O | O | O | O |
| Holds resistance for 5 seconds | | O | O | O | O | O | O |
| Performs assessment bilaterally | | O | O | O | O | O | O |
| **Identifies implications** | | **Y** | **N** | **Y** | **N** | **Y** | **N** |
| Correctly grades the MMT | | O | O | O | O | O | O |
| Total | | ____/11 | | ____/11 | | ____/11 | |
| Must achieve >7 to pass this examination | | P | F | P | F | P | F |

| Assessor: Date: | Test 1 Comments: |
|---|---|
| Assessor: Date: | Test 2 Comments: |
| Assessor: Date: | Test 3 Comments: |

**TEST ENVIRONMENTS**
**L:** Laboratory/Classroom
**C:** Clinical/Field Testing
**P:** Practicum
**A:** Assessment/Mock Exam

**TEST INFORMATION**
**Test Statistics:** N/A
**Reference(s):**    Hislop & Montgomery (2007)
                     Kendall et al. (2005)

## MUSCULOSKELETAL SYSTEM—REGION 7: SHOULDER
# MANUAL MUSCLE TESTING

| NATA EC 5th | BOC RD6 | SKILL |
|---|---|---|
| CE-21c | D2-0203 | MMT: Trapezius (Middle) |

**Supplies Needed:** Table

*This problem allows you the opportunity to demonstrate a* **manual muscle test** *for the* **trapezius (middle) muscle**.
*You have 2 minutes to complete this task.*

| MMT: Trapezius (Middle) | Course or Site Assessor Environment | | | | | |
|---|---|---|---|---|---|---|
| | | Test 1 | | Test 2 | | Test 3 |
| | | Y | N | Y | N | Y | N |
| **Tester places patient and limb in appropriate position** | | Y | N | Y | N | Y | N |
| Prone (shoulder at edge of table) | | ○ | ○ | ○ | ○ | ○ | ○ |
| Shoulder abducted to approximately 90 degrees | | ○ | ○ | ○ | ○ | ○ | ○ |
| Shoulder laterally rotated with thumb pointing upward | | ○ | ○ | ○ | ○ | ○ | ○ |
| **Tester placed in proper position** | | Y | N | Y | N | Y | N |
| Stands at side of the patient, facing the patient | | ○ | ○ | ○ | ○ | ○ | ○ |
| Places one hand on the opposite scapula | | ○ | ○ | ○ | ○ | ○ | ○ |
| Places other hand against the distal forearm (radius/ulna) | | ○ | ○ | ○ | ○ | ○ | ○ |
| **Tester performs test according to accepted guidelines** | | Y | N | Y | N | Y | N |
| Instructs the patient to actively horizontally extend the shoulder | | ○ | ○ | ○ | ○ | ○ | ○ |
| Applies resistance in a downward direction of horizontal flexion | | ○ | ○ | ○ | ○ | ○ | ○ |
| Holds resistance for 5 seconds | | ○ | ○ | ○ | ○ | ○ | ○ |
| Performs assessment bilaterally | | ○ | ○ | ○ | ○ | ○ | ○ |
| **Identifies implications** | | Y | N | Y | N | Y | N |
| Correctly grades the MMT | | ○ | ○ | ○ | ○ | ○ | ○ |
| Total | | ___/11 | | ___/11 | | ___/11 | |
| Must achieve >7 to pass this examination | | Ⓟ | Ⓕ | Ⓟ | Ⓕ | Ⓟ | Ⓕ |
| Assessor: Date: | Test 1 Comments: | | | | | |
| Assessor: Date: | Test 2 Comments: | | | | | |
| Assessor: Date: | Test 3 Comments: | | | | | |

**TEST ENVIRONMENTS**
**L:** Laboratory/Classroom
**C:** Clinical/Field Testing
**P:** Practicum
**A:** Assessment/Mock Exam

**TEST INFORMATION**
**Test Statistics:** N/A
**Reference(s):** Hislop & Montgomery (2007)
Kendall et al. (2005)

# MANUAL MUSCLE TESTING

| NATA EC 5th | BOC RD6 | SKILL |
|---|---|---|
| CE-21c | D2-0203 | MMT: Trapezius (Upper) |

**Supplies Needed:** Table or chair

*This problem allows you the opportunity to demonstrate a* **manual muscle test** *for the* **trapezius (upper) muscle***. You have 2 minutes to complete this task.*

| MMT: Trapezius (Upper) | Course or Site Assessor Environment | Test 1 | | Test 2 | | Test 3 | |
|---|---|---|---|---|---|---|---|
| **Tester places patient and limb in appropriate position** | | **Y** | **N** | **Y** | **N** | **Y** | **N** |
| Seated | | O | O | O | O | O | O |
| Hands relaxed in lap of the patient | | O | O | O | O | O | O |
| Elevates acromial end of clavicle toward the head | | O | O | O | O | O | O |
| Laterally rotates head toward opposite side | | O | O | O | O | O | O |
| **Tester placed in proper position** | | **Y** | **N** | **Y** | **N** | **Y** | **N** |
| Stands facing back of the patient | | O | O | O | O | O | O |
| Places one hand on the side of head | | O | O | O | O | O | O |
| Places other hand against superior aspect of shoulder | | O | O | O | O | O | O |
| **Tester performs test according to accepted guidelines** | | **Y** | **N** | **Y** | **N** | **Y** | **N** |
| Instructs the patient to hold the position | | O | O | O | O | O | O |
| Applies resistance in direction of lateral flexion to opposite side | | O | O | O | O | O | O |
| Applies downward resistance against shoulder elevation | | O | O | O | O | O | O |
| Holds resistance for 5 seconds | | O | O | O | O | O | O |
| Performs assessment bilaterally | | O | O | O | O | O | O |
| **Identifies implications** | | **Y** | **N** | **Y** | **N** | **Y** | **N** |
| Correctly grades the MMT | | O | O | O | O | O | O |
| | Total | ___/13 | | ___/13 | | ___/13 | |
| | Must achieve >9 to pass this examination | Ⓟ | Ⓕ | Ⓟ | Ⓕ | Ⓟ | Ⓕ |

| Assessor: Date: | **Test 1 Comments:** |
|---|---|
| Assessor: Date: | **Test 2 Comments:** |
| Assessor: Date: | **Test 3 Comments:** |

**TEST ENVIRONMENTS**
**L:** Laboratory/Classroom
**C:** Clinical/Field Testing
**P:** Practicum
**A:** Assessment/Mock Exam

**TEST INFORMATION**
**Test Statistics:** N/A
**Reference(s):** Kendall et al. (2005)

MUSCULOSKELETAL SYSTEM—REGION 7: SHOULDER
# OSTEOKINEMATIC JOINT MOTION

| NATA EC 5th | BOC RD6 | SKILL |
|---|---|---|
| CE-21d | D2-0203 | Goniometric Assessment: Glenohumeral Joint (Flexion) |

**Supplies Needed:** Table, large goniometer

*This problem allows you the opportunity to demonstrate how to measure a patient's shoulder* **range of motion** *for* **flexion** *at the* **glenohumeral joint**. You *have 2 minutes to complete this task.*

| Goniometric Assessment: Glenohumeral Joint (Flexion) | Course or Site Assessor Environment | Test 1 | | Test 2 | | Test 3 | |
|---|---|---|---|---|---|---|---|
| **Tester places patient and limb in appropriate position** | | **Y** | **N** | **Y** | **N** | **Y** | **N** |
| Supine | | ○ | ○ | ○ | ○ | ○ | ○ |
| Elbow flexed to 90 degrees | | ○ | ○ | ○ | ○ | ○ | ○ |
| Shoulder adducted to 0 degrees | | ○ | ○ | ○ | ○ | ○ | ○ |
| **Tester and goniometer placed in proper position** | | **Y** | **N** | **Y** | **N** | **Y** | **N** |
| Fulcrum (axis): Lateral to acromion process | | ○ | ○ | ○ | ○ | ○ | ○ |
| Stationary arm: Mid axillary line of thorax | | ○ | ○ | ○ | ○ | ○ | ○ |
| Moving arm: Lateral midline of the humerus (lateral epicondyle) | | ○ | ○ | ○ | ○ | ○ | ○ |
| The tester on side of the patient, scapula stabilized, palm against body | | ○ | ○ | ○ | ○ | ○ | ○ |
| **Tester performs test according to accepted guidelines** | | **Y** | **N** | **Y** | **N** | **Y** | **N** |
| Performs the measurement where the scapula begins to move | | ○ | ○ | ○ | ○ | ○ | ○ |
| Takes proper goniometric measurement | | ○ | ○ | ○ | ○ | ○ | ○ |
| Performs assessment bilaterally | | ○ | ○ | ○ | ○ | ○ | ○ |
| **Identifies implications** | | **Y** | **N** | **Y** | **N** | **Y** | **N** |
| Identifies normal ranges (GH flexion = 0 to 120 degrees) | | ○ | ○ | ○ | ○ | ○ | ○ |
| **Total** | | ___/11 | | ___/11 | | ___/11 | |
| **Must achieve >7 to pass this examination** | | Ⓟ | Ⓕ | Ⓟ | Ⓕ | Ⓟ | Ⓕ |

| Assessor: Date: | Test 1 Comments: |
|---|---|
| Assessor: Date: | Test 2 Comments: |
| Assessor: Date: | Test 3 Comments: |

**TEST ENVIRONMENTS**
L: Laboratory/Classroom
C: Clinical/Field Testing
P: Practicum
A: Assessment/Mock Exam

**TEST INFORMATION**
**Test Statistics:** N/A
**Reference(s):**  Norkin & White (2009)
Starkey & Brown (2015)

**MUSCULOSKELETAL SYSTEM—REGION 7: SHOULDER**
# OSTEOKINEMATIC JOINT MOTION

| NATA EC 5th | BOC RD6 | SKILL |
|---|---|---|
| CE-21d | D2-0203 | Goniometric Assessment:<br>Glenohumeral Joint (Extension) |

**Supplies Needed:** Table, large goniometer

*This problem allows you the opportunity to demonstrate how to measure a patient's shoulder* **range of motion** *for* **extension** *at the* **glenohumeral joint**. *You have 2 minutes to complete this task.*

| Goniometric Assessment:<br>Glenohumeral Joint (Extension) | Course or Site<br>Assessor<br>Environment | | Test 1 | | Test 2 | | Test 3 | |
|---|---|---|---|---|---|---|---|---|
| **Tester places patient and limb in appropriate position** | | **Y** | **N** | **Y** | **N** | **Y** | **N** | |
| Prone | | ○ | ○ | ○ | ○ | ○ | ○ | |
| Turns head away from involved shoulder | | ○ | ○ | ○ | ○ | ○ | ○ | |
| Shoulder adducted in 0 degrees | | ○ | ○ | ○ | ○ | ○ | ○ | |
| Places elbow in slight flexion | | ○ | ○ | ○ | ○ | ○ | ○ | |
| **Tester and goniometer placed in proper position** | | **Y** | **N** | **Y** | **N** | **Y** | **N** | |
| Stabilizes scapula | | ○ | ○ | ○ | ○ | ○ | ○ | |
| Fulcrum (axis): Aligned lateral to the acromion process | | ○ | ○ | ○ | ○ | ○ | ○ | |
| Stationary arm: Mid axillary line of the thorax | | ○ | ○ | ○ | ○ | ○ | ○ | |
| Moving arm: Lateral midline of the humerus (lateral epicondyle) | | ○ | ○ | ○ | ○ | ○ | ○ | |
| **Tester performs test according to accepted guidelines** | | **Y** | **N** | **Y** | **N** | **Y** | **N** | |
| Stabilizes the scapula on posterior surface | | ○ | ○ | ○ | ○ | ○ | ○ | |
| Takes proper goniometric measurement | | ○ | ○ | ○ | ○ | ○ | ○ | |
| Performs assessment bilaterally | | ○ | ○ | ○ | ○ | ○ | ○ | |
| **Identifies implications** | | **Y** | **N** | **Y** | **N** | **Y** | **N** | |
| Identifies normal ranges (GH extension = 60 degrees) | | ○ | ○ | ○ | ○ | ○ | ○ | |
| **Total** | | ___/12 | | ___/12 | | ___/12 | | |
| **Must achieve >8 to pass this examination** | | Ⓟ | Ⓕ | Ⓟ | Ⓕ | Ⓟ | Ⓕ | |

| Assessor:<br>Date: | **Test 1 Comments:** |
|---|---|
| Assessor:<br>Date: | **Test 2 Comments:** |
| Assessor:<br>Date: | **Test 3 Comments:** |

**TEST ENVIRONMENTS**
**L:** Laboratory/Classroom
**C:** Clinical/Field Testing
**P:** Practicum
**A:** Assessment/Mock Exam

**TEST INFORMATION**
**Test Statistics:** N/A
**Reference(s):** Norkin & White (2009)
Starkey & Brown (2015)

## MUSCULOSKELETAL SYSTEM—REGION 7: SHOULDER
# OSTEOKINEMATIC JOINT MOTION

| NATA EC 5th | BOC RD6 | SKILL |
|:---:|:---:|:---:|
| CE-21d | D2-0203 | Goniometric Assessment: Glenohumeral Joint (Internal/External Rotation) |

**Supplies Needed:** Table, large goniometer, pad or towel

*This problem allows you the opportunity to demonstrate how to measure a patient's shoulder* **range of motion** *for* **internal/external rotation** *at the* **glenohumeral joint**. *You have 2 minutes to complete this task.*

| Goniometric Assessment: Glenohumeral Joint (Internal/External Rotation) | Course or Site Assessor Environment ___ ___ ___ | | | | | |
|---|:---:|:---:|:---:|:---:|:---:|:---:|
| | Test 1 | | Test 2 | | Test 3 | |
| **Tester places patient and limb in appropriate position** | Y | N | Y | N | Y | N |
| Supine | O | O | O | O | O | O |
| Shoulder abducted to 90 degrees | O | O | O | O | O | O |
| Forearm maintained at 0 degrees | O | O | O | O | O | O |
| Pad/towel placed under the humerus | O | O | O | O | O | O |
| **Tester and goniometer placed in proper position** | Y | N | Y | N | Y | N |
| Provides appropriate scapular stabilization | O | O | O | O | O | O |
| Fulcrum (axis): Centered lateral to olecranon process | O | O | O | O | O | O |
| Stationary arm: Parallel or perpendicular to floor/table | O | O | O | O | O | O |
| Moving arm: Centered over long axis of the ulna (ulnar styloid) | O | O | O | O | O | O |
| **Tester performs test according to accepted guidelines** | Y | N | Y | N | Y | N |
| Takes measurement when scapula begins to move | O | O | O | O | O | O |
| Takes proper goniometric measurement | O | O | O | O | O | O |
| Performs assessment bilaterally | O | O | O | O | O | O |
| **Identifies implications** | Y | N | Y | N | Y | N |
| Identifies normal ranges (GH internal rotation = 90 degrees; GH external rotation = 90 degrees) | O | O | O | O | O | O |
| **Total** | ___/12 | | ___/12 | | ___/12 | |
| **Must achieve >8 to pass this examination** | Ⓟ | Ⓕ | Ⓟ | Ⓕ | Ⓟ | Ⓕ |

| Assessor: Date: | Test 1 Comments: |
|---|---|
| Assessor: Date: | Test 2 Comments: |
| Assessor: Date: | Test 3 Comments: |

**TEST ENVIRONMENTS**
**L:** Laboratory/Classroom
**C:** Clinical/Field Testing
**P:** Practicum
**A:** Assessment/Mock Exam

**TEST INFORMATION**
**Test Statistics:** N/A
**Reference(s):**   Norkin & White (2009)
                    Starkey & Brown (2015)

**MUSCULOSKELETAL SYSTEM—REGION 7: SHOULDER**
# OSTEOKINEMATIC JOINT MOTION

| NATA EC 5th | BOC RD6 | SKILL |
|---|---|---|
| CE-21d | D2-0203 | Goniometric Assessment: Glenohumeral Joint (Abduction) |

**Supplies Needed:** Table, large goniometer

*This problem allows you the opportunity to demonstrate how to measure a patient's shoulder* **range of motion** *for* **abduction** *at the* **glenohumeral joint**. *You* have 2 minutes to complete this task.

| Goniometric Assessment: Glenohumeral Joint (Abduction) | Course or Site / Assessor / Environment | | Test 1 | | Test 2 | | Test 3 | |
|---|---|---|---|---|---|---|---|---|
| **Tester places patient and limb in appropriate position** | | | Y | N | Y | N | Y | N |
| Supine or seated | | | O | O | O | O | O | O |
| Shoulder resting at the patient's side | | | O | O | O | O | O | O |
| **Tester and goniometer placed in proper position** | | | Y | N | Y | N | Y | N |
| The tester provides appropriate scapular stabilization | | | O | O | O | O | O | O |
| Fulcrum (axis): Anterior to the acromion process | | | O | O | O | O | O | O |
| Stationary arm: Aligned parallel to long axis of thorax | | | O | O | O | O | O | O |
| Moving arm: Centered over midline of the humerus | | | O | O | O | O | O | O |
| **Tester performs test according to accepted guidelines** | | | Y | N | Y | N | Y | N |
| Takes measurement when scapula begins to move | | | O | O | O | O | O | O |
| Takes proper goniometric measurement | | | O | O | O | O | O | O |
| Performs assessment bilaterally | | | O | O | O | O | O | O |
| **Identifies implications** | | | Y | N | Y | N | Y | N |
| Identifies normal ranges (GH abduction = 120 degrees) | | | O | O | O | O | O | O |
| | | Total | ___/10 | | ___/10 | | ___/10 | |
| | **Must achieve >6 to pass this examination** | | Ⓟ | Ⓕ | Ⓟ | Ⓕ | Ⓟ | Ⓕ |

| Assessor: Date: | Test 1 Comments: |
|---|---|
| Assessor: Date: | Test 2 Comments: |
| Assessor: Date: | Test 3 Comments: |

**TEST ENVIRONMENTS**
**L:** Laboratory/Classroom
**C:** Clinical/Field Testing
**P:** Practicum
**A:** Assessment/Mock Exam

**TEST INFORMATION**
**Test Statistics:** N/A
**Reference(s):** Norkin & White (2009)
Starkey & Brown (2015)

## MUSCULOSKELETAL SYSTEM—REGION 7: SHOULDER
# CAPSULAR AND LIGAMENTOUS STRESS TESTING

| NATA EC 5th | BOC RD6 | SKILL |
|---|---|---|
| CE-21e | D2-0203 | Acromioclavicular Joint Compression Test (Shear Test) |

**Supplies Needed:** Table

*This problem allows you the opportunity to demonstrate an* **orthopedic test** *known as the* **acromioclavicular joint compression test (shear test)**. *You have 2 minutes to complete this task.*

| Acromioclavicular Joint Compression Test (Shear Test) | Course or Site Assessor Environment | | Test 1 | | Test 2 | | Test 3 |
|---|---|---|---|---|---|---|---|
| **Tester places patient and limb in appropriate position** | | **Y** | **N** | **Y** | **N** | **Y** | **N** |
| Seated or standing | | ○ | ○ | ○ | ○ | ○ | ○ |
| Arm hanging at side (relaxed, natural position) | | ○ | ○ | ○ | ○ | ○ | ○ |
| **Tester placed in proper position** | | **Y** | **N** | **Y** | **N** | **Y** | **N** |
| Stands on the involved side | | ○ | ○ | ○ | ○ | ○ | ○ |
| Places one hand on the patient's clavicle | | ○ | ○ | ○ | ○ | ○ | ○ |
| Places other hand on the spine of the scapula | | ○ | ○ | ○ | ○ | ○ | ○ |
| **Tester performs test according to accepted guidelines** | | **Y** | **N** | **Y** | **N** | **Y** | **N** |
| Gently squeezes hands together (cupping motion) | | ○ | ○ | ○ | ○ | ○ | ○ |
| Maintains relaxation of limb | | ○ | ○ | ○ | ○ | ○ | ○ |
| Performs assessment bilaterally | | ○ | ○ | ○ | ○ | ○ | ○ |
| **Identifies positive findings and implications** | | **Y** | **N** | **Y** | **N** | **Y** | **N** |
| Pain at AC joint | | ○ | ○ | ○ | ○ | ○ | ○ |
| Excursion of clavicle over the acromion process | | ○ | ○ | ○ | ○ | ○ | ○ |
| Total | | /10 | | /10 | | /10 | |
| Must achieve >7 to pass this examination | | Ⓟ | Ⓕ | Ⓟ | Ⓕ | Ⓟ | Ⓕ |

| Assessor: Date: | Test 1 Comments: |
|---|---|
| Assessor: Date: | Test 2 Comments: |
| Assessor: Date: | Test 3 Comments: |

**TEST ENVIRONMENTS**
**L:** Laboratory/Classroom
**C:** Clinical/Field Testing
**P:** Practicum
**A:** Assessment/Mock Exam

**TEST INFORMATION**
**Test Statistics:** (+) LR 1.6
(-) LR .42
**Reference(s):** Konin et al. (2016)
Starkey & Brown (2015)

**MUSCULOSKELETAL SYSTEM—REGION 7: SHOULDER**
# CAPSULAR AND LIGAMENTOUS STRESS TESTING

| NATA EC 5th | BOC RD6 | SKILL |
|---|---|---|
| CE-21e | D2-0203 | Acromioclavicular Joint Distraction Test |

**Supplies Needed:** Table

*This problem allows you the opportunity to demonstrate an* **orthopedic test** *known as the* **acromioclavicular joint distraction test.** *You have 2 minutes to complete this task.*

| Acromioclavicular Joint Distraction Test | Course or Site Assessor Environment | | | | | |
|---|---|---|---|---|---|---|
| | | Test 1 | | Test 2 | | Test 3 |
| **Tester places patient and limb in appropriate position** | | Y | N | Y | N | Y | N |
| Seated or standing | | ○ | ○ | ○ | ○ | ○ | ○ |
| Arm hanging at side (relaxed, natural position) | | ○ | ○ | ○ | ○ | ○ | ○ |
| **Tester placed in proper position** | | Y | N | Y | N | Y | N |
| Stands on the involved side | | ○ | ○ | ○ | ○ | ○ | ○ |
| Holds the patient's arm (humerus) proximal to elbow | | ○ | ○ | ○ | ○ | ○ | ○ |
| Places other hand over the patient's AC joint, palpates joint | | ○ | ○ | ○ | ○ | ○ | ○ |
| **Tester performs test according to accepted guidelines** | | Y | N | Y | N | Y | N |
| Applies gentle downward traction/pressure on the humerus | | ○ | ○ | ○ | ○ | ○ | ○ |
| Maintains relaxation of limb | | ○ | ○ | ○ | ○ | ○ | ○ |
| Performs assessment bilaterally | | ○ | ○ | ○ | ○ | ○ | ○ |
| **Identifies positive findings and implications** | | Y | N | Y | N | Y | N |
| Pain at AC joint and/or | | ○ | ○ | ○ | ○ | ○ | ○ |
| Humerus and scapula move inferior causing "step deformity" | | ○ | ○ | ○ | ○ | ○ | ○ |
| Total | | ___/10 | | ___/10 | | ___/10 | |
| **Must achieve >7 to pass this examination** | | Ⓟ | Ⓕ | Ⓟ | Ⓕ | Ⓟ | Ⓕ |

| Assessor: Date: | Test 1 Comments: |
|---|---|
| Assessor: Date: | Test 2 Comments: |
| Assessor: Date: | Test 3 Comments: |

**TEST ENVIRONMENTS**
**L:** Laboratory/Classroom
**C:** Clinical/Field Testing
**P:** Practicum
**A:** Assessment/Mock Exam

**TEST INFORMATION**
**Test Statistics:** No data available
**Reference(s):** Konin et al. (2016)
Starkey & Brown (2015)

MUSCULOSKELETAL SYSTEM—REGION 7: SHOULDER
# CAPSULAR AND LIGAMENTOUS STRESS TESTING

| NATA EC 5th | BOC RD6 | SKILL |
|---|---|---|
| CE-21e | D2-0203 | Anterior Drawer Test for the Shoulder |

**Supplies Needed:** Table

*This problem allows you the opportunity to demonstrate an* **orthopedic test** *known as the* **anterior drawer test for the shoulder**. *You have 2 minutes to complete this task.*

| Anterior Drawer Test for the Shoulder | Course or Site / Assessor / Environment | Test 1 | | Test 2 | | Test 3 | |
|---|---|---|---|---|---|---|---|
| | | Y | N | Y | N | Y | N |
| **Tester places patient and limb in appropriate position** | | Y | N | Y | N | Y | N |
| Supine | | ○ | ○ | ○ | ○ | ○ | ○ |
| Arm placed in abduction (80 to 120 degrees), flexion (0 to 20 degrees), external rotation (0 to 30 degrees) | | ○ | ○ | ○ | ○ | ○ | ○ |
| **Tester placed in proper position** | | Y | N | Y | N | Y | N |
| Stands one hand in the patient's axilla area (holds arm) | | ○ | ○ | ○ | ○ | ○ | ○ |
| Stabilizes scapula with the opposite hand | | ○ | ○ | ○ | ○ | ○ | ○ |
| Applies counterpressure with thumb to the patient's coracoid process | | ○ | ○ | ○ | ○ | ○ | ○ |
| **Tester performs test according to accepted guidelines** | | Y | N | Y | N | Y | N |
| Instructs the patient to relax | | ○ | ○ | ○ | ○ | ○ | ○ |
| Applies appropriate pressure (forward displacement of the humerus) | | ○ | ○ | ○ | ○ | ○ | ○ |
| Performs assessment bilaterally | | ○ | ○ | ○ | ○ | ○ | ○ |
| **Identifies positive findings and implications** | | Y | N | Y | N | Y | N |
| Pain at GH joint and/or | | ○ | ○ | ○ | ○ | ○ | ○ |
| Excess excursion of humerus; grinding and/or apprehension | | ○ | ○ | ○ | ○ | ○ | ○ |
| Total | | ___/10 | | ___/10 | | ___/10 | |
| Must achieve >6 to pass this examination | | Ⓟ | Ⓕ | Ⓟ | Ⓕ | Ⓟ | Ⓕ |

| Assessor: Date: | Test 1 Comments: |
|---|---|
| Assessor: Date: | Test 2 Comments: |
| Assessor: Date: | Test 3 Comments: |

**TEST ENVIRONMENTS**
L: Laboratory/Classroom
C: Clinical/Field Testing
P: Practicum
A: Assessment/Mock Exam

**TEST INFORMATION**
**Test Statistics:** No data available
**Reference(s):** Konin et al. (2016)
Reider (2004)
Starkey & Brown (2015)

**MUSCULOSKELETAL SYSTEM—REGION 7: SHOULDER**
# CAPSULAR AND LIGAMENTOUS STRESS TESTING

| NATA EC 5th | BOC RD6 | SKILL |
|---|---|---|
| CE-21e | D2-0203 | Apprehension Test (Crank Test) |

**Supplies Needed:** Table

*This problem allows you the opportunity to demonstrate an* **orthopedic test** *known as the* **apprehension test (crank test)** *for the shoulder. You have 2 minutes to complete this task.*

| Apprehension Test (Crank Test) | Course or Site<br>Assessor<br>Environment<br>Test 1 | | Test 2 | | Test 3 | |
|---|---|---|---|---|---|---|
| **Tester places patient and limb in appropriate position** | **Y** | **N** | **Y** | **N** | **Y** | **N** |
| Supine (also standing or seated) | O | O | O | O | O | O |
| Shoulder abducted to 90 degrees | O | O | O | O | O | O |
| Elbow flexed to 90 degrees | O | O | O | O | O | O |
| **Tester placed in proper position** | **Y** | **N** | **Y** | **N** | **Y** | **N** |
| Stands on the involved side or in front of the patient | O | O | O | O | O | O |
| One hand grasps the forearm just proximal to wrist | O | O | O | O | O | O |
| Places other hand under distal humerus or at midshaft | O | O | O | O | O | O |
| **Tester performs test according to accepted guidelines** | **Y** | **N** | **Y** | **N** | **Y** | **N** |
| Applies pressure slowly to anterior forearm | O | O | O | O | O | O |
| Passively moves shoulder into external rotation | O | O | O | O | O | O |
| Maintains relaxation of limb | O | O | O | O | O | O |
| Performs assessment bilaterally | O | O | O | O | O | O |
| **Identifies positive findings and implications** | **Y** | **N** | **Y** | **N** | **Y** | **N** |
| Patient displays apprehension that GH joint may dislocate | O | O | O | O | O | O |
| Pain | O | O | O | O | O | O |
| Implications include internal impingement, rotator cuff pathology, and capsular and/or labral involvement | O | O | O | O | O | O |
| **Total** | __/13 | | __/13 | | __/13 | |
| **Must achieve >9 to pass this examination** | Ⓟ | Ⓕ | Ⓟ | Ⓕ | Ⓟ | Ⓕ |

| Assessor:<br>Date: | **Test 1 Comments:** |
|---|---|
| Assessor:<br>Date: | **Test 2 Comments:** |
| Assessor:<br>Date: | **Test 3 Comments:** |

**TEST ENVIRONMENTS**
**L:** Laboratory/Classroom
**C:** Clinical/Field Testing
**P:** Practicum
**A:** Assessment/Mock Exam

**TEST INFORMATION**
**Test Statistics:** (+) LR 18–48.18
(-) LR .3–.48
**Reference(s):** Konin et al. (2016)
Starkey & Brown (2015)

## Musculoskeletal System—Region 7: Shoulder
# Capsular and Ligamentous Stress Testing

| NATA EC 5th | BOC RD6 | SKILL |
|:---:|:---:|:---:|
| CE-21e | D2-0203 | Feagin Test |

**Supplies Needed:** Table

*This problem allows you the opportunity to demonstrate an* **orthopedic test** *known as the* **Feagin test** *for the shoulder. You have 2 minutes to complete this task.*

| Feagin Test | Course or Site / Assessor / Environment | | | | | |
|---|:---:|:---:|:---:|:---:|:---:|:---:|
| | Test 1 | | Test 2 | | Test 3 | |
| **Tester places patient and limb in appropriate position** | **Y** | **N** | **Y** | **N** | **Y** | **N** |
| Standing | ○ | ○ | ○ | ○ | ○ | ○ |
| Shoulder abducted to 90 degrees, elbow fully extended | ○ | ○ | ○ | ○ | ○ | ○ |
| **Tester placed in proper position** | **Y** | **N** | **Y** | **N** | **Y** | **N** |
| Positioned to the side of the patient; faces the patient | ○ | ○ | ○ | ○ | ○ | ○ |
| Hands clasped around upper and middle third of humerus | ○ | ○ | ○ | ○ | ○ | ○ |
| **Tester performs test according to accepted guidelines** | **Y** | **N** | **Y** | **N** | **Y** | **N** |
| Pushes humerus down and forward | ○ | ○ | ○ | ○ | ○ | ○ |
| Maintains relaxation of limb | ○ | ○ | ○ | ○ | ○ | ○ |
| Performs assessment bilaterally | ○ | ○ | ○ | ○ | ○ | ○ |
| **Identifies positive findings and implications** | **Y** | **N** | **Y** | **N** | **Y** | **N** |
| Sulcus may appear above the coracoid process | ○ | ○ | ○ | ○ | ○ | ○ |
| Patient apprehension | ○ | ○ | ○ | ○ | ○ | ○ |
| Capsular instability | ○ | ○ | ○ | ○ | ○ | ○ |
| **Total** | __/10 | | __/10 | | __/10 | |
| **Must achieve >6 to pass this examination** | Ⓟ | Ⓕ | Ⓟ | Ⓕ | Ⓟ | Ⓕ |

| Assessor: Date: | **Test 1 Comments:** |
|---|---|
| Assessor: Date: | **Test 2 Comments:** |
| Assessor: Date: | **Test 3 Comments:** |

**TEST ENVIRONMENTS**
**L:** Laboratory/Classroom
**C:** Clinical/Field Testing
**P:** Practicum
**A:** Assessment/Mock Exam

**TEST INFORMATION**
**Test Statistics:** No data available
**Reference(s):** Konin et al. (2016)
Starkey & Brown (2015)

# CAPSULAR AND LIGAMENTOUS STRESS TESTING

| NATA EC 5th | BOC RD6 | SKILL |
|---|---|---|
| CE-21e | D2-0203 | Jerk Test (Clunk Test) |

**Supplies Needed:** Table

*This problem allows you the opportunity to demonstrate an* **orthopedic test** *known as the* **jerk test (clunk test)** *for* **labral tears**. *You have 2 minutes to complete this task.*

| Jerk Test (Clunk Test) | Course or Site Assessor Environment | | Test 1 | | Test 2 | | Test 3 | |
|---|---|---|---|---|---|---|---|---|
| **Tester places patient and limb in appropriate position** | | | **Y** | **N** | **Y** | **N** | **Y** | **N** |
| Supine or seated (improved scapular stabilization in supine) | | | O | O | O | O | O | O |
| Arm abducted to 90 degrees, flexed 90 degrees, internal rotation 10 degrees | | | O | O | O | O | O | O |
| **Tester placed in proper position** | | | **Y** | **N** | **Y** | **N** | **Y** | **N** |
| Positioned behind the patient (or to side) | | | O | O | O | O | O | O |
| Stabilizes scapula with one hand | | | O | O | O | O | O | O |
| Shoulder held at 90 degrees flexion and internal rotation by other hand | | | O | O | O | O | O | O |
| **Tester performs test according to accepted guidelines** | | | **Y** | **N** | **Y** | **N** | **Y** | **N** |
| Passively moves arm into horizontal adduction while axial load is applied to the humerus | | | O | O | O | O | O | O |
| Maintains relaxation of limb | | | O | O | O | O | O | O |
| Performs assessment bilaterally | | | O | O | O | O | O | O |
| **Identifies positive findings and implications** | | | **Y** | **N** | **Y** | **N** | **Y** | **N** |
| Painful clunk (surgical treatment) | | | O | O | O | O | O | O |
| Painless clunk (nonsurgical treatment) | | | O | O | O | O | O | O |
| Labral pathology | | | O | O | O | O | O | O |
| | Total | | ___/11 | | ___/11 | | ___/11 | |
| | Must achieve >7 to pass this examination | | Ⓟ | Ⓕ | Ⓟ | Ⓕ | Ⓟ | Ⓕ |

| Assessor: Date: | Test 1 Comments: |
|---|---|
| Assessor: Date: | Test 2 Comments: |
| Assessor: Date: | Test 3 Comments: |

**TEST ENVIRONMENTS**
**L:** Laboratory/Classroom
**C:** Clinical/Field Testing
**P:** Practicum
**A:** Assessment/Mock Exam

**TEST INFORMATION**
**Test Statistics:** (+) LR 36.5
(-) LR .28
**Reference(s):** Konin et al. (2016)
Starkey & Brown (2015)

## MUSCULOSKELETAL SYSTEM—REGION 7: SHOULDER
# CAPSULAR AND LIGAMENTOUS STRESS TESTING

| NATA EC 5th | BOC RD6 | SKILL |
|---|---|---|
| CE-21e | D2-0203 | Posterior Apprehension (Stress) Test |

**Supplies Needed:** Table

*This problem allows you the opportunity to demonstrate an* **orthopedic test** *known as the* **posterior apprehension (stress) test** *for the shoulder. You have 2 minutes to complete this task.*

| Posterior Apprehension (Stress) Test | Course or Site Assessor Environment | | Test 1 | | Test 2 | | Test 3 | |
|---|---|---|---|---|---|---|---|---|
| **Tester places patient and limb in appropriate position** | | | **Y** | **N** | **Y** | **N** | **Y** | **N** |
| Supine (also seated) | | | ○ | ○ | ○ | ○ | ○ | ○ |
| Shoulder positioned in 90 degrees of flexion | | | ○ | ○ | ○ | ○ | ○ | ○ |
| Elbow positioned in 90 degrees of flexion | | | ○ | ○ | ○ | ○ | ○ | ○ |
| GH joint being tested is off side of table | | | ○ | ○ | ○ | ○ | ○ | ○ |
| **Tester placed in proper position** | | | **Y** | **N** | **Y** | **N** | **Y** | **N** |
| Stands (or sits) beside the patient | | | ○ | ○ | ○ | ○ | ○ | ○ |
| Stabilizes shoulder with one hand at posterior scapula | | | ○ | ○ | ○ | ○ | ○ | ○ |
| Other hand grasps the elbow or forearm | | | ○ | ○ | ○ | ○ | ○ | ○ |
| **Tester performs test according to accepted guidelines** | | | **Y** | **N** | **Y** | **N** | **Y** | **N** |
| Holds shoulder in internal rotation as force is applied | | | ○ | ○ | ○ | ○ | ○ | ○ |
| Applies posterior force through the long axis of humerus | | | ○ | ○ | ○ | ○ | ○ | ○ |
| Maintains relaxation of limb | | | ○ | ○ | ○ | ○ | ○ | ○ |
| Performs assessment bilaterally | | | ○ | ○ | ○ | ○ | ○ | ○ |
| **Identifies positive findings and implications** | | | **Y** | **N** | **Y** | **N** | **Y** | **N** |
| Apprehension, guarding, and/or pain | | | ○ | ○ | ○ | ○ | ○ | ○ |
| Laxity in the posterior capsule, torn posterior labrum | | | ○ | ○ | ○ | ○ | ○ | ○ |
| | | Total | \_\_\_\_/13 | | \_\_\_\_/13 | | \_\_\_\_/13 | |
| | Must achieve >9 to pass this examination | | Ⓟ | Ⓕ | Ⓟ | Ⓕ | Ⓟ | Ⓕ |
| **Assessor:** **Date:** | Test 1 Comments: | | | | | | | |
| **Assessor:** **Date:** | Test 2 Comments: | | | | | | | |
| **Assessor:** **Date:** | Test 3 Comments: | | | | | | | |

**TEST ENVIRONMENTS**
**L:** Laboratory/Classroom
**C:** Clinical/Field Testing
**P:** Practicum
**A:** Assessment/Mock Exam

**TEST INFORMATION**
**Test Statistics:** No data available
**Reference(s):** Konin et al. (2016)
Starkey & Brown (2015)

**MUSCULOSKELETAL SYSTEM—REGION 7: SHOULDER**
# CAPSULAR AND LIGAMENTOUS STRESS TESTING

| NATA EC 5th | BOC RD6 | SKILL |
|---|---|---|
| CE-21e | D2-0203 | Posterior Drawer Test for the Shoulder |

**Supplies Needed:** Table

*This problem allows you the opportunity to demonstrate an* **orthopedic test** *known as the* **posterior drawer test for the shoulder**. *You have 2 minutes to complete this task.*

| Posterior Drawer Test for the Shoulder | Course or Site Assessor Environment | | | | | |
|---|---|---|---|---|---|---|
| | | Test 1 | | Test 2 | | Test 3 |
| **Tester places patient and limb in appropriate position** | | Y | N | Y | N | Y | N |
| Seated or supine (preferred) | | ○ | ○ | ○ | ○ | ○ | ○ |
| Shoulder flexed to 90 degrees, elbow flexed to 90 degrees | | ○ | ○ | ○ | ○ | ○ | ○ |
| GH joint being tested is positioned off side of the table | | ○ | ○ | ○ | ○ | ○ | ○ |
| **Tester placed in proper position** | | Y | N | Y | N | Y | N |
| Stands on the involved side | | ○ | ○ | ○ | ○ | ○ | ○ |
| One hand grasps the forearm/distal humerus | | ○ | ○ | ○ | ○ | ○ | ○ |
| Other hand placed posteriorly to shoulder to stabilize scapula | | ○ | ○ | ○ | ○ | ○ | ○ |
| Thumbs placed on the coracoid process | | ○ | ○ | ○ | ○ | ○ | ○ |
| **Tester performs test according to accepted guidelines** | | Y | N | Y | N | Y | N |
| Applies longitudinal force to humeral shaft | | ○ | ○ | ○ | ○ | ○ | ○ |
| Encourages (forces) humeral head posteriorly | | ○ | ○ | ○ | ○ | ○ | ○ |
| Maintains relaxation of limb | | ○ | ○ | ○ | ○ | ○ | ○ |
| Performs assessment bilaterally | | ○ | ○ | ○ | ○ | ○ | ○ |
| **Identifies positive findings and implications** | | Y | N | Y | N | Y | N |
| Apprehension | | ○ | ○ | ○ | ○ | ○ | ○ |
| Muscle guarding | | ○ | ○ | ○ | ○ | ○ | ○ |
| Posterior laxity – instability of humeral head (laxity in the posterior GH capsule, torn posterior labrum) | | ○ | ○ | ○ | ○ | ○ | ○ |
| Total | | ___/14 | | ___/14 | | ___/14 |
| **Must achieve >9 to pass this examination** | | Ⓟ | Ⓕ | Ⓟ | Ⓕ | Ⓟ | Ⓕ |

| Assessor:<br>Date: | Test 1 Comments: |
|---|---|
| Assessor:<br>Date: | Test 2 Comments: |
| Assessor:<br>Date: | Test 3 Comments: |

**TEST ENVIRONMENTS**
**L:** Laboratory/Classroom
**C:** Clinical/Field Testing
**P:** Practicum
**A:** Assessment/Mock Exam

**TEST INFORMATION**
**Test Statistics:** No data available
**Reference(s):** Konin et al. (2016)
Starkey & Brown (2015)

# CAPSULAR AND LIGAMENTOUS STRESS TESTING

| NATA EC 5th | BOC RD6 | SKILL |
|---|---|---|
| CE-21e | D2-0203 | Relocation Test (Jobe's Test) |

**Supplies Needed:** Table

*This problem allows you the opportunity to demonstrate an* **orthopedic test** *known as the* **relocation test (Jobe's test)** *for the shoulder. You have 2 minutes to complete this task.*

| Relocation Test (Jobe's Test) | Course or Site / Assessor / Environment | | | | | |
|---|---|---|---|---|---|---|
| | | Test 1 | | Test 2 | | Test 3 |
| **Tester places patient and limb in appropriate position** | | Y | N | Y | N | Y | N |
| Supine | | ○ | ○ | ○ | ○ | ○ | ○ |
| Shoulder abducted to 90 degrees | | ○ | ○ | ○ | ○ | ○ | ○ |
| Elbow flexed to 90 degrees | | ○ | ○ | ○ | ○ | ○ | ○ |
| **Tester placed in proper position** | | Y | N | Y | N | Y | N |
| Stands on the involved side, inferior to the patient | | ○ | ○ | ○ | ○ | ○ | ○ |
| One hand grasps the forearm just proximal to wrist | | ○ | ○ | ○ | ○ | ○ | ○ |
| Other hand placed over humeral head (anterior) | | ○ | ○ | ○ | ○ | ○ | ○ |
| **Tester performs test according to accepted guidelines** | | Y | N | Y | N | Y | N |
| Applies posterior force to humeral head | | ○ | ○ | ○ | ○ | ○ | ○ |
| Applies passive external rotation to shoulder | | ○ | ○ | ○ | ○ | ○ | ○ |
| Maintains relaxation of limb | | ○ | ○ | ○ | ○ | ○ | ○ |
| Performs assessment bilaterally | | ○ | ○ | ○ | ○ | ○ | ○ |
| **Identifies positive findings and implications** | | Y | N | Y | N | Y | N |
| Decreased pain and/or increased range of motion – compared to the anterior apprehension test | | ○ | ○ | ○ | ○ | ○ | ○ |
| Increased laxity in anterior and capsular structure/labral tears | | ○ | ○ | ○ | ○ | ○ | ○ |
| Total | | __/12 | | __/12 | | __/12 | |
| Must achieve >8 to pass this examination | | Ⓟ | Ⓕ | Ⓟ | Ⓕ | Ⓟ | Ⓕ |

| Assessor: Date: | Test 1 Comments: |
|---|---|
| Assessor: Date: | Test 2 Comments: |
| Assessor: Date: | Test 3 Comments: |

**TEST ENVIRONMENTS**
**L:** Laboratory/Classroom
**C:** Clinical/Field Testing
**P:** Practicum
**A:** Assessment/Mock Exam

**TEST INFORMATION**
**Test Statistics:** (+) LR 3.3–10
　　　　　　　　(-) LR .65–.33
**Reference(s):** Konin et al. (2016)
　　　　　　　　Starkey & Brown (2015)

## MUSCULOSKELETAL SYSTEM—REGION 7: SHOULDER
# CAPSULAR AND LIGAMENTOUS STRESS TESTING

| NATA EC 5th | BOC RD6 | SKILL |
|---|---|---|
| CE-21e | D2-0203 | Sternoclavicular Joint Stress Test |

**Supplies Needed:** Table

*This problem allows you the opportunity to demonstrate an* **orthopedic test** *known as the* **sternoclavicular joint stress test***. You have 2 minutes to complete this task.*

| Sternoclavicular Joint Stress Test | Course or Site / Assessor / Environment | | Test 1 | | Test 2 | | Test 3 | |
|---|---|---|---|---|---|---|---|---|
| | | | Y | N | Y | N | Y | N |
| **Tester places patient and limb in appropriate position** | | | **Y** | **N** | **Y** | **N** | **Y** | **N** |
| Seated or standing (or supine) | | | ○ | ○ | ○ | ○ | ○ | ○ |
| Arm relaxed at side | | | ○ | ○ | ○ | ○ | ○ | ○ |
| **Tester placed in proper position** | | | **Y** | **N** | **Y** | **N** | **Y** | **N** |
| Positioned in front of the patient | | | ○ | ○ | ○ | ○ | ○ | ○ |
| Places both thumbs over anterior, medial clavicle | | | ○ | ○ | ○ | ○ | ○ | ○ |
| **Tester performs test according to accepted guidelines** | | | **Y** | **N** | **Y** | **N** | **Y** | **N** |
| Applies gliding pressure downward and inward on the clavicle | | | ○ | ○ | ○ | ○ | ○ | ○ |
| Notes any movement of the SC joint | | | ○ | ○ | ○ | ○ | ○ | ○ |
| Maintains relaxation of limb | | | ○ | ○ | ○ | ○ | ○ | ○ |
| Performs assessment bilaterally | | | ○ | ○ | ○ | ○ | ○ | ○ |
| **Identifies positive findings and implications** | | | **Y** | **N** | **Y** | **N** | **Y** | **N** |
| Pain | | | ○ | ○ | ○ | ○ | ○ | ○ |
| Hypomobility – joint adhesions | | | ○ | ○ | ○ | ○ | ○ | ○ |
| Hypermobility – ligamentous sprain (inferior: interclavicular, superior: costoclavicular, anterior: SC posterior ligament fibers, posterior: SC ligament anterior fibers) | | | ○ | ○ | ○ | ○ | ○ | ○ |
| Total | | | ___/11 | | ___/11 | | ___/11 | |
| Must achieve >7 to pass this examination | | | Ⓟ | Ⓕ | Ⓟ | Ⓕ | Ⓟ | Ⓕ |

| Assessor: Date: | Test 1 Comments: |
|---|---|
| Assessor: Date: | Test 2 Comments: |
| Assessor: Date: | Test 3 Comments: |

**TEST ENVIRONMENTS**
L: Laboratory/Classroom
C: Clinical/Field Testing
P: Practicum
A: Assessment/Mock Exam

**TEST INFORMATION**
**Test Statistics:** No data available
**Reference(s):** Konin et al. (2016)
Starkey & Brown (2015)

## MUSCULOSKELETAL SYSTEM—REGION 7: SHOULDER
# CAPSULAR AND LIGAMENTOUS STRESS TESTING

| NATA EC 5th | BOC RD6 | SKILL |
|---|---|---|
| CE-21e | D2-0203 | Sulcus Sign |

**Supplies Needed:** Table

*This problem allows you the opportunity to demonstrate an* **orthopedic test** *known as the* **sulcus sign** *for the shoulder. You have 2 minutes to complete this task.*

| Sulcus Sign | Course or Site Assessor Environment | | Test 1 | | Test 2 | | Test 3 |
|---|---|---|---|---|---|---|---|
| | | **Y** | **N** | **Y** | **N** | **Y** | **N** |
| **Tester places patient and limb in appropriate position** | | **Y** | **N** | **Y** | **N** | **Y** | **N** |
| Seated (also standing) | | ○ | ○ | ○ | ○ | ○ | ○ |
| Arms relaxed at the side | | ○ | ○ | ○ | ○ | ○ | ○ |
| **Tester placed in proper position** | | **Y** | **N** | **Y** | **N** | **Y** | **N** |
| Stands (or sits) lateral/perpendicular to the patient | | ○ | ○ | ○ | ○ | ○ | ○ |
| Places one hand on the scapula | | ○ | ○ | ○ | ○ | ○ | ○ |
| Other hand grasps the forearm just proximal to wrist | | ○ | ○ | ○ | ○ | ○ | ○ |
| **Tester performs test according to accepted guidelines** | | **Y** | **N** | **Y** | **N** | **Y** | **N** |
| Applies pressure inferiorly distracting the humerus distally | | ○ | ○ | ○ | ○ | ○ | ○ |
| Scapular stabilization is maintained | | ○ | ○ | ○ | ○ | ○ | ○ |
| Maintains relaxation of limb | | ○ | ○ | ○ | ○ | ○ | ○ |
| Performs assessment bilaterally | | ○ | ○ | ○ | ○ | ○ | ○ |
| **Identifies positive findings and implications** | | **Y** | **N** | **Y** | **N** | **Y** | **N** |
| Patient displays "step-off" deformity, sunken area (sulcus) | | ○ | ○ | ○ | ○ | ○ | ○ |
| Pain | | ○ | ○ | ○ | ○ | ○ | ○ |
| Implications include laxity of the superior GH ligament and widening of the subacromial space | | ○ | ○ | ○ | ○ | ○ | ○ |
| **Total** | | ____/12 | | ____/12 | | ____/12 | |
| **Must achieve >8 to pass this examination** | | Ⓟ | Ⓕ | Ⓟ | Ⓕ | Ⓟ | Ⓕ |

| Assessor: Date: | Test 1 Comments: |
|---|---|
| Assessor: Date: | Test 2 Comments: |
| Assessor: Date: | Test 3 Comments: |

**TEST ENVIRONMENTS**
L:  Laboratory/Classroom
C:  Clinical/Field Testing
P:  Practicum
A:  Assessment/Mock Exam

**TEST INFORMATION**
**Test Statistics:**  (+) LR <3
    (-) LR .2
**Reference(s):**  Konin et al. (2016)
    Starkey & Brown (2015)

## MUSCULOSKELETAL SYSTEM—REGION 7: SHOULDER
## CAPSULAR AND LIGAMENTOUS STRESS TESTING

| NATA EC 5th | BOC RD6 | SKILL |
|---|---|---|
| CE-21e | D2-0203 | Surprise Test (Anterior Release Test) |

**Supplies Needed:** Table

*This problem allows you the opportunity to demonstrate an* **orthopedic test** *known as the* **surprise test (anterior release test)** *for the shoulder. You have 2 minutes to complete this task.*

| Surprise Test (Anterior Release Test) | Course or Site Assessor Environment | | Test 1 | | Test 2 | | Test 3 | |
|---|---|---|---|---|---|---|---|---|
| **Tester places patient and limb in appropriate position** | | **Y** | **N** | **Y** | **N** | **Y** | **N** | |
| Supine | | ○ | ○ | ○ | ○ | ○ | ○ | |
| Shoulder abducted to 90 degrees | | ○ | ○ | ○ | ○ | ○ | ○ | |
| Elbow flexed to 90 degrees | | ○ | ○ | ○ | ○ | ○ | ○ | |
| **Tester placed in proper position** | | **Y** | **N** | **Y** | **N** | **Y** | **N** | |
| Stands on the involved side, inferior to the patient | | ○ | ○ | ○ | ○ | ○ | ○ | |
| One hand grasps the forearm just proximal to wrist | | ○ | ○ | ○ | ○ | ○ | ○ | |
| Other hand placed over humeral head (anterior) | | ○ | ○ | ○ | ○ | ○ | ○ | |
| **Tester performs test according to accepted guidelines** | | **Y** | **N** | **Y** | **N** | **Y** | **N** | |
| Applies posterior force to the humeral head | | ○ | ○ | ○ | ○ | ○ | ○ | |
| Applies passive external rotation to shoulder and then removes hand | | ○ | ○ | ○ | ○ | ○ | ○ | |
| Maintains relaxation of limb | | ○ | ○ | ○ | ○ | ○ | ○ | |
| Performs assessment bilaterally | | ○ | ○ | ○ | ○ | ○ | ○ | |
| **Identifies positive findings and implications** | | **Y** | **N** | **Y** | **N** | **Y** | **N** | |
| Apprehension and/or pain when pressure is removed | | ○ | ○ | ○ | ○ | ○ | ○ | |
| Total | | ___/11 | | ___/11 | | ___/11 | | |
| **Must achieve >7 to pass this examination** | | Ⓟ | Ⓕ | Ⓟ | Ⓕ | Ⓟ | Ⓕ | |

| Assessor: Date: | Test 1 Comments: |
|---|---|
| Assessor: Date: | Test 2 Comments: |
| Assessor: Date: | Test 3 Comments: |

**TEST ENVIRONMENTS**
**L:** Laboratory/Classroom
**C:** Clinical/Field Testing
**P:** Practicum
**A:** Assessment/Mock Exam

**TEST INFORMATION**
**Test Statistics:** (+) LR 8.5–58.09
(-) LR .37–.09
**Reference(s):** Konin et al. (2016)
Starkey & Brown (2015)

## MUSCULOSKELETAL SYSTEM—REGION 7: SHOULDER
# JOINT PLAY (ARTHROKINEMATICS)

| NATA EC 5th | BOC RD6 | SKILL |
|---|---|---|
| CE-21f | D2-0203 | Acromioclavicular Joint Play |

**Supplies Needed:** Table or chair

*This problem allows you the opportunity to demonstrate an* **orthopedic assessment** *known as* **acromioclavicular joint play**. *You have 2 minutes to complete this task.*

| Acromioclavicular Joint Play | Course or Site / Assessor / Environment | | Test 1 | | Test 2 | | Test 3 | |
|---|---|---|---|---|---|---|---|---|
| | | | Y | N | Y | N | Y | N |
| **Tester places patient and limb in appropriate position** | | | Y | N | Y | N | Y | N |
| Seated or supine position | | | ○ | ○ | ○ | ○ | ○ | ○ |
| Arms placed at the patient's side | | | ○ | ○ | ○ | ○ | ○ | ○ |
| **Tester placed in proper position** | | | Y | N | Y | N | Y | N |
| Stands to the side of the patient on the involved side | | | ○ | ○ | ○ | ○ | ○ | ○ |
| Grasps distal portion of clavicle just proximal to AC joint | | | ○ | ○ | ○ | ○ | ○ | ○ |
| Opposite hand stabilizes the shoulder | | | ○ | ○ | ○ | ○ | ○ | ○ |
| **Tester performs test according to accepted guidelines** | | | Y | N | Y | N | Y | N |
| Force is applied to move the distal clavicle downward | | | ○ | ○ | ○ | ○ | ○ | ○ |
| Force is applied to move the distal clavicle upward | | | ○ | ○ | ○ | ○ | ○ | ○ |
| Force is applied to move the distal clavicle anteriorly | | | ○ | ○ | ○ | ○ | ○ | ○ |
| Force is applied to move the distal clavicle posteriorly | | | ○ | ○ | ○ | ○ | ○ | ○ |
| Performs assessment bilaterally | | | ○ | ○ | ○ | ○ | ○ | ○ |
| **Identifies positive findings and implications** | | | Y | N | Y | N | Y | N |
| Pain | | | ○ | ○ | ○ | ○ | ○ | ○ |
| Hypomobility can be associated with joint adhesions | | | ○ | ○ | ○ | ○ | ○ | ○ |
| Hypermobility can be associated with laxity of the corresponding ligamentous structures | | | ○ | ○ | ○ | ○ | ○ | ○ |
| Total | | | ___/13 | | ___/13 | | ___/13 | |
| Must achieve >9 to pass this examination | | | Ⓟ | Ⓕ | Ⓟ | Ⓕ | Ⓟ | Ⓕ |

| Assessor: Date: | Test 1 Comments: |
|---|---|
| Assessor: Date: | Test 2 Comments: |
| Assessor: Date: | Test 3 Comments: |

**TEST ENVIRONMENTS**
L: Laboratory/Classroom
C: Clinical/Field Testing
P: Practicum
A: Assessment/Mock Exam

**TEST INFORMATION**
**Test Statistics:** No data available
**Reference(s):** Starkey & Brown (2015)

## MUSCULOSKELETAL SYSTEM—REGION 7: SHOULDER
# JOINT PLAY (ARTHROKINEMATICS)

| NATA EC 5th | BOC RD6 | SKILL |
|---|---|---|
| CE-21f | D2-0203 | Glenohumeral Joint Play |

**Supplies Needed:** Table or chair

*This problem allows you the opportunity to demonstrate an* **orthopedic assessment** *known as* **glenohumeral joint play***. You have 2 minutes to complete this task.*

| Glenohumeral Joint Play | Course or Site Assessor Environment ———— ———— ———— | | Test 1 | | Test 2 | | Test 3 | |
|---|---|---|---|---|---|---|---|---|
| **Tester places patient and limb in appropriate position** | | **Y** | **N** | **Y** | **N** | **Y** | **N** | |
| Seated or supine position | | ○ | ○ | ○ | ○ | ○ | ○ | |
| Shoulder placed in 55 degrees abduction and 30 degrees flexion | | ○ | ○ | ○ | ○ | ○ | ○ | |
| Arm is supported to maintain relaxation | | ○ | ○ | ○ | ○ | ○ | ○ | |
| **Tester placed in proper position** | | **Y** | **N** | **Y** | **N** | **Y** | **N** | |
| Stands to the side of the patient on the involved side | | ○ | ○ | ○ | ○ | ○ | ○ | |
| Grasps humerus from mid-shaft to proximal third | | ○ | ○ | ○ | ○ | ○ | ○ | |
| Opposite hand stabilizes the scapula | | ○ | ○ | ○ | ○ | ○ | ○ | |
| **Tester performs test according to accepted guidelines** | | **Y** | **N** | **Y** | **N** | **Y** | **N** | |
| Inferior glide | | | | | | | | |
|   Opposite hand is placed over the superior humerus | | ○ | ○ | ○ | ○ | ○ | ○ | |
|   Force is applied inferiorly | | ○ | ○ | ○ | ○ | ○ | ○ | |
| Anterior glide | | | | | | | | |
|   Opposite hand applies force at the posterior humerus | | ○ | ○ | ○ | ○ | ○ | ○ | |
|   Force is applied anteriorly | | ○ | ○ | ○ | ○ | ○ | ○ | |
| Posterior glide | | | | | | | | |
|   Opposite hand applies force at the anterior humerus head | | ○ | ○ | ○ | ○ | ○ | ○ | |
|   Force is applied posteriorly | | ○ | ○ | ○ | ○ | ○ | ○ | |
| Performs assessment bilaterally | | ○ | ○ | ○ | ○ | ○ | ○ | |
| **Identifies positive findings and implications** | | **Y** | **N** | **Y** | **N** | **Y** | **N** | |
| Pain | | ○ | ○ | ○ | ○ | ○ | ○ | |
| Hypomobility can be associated with joint capsule adhesions | | ○ | ○ | ○ | ○ | ○ | ○ | |
| Hypermobility can be associated with laxity of the corresponding ligamentous structures | | ○ | ○ | ○ | ○ | ○ | ○ | |
| **Total** | | \_\_\_\_ /16 | | \_\_\_\_ /16 | | \_\_\_\_ /16 | | |
| **Must achieve >11 to pass this examination** | | Ⓟ | Ⓕ | Ⓟ | Ⓕ | Ⓟ | Ⓕ | |

| Assessor: Date: | Test 1 Comments: |
|---|---|
| Assessor: Date: | Test 2 Comments: |
| Assessor: Date: | Test 3 Comments: |

**TEST ENVIRONMENTS**
**L:** Laboratory/Classroom
**C:** Clinical/Field Testing
**P:** Practicum
**A:** Assessment/Mock Exam

**TEST INFORMATION**
**Test Statistics:** No data available
**Reference(s):** Starkey & Brown (2015)

MUSCULOSKELETAL SYSTEM—REGION 7: SHOULDER
# JOINT PLAY (ARTHROKINEMATICS)

| NATA EC 5th | BOC RD6 | SKILL |
|---|---|---|
| CE-21f | D2-0203 | Sternoclavicular Joint Play |

**Supplies Needed:** Table or chair

*This problem allows you the opportunity to demonstrate an* **orthopedic assessment** *known as* **sternoclavicular joint play**. *You have 2 minutes to complete this task.*

| Sternoclavicular Joint Play | Course or Site<br>Assessor<br>Environment | | | | | |
|---|---|---|---|---|---|---|
| | | Test 1 | | Test 2 | | Test 3 |
| **Tester places patient and limb in appropriate position** | | Y | N | Y | N | Y | N |
| Seated or supine | | ○ | ○ | ○ | ○ | ○ | ○ |
| Arms placed at the patient's side | | ○ | ○ | ○ | ○ | ○ | ○ |
| **Tester placed in proper position** | | Y | N | Y | N | Y | N |
| Stands to the side of the patient on the involved side | | ○ | ○ | ○ | ○ | ○ | ○ |
| Grasps proximal portion of clavicle just distal to SC joint | | ○ | ○ | ○ | ○ | ○ | ○ |
| Opposite hand stabilizes the body/chest | | ○ | ○ | ○ | ○ | ○ | ○ |
| **Tester performs test according to accepted guidelines** | | Y | N | Y | N | Y | N |
| Force is applied to move the medial clavicle inferior | | ○ | ○ | ○ | ○ | ○ | ○ |
| Force is applied to move the medial clavicle superior | | ○ | ○ | ○ | ○ | ○ | ○ |
| Force is applied to move the medial clavicle anteriorly | | ○ | ○ | ○ | ○ | ○ | ○ |
| Force is applied to move the medial clavicle posteriorly | | ○ | ○ | ○ | ○ | ○ | ○ |
| Performs assessment bilaterally | | ○ | ○ | ○ | ○ | ○ | ○ |
| **Identifies positive findings and implications** | | Y | N | Y | N | Y | N |
| Pain | | ○ | ○ | ○ | ○ | ○ | ○ |
| Hypomobility can be associated with joint adhesions | | ○ | ○ | ○ | ○ | ○ | ○ |
| Hypermobility can be associated with laxity of the corresponding ligamentous structures/sprain | | ○ | ○ | ○ | ○ | ○ | ○ |
| Total | | ___/13 | | ___/13 | | ___/13 | |
| **Must achieve >9 to pass this examination** | | Ⓟ | Ⓕ | Ⓟ | Ⓕ | Ⓟ | Ⓕ |

| Assessor:<br>Date: | Test 1 Comments: |
|---|---|
| Assessor:<br>Date: | Test 2 Comments: |
| Assessor:<br>Date: | Test 3 Comments: |

**TEST ENVIRONMENTS**
**L:** Laboratory/Classroom
**C:** Clinical/Field Testing
**P:** Practicum
**A:** Assessment/Mock Exam

**TEST INFORMATION**
**Test Statistics:** No data available
**Reference(s):** Starkey & Brown (2015)

**MUSCULOSKELETAL SYSTEM—REGION 7: SHOULDER**
# SPECIAL TESTS

| NATA EC 5th | BOC RD6 | SKILL |
|---|---|---|
| CE-21g, CE-20e | D2-0203 | Active Compression Test (O'Brien Test) |

**Supplies Needed:** Table

*This problem allows you the opportunity to demonstrate an* **orthopedic special test** *known as the* **active compression test (O'Brien test)** *to rule out possible* **SLAP and AC joint lesions** *of the shoulder. You have 2 minutes to complete this task.*

| Active Compression Test (O'Brien Test) | Course or Site Assessor Environment | | Test 1 | | Test 2 | | Test 3 | |
|---|---|---|---|---|---|---|---|---|
| **Tester places patient and limb in appropriate position** | | **Y** | **N** | **Y** | **N** | **Y** | **N** | |
| Standing | | ○ | ○ | ○ | ○ | ○ | ○ | |
| Shoulder flexed to 90 degrees and horizontally flexed to 15 degrees | | ○ | ○ | ○ | ○ | ○ | ○ | |
| Humerus placed in full internal rotation | | ○ | ○ | ○ | ○ | ○ | ○ | |
| Elbow extended and forearm pronated | | ○ | ○ | ○ | ○ | ○ | ○ | |
| **Tester placed in proper position** | | **Y** | **N** | **Y** | **N** | **Y** | **N** | |
| Stands facing the patient | | ○ | ○ | ○ | ○ | ○ | ○ | |
| Places one hand under the elbow (or grasps the elbow) | | ○ | ○ | ○ | ○ | ○ | ○ | |
| Places other hand over the superior aspect of the distal forearm | | ○ | ○ | ○ | ○ | ○ | ○ | |
| **Tester performs test according to accepted guidelines** | | **Y** | **N** | **Y** | **N** | **Y** | **N** | |
| Patient isometrically resists the downward force of the tester | | ○ | ○ | ○ | ○ | ○ | ○ | |
| The tester repeats test with the shoulder in external rotation and the forearm supinated | | ○ | ○ | ○ | ○ | ○ | ○ | |
| Performs assessment bilaterally | | ○ | ○ | ○ | ○ | ○ | ○ | |
| **Identifies positive findings and implications** | | **Y** | **N** | **Y** | **N** | **Y** | **N** | |
| Pain and/or clicking in GH joint – possible tear of labrum | | ○ | ○ | ○ | ○ | ○ | ○ | |
| Pain at AC joint suggests possible AC joint pathology | | ○ | ○ | ○ | ○ | ○ | ○ | |
| **Total** | | \_\_\_\_/12 | | \_\_\_\_/12 | | \_\_\_\_/12 | | |
| **Must achieve >8 to pass this examination** | | Ⓟ | Ⓕ | Ⓟ | Ⓕ | Ⓟ | Ⓕ | |

| Assessor: Date: | Test 1 Comments: |
|---|---|
| Assessor: Date: | Test 2 Comments: |
| Assessor: Date: | Test 3 Comments: |

**TEST ENVIRONMENTS**
**L:** Laboratory/Classroom
**C:** Clinical/Field Testing
**P:** Practicum
**A:** Assessment/Mock Exam

**TEST INFORMATION**
**Test Statistics:** IRR .22 (poor)
AC joint (+) LR 29.41
(-) LR 0–.6
SLAP PLR 1.2
NLR .72–.91
Labrum PLR .7
NLR: 1.0
**Reference(s):** Starkey & Brown (2015)

© SLACK Incorporated, 2016. Hauth, J. M., Gloyeske, B. M., & Amato, H. K. (2016). *Clinical Skills Documentation Guide for Athletic Training, Third Edition.* Thorofare, NJ: SLACK Incorporated.

## MUSCULOSKELETAL SYSTEM—REGION 7: SHOULDER
## SPECIAL TESTS

| NATA EC 5th | BOC RD6 | SKILL |
|---|---|---|
| CE-21g, CE-20e | D2-0203 | Apley's Scratch Test |

**Supplies Needed:** Table or chair

*This problem allows you the opportunity to demonstrate an* **orthopedic special test** *known as* **Apley's scratch test** *for* **general shoulder flexibility***. You have 2 minutes to complete this task.*

| Apley's Scratch Test | Course or Site Assessor Environment | Test 1 | | Test 2 | | Test 3 | |
|---|---|---|---|---|---|---|---|
| | | **Y** | **N** | **Y** | **N** | **Y** | **N** |
| **Tester places patient and limb in appropriate position** | | Y | N | Y | N | Y | N |
| Seated or standing | | ○ | ○ | ○ | ○ | ○ | ○ |
| Arm placed at the patient's side | | ○ | ○ | ○ | ○ | ○ | ○ |
| **Tester placed in proper position** | | Y | N | Y | N | Y | N |
| Stands facing the patient (observe only) | | ○ | ○ | ○ | ○ | ○ | ○ |
| **Tester performs test according to accepted guidelines** | | Y | N | Y | N | Y | N |
| Instructs the patient to touch the opposite shoulder | | ○ | ○ | ○ | ○ | ○ | ○ |
| Instructs the patient to touch the opposite shoulder behind head | | ○ | ○ | ○ | ○ | ○ | ○ |
| Instructs the patient to reach behind the back and touch the opposite scapula | | ○ | ○ | ○ | ○ | ○ | ○ |
| Performs assessment bilaterally | | ○ | ○ | ○ | ○ | ○ | ○ |
| **Identifies positive findings and implications** | | Y | N | Y | N | Y | N |
| Positive finding is the inability to touch the opposite shoulder | | ○ | ○ | ○ | ○ | ○ | ○ |
| Restriction in range of motion involving structures around the GH joint | | ○ | ○ | ○ | ○ | ○ | ○ |
| **Total** | | __/9 | | __/9 | | __/9 | |
| **Must achieve >6 to pass this examination** | | Ⓟ | Ⓕ | Ⓟ | Ⓕ | Ⓟ | Ⓕ |

| Assessor: Date: | Test 1 Comments: |
|---|---|
| Assessor: Date: | Test 2 Comments: |
| Assessor: Date: | Test 3 Comments: |

**TEST ENVIRONMENTS**
**L:** Laboratory/Classroom
**C:** Clinical/Field Testing
**P:** Practicum
**A:** Assessment/Mock Exam

**TEST INFORMATION**
**Test Statistics:** No data available
**Reference(s):** Konin et al. (2016)
Starkey & Brown (2015)

## MUSCULOSKELETAL SYSTEM—REGION 7: SHOULDER
## SPECIAL TESTS

| NATA EC 5th | BOC RD6 | SKILL |
|---|---|---|
| CE-21g, CE-20e | D2-0203 | Drop Arm Test (Codman's Test) |

**Supplies Needed:** Table or chair

*This problem allows you the opportunity to demonstrate an* **orthopedic special test** *known as the* **drop arm test (Codman's test)** *to rule out a possible* **rotator cuff lesion**. *You have 2 minutes to complete this task.*

| Drop Arm Test (Codman's Test) | Course or Site Assessor Environment | | | | | |
|---|---|---|---|---|---|---|
| | | Test 1 | | Test 2 | | Test 3 |
| **Tester places patient and limb in appropriate position** | | Y | N | Y | N | Y | N |
| Seated or standing | | ○ | ○ | ○ | ○ | ○ | ○ |
| Arm rests at side | | ○ | ○ | ○ | ○ | ○ | ○ |
| Shoulder internally rotated, elbow pronated | | ○ | ○ | ○ | ○ | ○ | ○ |
| **Tester placed in proper position** | | Y | N | Y | N | Y | N |
| Stands in front of the patient (alternate – behind the patient) | | ○ | ○ | ○ | ○ | ○ | ○ |
| Places one hand on the forearm just proximal to the wrist | | ○ | ○ | ○ | ○ | ○ | ○ |
| **Tester performs test according to accepted guidelines** | | Y | N | Y | N | Y | N |
| Passively abducts shoulder to 90 degrees and releases the arm | | ○ | ○ | ○ | ○ | ○ | ○ |
| Instructs the patient to slowly lower the arm to the side | | ○ | ○ | ○ | ○ | ○ | ○ |
| Performs assessment bilaterally | | ○ | ○ | ○ | ○ | ○ | ○ |
| **Identifies positive findings and implications** | | Y | N | Y | N | Y | N |
| Pain | | ○ | ○ | ○ | ○ | ○ | ○ |
| Inability to slowly return arm to side (adduct) | | ○ | ○ | ○ | ○ | ○ | ○ |
| Total | | /10 | | /10 | | /10 | |
| Must achieve >6 to pass this examination | | Ⓟ | Ⓕ | Ⓟ | Ⓕ | Ⓟ | Ⓕ |

| Assessor: Date: | Test 1 Comments: |
|---|---|
| Assessor: Date: | Test 2 Comments: |
| Assessor: Date: | Test 3 Comments: |

**TEST ENVIRONMENTS**
**L:** Laboratory/Classroom
**C:** Clinical/Field Testing
**P:** Practicum
**A:** Assessment/Mock Exam

**TEST INFORMATION**
**Test Statistics:** No data available
**Reference(s):** Konin et al. (2016)

## MUSCULOSKELETAL SYSTEM—REGION 7: SHOULDER
# SPECIAL TESTS

| NATA EC 5th | BOC RD6 | SKILL |
|---|---|---|
| CE-21g, CE-20e | D2-0203 | Empty Can Test (Supraspinatus Test) |

**Supplies Needed:** Table or chair

*This problem allows you the opportunity to demonstrate an* **orthopedic special test** *known as the* **empty can test (supraspinatus test)** *to rule out a possible* **supraspinatus lesion**. *You have 2 minutes to complete this task.*

| Empty Can Test (Supraspinatus Test) | Course or Site Assessor Environment | | | | | |
|---|---|---|---|---|---|---|
| | | Test 1 | | Test 2 | | Test 3 |
| **Tester places patient and limb in appropriate position** | | Y | N | Y | N | Y | N |
| Seated or standing | | ○ | ○ | ○ | ○ | ○ | ○ |
| Shoulder abducted to 90 degrees, internally rotated (thumb down) | | ○ | ○ | ○ | ○ | ○ | ○ |
| Shoulder horizontally flexed to 30 degrees | | ○ | ○ | ○ | ○ | ○ | ○ |
| Elbow fully extended (alternate – "full can test" – less painful and similar accuracy) | | ○ | ○ | ○ | ○ | ○ | ○ |
| **Tester placed in proper position** | | Y | N | Y | N | Y | N |
| Stands facing the patient | | ○ | ○ | ○ | ○ | ○ | ○ |
| Places one hand on the distal third of the forearm | | ○ | ○ | ○ | ○ | ○ | ○ |
| **Tester performs test according to accepted guidelines** | | Y | N | Y | N | Y | N |
| Instructs the patient to hold arm in this position | | ○ | ○ | ○ | ○ | ○ | ○ |
| Applies downward pressure (resists abduction) | | ○ | ○ | ○ | ○ | ○ | ○ |
| Performs assessment bilaterally | | ○ | ○ | ○ | ○ | ○ | ○ |
| **Identifies positive findings and implications** | | Y | N | Y | N | Y | N |
| Pain and/or weakness with testing | | ○ | ○ | ○ | ○ | ○ | ○ |
| Inability to hold arm in abduction/flexion | | ○ | ○ | ○ | ○ | ○ | ○ |
| Total | | ___/11 | | ___/11 | | ___/11 | |
| Must achieve >7 to pass this examination | | Ⓟ | Ⓕ | Ⓟ | Ⓕ | Ⓟ | Ⓕ |

| Assessor: Date: | Test 1 Comments: |
|---|---|
| Assessor: Date: | Test 2 Comments: |
| Assessor: Date: | Test 3 Comments: |

**TEST ENVIRONMENTS**
**L:** Laboratory/Classroom
**C:** Clinical/Field Testing
**P:** Practicum
**A:** Assessment/Mock Exam

**TEST INFORMATION**
**Test Statistics:** (+) LR 1.8–3.0
(-) LR .18–.21
**Reference(s):** Konin et al. (2016)
Starkey & Brown (2015)

## MUSCULOSKELETAL SYSTEM—REGION 7: SHOULDER
## SPECIAL TESTS

| NATA EC 5th | BOC RD6 | SKILL |
|---|---|---|
| CE-21g, CE-20e | D2-0203 | Hawkins-Kennedy Test |

**Supplies Needed:** Table or chair

*This problem allows you the opportunity to demonstrate an* **orthopedic special test** *known as the* **Hawkins-Kennedy test** *to rule out a possible* **impingement** *of the shoulder. You have 2 minutes to complete this task.*

| Hawkins-Kennedy Test | Course or Site Assessor Environment | | Test 1 | | Test 2 | | Test 3 | |
|---|---|---|---|---|---|---|---|---|
| **Tester places patient and limb in appropriate position** | | **Y** | **N** | **Y** | **N** | **Y** | **N** | |
| Seated or standing | | ○ | ○ | ○ | ○ | ○ | ○ | |
| Shoulder horizontally flexed to 90 degrees (forward flexion) | | ○ | ○ | ○ | ○ | ○ | ○ | |
| Elbow flexed to 90 degrees | | ○ | ○ | ○ | ○ | ○ | ○ | |
| Forearm is fully pronated | | ○ | ○ | ○ | ○ | ○ | ○ | |
| **Tester placed in proper position** | | **Y** | **N** | **Y** | **N** | **Y** | **N** | |
| Stands facing the patient | | ○ | ○ | ○ | ○ | ○ | ○ | |
| Places one hand under the elbow (or grasps the elbow) | | ○ | ○ | ○ | ○ | ○ | ○ | |
| Places the other hand over the distal forearm just above the wrist | | ○ | ○ | ○ | ○ | ○ | ○ | |
| **Tester performs test according to accepted guidelines** | | **Y** | **N** | **Y** | **N** | **Y** | **N** | |
| Maintains elbow and shoulder flexion | | ○ | ○ | ○ | ○ | ○ | ○ | |
| Applies passive internal rotation | | ○ | ○ | ○ | ○ | ○ | ○ | |
| Performs assessment bilaterally | | ○ | ○ | ○ | ○ | ○ | ○ | |
| **Identifies positive findings and implications** | | **Y** | **N** | **Y** | **N** | **Y** | **N** | |
| Pain with testing (pain before scapular rotation occurs) | | ○ | ○ | ○ | ○ | ○ | ○ | |
| Pain at end or range implicates rotator cuff, biceps tendon | | ○ | ○ | ○ | ○ | ○ | ○ | |
| **Total** | | ___/12 | | ___/12 | | ___/12 | | |
| **Must achieve >8 to pass this examination** | | Ⓟ | Ⓕ | Ⓟ | Ⓕ | Ⓟ | Ⓕ | |

| Assessor:<br>Date: | Test 1 Comments: |
|---|---|
| Assessor:<br>Date: | Test 2 Comments: |
| Assessor:<br>Date: | Test 3 Comments: |

**TEST ENVIRONMENTS**
**L:** Laboratory/Classroom
**C:** Clinical/Field Testing
**P:** Practicum
**A:** Assessment/Mock Exam

**TEST INFORMATION**
**Test Statistics:** (+) LR 1.9
(-) LR .37
**Reference(s):** Konin et al. (2016)
Starkey & Brown (2015)

## MUSCULOSKELETAL SYSTEM—REGION 7: SHOULDER
## SPECIAL TESTS

| NATA EC 5th | BOC RD6 | SKILL |
|---|---|---|
| CE-21g, CE-20e | D2-0203 | Neer Impingement Test |

**Supplies Needed:** Table or chair

*This problem allows you the opportunity to demonstrate an* **orthopedic special test** *known as the* **Neer impingement test** *to rule out a possible* **vascular compromise** *or* **thoracic outlet syndrome**. *You have 2 minutes to complete this task.*

| Neer Impingement Test | Course or Site<br>Assessor<br>Environment | | | | | |
|---|---|---|---|---|---|---|
| | | Test 1 | | Test 2 | | Test 3 |
| **Tester places patient and limb in appropriate position** | | Y | N | Y | N | Y | N |
| Seated or standing | | ○ | ○ | ○ | ○ | ○ | ○ |
| Head faces forward | | ○ | ○ | ○ | ○ | ○ | ○ |
| Arm rests at side | | ○ | ○ | ○ | ○ | ○ | ○ |
| Shoulder internally rotated, forearm pronated fully | | ○ | ○ | ○ | ○ | ○ | ○ |
| **Tester placed in proper position** | | Y | N | Y | N | Y | N |
| Stands to side, facing the patient | | ○ | ○ | ○ | ○ | ○ | ○ |
| Places one hand on scapula | | ○ | ○ | ○ | ○ | ○ | ○ |
| Opposite hand grasps forearm below the elbow | | ○ | ○ | ○ | ○ | ○ | ○ |
| **Tester performs test according to accepted guidelines** | | Y | N | Y | N | Y | N |
| Passively moves the shoulder into full flexion | | ○ | ○ | ○ | ○ | ○ | ○ |
| Pushes the greater tuberosity into the acromial border | | ○ | ○ | ○ | ○ | ○ | ○ |
| Maintains relaxation of the limb | | ○ | ○ | ○ | ○ | ○ | ○ |
| Performs assessment bilaterally | | ○ | ○ | ○ | ○ | ○ | ○ |
| **Identifies positive findings and implications** | | Y | N | Y | N | Y | N |
| Pain in the anterior/lateral shoulder with movement | | ○ | ○ | ○ | ○ | ○ | ○ |
| Rotator cuff (supraspinatus) and/or long head of biceps | | ○ | ○ | ○ | ○ | ○ | ○ |
| | Total | ___/13 | | ___/13 | | ___/13 |
| | Must achieve >9 to pass this examination | Ⓟ | Ⓕ | Ⓟ | Ⓕ | Ⓟ | Ⓕ |

| Assessor:<br>Date: | Test 1 Comments: |
|---|---|
| Assessor:<br>Date: | Test 2 Comments: |
| Assessor:<br>Date: | Test 3 Comments: |

**TEST ENVIRONMENTS**
**L:** Laboratory/Classroom
**C:** Clinical/Field Testing
**P:** Practicum
**A:** Assessment/Mock Exam

**TEST INFORMATION**
**Test Statistics:** (+) LR 1.8
(-) LR .4
**Reference(s):** Konin et al. (2016)
Starkey & Brown (2015)

**MUSCULOSKELETAL SYSTEM—REGION 7: SHOULDER**
## SPECIAL TESTS

| NATA EC 5th | BOC RD6 | SKILL |
|---|---|---|
| CE-21g, CE-20e | D2-0203 | Pectoralis Major Contracture Test |

**Supplies Needed:** Table

*This problem allows you the opportunity to demonstrate an* **orthopedic special test** *known as the* **pectoralis major contracture test** *to examine muscle* **flexibility**. *You have 2 minutes to complete this task.*

| Pectoralis Major Contracture Test | Course or Site Assessor Environment | | | | | |
|---|---|---|---|---|---|---|
| | | Test 1 | | Test 2 | | Test 3 |
| **Tester places patient and limb in appropriate position** | | Y | N | Y | N | Y | N |
| Supine | | ○ | ○ | ○ | ○ | ○ | ○ |
| The patient clasps both hands behind the head with fingers interlocked | | ○ | ○ | ○ | ○ | ○ | ○ |
| **Tester placed in proper position** | | Y | N | Y | N | Y | N |
| Stands behind the patient's head | | ○ | ○ | ○ | ○ | ○ | ○ |
| **Tester performs test according to accepted guidelines** | | Y | N | Y | N | Y | N |
| Instructs the patient to relax arms | | ○ | ○ | ○ | ○ | ○ | ○ |
| Passively forces the patient's elbows to the table (hyperextension of the shoulder) | | ○ | ○ | ○ | ○ | ○ | ○ |
| Compares assessment bilaterally | | ○ | ○ | ○ | ○ | ○ | ○ |
| **Identifies positive findings and implications** | | Y | N | Y | N | Y | N |
| Elbows unable to touch table surface | | ○ | ○ | ○ | ○ | ○ | ○ |
| Contracture/shortening of the pectoralis major muscle(s) | | ○ | ○ | ○ | ○ | ○ | ○ |
| | Total | ___/8 | | ___/8 | | ___/8 |
| **Must achieve >5 to pass this examination** | | Ⓟ | Ⓕ | Ⓟ | Ⓕ | Ⓟ | Ⓕ |

| Assessor: Date: | **Test 1 Comments:** |
|---|---|
| Assessor: Date: | **Test 2 Comments:** |
| Assessor: Date: | **Test 3 Comments:** |

**TEST ENVIRONMENTS**
**L:** Laboratory/Classroom
**C:** Clinical/Field Testing
**P:** Practicum
**A:** Assessment/Mock Exam

**TEST INFORMATION**
**Test Statistics:** No data available
**Reference(s):** Magee (2005)

## MUSCULOSKELETAL SYSTEM—REGION 7: SHOULDER
## SPECIAL TESTS

| NATA EC 5th | BOC RD6 | SKILL |
|---|---|---|
| CE-21g, CE-20e | D2-0203 | Speed's Test (Straight Arm Test) |

**Supplies Needed:** Table or chair

*This problem allows you the opportunity to demonstrate an* **orthopedic special test** *known as* **Speed's test (straight arm test)** *to rule out a possible involvement of the* **long head of the biceps**. *You have 2 minutes to complete this task.*

| Speed's Test (Straight Arm Test) | Course or Site Assessor Environment | | | | | |
|---|---|---|---|---|---|---|
| | | Test 1 | | Test 2 | | Test 3 |
| **Tester places patient and limb in appropriate position** | | Y | N | Y | N | Y | N |
| Seated or standing | | ○ | ○ | ○ | ○ | ○ | ○ |
| Shoulder placed in anatomical position (or slightly extended) | | ○ | ○ | ○ | ○ | ○ | ○ |
| Elbow extended and in anatomical position (palm out) | | ○ | ○ | ○ | ○ | ○ | ○ |
| Arm rests at side | | ○ | ○ | ○ | ○ | ○ | ○ |
| **Tester placed in proper position** | | Y | N | Y | N | Y | N |
| Stands to the side and faces the patient | | ○ | ○ | ○ | ○ | ○ | ○ |
| Palpates and places fingers over the bicipital groove | | ○ | ○ | ○ | ○ | ○ | ○ |
| Stabilizes forearm just proximal to the wrist | | ○ | ○ | ○ | ○ | ○ | ○ |
| **Tester performs test according to accepted guidelines** | | Y | N | Y | N | Y | N |
| Resists shoulder flexion to 90 degrees | | ○ | ○ | ○ | ○ | ○ | ○ |
| Palpates for tenderness over the bicipital groove | | ○ | ○ | ○ | ○ | ○ | ○ |
| Performs break test at 90 degrees | | ○ | ○ | ○ | ○ | ○ | ○ |
| Performs assessment bilaterally | | ○ | ○ | ○ | ○ | ○ | ○ |
| **Identifies positive findings and implications** | | Y | N | Y | N | Y | N |
| Pain along bicipital groove, transverse humeral ligament | | ○ | ○ | ○ | ○ | ○ | ○ |
| Tenderness – long head of biceps brachii, SLAP lesion | | ○ | ○ | ○ | ○ | ○ | ○ |
| **Total** | | ___/13 | | ___/13 | | ___/13 | |
| **Must achieve >9 to pass this examination** | | Ⓟ | Ⓕ | Ⓟ | Ⓕ | Ⓟ | Ⓕ |

| Assessor: Date: | Test 1 Comments: |
|---|---|
| Assessor: Date: | Test 2 Comments: |
| Assessor: Date: | Test 3 Comments: |

**TEST ENVIRONMENTS**
**L:** Laboratory/Classroom
**C:** Clinical/Field Testing
**P:** Practicum
**A:** Assessment/Mock Exam

**TEST INFORMATION**
**Test Statistics:** SLAP (+) LR .9
(-) LR 1.0
BTP (+) LR 1.3
(-) LR .72–.9
**Reference(s):** Konin et al. (2016)
Starkey & Brown (2015)

| NATA EC 5th | BOC RD6 | SKILL |
|---|---|---|
| CE-21g, CE-20e | D2-0203 | Yergason's Test |

**Supplies Needed:** Table or chair

*This problem allows you the opportunity to demonstrate an* **orthopedic special test** *known as* **Yergason's test** *to rule out a possible involvement of the* **long head of the biceps, SLAP legion**. *You have 2 minutes to complete this task.*

| Yergason's Test | Course or Site Assessor Environment | | Test 1 | | Test 2 | | Test 3 | |
|---|---|---|---|---|---|---|---|---|
| **Tester places patient and limb in appropriate position** | | | Y | N | Y | N | Y | N |
| Seated or standing | | | ○ | ○ | ○ | ○ | ○ | ○ |
| Shoulder placed in anatomical position | | | ○ | ○ | ○ | ○ | ○ | ○ |
| Elbow flexed to 90 degrees | | | ○ | ○ | ○ | ○ | ○ | ○ |
| Forearm is fully pronated | | | ○ | ○ | ○ | ○ | ○ | ○ |
| **Tester placed in proper position** | | | Y | N | Y | N | Y | N |
| Stands to the side and faces the patient | | | ○ | ○ | ○ | ○ | ○ | ○ |
| Palpates and places fingers over the bicipital groove | | | ○ | ○ | ○ | ○ | ○ | ○ |
| Places hand around the distal forearm | | | ○ | ○ | ○ | ○ | ○ | ○ |
| Stabilizes the elbow close to the thorax | | | ○ | ○ | ○ | ○ | ○ | ○ |
| **Tester performs test according to accepted guidelines** | | | Y | N | Y | N | Y | N |
| The tester guides the shoulder into external rotation; the patient resists | | | ○ | ○ | ○ | ○ | ○ | ○ |
| Patient resists supination of the forearm through full range of motion | | | ○ | ○ | ○ | ○ | ○ | ○ |
| Palpates bicipital groove throughout | | | ○ | ○ | ○ | ○ | ○ | ○ |
| Performs assessment bilaterally | | | ○ | ○ | ○ | ○ | ○ | ○ |
| **Identifies positive findings and implications** | | | Y | N | Y | N | Y | N |
| Pain along bicipital groove, transverse humeral ligament | | | ○ | ○ | ○ | ○ | ○ | ○ |
| Snapping/popping – long head of biceps brachii, SLAP lesion | | | ○ | ○ | ○ | ○ | ○ | ○ |
| **Total** | | | ___/14 | | ___/14 | | ___/14 | |
| **Must achieve >9 to pass this examination** | | | Ⓟ | Ⓕ | Ⓟ | Ⓕ | Ⓟ | Ⓕ |
| Assessor: Date: | Test 1 Comments: | | | | | | | |
| Assessor: Date: | Test 2 Comments: | | | | | | | |
| Assessor: Date: | Test 3 Comments: | | | | | | | |

**TEST ENVIRONMENTS**
**L:** Laboratory/Classroom
**C:** Clinical/Field Testing
**P:** Practicum
**A:** Assessment/Mock Exam

**TEST INFORMATION**
**Test Statistics:** SLAP (+) LR 1.2
   (-) LR .94
   BTP (+) LR 1.9
   (-) LR .94
**Reference(s):** Konin et al. (2016)
   Starkey & Brown (2015)

# 11

# MUSCULOSKELETAL SYSTEM— REGION 8: ELBOW

Hauth, J. M., Gloyeske, B. M., & Amato, H. K.
*Clinical Skills Documentation Guide for Athletic Training, Third Edition* (pp. 344-366).
© 2016 SLACK Incorporated.

## MUSCULOSKELETAL SYSTEM—REGION 8: ELBOW
# KNOWLEDGE AND SKILLS

| *Musculoskeletal System—Region 8: Elbow* | | | | *Skill: Acquisition, Reinforcement, Proficiency* | | |
|---|---|---|---|---|---|---|
| **NATA EC 5th** | **BOC RD6** | **Palpation** | **Page #** | | | |
| CE-21b, CE-20c | D2-0202 | Palpation: Elbow – 01 | 346 | | | |
| CE-21b, CE-20c | D2-0202 | Palpation: Elbow – 02 | 347 | | | |
| CE-21b, CE-20c | D2-0202 | Palpation: Elbow – 03 | 348 | | | |
| **NATA EC 5th** | **BOC RD6** | **Manual Muscle Testing** | **Page #** | | | |
| CE-21c | D2-0203 | MMT: Anconeus | 349 | | | |
| CE-21c | D2-0203 | MMT: Biceps Brachii | 350 | | | |
| CE-21c | D2-0203 | MMT: Brachialis | 351 | | | |
| CE-21c | D2-0203 | MMT: Brachioradialis | 352 | | | |
| CE-21c | D2-0203 | MMT: Pronator Quadratus | 353 | | | |
| CE-21c | D2-0203 | MMT: Supinator | 354 | | | |
| CE-21c | D2-0203 | MMT: Triceps Brachii | 355 | | | |
| **NATA EC 5th** | **BOC RD6** | **Osteokinematic Joint Motion** | **Page #** | | | |
| CE-21d | D2-0203 | Goniometric Assessment: Humeroulnar Joint (Flexion) | 356 | | | |
| CE-21d | D2-0203 | Goniometric Assessment: Humeroulnar Joint (Extension) | 357 | | | |
| CE-21d | D2-0203 | Goniometric Assessment: Radioulnar Joint (Pronation) | 358 | | | |
| CE-21d | D2-0203 | Goniometric Assessment: Radioulnar Joint (Supination) | 359 | | | |
| **NATA EC 5th** | **BOC RD6** | **Capsular and Ligamentous Stress Testing** | **Page #** | | | |
| CE-21e | D2-0203 | Valgus Stress Test for the Elbow | 360 | | | |
| CE-21e | D2-0203 | Varus Stress Test for the Elbow | 361 | | | |
| CE-21e | D2-0203 | Moving Valgus Stress Test for the Elbow | 362 | | | |
| **NATA EC 5th** | **BOC RD6** | **Special Tests** | **Page #** | | | |
| CE-21g, CE-20e | D2-0203 | Cozen's Sign (Active Lateral Epicondyle Test) | 363 | | | |
| CE-21g, CE-20e | D2-0203 | Elbow Flexion Test | 364 | | | |
| CE-21g, CE-20e | D2-0203 | Passive Tennis Elbow Test | 365 | | | |
| CE-21g, CE-20e | D2-0203 | Tinel's Sign | 366 | | | |

## MUSCULOSKELETAL SYSTEM—REGION 8: ELBOW
# PALPATION

| NATA EC 5th | BOC RD6 | SKILL |
|---|---|---|
| CE-21b, CE-20c | D2-0202 | Palpation: Elbow – 01 |

**Supplies Needed:** Table

*This problem allows you the opportunity to demonstrate your ability to* **palpate** *the* **elbow**.
*You have 2 minutes to complete this task.*

| Palpation: Elbow – 01 | Course or Site Assessor Environment | Test 1 | | Test 2 | | Test 3 | |
|---|---|---|---|---|---|---|---|
| | | Y | N | Y | N | Y | N |
| Ulnar collateral ligament | | ○ | ○ | ○ | ○ | ○ | ○ |
| Radial head | | ○ | ○ | ○ | ○ | ○ | ○ |
| Brachialis muscle | | ○ | ○ | ○ | ○ | ○ | ○ |
| Medial epicondyle | | ○ | ○ | ○ | ○ | ○ | ○ |
| Cubital fossa | | ○ | ○ | ○ | ○ | ○ | ○ |
| Olecranon process | | ○ | ○ | ○ | ○ | ○ | ○ |
| Annular ligament | | ○ | ○ | ○ | ○ | ○ | ○ |
| | Total | ___/7 | | ___/7 | | ___/7 | |
| | Must achieve >4 to pass this examination | Ⓟ | Ⓕ | Ⓟ | Ⓕ | Ⓟ | Ⓕ |
| Assessor: Date: | Test 1 Comments: | | | | | | |
| Assessor: Date: | Test 2 Comments: | | | | | | |
| Assessor: Date: | Test 3 Comments: | | | | | | |

**TEST ENVIRONMENTS**
**L:** Laboratory/Classroom
**C:** Clinical/Field Testing
**P:** Practicum
**A:** Assessment/Mock Exam

**TEST INFORMATION**
**Test Statistics:** N/A
**Reference(s):** Starkey & Brown (2015)

## MUSCULOSKELETAL SYSTEM—REGION 8: ELBOW
## PALPATION

| NATA EC 5th | BOC RD6 | SKILL |
|---|---|---|
| CE-21b, CE-20c | D2-0202 | Palpation: Elbow – 02 |

**Supplies Needed:** Table

*This problem allows you the opportunity to demonstrate your ability to* **palpate** *the* **elbow**.
*You have 2 minutes to complete this task.*

| Palpation: Elbow – 02 | Course or Site / Assessor / Environment | Test 1 | | Test 2 | | Test 3 | |
|---|---|---|---|---|---|---|---|
| | | Y | N | Y | N | Y | N |
| Radial head | | ○ | ○ | ○ | ○ | ○ | ○ |
| Triceps brachii insertion | | ○ | ○ | ○ | ○ | ○ | ○ |
| Lateral epicondyle | | ○ | ○ | ○ | ○ | ○ | ○ |
| Olecranon fossa | | ○ | ○ | ○ | ○ | ○ | ○ |
| Radial collateral ligament | | ○ | ○ | ○ | ○ | ○ | ○ |
| Ulnar nerve | | ○ | ○ | ○ | ○ | ○ | ○ |
| Brachioradialis muscle | | ○ | ○ | ○ | ○ | ○ | ○ |
| Total | | __/7 | | __/7 | | __/7 | |
| Must achieve >4 to pass this examination | | Ⓟ | Ⓕ | Ⓟ | Ⓕ | Ⓟ | Ⓕ |

| Assessor:<br>Date: | Test 1 Comments: |
|---|---|
| Assessor:<br>Date: | Test 2 Comments: |
| Assessor:<br>Date: | Test 3 Comments: |

**TEST ENVIRONMENTS**
**L:** Laboratory/Classroom
**C:** Clinical/Field Testing
**P:** Practicum
**A:** Assessment/Mock Exam

**TEST INFORMATION**
**Test Statistics:** N/A
**Reference(s):** Starkey & Brown (2015)

# PALPATION

| NATA EC 5th | BOC RD6 | SKILL |
|---|---|---|
| CE-21b, CE-20c | D2-0202 | Palpation: Elbow – 03 |

**Supplies Needed:** Table

*This problem allows you the opportunity to demonstrate your ability to* **palpate** *the* **elbow**.
*You have 2 minutes to complete this task.*

| Palpation: Elbow – 03 | Course or Site Assessor Environment | Test 1 | | Test 2 | | Test 3 | |
|---|---|---|---|---|---|---|---|
| | | Y | N | Y | N | Y | N |
| Brachialis muscle | | ○ | ○ | ○ | ○ | ○ | ○ |
| Ulnar collateral ligament | | ○ | ○ | ○ | ○ | ○ | ○ |
| Radial head | | ○ | ○ | ○ | ○ | ○ | ○ |
| Ulnar nerve | | ○ | ○ | ○ | ○ | ○ | ○ |
| Olecranon fossa | | ○ | ○ | ○ | ○ | ○ | ○ |
| Radial collateral ligament | | ○ | ○ | ○ | ○ | ○ | ○ |
| Medial epicondyle | | ○ | ○ | ○ | ○ | ○ | ○ |
| Total | | ___/7 | | ___/7 | | ___/7 | |
| Must achieve >4 to pass this examination | | Ⓟ | Ⓕ | Ⓟ | Ⓕ | Ⓟ | Ⓕ |
| Assessor: Date: | Test 1 Comments: | | | | | | |
| Assessor: Date: | Test 2 Comments: | | | | | | |
| Assessor: Date: | Test 3 Comments: | | | | | | |

**TEST ENVIRONMENTS**
**L:** Laboratory/Classroom
**C:** Clinical/Field Testing
**P:** Practicum
**A:** Assessment/Mock Exam

**TEST INFORMATION**
**Test Statistics:** N/A
**Reference(s):** Starkey & Brown (2015)

# MANUAL MUSCLE TESTING

| NATA EC 5th | BOC RD6 | SKILL |
|---|---|---|
| CE-21c | D2-0203 | MMT: Anconeus |

**Supplies Needed:** Table

*This problem allows you the opportunity to demonstrate a* **manual muscle test** *for the* **anconeus.**
*You have 2 minutes to complete this task.*

| MMT: Anconeus | Course or Site Assessor Environment | | | | | |
|---|---|---|---|---|---|---|
| | | Test 1 | | Test 2 | | Test 3 |
| **Tester places patient and limb in appropriate position** | | Y | N | Y | N | Y | N |
| Supine, with shoulder in at least 90 degrees of abduction | | O | O | O | O | O | O |
| Elbow in 10 degrees of flexion to eliminate triceps brachii | | O | O | O | O | O | O |
| **Tester placed in proper position** | | Y | N | Y | N | Y | N |
| Places one hand around the biceps brachii belly to prevent excessive shoulder flexion | | O | O | O | O | O | O |
| **Tester performs test according to accepted guidelines** | | Y | N | Y | N | Y | N |
| Instructs the patient to actively extend elbow against pressure | | O | O | O | O | O | O |
| Applies resistance to the forearm into elbow flexion | | O | O | O | O | O | O |
| Holds resistance for 5 seconds | | O | O | O | O | O | O |
| Performs assessment bilaterally | | O | O | O | O | O | O |
| **Identifies implications** | | Y | N | Y | N | Y | N |
| Correctly grades the MMT | | O | O | O | O | O | O |
| Total | | ____/8 | | ____/8 | | ____/8 |
| Must achieve >5 to pass this examination | | Ⓟ | Ⓕ | Ⓟ | Ⓕ | Ⓟ | Ⓕ |

| Assessor: Date: | Test 1 Comments: |
|---|---|
| Assessor: Date: | Test 2 Comments: |
| Assessor: Date: | Test 3 Comments: |

**TEST ENVIRONMENTS**
**L:** Laboratory/Classroom
**C:** Clinical/Field Testing
**P:** Practicum
**A:** Assessment/Mock Exam

**TEST INFORMATION**
**Test Statistics:** No data available
**Reference(s):** Kendall et al. (2005)

## MUSCULOSKELETAL SYSTEM—REGION 8: ELBOW
# MANUAL MUSCLE TESTING

| NATA EC 5th | BOC RD6 | SKILL |
|---|---|---|
| CE-21c | D2-0203 | MMT: Biceps Brachii |

**Supplies Needed:** Table

*This problem allows you the opportunity to demonstrate a* **manual muscle test** *for the* **biceps brachii***. You have 2 minutes to complete this task.*

| MMT: Biceps Brachii | Course or Site Assessor Environment | | Test 1 | | Test 2 | | Test 3 | |
|---|---|---|---|---|---|---|---|---|
| **Tester places patient and limb in appropriate position** | | | **Y** | **N** | **Y** | **N** | **Y** | **N** |
| Supine or seated, with shoulder at side and elbow in slight flexion | | | ○ | ○ | ○ | ○ | ○ | ○ |
| Forearm in supination | | | ○ | ○ | ○ | ○ | ○ | ○ |
| **Tester placed in proper position** | | | **Y** | **N** | **Y** | **N** | **Y** | **N** |
| Places one hand under the elbow to cushion it from table pressure | | | ○ | ○ | ○ | ○ | ○ | ○ |
| **Tester performs test according to accepted guidelines** | | | **Y** | **N** | **Y** | **N** | **Y** | **N** |
| Instructs the patient to actively flex the elbow against resistance | | | ○ | ○ | ○ | ○ | ○ | ○ |
| Applies resistance against the lower forearm into extension | | | ○ | ○ | ○ | ○ | ○ | ○ |
| Holds resistance for 5 seconds | | | ○ | ○ | ○ | ○ | ○ | ○ |
| Performs assessment bilaterally | | | ○ | ○ | ○ | ○ | ○ | ○ |
| **Identifies implications** | | | **Y** | **N** | **Y** | **N** | **Y** | **N** |
| Correctly grades the MMT | | | ○ | ○ | ○ | ○ | ○ | ○ |
| **Total** | | | ___/8 | | ___/8 | | ___/8 | |
| **Must achieve >5 to pass this examination** | | | Ⓟ | Ⓕ | Ⓟ | Ⓕ | Ⓟ | Ⓕ |

| Assessor:<br>Date: | Test 1 Comments: |
|---|---|
| Assessor:<br>Date: | Test 2 Comments: |
| Assessor:<br>Date: | Test 3 Comments: |

**TEST ENVIRONMENTS**
**L:** Laboratory/Classroom
**C:** Clinical/Field Testing
**P:** Practicum
**A:** Assessment/Mock Exam

**TEST INFORMATION**
**Test Statistics:** No data available
**Reference(s):** Kendall et al. (2005)

# MANUAL MUSCLE TESTING

| NATA EC 5th | BOC RD6 | SKILL |
|---|---|---|
| CE-21c | D2-0203 | MMT: Brachialis |

**Supplies Needed:** Table

*This problem allows you the opportunity to demonstrate a* **manual muscle test** *for the* **brachialis**.
*You have 2 minutes to complete this task.*

| MMT: Brachialis | Course or Site Assessor Environment | Test 1 | | Test 2 | | Test 3 | |
|---|---|---|---|---|---|---|---|
| | | Y | N | Y | N | Y | N |
| **Tester places patient and limb in appropriate position** | | Y | N | Y | N | Y | N |
| Supine or seated, with shoulder at side and elbow in slight flexion | | O | O | O | O | O | O |
| Forearm in pronation | | O | O | O | O | O | O |
| **Tester placed in proper position** | | Y | N | Y | N | Y | N |
| Places one hand under the elbow to cushion it from table pressure | | O | O | O | O | O | O |
| **Tester performs test according to accepted guidelines** | | Y | N | Y | N | Y | N |
| Instructs the patient to actively flex the elbow against resistance | | O | O | O | O | O | O |
| Applies resistance against the lower forearm into extension | | O | O | O | O | O | O |
| Holds resistance for 5 seconds | | O | O | O | O | O | O |
| Performs assessment bilaterally | | O | O | O | O | O | O |
| **Identifies implications** | | Y | N | Y | N | Y | N |
| Correctly grades the MMT | | O | O | O | O | O | O |
| **Total** | | ___/8 | | ___/8 | | ___/8 | |
| **Must achieve >5 to pass this examination** | | Ⓟ | Ⓕ | Ⓟ | Ⓕ | Ⓟ | Ⓕ |

| Assessor: Date: | Test 1 Comments: |
|---|---|
| Assessor: Date: | Test 2 Comments: |
| Assessor: Date: | Test 3 Comments: |

**TEST ENVIRONMENTS**
**L:** Laboratory/Classroom
**C:** Clinical/Field Testing
**P:** Practicum
**A:** Assessment/Mock Exam

**TEST INFORMATION**
**Test Statistics:** No data available
**Reference(s):** Kendall et al. (2005)

MUSCULOSKELETAL SYSTEM—REGION 8: ELBOW
# MANUAL MUSCLE TESTING

| NATA EC 5th | BOC RD6 | SKILL |
|---|---|---|
| CE-21c | D2-0203 | MMT: Brachioradialis |

**Supplies Needed:** Table

*This problem allows you the opportunity to demonstrate a* **manual muscle test** *for the* **brachioradialis**. *You have 2 minutes to complete this task.*

| MMT: Brachioradialis | Course or Site Assessor Environment | | Test 1 | | Test 2 | | Test 3 |
|---|---|---|---|---|---|---|---|
| **Tester places patient and limb in appropriate position** | | Y | N | Y | N | Y | N |
| Supine or seated, with elbow in neutral position and slight flexion | | ○ | ○ | ○ | ○ | ○ | ○ |
| **Tester placed in proper position** | | Y | N | Y | N | Y | N |
| Places one hand under the elbow to cushion it from table pressure | | ○ | ○ | ○ | ○ | ○ | ○ |
| **Tester performs test according to accepted guidelines** | | Y | N | Y | N | Y | N |
| Instructs the patient to actively flex the elbow against resistance | | ○ | ○ | ○ | ○ | ○ | ○ |
| Applies resistance against the lower forearm into extension | | ○ | ○ | ○ | ○ | ○ | ○ |
| Holds resistance for 5 seconds | | ○ | ○ | ○ | ○ | ○ | ○ |
| Performs assessment bilaterally | | ○ | ○ | ○ | ○ | ○ | ○ |
| **Identifies implications** | | Y | N | Y | N | Y | N |
| Correctly grades the MMT | | ○ | ○ | ○ | ○ | ○ | ○ |
| Total | | __/7 | | __/7 | | __/7 | |
| **Must achieve >4 to pass this examination** | | Ⓟ | Ⓕ | Ⓟ | Ⓕ | Ⓟ | Ⓕ |

| Assessor: Date: | Test 1 Comments: |
|---|---|
| Assessor: Date: | Test 2 Comments: |
| Assessor: Date: | Test 3 Comments: |

**TEST ENVIRONMENTS**
L: Laboratory/Classroom
C: Clinical/Field Testing
P: Practicum
A: Assessment/Mock Exam

**TEST INFORMATION**
**Test Statistics:** No data available
**Reference(s):** Kendall et al. (2005)

**MUSCULOSKELETAL SYSTEM—REGION 8: ELBOW**
# MANUAL MUSCLE TESTING

| NATA EC 5th | BOC RD6 | SKILL |
|---|---|---|
| CE-21c | D2-0203 | MMT: Pronator Quadratus |

**Supplies Needed:** Table

*This problem allows you the opportunity to demonstrate a* **manual muscle test** *for the* **pronator quadratus.**
*You have 2 minutes to complete this task.*

| MMT: Pronator Quadratus | Course or Site<br>Assessor<br>Environment | | Test 1 | | Test 2 | | Test 3 |
|---|---|---|---|---|---|---|---|
| | | Y | N | Y | N | Y | N |
| **Tester places patient and limb in appropriate position** | | Y | N | Y | N | Y | N |
| Supine or seated, with elbow held against the patient's side, and flexed to its end range | | ○ | ○ | ○ | ○ | ○ | ○ |
| **Tester placed in proper position** | | Y | N | Y | N | Y | N |
| Stabilizes the elbow against the body | | ○ | ○ | ○ | ○ | ○ | ○ |
| **Tester performs test according to accepted guidelines** | | Y | N | Y | N | Y | N |
| Instructs the patient to actively pronate the elbow against resistance | | ○ | ○ | ○ | ○ | ○ | ○ |
| Applies resistance above the wrist into supination | | ○ | ○ | ○ | ○ | ○ | ○ |
| Holds resistance for 5 seconds | | ○ | ○ | ○ | ○ | ○ | ○ |
| Performs assessment bilaterally | | ○ | ○ | ○ | ○ | ○ | ○ |
| **Identifies implications** | | Y | N | Y | N | Y | N |
| Correctly grades the MMT | | ○ | ○ | ○ | ○ | ○ | ○ |
| Total | | __/7 | | __/7 | | __/7 | |
| Must achieve >4 to pass this examination | | Ⓟ | Ⓕ | Ⓟ | Ⓕ | Ⓟ | Ⓕ |

| Assessor:<br>Date: | Test 1 Comments: |
|---|---|
| Assessor:<br>Date: | Test 2 Comments: |
| Assessor:<br>Date: | Test 3 Comments: |

**TEST ENVIRONMENTS**
**L:** Laboratory/Classroom
**C:** Clinical/Field Testing
**P:** Practicum
**A:** Assessment/Mock Exam

**TEST INFORMATION**
**Test Statistics:** No data available
**Reference(s):** Kendall et al. (2005)

## MUSCULOSKELETAL SYSTEM—REGION 8: ELBOW
# MANUAL MUSCLE TESTING

| NATA EC 5th | BOC RD6 | SKILL |
|---|---|---|
| CE-21c | D2-0203 | MMT: Supinator |

**Supplies Needed:** Table

*This problem allows you the opportunity to demonstrate a* **manual muscle test** *for the* **supinator**.
*You have 2 minutes to complete this task.*

| MMT: Supinator | Course or Site<br>Assessor<br>Environment | | | | | | |
|---|---|---|---|---|---|---|---|
| | | Test 1 | | Test 2 | | Test 3 | |
| **Tester places patient and limb in appropriate position** | | **Y** | **N** | **Y** | **N** | **Y** | **N** |
| Supine, with shoulder flexed to 90 degrees and elbow flexed to its end range | | ○ | ○ | ○ | ○ | ○ | ○ |
| **Tester placed in proper position** | | **Y** | **N** | **Y** | **N** | **Y** | **N** |
| Places one hand under the elbow to cushion it from table pressure | | ○ | ○ | ○ | ○ | ○ | ○ |
| **Tester performs test according to accepted guidelines** | | **Y** | **N** | **Y** | **N** | **Y** | **N** |
| Instructs the patient to actively supinate the forearm against resistance | | ○ | ○ | ○ | ○ | ○ | ○ |
| Applies resistance against the lower forearm into extension | | ○ | ○ | ○ | ○ | ○ | ○ |
| Holds resistance for 5 seconds | | ○ | ○ | ○ | ○ | ○ | ○ |
| Performs assessment bilaterally | | ○ | ○ | ○ | ○ | ○ | ○ |
| **Identifies implications** | | **Y** | **N** | **Y** | **N** | **Y** | **N** |
| Correctly grades the MMT | | ○ | ○ | ○ | ○ | ○ | ○ |
| **Total** | | ___/7 | | ___/7 | | ___/7 | |
| **Must achieve >4 to pass this examination** | | Ⓟ | Ⓕ | Ⓟ | Ⓕ | Ⓟ | Ⓕ |

| Assessor:<br>Date: | Test 1 Comments: |
|---|---|
| Assessor:<br>Date: | Test 2 Comments: |
| Assessor:<br>Date: | Test 3 Comments: |

**TEST ENVIRONMENTS**
**L:** Laboratory/Classroom
**C:** Clinical/Field Testing
**P:** Practicum
**A:** Assessment/Mock Exam

**TEST INFORMATION**
**Test Statistics:** No data available
**Reference(s):**   Kendall et al. (2005)

MUSCULOSKELETAL SYSTEM—REGION 8: ELBOW
# MANUAL MUSCLE TESTING

| NATA EC 5th | BOC RD6 | SKILL |
|---|---|---|
| CE-21c | D2-0203 | MMT: Triceps Brachii |

**Supplies Needed:** Table

*This problem allows you the opportunity to demonstrate a* **manual muscle test** *for the* **triceps brachii**. *You have 2 minutes to complete this task.*

| MMT: Triceps Brachii | Course or Site Assessor Environment | | Test 1 | | Test 2 | | Test 3 | |
|---|---|---|---|---|---|---|---|---|
| **Tester places patient and limb in appropriate position** | | Y | N | Y | N | Y | N |
| Prone, with shoulder abducted to 90 degrees | | O | O | O | O | O | O |
| **Tester placed in proper position** | | Y | N | Y | N | Y | N |
| Places one hand under the arm near the elbow to cushion against table pressure | | O | O | O | O | O | O |
| **Tester performs test according to accepted guidelines** | | Y | N | Y | N | Y | N |
| Instructs the patient to actively extend the elbow | | O | O | O | O | O | O |
| Applies resistance against the forearm into flexion | | O | O | O | O | O | O |
| Holds resistance for 5 seconds | | O | O | O | O | O | O |
| Performs assessment bilaterally | | O | O | O | O | O | O |
| **Identifies implications** | | Y | N | Y | N | Y | N |
| Correctly grades the MMT | | O | O | O | O | O | O |
| **Total** | | ___/7 | | ___/7 | | ___/7 | |
| **Must achieve >4 to pass this examination** | | ⓟ | Ⓕ | ⓟ | Ⓕ | ⓟ | Ⓕ |

| Assessor: Date: | Test 1 Comments: |
|---|---|
| Assessor: Date: | Test 2 Comments: |
| Assessor: Date: | Test 3 Comments: |

**TEST ENVIRONMENTS**
**L:** Laboratory/Classroom
**C:** Clinical/Field Testing
**P:** Practicum
**A:** Assessment/Mock Exam

**TEST INFORMATION**
**Test Statistics:** No data available
**Reference(s):** Kendall et al. (2005)

**MUSCULOSKELETAL SYSTEM—REGION 8: ELBOW**
# OSTEOKINEMATIC JOINT MOTION

| NATA EC 5th | BOC RD6 | SKILL |
|---|---|---|
| CE-21d | D2-0203 | Goniometric Assessment: Humeroulnar Joint (Flexion) |

**Supplies Needed:** Table, large goniometer, pad or towel

*This problem allows you the opportunity to demonstrate a* **goniometric assessment** *for the* **humeroulnar joint (flexion)**. *You have 2 minutes to complete this task.*

| Goniometric Assessment: Humeroulnar Joint (Flexion) | Course or Site _____ Assessor _____ Environment _____ | | | | | |
|---|---|---|---|---|---|---|
| | | Test 1 | | Test 2 | | Test 3 |
| **Tester places patient and limb in appropriate position** | | Y | N | Y | N | Y | N |
| Supine, with the shoulder in neutral position, close to the body | | O | O | O | O | O | O |
| Places a pad or towel roll under the distal humerus to allow full elbow extension | | O | O | O | O | O | O |
| **Tester and goniometer placed in proper position** | | Y | N | Y | N | Y | N |
| Stabilizes the humerus to prevent flexion of the shoulder | | O | O | O | O | O | O |
| Places fulcrum over the lateral epicondyle of the humerus | | O | O | O | O | O | O |
| Aligns fixed arm with the lateral midline of the humerus, in line with the acromion process | | O | O | O | O | O | O |
| Aligns moving arm with the radius, using the radial head and radial styloid process for reference | | O | O | O | O | O | O |
| **Tester performs test according to accepted guidelines** | | Y | N | Y | N | Y | N |
| Passively flexes the elbow to its end feel | | O | O | O | O | O | O |
| Forearm is maintained in supination through the full range | | O | O | O | O | O | O |
| Records correct goniometric measurement | | O | O | O | O | O | O |
| Performs bilateral assessment | | O | O | O | O | O | O |
| **Identifies implications** | | Y | N | Y | N | Y | N |
| Identifies normal ranges (flexion = 140 to 150 degrees) | | O | O | O | O | O | O |
| Total | | ___/11 | | ___/11 | | ___/11 | |
| Must achieve >7 to pass this examination | | P | F | P | F | P | F |
| Assessor: Date: | Test 1 Comments: | | | | | |
| Assessor: Date: | Test 2 Comments: | | | | | |
| Assessor: Date: | Test 3 Comments: | | | | | |

**TEST ENVIRONMENTS**
L: Laboratory/Classroom
C: Clinical/Field Testing
P: Practicum
A: Assessment/Mock Exam

**TEST INFORMATION**
**Test Statistics:** N/A
**Reference(s):** Norkin & White (2009)

**MUSCULOSKELETAL SYSTEM—REGION 8: ELBOW**
# OSTEOKINEMATIC JOINT MOTION

| NATA EC 5th | BOC RD6 | SKILL |
|---|---|---|
| CE-21d | D2-0203 | Goniometric Assessment: Humeroulnar Joint (Extension) |

**Supplies Needed:** Table, large goniometer, pad or towel

*This problem allows you the opportunity to demonstrate a* **goniometric assessment** *for the* **humeroulnar joint (extension)***. You have 2 minutes to complete this task.*

| Goniometric Assessment: Humeroulnar Joint (Extension) | Course or Site Assessor Environment | | Test 1 | | Test 2 | | Test 3 |
|---|---|---|---|---|---|---|---|
| | | Y | N | Y | N | Y | N |
| **Tester places patient and limb in appropriate position** | | Y | N | Y | N | Y | N |
| Supine, with the shoulder in neutral position, close to the body | | O | O | O | O | O | O |
| Places a pad or towel roll under the distal humerus to allow full elbow extension | | O | O | O | O | O | O |
| **Tester and goniometer placed in proper position** | | Y | N | Y | N | Y | N |
| Stabilizes the humerus to prevent flexion of the shoulder | | O | O | O | O | O | O |
| Places fulcrum over the lateral epicondyle of the humerus | | O | O | O | O | O | O |
| Aligns fixed arm with the lateral midline of the humerus, in line with the acromion process | | O | O | O | O | O | O |
| Aligns moving arm with the radius, using the radial head and radial styloid process for reference | | O | O | O | O | O | O |
| **Tester performs test according to accepted guidelines** | | Y | N | Y | N | Y | N |
| Passively extends the elbow to its end feel | | O | O | O | O | O | O |
| Forearm is maintained in supination through the full range | | O | O | O | O | O | O |
| Records correct goniometric measurement | | O | O | O | O | O | O |
| Performs bilateral assessment | | O | O | O | O | O | O |
| **Identifies implications** | | Y | N | Y | N | Y | N |
| Identifies normal ranges (extension = 0) | | O | O | O | O | O | O |
| Total | | __/11 | | __/11 | | __/11 | |
| Must achieve >7 to pass this examination | | P | F | P | F | P | F |

| Assessor: Date: | Test 1 Comments: |
|---|---|
| Assessor: Date: | Test 2 Comments: |
| Assessor: Date: | Test 3 Comments: |

**TEST ENVIRONMENTS**
**L:** Laboratory/Classroom
**C:** Clinical/Field Testing
**P:** Practicum
**A:** Assessment/Mock Exam

**TEST INFORMATION**
**Test Statistics:** N/A
**Reference(s):** Norkin & White (2009)

MUSCULOSKELETAL SYSTEM—REGION 8: ELBOW
# OSTEOKINEMATIC JOINT MOTION

| NATA EC 5th | BOC RD6 | SKILL |
|---|---|---|
| CE-21d | D2-0203 | Goniometric Assessment: Radioulnar Joint (Pronation) |

**Supplies Needed:** Table, small goniometer

*This problem allows you the opportunity to demonstrate a **goniometric assessment** for the **radioulnar joint (pronation)**. You have 2 minutes to complete this task.*

| Goniometric Assessment: Radioulnar Joint (Pronation) | Course or Site Assessor Environment | | Test 1 | | Test 2 | | Test 3 | |
|---|---|---|---|---|---|---|---|---|
| **Tester places patient and limb in appropriate position** | | Y | N | Y | N | Y | N | |
| Seated with the shoulder in neutral position, elbow flexed to 90 degrees | | O | O | O | O | O | O | |
| The tester positions the patient's forearm midway between supination and pronation so the thumb is pointed to the ceiling | | O | O | O | O | O | O | |
| **Tester and goniometer placed in proper position** | | Y | N | Y | N | Y | N | |
| Stabilizes the distal humerus to prevent medial rotation and abduction of the shoulder | | O | O | O | O | O | O | |
| Places fulcrum lateral and proximal to the ulnar styloid process | | O | O | O | O | O | O | |
| Aligns fixed arm with the anterior midline of the humerus | | O | O | O | O | O | O | |
| Places moving arm across dorsal aspect of the forearm, just proximal to the ulnar and radial styloid processes | | O | O | O | O | O | O | |
| **Tester performs test according to accepted guidelines** | | Y | N | Y | N | Y | N | |
| Pronates the forearm by moving the distal radius volarly | | O | O | O | O | O | O | |
| Records correct goniometric measurement | | O | O | O | O | O | O | |
| Performs bilateral assessment | | O | O | O | O | O | O | |
| **Identifies implications** | | Y | N | Y | N | Y | N | |
| Identifies normal ranges (pronation = 75 to 85 degrees) | | O | O | O | O | O | O | |
| Total | | /10 | | /10 | | /10 | | |
| Must achieve >6 to pass this examination | | P | F | P | F | P | F | |

| Assessor: Date: | Test 1 Comments: |
|---|---|
| Assessor: Date: | Test 2 Comments: |
| Assessor: Date: | Test 3 Comments: |

**TEST ENVIRONMENTS**
L: Laboratory/Classroom
C: Clinical/Field Testing
P: Practicum
A: Assessment/Mock Exam

**TEST INFORMATION**
**Test Statistics:** N/A
**Reference(s):** Norkin & White (2009)

## MUSCULOSKELETAL SYSTEM—REGION 8: ELBOW
# OSTEOKINEMATIC JOINT MOTION

| NATA EC 5th | BOC RD6 | SKILL |
|---|---|---|
| CE-21d | D2-0203 | Goniometric Assessment: Radioulnar Joint (Supination) |

**Supplies Needed:** Table, small goniometer

*This problem allows you the opportunity to demonstrate a* **goniometric assessment** *for the* **radioulnar joint (supination)**. *You have 2 minutes to complete this task.*

| Goniometric Assessment: Radioulnar Joint (Supination) | Course or Site Assessor Environment | | Test 1 | | Test 2 | | Test 3 | |
|---|---|---|---|---|---|---|---|---|
| **Tester places patient and limb in appropriate position** | | **Y** | **N** | **Y** | **N** | **Y** | **N** | |
| Seated with the shoulder in neutral position, elbow flexed to 90 degrees | | ○ | ○ | ○ | ○ | ○ | ○ | |
| Positions the patient's forearm midway between supination and pronation so the thumb is pointed to the ceiling | | ○ | ○ | ○ | ○ | ○ | ○ | |
| **Tester and goniometer placed in proper position** | | **Y** | **N** | **Y** | **N** | **Y** | **N** | |
| Stabilizes the distal humerus to prevent lateral rotation and adduction of the shoulder | | ○ | ○ | ○ | ○ | ○ | ○ | |
| Places fulcrum medial and proximal to the ulnar styloid process | | ○ | ○ | ○ | ○ | ○ | ○ | |
| Aligns fixed arm with the anterior midline of the humerus | | ○ | ○ | ○ | ○ | ○ | ○ | |
| Places moving arm across ventral aspect of the forearm, just proximal to the ulnar and radial styloid processes | | ○ | ○ | ○ | ○ | ○ | ○ | |
| **Tester performs test according to accepted guidelines** | | **Y** | **N** | **Y** | **N** | **Y** | **N** | |
| Supinates the forearm by moving the distal radius volarly | | ○ | ○ | ○ | ○ | ○ | ○ | |
| Records correct goniometric measurement | | ○ | ○ | ○ | ○ | ○ | ○ | |
| Performs bilateral assessment | | ○ | ○ | ○ | ○ | ○ | ○ | |
| **Identifies implications** | | **Y** | **N** | **Y** | **N** | **Y** | **N** | |
| Identifies normal ranges (supination = 80 to 90 degrees) | | ○ | ○ | ○ | ○ | ○ | ○ | |
| **Total** | | \_\_\_\_/10 | | \_\_\_\_/10 | | \_\_\_\_/10 | | |
| **Must achieve >6 to pass this examination** | | Ⓟ | Ⓕ | Ⓟ | Ⓕ | Ⓟ | Ⓕ | |

| Assessor: Date: | Test 1 Comments: |
|---|---|
| Assessor: Date: | Test 2 Comments: |
| Assessor: Date: | Test 3 Comments: |

**TEST ENVIRONMENTS**
**L:** Laboratory/Classroom
**C:** Clinical/Field Testing
**P:** Practicum
**A:** Assessment/Mock Exam

**TEST INFORMATION**
**Test Statistics:** N/A
**Reference(s):** Norkin & White (2009)

# CAPSULAR AND LIGAMENTOUS STRESS TESTING

| NATA EC 5th | BOC RD6 | SKILL |
|---|---|---|
| CE-21e | D2-0203 | Valgus Stress Test for the Elbow |

**Supplies Needed:** Table

*This problem allows you the opportunity to demonstrate an* **orthopedic test** *known as the* **valgus stress test for the elbow.** *You have 2 minutes to complete this task.*

| Valgus Stress Test for the Elbow | Course or Site Assessor Environment | | Test 1 | | Test 2 | | Test 3 |
|---|---|---|---|---|---|---|---|
| | | **Y** | **N** | **Y** | **N** | **Y** | **N** |
| **Tester places patient and limb in appropriate position** | | **Y** | **N** | **Y** | **N** | **Y** | **N** |
| Standing, seated, or supine | | ○ | ○ | ○ | ○ | ○ | ○ |
| Elbow flexed to 10 to 25 degrees and humerus internally rotated | | ○ | ○ | ○ | ○ | ○ | ○ |
| **Tester placed in proper position** | | **Y** | **N** | **Y** | **N** | **Y** | **N** |
| Stands lateral to the joint being tested | | ○ | ○ | ○ | ○ | ○ | ○ |
| One hand supports lateral elbow while palpating the medial joint | | ○ | ○ | ○ | ○ | ○ | ○ |
| Opposite hand grasps distal forearm | | ○ | ○ | ○ | ○ | ○ | ○ |
| **Tester performs test according to accepted guidelines** | | **Y** | **N** | **Y** | **N** | **Y** | **N** |
| Applies a valgus force to the joint | | ○ | ○ | ○ | ○ | ○ | ○ |
| Procedure is repeated in 0 and 20 degrees of elbow flexion | | ○ | ○ | ○ | ○ | ○ | ○ |
| **Identifies positive findings and implications** | | **Y** | **N** | **Y** | **N** | **Y** | **N** |
| Increased laxity or pain compared to the opposite side | | ○ | ○ | ○ | ○ | ○ | ○ |
| Sprain of the ulnar collateral ligament | | ○ | ○ | ○ | ○ | ○ | ○ |
| Total | | ___/9 | | ___/9 | | ___/9 | |
| Must achieve >6 to pass this examination | | Ⓟ | Ⓕ | Ⓟ | Ⓕ | Ⓟ | Ⓕ |

| Assessor: Date: | Test 1 Comments: |
|---|---|
| Assessor: Date: | Test 2 Comments: |
| Assessor: Date: | Test 3 Comments: |

**TEST ENVIRONMENTS**
L: Laboratory/Classroom
C: Clinical/Field Testing
P: Practicum
A: Assessment/Mock Exam

**TEST INFORMATION**
**Test Statistics:** No data available
**Reference(s):** Starkey & Brown (2015)

## MUSCULOSKELETAL SYSTEM—REGION 8: ELBOW
# CAPSULAR AND LIGAMENTOUS STRESS TESTING

| NATA EC 5th | BOC RD6 | SKILL |
|---|---|---|
| CE-21e | D2-0203 | Varus Stress Test for the Elbow |

**Supplies Needed:** Table

*This problem allows you the opportunity to demonstrate an* **orthopedic test** *known as the* **varus stress test for the elbow.** *You have 2 minutes to complete this task.*

| Varus Stress Test for the Elbow | Course or Site Assessor Environment | | Test 1 | | Test 2 | | Test 3 | |
|---|---|---|---|---|---|---|---|---|
| | | **Y** | **N** | **Y** | **N** | **Y** | **N** |
| **Tester places patient and limb in appropriate position** | | Y | N | Y | N | Y | N |
| Standing, seated, or supine | | ○ | ○ | ○ | ○ | ○ | ○ |
| Elbow flexed to 25 degrees and humerus in neutral position | | ○ | ○ | ○ | ○ | ○ | ○ |
| **Tester placed in proper position** | | Y | N | Y | N | Y | N |
| Stands medial to the joint being tested | | ○ | ○ | ○ | ○ | ○ | ○ |
| One hand supports medial elbow, while palpating the lateral joint | | ○ | ○ | ○ | ○ | ○ | ○ |
| Opposite hand grasps distal forearm | | ○ | ○ | ○ | ○ | ○ | ○ |
| **Tester performs test according to accepted guidelines** | | Y | N | Y | N | Y | N |
| Applies a varus force to the joint | | ○ | ○ | ○ | ○ | ○ | ○ |
| The procedure is repeated in 0 and 20 degrees of elbow flexion | | ○ | ○ | ○ | ○ | ○ | ○ |
| **Identifies positive findings and implications** | | Y | N | Y | N | Y | N |
| Increased laxity or pain compared to the opposite side | | ○ | ○ | ○ | ○ | ○ | ○ |
| Sprain of the radial collateral ligament, annular, or accessory LCL | | ○ | ○ | ○ | ○ | ○ | ○ |
| **Total** | | /9 | | /9 | | /9 | |
| **Must achieve >6 to pass this examination** | | Ⓟ | Ⓕ | Ⓟ | Ⓕ | Ⓟ | Ⓕ |

| Assessor: Date: | Test 1 Comments: |
|---|---|
| Assessor: Date: | Test 2 Comments: |
| Assessor: Date: | Test 3 Comments: |

**TEST ENVIRONMENTS**
**L:** Laboratory/Classroom
**C:** Clinical/Field Testing
**P:** Practicum
**A:** Assessment/Mock Exam

**TEST INFORMATION**
**Test Statistics:** No data available
**Reference(s):** Starkey & Brown (2015)

# CAPSULAR AND LIGAMENTOUS STRESS TESTING

| NATA EC 5th | BOC RD6 | SKILL |
|---|---|---|
| CE-21e | D2-0203 | Moving Valgus Stress Test for the Elbow |

**Supplies Needed:** Table

*This problem allows you the opportunity to demonstrate an* **orthopedic test** *known as the* **moving valgus stress test for the elbow**. *You have 2 minutes to complete this task.*

| Moving Valgus Stress Test for the Elbow | Course or Site Assessor Environment | | Test 1 | | Test 2 | | Test 3 |
|---|---|---|---|---|---|---|---|
| **Tester places patient and limb in appropriate position** | | **Y** | **N** | **Y** | **N** | **Y** | **N** |
| Seated | | ○ | ○ | ○ | ○ | ○ | ○ |
| Shoulder abducted to 90 degrees and elbow flexed to its end range of motion | | ○ | ○ | ○ | ○ | ○ | ○ |
| **Tester placed in proper position** | | **Y** | **N** | **Y** | **N** | **Y** | **N** |
| Stands medial to the joint being tested | | ○ | ○ | ○ | ○ | ○ | ○ |
| One hand supports medial elbow, while palpating the lateral joint | | ○ | ○ | ○ | ○ | ○ | ○ |
| Opposite hand grasps distal forearm | | ○ | ○ | ○ | ○ | ○ | ○ |
| **Tester performs test according to accepted guidelines** | | **Y** | **N** | **Y** | **N** | **Y** | **N** |
| Applies valgus force on elbow while externally rotating humerus | | ○ | ○ | ○ | ○ | ○ | ○ |
| Extends elbow to approximately 30 degrees while maintaining valgus force | | ○ | ○ | ○ | ○ | ○ | ○ |
| Moves elbow into flexion while maintaining a valgus stress on the joint | | ○ | ○ | ○ | ○ | ○ | ○ |
| **Identifies positive findings and implications** | | **Y** | **N** | **Y** | **N** | **Y** | **N** |
| Pain at medial elbow sometimes accompanied by apprehension | | ○ | ○ | ○ | ○ | ○ | ○ |
| Pain that occurs between 120 and 70 degrees | | ○ | ○ | ○ | ○ | ○ | ○ |
| **Total** | | ___/10 | | ___/10 | | ___/10 | |
| **Must achieve >6 to pass this examination** | | Ⓟ | Ⓕ | Ⓟ | Ⓕ | Ⓟ | Ⓕ |

| **Assessor:** **Date:** | **Test 1 Comments:** |
|---|---|
| **Assessor:** **Date:** | **Test 2 Comments:** |
| **Assessor:** **Date:** | **Test 3 Comments:** |

**TEST ENVIRONMENTS**
**L:** Laboratory/Classroom
**C:** Clinical/Field Testing
**P:** Practicum
**A:** Assessment/Mock Exam

**TEST INFORMATION**
**Test Statistics:** Sensitivity 1
Specificity .75
**Reference(s):** Cook & Hegedus (2013)
Starkey & Brown (2015)

**MUSCULOSKELETAL SYSTEM—REGION 8: ELBOW**
# SPECIAL TESTS

| NATA EC 5th | BOC RD6 | SKILL |
|---|---|---|
| CE-21g, CE-20e | D2-0203 | Cozen's Sign (Active Lateral Epicondyle Test) |

**Supplies Needed:** Table

*This problem allows you the opportunity to demonstrate an* **orthopedic test** *known as* **Cozen's sign (active lateral epicondyle test)** *to rule out a* **lateral epicondylitis.** *You have 2 minutes to complete this task.*

| Cozen's Sign (Active Lateral Epicondyle Test) | Course or Site Assessor Environment | | | | | |
|---|---|---|---|---|---|---|
| | | Test 1 | | Test 2 | | Test 3 |
| **Tester places patient and limb in appropriate position** | | Y | N | Y | N | Y | N |
| Seated | | O | O | O | O | O | O |
| Arms and shoulders in anatomical position | | O | O | O | O | O | O |
| **Tester placed in proper position** | | Y | N | Y | N | Y | N |
| Stands on the side being tested | | O | O | O | O | O | O |
| Holds the patient's arm at the distal radiocarpal joint in 90 degrees of elbow flexion | | O | O | O | O | O | O |
| **Tester performs test according to accepted guidelines** | | Y | N | Y | N | Y | N |
| Palpates the lateral epicondyle with his/her thumb | | O | O | O | O | O | O |
| Applies manual resistance against wrist extension | | O | O | O | O | O | O |
| **Identifies positive findings and implications** | | Y | N | Y | N | Y | N |
| Reproduction of pain in lateral epicondyle | | O | O | O | O | O | O |
| | Total | __/7 | | __/7 | | __/7 |
| | Must achieve >4 to pass this examination | Ⓟ | Ⓕ | Ⓟ | Ⓕ | Ⓟ | Ⓕ |

| Assessor:<br>Date: | Test 1 Comments: |
|---|---|
| Assessor:<br>Date: | Test 2 Comments: |
| Assessor:<br>Date: | Test 3 Comments: |

**TEST ENVIRONMENTS**
**L:** Laboratory/Classroom
**C:** Clinical/Field Testing
**P:** Practicum
**A:** Assessment/Mock Exam

**TEST INFORMATION**
**Test Statistics:** No data available
**Reference(s):** Cook & Hegedus (2013)

## MUSCULOSKELETAL SYSTEM—REGION 8: ELBOW
# SPECIAL TESTS

| NATA EC 5th | BOC RD6 | SKILL |
|---|---|---|
| CE-21g, CE-20e | D2-0203 | Elbow Flexion Test |

**Supplies Needed:** Table

*This problem allows you the opportunity to demonstrate an* **orthopedic test** *known as the* **elbow flexion test** *to rule out* **ulnar nerve entrapment.** *You have 2 minutes to complete this task.*

| Elbow Flexion Test | Course or Site Assessor Environment | | Test 1 | | Test 2 | | Test 3 | |
|---|---|---|:---:|:---:|:---:|:---:|:---:|:---:|
| | | | Y | N | Y | N | Y | N |
| **Tester places patient and limb in appropriate position** | | | Y | N | Y | N | Y | N |
| Seated | | | ○ | ○ | ○ | ○ | ○ | ○ |
| Arms and shoulders in anatomical position | | | ○ | ○ | ○ | ○ | ○ | ○ |
| **Tester placed in proper position** | | | Y | N | Y | N | Y | N |
| Stands in front of the patient | | | ○ | ○ | ○ | ○ | ○ | ○ |
| **Tester performs test according to accepted guidelines** | | | Y | N | Y | N | Y | N |
| Instructs the patient to fully flex the elbows and fully extend the wrists | | | ○ | ○ | ○ | ○ | ○ | ○ |
| Instructs the patient to hold position for 3 minutes | | | ○ | ○ | ○ | ○ | ○ | ○ |
| **Identifies positive findings and implications** | | | Y | N | Y | N | Y | N |
| Reproduction of pain, tingling, or numbness along the ulnar nerve distribution | | | ○ | ○ | ○ | ○ | ○ | ○ |
| Total | | | ___/6 | | ___/6 | | ___/6 | |
| Must achieve >4 to pass this examination | | | Ⓟ | Ⓕ | Ⓟ | Ⓕ | Ⓟ | Ⓕ |
| **Assessor:** **Date:** | **Test 1 Comments:** | | | | | | | |
| **Assessor:** **Date:** | **Test 2 Comments:** | | | | | | | |
| **Assessor:** **Date:** | **Test 3 Comments:** | | | | | | | |

**TEST ENVIRONMENTS**
**L:** Laboratory/Classroom
**C:** Clinical/Field Testing
**P:** Practicum
**A:** Assessment/Mock Exam

**TEST INFORMATION**
**Test Statistics:** Specificity .13
**Reference(s):** Cook & Hegedus (2013)

| NATA EC 5th | BOC RD6 | SKILL |
|---|---|---|
| CE-21g, CE-20e | D2-0203 | Passive Tennis Elbow Test |

**Supplies Needed:** Table

*This problem allows you the opportunity to demonstrate an* **orthopedic test** *known as the* **passive tennis elbow test** *to rule out a* **lateral epicondylitis**. *You have 2 minutes to complete this task.*

| Passive Tennis Elbow Test | Course or Site Assessor Environment | | Test 1 | | Test 2 | | Test 3 | |
|---|---|---|---|---|---|---|---|---|
| | | | Y | N | Y | N | Y | N |
| **Tester places patient and limb in appropriate position** | | | Y | N | Y | N | Y | N |
| Seated | | | ○ | ○ | ○ | ○ | ○ | ○ |
| Arms and shoulders in anatomical position | | | ○ | ○ | ○ | ○ | ○ | ○ |
| **Tester placed in proper position** | | | Y | N | Y | N | Y | N |
| Stands on the side being tested | | | ○ | ○ | ○ | ○ | ○ | ○ |
| Holds the patient's arm at the distal radiocarpal joint in 90 degrees of elbow flexion | | | ○ | ○ | ○ | ○ | ○ | ○ |
| **Tester performs test according to accepted guidelines** | | | Y | N | Y | N | Y | N |
| Palpates the lateral epicondyle with his/her thumb | | | ○ | ○ | ○ | ○ | ○ | ○ |
| Passively pronates the forearm and flexes the wrist to end range | | | ○ | ○ | ○ | ○ | ○ | ○ |
| **Identifies positive findings and implications** | | | Y | N | Y | N | Y | N |
| Reproduction of pain in lateral epicondyle | | | ○ | ○ | ○ | ○ | ○ | ○ |
| | | Total | ___/7 | | ___/7 | | ___/7 | |
| | Must achieve >4 to pass this examination | | Ⓟ | Ⓕ | Ⓟ | Ⓕ | Ⓟ | Ⓕ |

| Assessor: Date: | Test 1 Comments: |
|---|---|
| Assessor: Date: | Test 2 Comments: |
| Assessor: Date: | Test 3 Comments: |

**TEST ENVIRONMENTS**
**L:** Laboratory/Classroom
**C:** Clinical/Field Testing
**P:** Practicum
**A:** Assessment/Mock Exam

**TEST INFORMATION**
**Test Statistics:** No data available
**Reference(s):** Cook & Hegedus (2013)

## MUSCULOSKELETAL SYSTEM—REGION 8: ELBOW
# SPECIAL TESTS

| NATA EC 5th | BOC RD6 | SKILL |
|---|---|---|
| CE-21g, CE-20e | D2-0203 | Tinel's Sign |

**Supplies Needed:** Table

*This problem allows you the opportunity to demonstrate an* **orthopedic test** *known as* **Tinel's sign** *to rule out* **ulnar nerve entrapment.** *You have 2 minutes to complete this task.*

| Tinel's Sign | Course or Site Assessor Environment | | Test 1 | | Test 2 | | Test 3 | |
|---|---|---|---|---|---|---|---|---|
| **Tester places patient and limb in appropriate position** | | | Y | N | Y | N | Y | N |
| Seated | | | O | O | O | O | O | O |
| Arms and shoulders in anatomical position | | | O | O | O | O | O | O |
| **Tester placed in proper position** | | | Y | N | Y | N | Y | N |
| Stands in front of the patient | | | O | O | O | O | O | O |
| Cradles the patient's arm with 40 degrees of elbow flexion | | | O | O | O | O | O | O |
| **Tester performs test according to accepted guidelines** | | | Y | N | Y | N | Y | N |
| Firmly taps over area of cubital tunnel with two fingers | | | O | O | O | O | O | O |
| **Identifies positive findings and implications** | | | Y | N | Y | N | Y | N |
| Reproduction of tingling sensation | | | O | O | O | O | O | O |
| Total | | | __/6 | | __/6 | | __/6 | |
| Must achieve >4 to pass this examination | | | P | F | P | F | P | F |

| Assessor: Date: | Test 1 Comments: |
|---|---|
| Assessor: Date: | Test 2 Comments: |
| Assessor: Date: | Test 3 Comments: |

### TEST ENVIRONMENTS
**L:** Laboratory/Classroom
**C:** Clinical/Field Testing
**P:** Practicum
**A:** Assessment/Mock Exam

### TEST INFORMATION
**Test Statistics:** Sensitivity .54–.7
Specificity .24–.99
(+) LR 35–54
(-) LR .46–.31
**Reference(s):** Cook & Hegedus (2013)

# 12

# MUSCULOSKELETAL SYSTEM— REGION 9: WRIST AND HAND

Hauth, J. M., Gloyeske, B. M., & Amato, H. K.
*Clinical Skills Documentation Guide for Athletic Training, Third Edition* (pp. 367-414).
© 2016 SLACK Incorporated.

## MUSCULOSKELETAL SYSTEM—REGION 9: WRIST AND HAND
# KNOWLEDGE AND SKILLS

| Musculokeletal System—Region 9: Wrist and Hand | | | | Skill: Acquisition, Reinforcement, Proficiency | | |
|---|---|---|---|---|---|---|
| **NATA EC 5th** | **BOC RD6** | **Palpation** | **Page #** | | | |
| CE-21b, CE-20c | D2-0202 | Palpation: Wrist and Hand – 01 | 370 | | | |
| CE-21b, CE-20c | D2-0202 | Palpation: Wrist and Hand – 02 | 371 | | | |
| CE-21b, CE-20c | D2-0202 | Palpation: Wrist and Hand – 03 | 372 | | | |
| **NATA EC 5th** | **BOC RD6** | **Manual Muscle Testing** | **Page #** | | | |
| CE-21c | D2-0203 | MMT: Abductor Digiti Minimi (Abducts the Fifth Finger, Assists in Opposition) | 373 | | | |
| CE-21c | D2-0203 | MMT: Abductor Pollicis Brevis (First CMC and MCP Abduction, Assists in Opposition) | 374 | | | |
| CE-21c | D2-0203 | MMT: Abductor Pollicis Longus (First CMC Abduction and Extension, Assists in Radial Deviation) | 375 | | | |
| CE-21c | D2-0203 | MMT: Adductor Pollicis (First CMC Adduction, First MCP Adduction and Flexion, Assists in Opposition) | 376 | | | |
| CE-21c | D2-0203 | MMT: Extensor Carpi Radialis Brevis (Wrist Extension, Radial Deviation) | 377 | | | |
| CE-21c | D2-0203 | MMT: Extensor Carpi Radialis Longus (Wrist Extension, Radial Deviation) | 378 | | | |
| CE-21c | D2-0203 | MMT: Extensor Carpi Ulnaris (Wrist Extension, Ulnar Deviation) | 379 | | | |
| CE-21c | D2-0203 | MMT: Extensor Digitorum (Wrist Extension, MCP Extension, IP Extension, Radial Deviation) | 380 | | | |
| CE-21c | D2-0203 | MMT: Extensor Pollicis Brevis (First MCP Extension, First CMC Extension and Abduction, Assists Wrist Radial Deviation) | 381 | | | |
| CE-21c | D2-0203 | MMT: Extensor Pollicis Longus (First IP Extension, First MCP Extension, First CMC Extension, Assists Wrist Extension and Radial Deviation) | 382 | | | |
| CE-21c | D2-0203 | MMT: Flexor Carpi Radialis (Wrist Flexion, Forearm Pronation, Radial Deviation) | 383 | | | |
| CE-21c | D2-0203 | MMT: Flexor Carpi Ulnaris (Wrist Flexion, Ulnar Deviation) | 384 | | | |
| CE-21c | D2-0203 | MMT: Flexor Digiti Minimi (Fifth MCP Flexion, Assists in Opposition) | 385 | | | |
| CE-21c | D2-0203 | MMT: Flexor Digitorum Profundus (DIP Flexion, PIP Flexion, Wrist Flexion) | 386 | | | |
| CE-21c | D2-0203 | MMT: Flexor Pollicis Brevis (First MCP and CMC Flexion, Assists in Opposition) | 387 | | | |
| CE-21c | D2-0203 | MMT: Flexor Pollicis Longus (First IP and MCP Flexion, Assists in Wrist Flexion) | 388 | | | |
| CE-21c | D2-0203 | MMT: Opponens Digiti Minimi (Opposition of Fifth Finger) | 389 | | | |
| CE-21c | D2-0203 | MMT: Opponens Pollicis (Thumb Opposition) | 390 | | | |
| CE-21c | D2-0203 | MMT: Palmaris Longus (Wrist Flexion) | 391 | | | |

*(continued on the next page)*

## MUSCULOSKELETAL SYSTEM—REGION 9: WRIST AND HAND
# KNOWLEDGE AND SKILLS

| NATA EC 5th | BOC RD6 | Osteokinematic Joint Motion | Page # | | | |
|---|---|---|---|---|---|---|
| CE-21d | D2-0203 | Goniometric Assessment: Radiocarpal (Flexion) | 392 | | | |
| CE-21d | D2-0203 | Goniometric Assessment: Radiocarpal (Extension) | 393 | | | |
| CE-21d | D2-0203 | Goniometric Assessment: Radiocarpal (Radial Deviation) | 394 | | | |
| CE-21d | D2-0203 | Goniometric Assessment: Radiocarpal (Ulnar Deviation) | 395 | | | |
| **NATA EC 5th** | **BOC RD6** | **Capsular and Ligamentous Stress Testing** | **Page #** | | | |
| CE-21e | D2-0203 | Gamekeeper's Thumb Test (Ulnar Collateral Ligament Test) | 396 | | | |
| CE-21e | D2-0203 | Interphalangeal Joint Valgus Stress Test | 397 | | | |
| CE-21e | D2-0203 | Interphalangeal Joint Varus Stress Test | 398 | | | |
| CE-21e | D2-0203 | Radiocarpal Valgus Stress Test | 399 | | | |
| CE-21e | D2-0203 | Radiocarpal Varus Stress Test | 400 | | | |
| **NATA EC 5th** | **BOC RD6** | **Joint Play (Arthrokinematics)** | **Page #** | | | |
| CE-21f | D2-0203 | Intermetacarpal Glide | 401 | | | |
| CE-21f | D2-0203 | Carpometacarpal Glide | 402 | | | |
| CE-21f | D2-0203 | Radiocarpal Glide | 403 | | | |
| **NATA EC 5th** | **BOC RD6** | **Special Tests** | **Page #** | | | |
| CE-21g, CE-20e | D2-0203 | Allen's Test | 404 | | | |
| CE-21g, CE-20e | D2-0203 | Finkelstein's Test | 405 | | | |
| CE-21g, CE-20e | D2-0203 | Phalen's Test (Wrist Flexion Test) | 406 | | | |
| CE-21g, CE-20e | D2-0203 | Reagan's Test | 407 | | | |
| CE-21g, CE-20e | D2-0203 | Reverse Phalen's Test | 408 | | | |
| CE-21g, CE-20e | D2-0203 | Scaphoid Compression Test | 409 | | | |
| CE-21g, CE-20e | D2-0203 | Tinel's Sign (Median Nerve) | 410 | | | |
| CE-21g, CE-20e | D2-0203 | Watson's Test (Scapholunate Instability) | 411 | | | |
| **NATA EC 5th** | **BOC RD6** | **Neurological Assessment** | **Page #** | | | |
| CE-21h, CE-20f | D2-0203 | Median Nerve | 412 | | | |
| CE-21h, CE-20f | D2-0203 | Radial Nerve | 413 | | | |
| CE-21h, CE-20f | D2-0203 | Ulnar Nerve | 414 | | | |

## MUSCULOSKELETAL SYSTEM—REGION 9: WRIST AND HAND
# PALPATION

| NATA EC 5th | BOC RD6 | SKILL |
|---|---|---|
| CE-21b, CE-20c | D2-0202 | Palpation: Wrist and Hand – 01 |

**Supplies Needed:** Table

*This problem allows you the opportunity to demonstrate your ability to* **palpate** *the* **wrist and hand**.
*You have 2 minutes to complete this task.*

| Palpation: Wrist and Hand – 01 | Course or Site Assessor Environment | | Test 1 | | Test 2 | | Test 3 | |
|---|---|---|---|---|---|---|---|---|
| | | | Y | N | Y | N | Y | N |
| Trapezium carpal bone | | | ○ | ○ | ○ | ○ | ○ | ○ |
| Thenar eminence of the hand | | | ○ | ○ | ○ | ○ | ○ | ○ |
| Origin of flexor carpi radialis muscle | | | ○ | ○ | ○ | ○ | ○ | ○ |
| Radial collateral ligament of the wrist | | | ○ | ○ | ○ | ○ | ○ | ○ |
| Second proximal phalanx | | | ○ | ○ | ○ | ○ | ○ | ○ |
| Insertion of extensor digiti minimi | | | ○ | ○ | ○ | ○ | ○ | ○ |
| Extensor retinaculum | | | ○ | ○ | ○ | ○ | ○ | ○ |
| | Total | | __/7 | | __/7 | | __/7 | |
| Must achieve >4 to pass this examination | | | Ⓟ | Ⓕ | Ⓟ | Ⓕ | Ⓟ | Ⓕ |
| Assessor: Date: | Test 1 Comments: | | | | | | | |
| Assessor: Date: | Test 2 Comments: | | | | | | | |
| Assessor: Date: | Test 3 Comments: | | | | | | | |

**TEST ENVIRONMENTS**
**L:** Laboratory/Classroom
**C:** Clinical/Field Testing
**P:** Practicum
**A:** Assessment/Mock Exam

**TEST INFORMATION**
**Test Statistics:** N/A
**Reference(s):** Starkey & Brown (2015)

## MUSCULOSKELETAL SYSTEM—REGION 9: WRIST AND HAND
# PALPATION

| NATA EC 5th | BOC RD6 | SKILL |
|---|---|---|
| CE-21b, CE-20c | D2-0202 | Palpation: Wrist and Hand – 02 |

**Supplies Needed:** Table

*This problem allows you the opportunity to demonstrate your ability to **palpate** the **wrist and hand**. You have 2 minutes to complete this task.*

| Palpation: Wrist and Hand – 02 | Course or Site<br>Assessor<br>Environment | | | | | | |
|---|---|---|---|---|---|---|---|
| | | Test 1 | | Test 2 | | Test 3 | |
| | | Y | N | Y | N | Y | N |
| Hook of the hamate | | ○ | ○ | ○ | ○ | ○ | ○ |
| Hypothenar eminence of the hand | | ○ | ○ | ○ | ○ | ○ | ○ |
| Origin of flexor pollicis longus | | ○ | ○ | ○ | ○ | ○ | ○ |
| Dorsal radiocarpal ligament | | ○ | ○ | ○ | ○ | ○ | ○ |
| Fifth distal phalanx | | ○ | ○ | ○ | ○ | ○ | ○ |
| Insertion of extensor digitorum communis | | ○ | ○ | ○ | ○ | ○ | ○ |
| Ulnar collateral ligament of the wrist | | ○ | ○ | ○ | ○ | ○ | ○ |
| | Total | ___/7 | | ___/7 | | ___/7 | |
| | Must achieve >4 to pass this examination | Ⓟ | Ⓕ | Ⓟ | Ⓕ | Ⓟ | Ⓕ |

| Assessor:<br>Date: | Test 1 Comments: |
|---|---|
| Assessor:<br>Date: | Test 2 Comments: |
| Assessor:<br>Date: | Test 3 Comments: |

**TEST ENVIRONMENTS**
**L:** Laboratory/Classroom
**C:** Clinical/Field Testing
**P:** Practicum
**A:** Assessment/Mock Exam

**TEST INFORMATION**
**Test Statistics:** N/A
**Reference(s):**  Starkey & Brown (2015)

## Musculoskeletal System—Region 9: Wrist and Hand
# Palpation

| NATA EC 5th | BOC RD6 | SKILL |
|---|---|---|
| CE-21b, CE-20c | D2-0202 | Palpation: Wrist and Hand – 03 |

**Supplies Needed:** Table

*This problem allows you the opportunity to demonstrate your ability to* **palpate** *the* **wrist and hand**.
*You have 2 minutes to complete this task.*

| Palpation: Wrist and Hand – 03 | Course or Site Assessor Environment | | | | | |
|---|---|---|---|---|---|---|
| | | Test 1 | | Test 2 | | Test 3 |
| | | Y | N | Y | N | Y | N |
| Scaphoid carpal bone | | ○ | ○ | ○ | ○ | ○ | ○ |
| Carpal tunnel | | ○ | ○ | ○ | ○ | ○ | ○ |
| Insertion of abductor pollicis longus | | ○ | ○ | ○ | ○ | ○ | ○ |
| Triangular fibrocartilaginous complex | | ○ | ○ | ○ | ○ | ○ | ○ |
| Fourth middle phalanx | | ○ | ○ | ○ | ○ | ○ | ○ |
| Muscle belly of flexor carpi ulnaris | | ○ | ○ | ○ | ○ | ○ | ○ |
| Palmaris longus tendon | | ○ | ○ | ○ | ○ | ○ | ○ |
| **Total** | | __/7 | | __/7 | | __/7 | |
| **Must achieve >4 to pass this examination** | | Ⓟ | Ⓕ | Ⓟ | Ⓕ | Ⓟ | Ⓕ |

**Assessor:**
**Date:**     Test 1 Comments:

**Assessor:**
**Date:**     Test 2 Comments:

**Assessor:**
**Date:**     Test 3 Comments:

**TEST ENVIRONMENTS**
**L:** Laboratory/Classroom
**C:** Clinical/Field Testing
**P:** Practicum
**A:** Assessment/Mock Exam

**TEST INFORMATION**
**Test Statistics:** N/A
**Reference(s):** Starkey & Brown (2015)

## MUSCULOSKELETAL SYSTEM—REGION 9: WRIST AND HAND
# MANUAL MUSCLE TESTING

| NATA EC 5th | BOC RD6 | SKILL |
|---|---|---|
| CE-21c | D2-0203 | MMT: Abductor Digiti Minimi<br>(Abducts the Fifth Finger, Assists in Opposition) |

**Supplies Needed:** Table, chair

*This problem allows you the opportunity to demonstrate a* **manual muscle test** *for the* **abductor digiti minimi.** *You have 2 minutes to complete this task.*

| MMT: Abductor Digiti Minimi (Abducts the Fifth Finger, Assists in Opposition) | Course or Site Assessor Environment | Test 1 | | Test 2 | | Test 3 | |
|---|---|---|---|---|---|---|---|
| **Tester places patient and limb in appropriate position** | | **Y** | **N** | **Y** | **N** | **Y** | **N** |
| Seated with arm lying flat on table, forearm pronated | | O | O | O | O | O | O |
| Fingers start in extension and adduction | | O | O | O | O | O | O |
| **Tester placed in proper position** | | **Y** | **N** | **Y** | **N** | **Y** | **N** |
| Stands or sits next to or in front of the patient | | O | O | O | O | O | O |
| One hand supports wrist in neutral | | O | O | O | O | O | O |
| Other hand applies the resistance | | O | O | O | O | O | O |
| **Tester performs test according to accepted guidelines** | | **Y** | **N** | **Y** | **N** | **Y** | **N** |
| Instructs the patient to abduct the fifth finger away from ring finger | | O | O | O | O | O | O |
| Applies resistance to ulnar side of fifth finger | | O | O | O | O | O | O |
| Resistance is held for 5 seconds | | O | O | O | O | O | O |
| **Identifies implications** | | **Y** | **N** | **Y** | **N** | **Y** | **N** |
| Correctly grades the MMT | | O | O | O | O | O | O |
| **Total** | | ___/9 | | ___/9 | | ___/9 | |
| **Must achieve >6 to pass this examination** | | Ⓟ | Ⓕ | Ⓟ | Ⓕ | Ⓟ | Ⓕ |

| Assessor:<br>Date: | Test 1 Comments: |
|---|---|
| Assessor:<br>Date: | Test 2 Comments: |
| Assessor:<br>Date: | Test 3 Comments: |

**TEST ENVIRONMENTS**
**L:** Laboratory/Classroom
**C:** Clinical/Field Testing
**P:** Practicum
**A:** Assessment/Mock Exam

**TEST INFORMATION**
**Test Statistics:** N/A
**Reference(s):** Hislop & Montgomery (2007)
Starkey & Brown (2015)

MUSCULOSKELETAL SYSTEM—REGION 9: WRIST AND HAND
# MANUAL MUSCLE TESTING

| NATA EC 5th | BOC RD6 | SKILL |
|---|---|---|
| CE-21c | D2-0203 | MMT: Abductor Pollicis Brevis (First CMC and MCP Abduction, Assists in Opposition) |

**Supplies Needed:** Table, chair

*This problem allows you the opportunity to demonstrate a* **manual muscle test** *for the* **abductor pollicis brevis**. *You have 2 minutes to complete this task.*

| MMT: Abductor Pollicis Brevis (First CMC and MCP Abduction, Assists in Opposition) | Course or Site Assessor Environment | | Test 1 | | Test 2 | | Test 3 | |
|---|---|---|---|---|---|---|---|---|
| **Tester places patient and limb in appropriate position** | | | **Y** | **N** | **Y** | **N** | **Y** | **N** |
| Seated with forearm in supination on table, neutral wrist | | | O | O | O | O | O | O |
| Thumb relaxed, starting in adduction | | | O | O | O | O | O | O |
| **Tester placed in proper position** | | | **Y** | **N** | **Y** | **N** | **Y** | **N** |
| Stands or sits next to or in front of the patient | | | O | O | O | O | O | O |
| One hand stabilizes the metacarpals by placing hand over the patient's palm | | | O | O | O | O | O | O |
| Other hand applies resistance to lateral proximal phalanx of thumb | | | O | O | O | O | O | O |
| **Tester performs test according to accepted guidelines** | | | **Y** | **N** | **Y** | **N** | **Y** | **N** |
| Instructs the patient to abduct the thumb | | | O | O | O | O | O | O |
| Applies resistance to lateral thumb into adduction | | | O | O | O | O | O | O |
| Resistance is held for 5 seconds | | | O | O | O | O | O | O |
| **Identifies implications** | | | **Y** | **N** | **Y** | **N** | **Y** | **N** |
| Correctly grades the MMT | | | O | O | O | O | O | O |
| Total | | | ___/9 | | ___/9 | | ___/9 | |
| Must achieve >6 to pass this examination | | | Ⓟ | Ⓕ | Ⓟ | Ⓕ | Ⓟ | Ⓕ |

| Assessor: Date: | Test 1 Comments: |
|---|---|
| Assessor: Date: | Test 2 Comments: |
| Assessor: Date: | Test 3 Comments: |

**TEST ENVIRONMENTS**
**L:** Laboratory/Classroom
**C:** Clinical/Field Testing
**P:** Practicum
**A:** Assessment/Mock Exam

**TEST INFORMATION**
**Test Statistics:** N/A
**Reference(s):**  Hislop & Montgomery (2007)
Starkey & Brown (2015)

# MANUAL MUSCLE TESTING

| NATA EC 5th | BOC RD6 | SKILL |
|---|---|---|
| CE-21c | D2-0203 | MMT: Abductor Pollicis Longus (First CMC Abduction and Extension, Assists in Radial Deviation) |

**Supplies Needed:** Table, chair

*This problem allows you the opportunity to demonstrate a* **manual muscle test** *for the* **abductor pollicis longus**. *You have 2 minutes to complete this task.*

| MMT: Abductor Pollicis Longus (First CMC Abduction and Extension, Assists in Radial Deviation) | Course or Site Assessor Environment | | | | | |
|---|---|---|---|---|---|---|
| | | Test 1 | | Test 2 | | Test 3 |
| **Tester places patient and limb in appropriate position** | | Y | N | Y | N | Y | N |
| Seated with forearm supinated on table, wrist neutral | | O | O | O | O | O | O |
| Thumb relaxed, starting in adduction | | O | O | O | O | O | O |
| **Tester placed in proper position** | | Y | N | Y | N | Y | N |
| Stands or sits next to or in front of the patient | | O | O | O | O | O | O |
| One hand stabilizes the metacarpals and wrist | | O | O | O | O | O | O |
| Other hand applies resistance on distal phalanx of the thumb | | O | O | O | O | O | O |
| **Tester performs test according to accepted guidelines** | | Y | N | Y | N | Y | N |
| Instructs the patient to abduct the thumb away from hand | | O | O | O | O | O | O |
| Applies resistance over distal phalanx into adduction | | O | O | O | O | O | O |
| Resistance is held for 5 seconds | | O | O | O | O | O | O |
| Performs assessment bilaterally | | O | O | O | O | O | O |
| **Identifies implications** | | Y | N | Y | N | Y | N |
| Correctly grades the MMT | | O | O | O | O | O | O |
| Total | | __/10 | | __/10 | | __/10 |
| Must achieve >6 to pass this examination | | P | F | P | F | P | F |

| Assessor: Date: | Test 1 Comments: |
|---|---|
| Assessor: Date: | Test 2 Comments: |
| Assessor: Date: | Test 3 Comments: |

**TEST ENVIRONMENTS**
**L:** Laboratory/Classroom
**C:** Clinical/Field Testing
**P:** Practicum
**A:** Assessment/Mock Exam

**TEST INFORMATION**
**Test Statistics:** N/A
**Reference(s):** Hislop & Montgomery (2007)
Starkey & Brown (2015)

# Manual Muscle Testing

| NATA EC 5th | BOC RD6 | SKILL |
|---|---|---|
| CE-21c | D2-0203 | MMT: Adductor Pollicis (First CMC Adduction, First MCP Adduction and Flexion, Assists in Opposition) |

**Supplies Needed:** Table, chairs

*This problem allows you the opportunity to demonstrate a* **manual muscle test** *for the* **adductor pollicis.** *You have 2 minutes to complete this task.*

| MMT: Adductor Pollicis (First CMC Adduction, First MCP Adduction and Flexion, Assists in Opposition) | Course or Site Assessor Environment | | Test 1 | | Test 2 | | Test 3 | |
|---|---|---|---|---|---|---|---|---|
| **Tester places patient and limb in appropriate position** | | **Y** | **N** | **Y** | **N** | **Y** | **N** | |
| Seated with forearm pronated on table, wrist neutral | | ○ | ○ | ○ | ○ | ○ | ○ | |
| Thumb relaxed, hanging in abduction | | ○ | ○ | ○ | ○ | ○ | ○ | |
| **Tester placed in proper position** | | **Y** | **N** | **Y** | **N** | **Y** | **N** | |
| Stands or sits next to or in front of the patient | | ○ | ○ | ○ | ○ | ○ | ○ | |
| One hand stabilizes metacarpals by grasping hand around ulnar side | | ○ | ○ | ○ | ○ | ○ | ○ | |
| Other hand applies resistance on medial, proximal phalanx of the thumb | | ○ | ○ | ○ | ○ | ○ | ○ | |
| **Tester performs test according to accepted guidelines** | | **Y** | **N** | **Y** | **N** | **Y** | **N** | |
| Instructs the patient to adduct the thumb against resistance | | ○ | ○ | ○ | ○ | ○ | ○ | |
| Applies resistance into abduction of thumb | | ○ | ○ | ○ | ○ | ○ | ○ | |
| Resistance is held for 5 seconds | | ○ | ○ | ○ | ○ | ○ | ○ | |
| Performs assessment bilaterally | | ○ | ○ | ○ | ○ | ○ | ○ | |
| **Identifies implications** | | **Y** | **N** | **Y** | **N** | **Y** | **N** | |
| Correctly grades the MMT | | ○ | ○ | ○ | ○ | ○ | ○ | |
| **Total** | | ___/10 | | ___/10 | | ___/10 | | |
| **Must achieve >6 to pass this examination** | | Ⓟ | Ⓕ | Ⓟ | Ⓕ | Ⓟ | Ⓕ | |

| Assessor: Date: | Test 1 Comments: |
|---|---|
| Assessor: Date: | Test 2 Comments: |
| Assessor: Date: | Test 3 Comments: |

**TEST ENVIRONMENTS**
**L:** Laboratory/Classroom
**C:** Clinical/Field Testing
**P:** Practicum
**A:** Assessment/Mock Exam

**TEST INFORMATION**
**Test Statistics:** N/A
**Reference(s):** Hislop & Montgomery (2007)
Starkey & Brown (2015)

# MANUAL MUSCLE TESTING

| NATA EC 5th | BOC RD6 | SKILL |
|---|---|---|
| CE-21c | D2-0203 | MMT: Extensor Carpi Radialis Brevis (Wrist Extension, Radial Deviation) |

**Supplies Needed:** Table, chairs

*This problem allows you the opportunity to demonstrate a* **manual muscle test** *for the* **extensor carpi radialis brevis**. *You have 2 minutes to complete this task.*

| MMT: Extensor Carpi Radialis Brevis (Wrist Extension, Radial Deviation) | Course or Site Assessor Environment | | Test 1 | | Test 2 | | Test 3 | |
|---|---|---|---|---|---|---|---|---|
| **Tester places patient and limb in appropriate position** | | **Y** | **N** | **Y** | **N** | **Y** | **N** | |
| Seated with forearm pronated on table | | ○ | ○ | ○ | ○ | ○ | ○ | |
| To start, instructs the patient to radially deviate and extend wrist | | ○ | ○ | ○ | ○ | ○ | ○ | |
| **Tester placed in proper position** | | **Y** | **N** | **Y** | **N** | **Y** | **N** | |
| Stands or sits diagonal from the patient | | ○ | ○ | ○ | ○ | ○ | ○ | |
| One hand supports forearm | | ○ | ○ | ○ | ○ | ○ | ○ | |
| Other hand applies resistance over dorsal surface of the second and third metacarpals | | ○ | ○ | ○ | ○ | ○ | ○ | |
| **Tester performs test according to accepted guidelines** | | **Y** | **N** | **Y** | **N** | **Y** | **N** | |
| Instructs the patient to extend wrist in radial deviation against resistance | | ○ | ○ | ○ | ○ | ○ | ○ | |
| Applies resistance into flexion and ulnar deviation | | ○ | ○ | ○ | ○ | ○ | ○ | |
| Resistance is held for 5 seconds | | ○ | ○ | ○ | ○ | ○ | ○ | |
| Performs assessment bilaterally | | ○ | ○ | ○ | ○ | ○ | ○ | |
| **Identifies implications** | | **Y** | **N** | **Y** | **N** | **Y** | **N** | |
| Correctly grades the MMT | | ○ | ○ | ○ | ○ | ○ | ○ | |
| Total | | ___/10 | | ___/10 | | ___/10 | | |
| Must achieve >6 to pass this examination | | Ⓟ | Ⓕ | Ⓟ | Ⓕ | Ⓟ | Ⓕ | |

| Assessor: Date: | **Test 1 Comments:** |
|---|---|
| Assessor: Date: | **Test 2 Comments:** |
| Assessor: Date: | **Test 3 Comments:** |

**TEST ENVIRONMENTS**
**L:** Laboratory/Classroom
**C:** Clinical/Field Testing
**P:** Practicum
**A:** Assessment/Mock Exam

**TEST INFORMATION**
**Test Statistics:** N/A
**Reference(s):** Hislop & Montgomery (2007)
Starkey & Brown (2015)

## MUSCULOSKELETAL SYSTEM—REGION 9: WRIST AND HAND
# MANUAL MUSCLE TESTING

| NATA EC 5th | BOC RD6 | SKILL |
|---|---|---|
| CE-21c | D2-0203 | MMT: Extensor Carpi Radialis Longus (Wrist Extension, Radial Deviation) |

**Supplies Needed:** Table, chairs

*This problem allows you the opportunity to demonstrate a* **manual muscle test** *for the* **extensor carpi radialis longus**. *You have 2 minutes to complete this task.*

| MMT: Extensor Carpi Radialis Longus (Wrist Extension, Radial Deviation) | Course or Site Assessor Environment | | Test 1 | | Test 2 | | Test 3 |
|---|---|---|---|---|---|---|---|
| **Tester places patient and limb in appropriate position** | | **Y** | **N** | **Y** | **N** | **Y** | **N** |
| Seated with forearm pronated on table | | O | O | O | O | O | O |
| To start, instructs the patient to radially deviate and extend wrist | | O | O | O | O | O | O |
| **Tester placed in proper position** | | **Y** | **N** | **Y** | **N** | **Y** | **N** |
| Stands or sits diagonal from the patient | | O | O | O | O | O | O |
| One hand supports forearm | | O | O | O | O | O | O |
| Other hand applies resistance over dorsal surface of the second and third metacarpals | | O | O | O | O | O | O |
| **Tester performs test according to accepted guidelines** | | **Y** | **N** | **Y** | **N** | **Y** | **N** |
| Instructs the patient to extend wrist in radial deviation against resistance | | O | O | O | O | O | O |
| Applies resistance into flexion and ulnar deviation | | O | O | O | O | O | O |
| Resistance is held for 5 seconds | | O | O | O | O | O | O |
| Performs assessment bilaterally | | O | O | O | O | O | O |
| **Identifies implications** | | **Y** | **N** | **Y** | **N** | **Y** | **N** |
| Correctly grades the MMT | | O | O | O | O | O | O |
| | Total | | /10 | | /10 | | /10 |
| | Must achieve >6 to pass this examination | Ⓟ | Ⓕ | Ⓟ | Ⓕ | Ⓟ | Ⓕ |

| Assessor: Date: | Test 1 Comments: |
|---|---|
| Assessor: Date: | Test 2 Comments: |
| Assessor: Date: | Test 3 Comments: |

**TEST ENVIRONMENTS**
**L:** Laboratory/Classroom
**C:** Clinical/Field Testing
**P:** Practicum
**A:** Assessment/Mock Exam

**TEST INFORMATION**
**Test Statistics:** N/A
**Reference(s):** Hislop & Montgomery (2007)
Starkey & Brown (2015)

# MUSCULOSKELETAL SYSTEM—REGION 9: WRIST AND HAND
## MANUAL MUSCLE TESTING

| NATA EC 5th | BOC RD6 | SKILL |
|---|---|---|
| CE-21c | D2-0203 | MMT: Extensor Carpi Ulnaris (Wrist Extension, Ulnar Deviation) |

**Supplies Needed:** Table, chairs

*This problem allows you the opportunity to demonstrate a* **manual muscle test** *for the* **extensor carpi ulnaris.** *You have 2 minutes to complete this task.*

| MMT: Extensor Carpi Ulnaris (Wrist Extension, Ulnar Deviation) | Course or Site Assessor Environment | | Test 1 | | Test 2 | | Test 3 | |
|---|---|---|---|---|---|---|---|---|
| **Tester places patient and limb in appropriate position** | | **Y** | **N** | **Y** | **N** | **Y** | **N** | |
| Seated with forearm pronated on table | | O | O | O | O | O | O | |
| To start, instructs the patient to ulnarly deviate and extend wrist | | O | O | O | O | O | O | |
| **Tester placed in proper position** | | **Y** | **N** | **Y** | **N** | **Y** | **N** | |
| Stands or sits diagonal from the patient | | O | O | O | O | O | O | |
| One hand supports forearm | | O | O | O | O | O | O | |
| Other hand applies resistance over dorsal surface of fifth metacarpal | | O | O | O | O | O | O | |
| **Tester performs test according to accepted guidelines** | | **Y** | **N** | **Y** | **N** | **Y** | **N** | |
| Instructs the patient to extend wrist in ulnar deviation against resistance | | O | O | O | O | O | O | |
| Applies resistance into flexion and radial deviation | | O | O | O | O | O | O | |
| Resistance is held for 5 seconds | | O | O | O | O | O | O | |
| Performs assessment bilaterally | | O | O | O | O | O | O | |
| **Identifies implications** | | **Y** | **N** | **Y** | **N** | **Y** | **N** | |
| Correctly grades the MMT | | O | O | O | O | O | O | |
| **Total** | | ___/10 | | ___/10 | | ___/10 | | |
| **Must achieve >6 to pass this examination** | | Ⓟ | Ⓕ | Ⓟ | Ⓕ | Ⓟ | Ⓕ | |

| Assessor: Date: | Test 1 Comments: |
|---|---|
| Assessor: Date: | Test 2 Comments: |
| Assessor: Date: | Test 3 Comments: |

**TEST ENVIRONMENTS**
**L:** Laboratory/Classroom
**C:** Clinical/Field Testing
**P:** Practicum
**A:** Assessment/Mock Exam

**TEST INFORMATION**
**Test Statistics:** N/A
**Reference(s):** Hislop & Montgomery (2007)
Starkey & Brown (2015)

MUSCULOSKELETAL SYSTEM—REGION 9: WRIST AND HAND
# MANUAL MUSCLE TESTING

| NATA EC 5th | BOC RD6 | SKILL |
|---|---|---|
| CE-21c | D2-0203 | MMT: Extensor Digitorum (Wrist Extension, MCP Extension, IP Extension, Radial Deviation) |

**Supplies Needed:** Table, chairs

*This problem allows you the opportunity to demonstrate a* **manual muscle test** *for the* **extensor digitorum**. *You have 2 minutes to complete this task.*

| MMT: Extensor Digitorum (Wrist Extension, MCP Extension, IP Extension, Radial Deviation) | Course or Site Assessor Environment | | Test 1 | | Test 2 | | Test 3 |
|---|---|---|---|---|---|---|---|
| **Tester places patient and limb in appropriate position** | | Y | N | Y | N | Y | N |
| Seated with forearm pronated on table | | O | O | O | O | O | O |
| Wrist neutral, MP and IP joints relaxed in flexion | | O | O | O | O | O | O |
| **Tester placed in proper position** | | Y | N | Y | N | Y | N |
| Stands or sits in front of or next to the patient | | O | O | O | O | O | O |
| One hand supports forearm | | O | O | O | O | O | O |
| Other hand applies resistance with index finger over dorsal surface of all proximal phalanges | | O | O | O | O | O | O |
| **Tester performs test according to accepted guidelines** | | Y | N | Y | N | Y | N |
| Instructs the patient to extend MP joints, with IP joints in slight flexion | | O | O | O | O | O | O |
| Applies resistance into flexion | | O | O | O | O | O | O |
| Resistance is held for 5 seconds | | O | O | O | O | O | O |
| Performs assessment bilaterally | | O | O | O | O | O | O |
| **Identifies implications** | | Y | N | Y | N | Y | N |
| Correctly grades the MMT | | O | O | O | O | O | O |
| Total | | ___/10 | | ___/10 | | ___/10 | |
| **Must achieve >6 to pass this examination** | | Ⓟ | Ⓕ | Ⓟ | Ⓕ | Ⓟ | Ⓕ |

| Assessor: Date: | Test 1 Comments: |
|---|---|
| Assessor: Date: | Test 2 Comments: |
| Assessor: Date: | Test 3 Comments: |

**TEST ENVIRONMENTS**
**L:** Laboratory/Classroom
**C:** Clinical/Field Testing
**P:** Practicum
**A:** Assessment/Mock Exam

**TEST INFORMATION**
**Test Statistics:** N/A
**Reference(s):** Hislop & Montgomery (2007)
Starkey & Brown (2015)

# MANUAL MUSCLE TESTING

| NATA EC 5th | BOC RD6 | SKILL |
|---|---|---|
| CE-21c | D2-0203 | MMT: Extensor Pollicis Brevis (First MCP Extension, First CMC Extension and Abduction, Assists Wrist Radial Deviation) |

**Supplies Needed:** Table, chairs

*This problem allows you the opportunity to demonstrate a* **manual muscle test** *for the* **extensor pollicis brevis.** *You have 2 minutes to complete this task.*

| MMT: Extensor Pollicis Brevis (First MCP Extension, First CMC Extension and Abduction, Assists Wrist Radial Deviation) | Course or Site Assessor Environment | | Test 1 | | Test 2 | | Test 3 |
|---|---|---|---|---|---|---|---|
| **Tester places patient and limb in appropriate position** | | Y | N | Y | N | Y | N |
| Seated with forearm in mid-position on table | | O | O | O | O | O | O |
| Wrist neutral, thumb abducted and relaxed in flexion | | O | O | O | O | O | O |
| **Tester placed in proper position** | | Y | N | Y | N | Y | N |
| Stands or sits in front of or next to the patient | | O | O | O | O | O | O |
| One hand stabilizes the first metacarpal | | O | O | O | O | O | O |
| Other hand applies resistance with index finger over dorsal surface of proximal phalanx | | O | O | O | O | O | O |
| **Tester performs test according to accepted guidelines** | | Y | N | Y | N | Y | N |
| Instructs the patient to extend MP joint of thumb, with IP joint in slight flexion | | O | O | O | O | O | O |
| Applies resistance into flexion | | O | O | O | O | O | O |
| Resistance is held for 5 seconds | | O | O | O | O | O | O |
| Performs assessment bilaterally | | O | O | O | O | O | O |
| **Identifies implications** | | Y | N | Y | N | Y | N |
| Correctly grades the MMT | | O | O | O | O | O | O |
| Total | | __/10 | | __/10 | | __/10 | |
| Must achieve >7 to pass this examination | | Ⓟ | Ⓕ | Ⓟ | Ⓕ | Ⓟ | Ⓕ |

| Assessor: Date: | Test 1 Comments: |
|---|---|
| Assessor: Date: | Test 2 Comments: |
| Assessor: Date: | Test 3 Comments: |

**TEST ENVIRONMENTS**
**L:** Laboratory/Classroom
**C:** Clinical/Field Testing
**P:** Practicum
**A:** Assessment/Mock Exam

**TEST INFORMATION**
**Test Statistics:** N/A
**Reference(s):** Hislop & Montgomery (2007)
Starkey & Brown (2015)

## MUSCULOSKELETAL SYSTEM—REGION 9: WRIST AND HAND
# MANUAL MUSCLE TESTING

| NATA EC 5th | BOC RD6 | SKILL |
|---|---|---|
| CE-21c | D2-0203 | MMT: Extensor Pollicis Longus (First IP Extension, First MCP Extension, First CMC Extension, Assists Wrist Extension and Radial Deviation) |

**Supplies Needed:** Table, chairs

*This problem allows you the opportunity to demonstrate a* **manual muscle test** *for the* **extensor pollicis longus**. *You have 2 minutes to complete this task.*

| MMT: Extensor Pollicis Longus (First IP Extension, First MCP Extension, First CMC Extension, Assists Wrist Extension and Radial Deviation) | Test 1 | | Test 2 | | Test 3 | |
|---|---|---|---|---|---|---|
| **Tester places patient and limb in appropriate position** | Y | N | Y | N | Y | N |
| Seated with forearm in mid-position on table | ○ | ○ | ○ | ○ | ○ | ○ |
| Wrist neutral, ulnar side on table, thumb relaxed in flexion | ○ | ○ | ○ | ○ | ○ | ○ |
| **Tester placed in proper position** | Y | N | Y | N | Y | N |
| Stands or sits in front of or next to the patient | ○ | ○ | ○ | ○ | ○ | ○ |
| One hand stabilizes the first proximal phalanx | ○ | ○ | ○ | ○ | ○ | ○ |
| Other hand applies resistance over dorsal surface of distal phalanx | ○ | ○ | ○ | ○ | ○ | ○ |
| **Tester performs test according to accepted guidelines** | Y | N | Y | N | Y | N |
| Instructs the patient to extend IP joint of thumb | ○ | ○ | ○ | ○ | ○ | ○ |
| Applies resistance into flexion | ○ | ○ | ○ | ○ | ○ | ○ |
| Resistance is held for 5 seconds | ○ | ○ | ○ | ○ | ○ | ○ |
| Performs assessment bilaterally | ○ | ○ | ○ | ○ | ○ | ○ |
| **Identifies implications** | Y | N | Y | N | Y | N |
| Correctly grades the MMT | ○ | ○ | ○ | ○ | ○ | ○ |
| Total | __/10 | | __/10 | | __/10 | |
| Must achieve >6 to pass this examination | Ⓟ | Ⓕ | Ⓟ | Ⓕ | Ⓟ | Ⓕ |

| Assessor:<br>Date: | Test 1 Comments: |
|---|---|
| Assessor:<br>Date: | Test 2 Comments: |
| Assessor:<br>Date: | Test 3 Comments: |

**TEST ENVIRONMENTS**
**L:** Laboratory/Classroom
**C:** Clinical/Field Testing
**P:** Practicum
**A:** Assessment/Mock Exam

**TEST INFORMATION**
**Test Statistics:** N/A
**Reference(s):** Hislop & Montgomery (2007)
Starkey & Brown (2015)

# MANUAL MUSCLE TESTING

| NATA EC 5th | BOC RD6 | SKILL |
|---|---|---|
| CE-21c | D2-0203 | MMT: Flexor Carpi Radialis (Wrist Flexion, Forearm Pronation, Radial Deviation) |

**Supplies Needed:** Table, chairs

*This problem allows you the opportunity to demonstrate a* **manual muscle test** *for the* **flexor carpi radialis**. *You have 2 minutes to complete this task.*

| MMT: Flexor Carpi Radialis (Wrist Flexion, Forearm Pronation, Radial Deviation) | Course or Site Assessor Environment | | Test 1 | | Test 2 | | Test 3 | |
|---|---|---|---|---|---|---|---|---|
| **Tester places patient and limb in appropriate position** | | **Y** | **N** | **Y** | **N** | **Y** | **N** | |
| Seated with forearm in supination on table | | O | O | O | O | O | O | |
| To start, wrist is flexed and radially deviated | | O | O | O | O | O | O | |
| **Tester placed in proper position** | | **Y** | **N** | **Y** | **N** | **Y** | **N** | |
| Stands or sits in front of or next to the patient | | O | O | O | O | O | O | |
| One hand supports forearm under the wrist | | O | O | O | O | O | O | |
| Other hand applies resistance over the second metacarpal | | O | O | O | O | O | O | |
| **Tester performs test according to accepted guidelines** | | **Y** | **N** | **Y** | **N** | **Y** | **N** | |
| Instructs the patient to flex the wrist in radial deviation against resistance | | O | O | O | O | O | O | |
| Applies resistance into extension and ulnar deviation | | O | O | O | O | O | O | |
| Resistance is held for 5 seconds | | O | O | O | O | O | O | |
| Performs assessment bilaterally | | O | O | O | O | O | O | |
| **Identifies implications** | | **Y** | **N** | **Y** | **N** | **Y** | **N** | |
| Correctly grades the MMT | | O | O | O | O | O | O | |
| Total | | ___/10 | | ___/10 | | ___/10 | | |
| Must achieve >6 to pass this examination | | Ⓟ | Ⓕ | Ⓟ | Ⓕ | Ⓟ | Ⓕ | |

| Assessor: Date: | Test 1 Comments: |
|---|---|
| Assessor: Date: | Test 2 Comments: |
| Assessor: Date: | Test 3 Comments: |

**TEST ENVIRONMENTS**
**L:** Laboratory/Classroom
**C:** Clinical/Field Testing
**P:** Practicum
**A:** Assessment/Mock Exam

**TEST INFORMATION**
**Test Statistics:** N/A
**Reference(s):** Hislop & Montgomery (2007)
Starkey & Brown (2015)

MUSCULOSKELETAL SYSTEM—REGION 9: WRIST AND HAND
# MANUAL MUSCLE TESTING

| NATA EC 5th | BOC RD6 | SKILL |
|---|---|---|
| CE-21c | D2-0203 | MMT: Flexor Carpi Ulnaris (Wrist Flexion, Ulnar Deviation) |

**Supplies Needed:** Table, chairs

*This problem allows you the opportunity to demonstrate a* **manual muscle test** *for the* **flexor carpi ulnaris**. *You have 2 minutes to complete this task.*

| MMT: Flexor Carpi Ulnaris (Wrist Flexion, Ulnar Deviation) | Course or Site Assessor Environment | Test 1 | | Test 2 | | Test 3 | |
|---|---|---|---|---|---|---|---|
| **Tester places patient and limb in appropriate position** | | **Y** | **N** | **Y** | **N** | **Y** | **N** |
| Seated with forearm in supination on table | | ○ | ○ | ○ | ○ | ○ | ○ |
| To start, wrist is flexed and ulnarly deviated | | ○ | ○ | ○ | ○ | ○ | ○ |
| **Tester placed in proper position** | | **Y** | **N** | **Y** | **N** | **Y** | **N** |
| Stands or sits in front of or next to the patient | | ○ | ○ | ○ | ○ | ○ | ○ |
| One hand supports forearm under the wrist | | ○ | ○ | ○ | ○ | ○ | ○ |
| Other hand applies resistance over the fifth metacarpal | | ○ | ○ | ○ | ○ | ○ | ○ |
| **Tester performs test according to accepted guidelines** | | **Y** | **N** | **Y** | **N** | **Y** | **N** |
| Instructs the patient to flex the wrist in ulnar deviation against resistance | | ○ | ○ | ○ | ○ | ○ | ○ |
| Applies resistance into extension and radial deviation | | ○ | ○ | ○ | ○ | ○ | ○ |
| Resistance is held for 5 seconds | | ○ | ○ | ○ | ○ | ○ | ○ |
| Performs assessment bilaterally | | ○ | ○ | ○ | ○ | ○ | ○ |
| **Identifies implications** | | **Y** | **N** | **Y** | **N** | **Y** | **N** |
| Correctly grades the MMT | | ○ | ○ | ○ | ○ | ○ | ○ |
| | Total | ___/10 | | ___/10 | | ___/10 | |
| | Must achieve >6 to pass this examination | Ⓟ | Ⓕ | Ⓟ | Ⓕ | Ⓟ | Ⓕ |

| Assessor: Date: | Test 1 Comments: |
|---|---|
| Assessor: Date: | Test 2 Comments: |
| Assessor: Date: | Test 3 Comments: |

**TEST ENVIRONMENTS**
**L:** Laboratory/Classroom
**C:** Clinical/Field Testing
**P:** Practicum
**A:** Assessment/Mock Exam

**TEST INFORMATION**
**Test Statistics:** N/A
**Reference(s):**   Hislop & Montgomery (2007)
                    Starkey & Brown (2015)

MUSCULOSKELETAL SYSTEM—REGION 9: WRIST AND HAND
# MANUAL MUSCLE TESTING

| NATA EC 5th | BOC RD6 | SKILL |
|---|---|---|
| CE-21c | D2-0203 | MMT: Flexor Digiti Minimi (Fifth MCP Flexion, Assists in Opposition) |

**Supplies Needed:** Table, chairs

*This problem allows you the opportunity to demonstrate a* **manual muscle test** *for the* **flexor digiti minimi.** *You have 2 minutes to complete this task.*

| MMT: Flexor Digiti Minimi (Fifth MCP Flexion, Assists in Opposition) | Course or Site / Assessor / Environment | | Test 1 | | Test 2 | | Test 3 |
|---|---|---|---|---|---|---|---|
| **Tester places patient and limb in appropriate position** | | Y | N | Y | N | Y | N |
| Seated with forearm in pronation on table | | O | O | O | O | O | O |
| Wrist neutral and MP and IP joints relaxed in flexion | | O | O | O | O | O | O |
| **Tester placed in proper position** | | Y | N | Y | N | Y | N |
| Stands or sits in front of or next to the patient | | O | O | O | O | O | O |
| One hand stabilizes wrist | | O | O | O | O | O | O |
| Other hand applies resistance with index finger over dorsal surface of proximal phalanx of fifth metacarpal | | O | O | O | O | O | O |
| **Tester performs test according to accepted guidelines** | | Y | N | Y | N | Y | N |
| Instructs the patient to extend the MP joint of the fifth finger | | O | O | O | O | O | O |
| Applies resistance into flexion | | O | O | O | O | O | O |
| Resistance is held for 5 seconds | | O | O | O | O | O | O |
| Performs assessment bilaterally | | O | O | O | O | O | O |
| **Identifies implications** | | Y | N | Y | N | Y | N |
| Correctly grades the MMT | | O | O | O | O | O | O |
| **Total** | | ___/10 | | ___/10 | | ___/10 | |
| **Must achieve >6 to pass this examination** | | P | F | P | F | P | F |

Assessor: Date: — Test 1 Comments:

Assessor: Date: — Test 2 Comments:

Assessor: Date: — Test 3 Comments:

**TEST ENVIRONMENTS**
L: Laboratory/Classroom
C: Clinical/Field Testing
P: Practicum
A: Assessment/Mock Exam

**TEST INFORMATION**
**Test Statistics:** N/A
**Reference(s):** Hislop & Montgomery (2007)
Starkey & Brown (2015)

MUSCULOSKELETAL SYSTEM—REGION 9: WRIST AND HAND
# MANUAL MUSCLE TESTING

| NATA EC 5th | BOC RD6 | SKILL |
|---|---|---|
| CE-21c | D2-0203 | MMT: Flexor Digitorum Profundus (DIP Flexion, PIP Flexion, Wrist Flexion) |

**Supplies Needed:** Table, chairs

*This problem allows you the opportunity to demonstrate a* **manual muscle test** *for the* **flexor digitorum profundus.** *You have 2 minutes to complete this task.*

| MMT: Flexor Digitorum Profundus (DIP Flexion, PIP Flexion, Wrist Flexion) | Course or Site / Assessor / Environment | Test 1 | | Test 2 | | Test 3 | |
|---|---|---|---|---|---|---|---|
| Tester places patient and limb in appropriate position | | Y | N | Y | N | Y | N |
| Seated with forearm in supination on table | | O | O | O | O | O | O |
| Wrist neutral, PIP joint in extension | | O | O | O | O | O | O |
| Tester placed in proper position | | Y | N | Y | N | Y | N |
| Stands or sits in front of or next to the patient | | O | O | O | O | O | O |
| One hand stabilizes middle phalanx in extension | | O | O | O | O | O | O |
| Other hand applies resistance over distal phalanx | | O | O | O | O | O | O |
| Tester performs test according to accepted guidelines | | Y | N | Y | N | Y | N |
| Instructs the patient to flex the individual distal phalanx | | O | O | O | O | O | O |
| Applies resistance into extension | | O | O | O | O | O | O |
| Resistance is held for 5 seconds | | O | O | O | O | O | O |
| Performs assessment bilaterally | | O | O | O | O | O | O |
| Identifies implications | | Y | N | Y | N | Y | N |
| Correctly grades the MMT | | O | O | O | O | O | O |
| Total | | __/10 | | __/10 | | __/10 | |
| Must achieve >6 to pass this examination | | P | F | P | F | P | F |

| Assessor: Date: | Test 1 Comments: |
|---|---|
| Assessor: Date: | Test 2 Comments: |
| Assessor: Date: | Test 3 Comments: |

**TEST ENVIRONMENTS**
**L:** Laboratory/Classroom
**C:** Clinical/Field Testing
**P:** Practicum
**A:** Assessment/Mock Exam

**TEST INFORMATION**
**Test Statistics:** N/A
**Reference(s):** Hislop & Montgomery (2007)
Starkey & Brown (2015)

# MANUAL MUSCLE TESTING

| NATA EC 5th | BOC RD6 | SKILL |
|---|---|---|
| CE-21c | D2-0203 | MMT: Flexor Pollicis Brevis (First MCP and CMC Flexion, Assists in Opposition) |

**Supplies Needed:** Table, chairs

*This problem allows you the opportunity to demonstrate a* **manual muscle test** *for the* **flexor pollicis brevis.** *You have 2 minutes to complete this task.*

| MMT: Flexor Pollicis Brevis (First MCP and CMC Flexion, Assists in Opposition) | Course or Site Assessor Environment | | Test 1 | | Test 2 | | Test 3 |
|---|---|---|---|---|---|---|---|
| **Tester places patient and limb in appropriate position** | | Y | N | Y | N | Y | N |
| Seated with forearm in supination on table | | O | O | O | O | O | O |
| Wrist neutral, thumb in adduction | | O | O | O | O | O | O |
| **Tester placed in proper position** | | Y | N | Y | N | Y | N |
| Stands or sits in front of or next to the patient | | O | O | O | O | O | O |
| One hand supports first metacarpal | | O | O | O | O | O | O |
| Other hand applies resistance with one finger over proximal phalanx | | O | O | O | O | O | O |
| **Tester performs test according to accepted guidelines** | | Y | N | Y | N | Y | N |
| Instructs the patient to flex MP joint of thumb, keeping IP joint straight | | O | O | O | O | O | O |
| Applies resistance into extension | | O | O | O | O | O | O |
| Resistance is held for 5 seconds | | O | O | O | O | O | O |
| Performs assessment bilaterally | | O | O | O | O | O | O |
| **Identifies implications** | | Y | N | Y | N | Y | N |
| Correctly grades the MMT | | O | O | O | O | O | O |
| **Total** | | \_\_/10 | | \_\_/10 | | \_\_/10 | |
| **Must achieve >6 to pass this examination** | | Ⓟ | Ⓕ | Ⓟ | Ⓕ | Ⓟ | Ⓕ |

| Assessor: Date: | Test 1 Comments: |
|---|---|
| Assessor: Date: | Test 2 Comments: |
| Assessor: Date: | Test 3 Comments: |

**TEST ENVIRONMENTS**
**L:** Laboratory/Classroom
**C:** Clinical/Field Testing
**P:** Practicum
**A:** Assessment/Mock Exam

**TEST INFORMATION**
**Test Statistics:** N/A
**Reference(s):** Hislop & Montgomery (2007)
Starkey & Brown (2015)

MUSCULOSKELETAL SYSTEM—REGION 9: WRIST AND HAND
# MANUAL MUSCLE TESTING

| NATA EC 5th | BOC RD6 | SKILL |
|---|---|---|
| CE-21c | D2-0203 | MMT: Flexor Pollicis Longus (First IP and MCP Flexion, Assists in Wrist Flexion) |

**Supplies Needed:** Table, chairs

*This problem allows you the opportunity to demonstrate a* **manual muscle test** *for the* **flexor pollicis longus.** *You have 2 minutes to complete this task.*

| MMT: Flexor Pollicis Longus (First IP and MCP Flexion, Assists in Wrist Flexion) | Course or Site Assessor Environment | | | | | |
|---|---|---|---|---|---|---|
| | | Test 1 | | Test 2 | | Test 3 |
| **Tester places patient and limb in appropriate position** | | Y | N | Y | N | Y | N |
| Seated with forearm in supination on table | | O | O | O | O | O | O |
| Wrist neutral, MP joint of thumb in extension | | O | O | O | O | O | O |
| **Tester placed in proper position** | | Y | N | Y | N | Y | N |
| Stands or sits in front of or next to the patient | | O | O | O | O | O | O |
| One hand stabilizes MP joint in extension | | O | O | O | O | O | O |
| Other hand applies resistance over palmar surface of distal phalanx | | O | O | O | O | O | O |
| **Tester performs test according to accepted guidelines** | | Y | N | Y | N | Y | N |
| Instructs the patient to flex IP joint of thumb | | O | O | O | O | O | O |
| Applies resistance into extension | | O | O | O | O | O | O |
| Resistance is held for 5 seconds | | O | O | O | O | O | O |
| Performs assessment bilaterally | | O | O | O | O | O | O |
| **Identifies implications** | | Y | N | Y | N | Y | N |
| Correctly grades the MMT | | O | O | O | O | O | O |
| Total | | __/10 | | __/10 | | __/10 |
| Must achieve >6 to pass this examination | | P | F | P | F | P | F |

| Assessor: Date: | Test 1 Comments: |
|---|---|
| Assessor: Date: | Test 2 Comments: |
| Assessor: Date: | Test 3 Comments: |

**TEST ENVIRONMENTS**
**L:** Laboratory/Classroom
**C:** Clinical/Field Testing
**P:** Practicum
**A:** Assessment/Mock Exam

**TEST INFORMATION**
**Test Statistics:** N/A
**Reference(s):** Hislop & Montgomery (2007)
Starkey & Brown (2015)

# MANUAL MUSCLE TESTING

| NATA EC 5th | BOC RD6 | SKILL |
|---|---|---|
| CE-21c | D2-0203 | MMT: Opponens Digiti Minimi (Opposition of Fifth Finger) |

**Supplies Needed:** Table, chairs

*This problem allows you the opportunity to demonstrate a* **manual muscle test** *for the* **opponens digiti minimi.** *You have 2 minutes to complete this task.*

| MMT: Opponens Digiti Minimi (Opposition of Fifth Finger) | Course or Site Assessor Environment | | Test 1 | | Test 2 | | Test 3 |
|---|---|---|---|---|---|---|---|
| **Tester places patient and limb in appropriate position** | | Y | N | Y | N | Y | N |
| Seated with forearm in supination on table | | ○ | ○ | ○ | ○ | ○ | ○ |
| Wrist neutral, thumb in adduction with MP and IP flexion | | ○ | ○ | ○ | ○ | ○ | ○ |
| **Tester placed in proper position** | | Y | N | Y | N | Y | N |
| Stands or sits in front of or next to the patient | | ○ | ○ | ○ | ○ | ○ | ○ |
| One hand stabilizes by holding dorsal wrist | | ○ | ○ | ○ | ○ | ○ | ○ |
| Other hand applies resistance over palmar surface of fifth metacarpal | | ○ | ○ | ○ | ○ | ○ | ○ |
| **Tester performs test according to accepted guidelines** | | Y | N | Y | N | Y | N |
| Instructs the patient to bring thumb and fifth finger together | | ○ | ○ | ○ | ○ | ○ | ○ |
| Applies resistance into medial rotation (flatten out palm) | | ○ | ○ | ○ | ○ | ○ | ○ |
| Resistance is held for 5 seconds | | ○ | ○ | ○ | ○ | ○ | ○ |
| Performs assessment bilaterally | | ○ | ○ | ○ | ○ | ○ | ○ |
| **Identifies implications** | | Y | N | Y | N | Y | N |
| Correctly grades the MMT | | ○ | ○ | ○ | ○ | ○ | ○ |
| | Total | ___/10 | | ___/10 | | ___/10 | |
| | Must achieve >6 to pass this examination | Ⓟ | Ⓕ | Ⓟ | Ⓕ | Ⓟ | Ⓕ |

| Assessor: Date: | Test 1 Comments: |
|---|---|
| Assessor: Date: | Test 2 Comments: |
| Assessor: Date: | Test 3 Comments: |

**TEST ENVIRONMENTS**
**L:** Laboratory/Classroom
**C:** Clinical/Field Testing
**P:** Practicum
**A:** Assessment/Mock Exam

**TEST INFORMATION**
**Test Statistics:** N/A
**Reference(s):** Hislop & Montgomery (2007)
Starkey & Brown (2015)

MUSCULOSKELETAL SYSTEM—REGION 9: WRIST AND HAND
# MANUAL MUSCLE TESTING

| NATA EC 5th | BOC RD6 | SKILL |
|---|---|---|
| CE-21c | D2-0203 | MMT: Opponens Pollicis (Thumb Opposition) |

**Supplies Needed:** Table, chairs

*This problem allows you the opportunity to demonstrate a* **manual muscle test** *for the* **opponens pollicis**.
*You have 2 minutes to complete this task.*

| MMT: Opponens Pollicis (Thumb Opposition) | Course or Site Assessor Environment | | Test 1 | | Test 2 | | Test 3 | |
|---|---|---|---|---|---|---|---|---|
| **Tester places patient and limb in appropriate position** | | **Y** | **N** | **Y** | **N** | **Y** | **N** | |
| Seated with forearm in supination on table | | ◯ | ◯ | ◯ | ◯ | ◯ | ◯ | |
| Wrist neutral, thumb in adduction with MP and IP flexion | | ◯ | ◯ | ◯ | ◯ | ◯ | ◯ | |
| **Tester placed in proper position** | | **Y** | **N** | **Y** | **N** | **Y** | **N** | |
| Stands or sits in front of or next to the patient | | ◯ | ◯ | ◯ | ◯ | ◯ | ◯ | |
| One hand stabilizes by holding dorsal wrist | | ◯ | ◯ | ◯ | ◯ | ◯ | ◯ | |
| Other hand applies resistance over palmar surface of the head of the first metacarpal | | ◯ | ◯ | ◯ | ◯ | ◯ | ◯ | |
| **Tester performs test according to accepted guidelines** | | **Y** | **N** | **Y** | **N** | **Y** | **N** | |
| Instructs the patient to bring thumb and fifth finger together | | ◯ | ◯ | ◯ | ◯ | ◯ | ◯ | |
| Applies resistance of lateral rotation, extension, adduction (flatten out palm) | | ◯ | ◯ | ◯ | ◯ | ◯ | ◯ | |
| Resistance is held for 5 seconds | | ◯ | ◯ | ◯ | ◯ | ◯ | ◯ | |
| Performs assessment bilaterally | | ◯ | ◯ | ◯ | ◯ | ◯ | ◯ | |
| **Identifies implications** | | **Y** | **N** | **Y** | **N** | **Y** | **N** | |
| Correctly grades the MMT | | ◯ | ◯ | ◯ | ◯ | ◯ | ◯ | |
| Total | | ___/10 | | ___/10 | | ___/10 | | |
| Must achieve >6 to pass this examination | | Ⓟ | Ⓕ | Ⓟ | Ⓕ | Ⓟ | Ⓕ | |

| Assessor: Date: | Test 1 Comments: |
|---|---|
| Assessor: Date: | Test 2 Comments: |
| Assessor: Date: | Test 3 Comments: |

## TEST ENVIRONMENTS
**L:** Laboratory/Classroom
**C:** Clinical/Field Testing
**P:** Practicum
**A:** Assessment/Mock Exam

## TEST INFORMATION
**Test Statistics:** N/A
**Reference(s):** Hislop & Montgomery (2007)
Starkey & Brown (2015)

# MANUAL MUSCLE TESTING

| NATA EC 5th | BOC RD6 | SKILL |
|---|---|---|
| CE-21c | D2-0203 | MMT: Palmaris Longus (Wrist Flexion) |

**Supplies Needed:** Table, chairs

*This problem allows you the opportunity to demonstrate a* **manual muscle test** *for the* **palmaris longus.**
*You have 2 minutes to complete this task.*

| MMT: Palmaris Longus (Wrist Flexion) | Course or Site Assessor Environment | | Test 1 | | Test 2 | | Test 3 | |
|---|---|---|---|---|---|---|---|---|
| **Tester places patient and limb in appropriate position** | | **Y** | **N** | **Y** | **N** | **Y** | **N** | |
| Seated with forearm in supination on table | | O | O | O | O | O | O | |
| To start, wrist is flexed | | O | O | O | O | O | O | |
| **Tester placed in proper position** | | **Y** | **N** | **Y** | **N** | **Y** | **N** | |
| Stands or sits in front of or next to the patient | | O | O | O | O | O | O | |
| One hand supports forearm under the wrist | | O | O | O | O | O | O | |
| Other hand applies resistance over the palmar surface of metacarpals | | O | O | O | O | O | O | |
| **Tester performs test according to accepted guidelines** | | **Y** | **N** | **Y** | **N** | **Y** | **N** | |
| Instructs the patient to flex the wrist against resistance | | O | O | O | O | O | O | |
| Applies resistance into extension | | O | O | O | O | O | O | |
| Resistance is held for 5 seconds | | O | O | O | O | O | O | |
| Performs assessment bilaterally | | O | O | O | O | O | O | |
| **Identifies implications** | | **Y** | **N** | **Y** | **N** | **Y** | **N** | |
| Correctly grades the MMT | | O | O | O | O | O | O | |
| Total | | _/10 | | _/10 | | _/10 | | |
| Must achieve >6 to pass this examination | | Ⓟ | Ⓕ | Ⓟ | Ⓕ | Ⓟ | Ⓕ | |

| Assessor: Date: | Test 1 Comments: |
|---|---|
| Assessor: Date: | Test 2 Comments: |
| Assessor: Date: | Test 3 Comments: |

**TEST ENVIRONMENTS**
**L:** Laboratory/Classroom
**C:** Clinical/Field Testing
**P:** Practicum
**A:** Assessment/Mock Exam

**TEST INFORMATION**
**Test Statistics:** N/A
**Reference(s):** Hislop & Montgomery (2007)
Starkey & Brown (2015)

# OSTEOKINEMATIC JOINT MOTION

| NATA EC 5th | BOC RD6 | SKILL |
|---|---|---|
| CE-21d | D2-0203 | Goniometric Assessment: Radiocarpal (Flexion) |

**Supplies Needed:** Table, chairs, small or large goniometer

*This problem allows you the opportunity to demonstrate a* **goniometric assessment** *for* **radiocarpal (flexion)**. *You have 2 minutes to complete this task.*

| Goniometric Assessment: Radiocarpal (Flexion) | Course or Site _____ _____ _____<br>Assessor _____ _____ _____<br>Environment _____ _____ _____ | | | | | |
|---|---|---|---|---|---|---|
| | | **Test 1** | | **Test 2** | | **Test 3** |
| **Tester places patient and limb in appropriate position** | | **Y** | **N** | **Y** | **N** | **Y** | **N** |
| Seated with forearm on table, shoulder and elbow at 90 degrees | | ○ | ○ | ○ | ○ | ○ | ○ |
| Allow hand/wrist to lie off the edge of the table, palm down | | ○ | ○ | ○ | ○ | ○ | ○ |
| **Tester and goniometer placed in proper position** | | **Y** | **N** | **Y** | **N** | **Y** | **N** |
| Sits or stands next to or in front of the patient | | ○ | ○ | ○ | ○ | ○ | ○ |
| Places center of fulcrum over triquetrum on lateral aspect of wrist | | ○ | ○ | ○ | ○ | ○ | ○ |
| Stationary arm aligned with lateral midline of ulna | | ○ | ○ | ○ | ○ | ○ | ○ |
| Moving arm aligned with lateral midline of fifth metacarpal | | ○ | ○ | ○ | ○ | ○ | ○ |
| **Tester performs test according to accepted guidelines** | | **Y** | **N** | **Y** | **N** | **Y** | **N** |
| Instructs the patient to flex the wrist as far as possible | | ○ | ○ | ○ | ○ | ○ | ○ |
| Takes proper goniometric measurement once the patient reaches end range | | ○ | ○ | ○ | ○ | ○ | ○ |
| **Identifies implications** | | **Y** | **N** | **Y** | **N** | **Y** | **N** |
| Identifies normal ranges (radiocarpal flexion = 60 to 80 degrees) | | ○ | ○ | ○ | ○ | ○ | ○ |
| **Total** | | ____/9 | | ____/9 | | ____/9 |
| **Must achieve >6 to pass this examination** | | Ⓟ | Ⓕ | Ⓟ | Ⓕ | Ⓟ | Ⓕ |

| Assessor:<br>Date: | Test 1 Comments: |
|---|---|
| Assessor:<br>Date: | Test 2 Comments: |
| Assessor:<br>Date: | Test 3 Comments: |

**TEST ENVIRONMENTS**
**L:** Laboratory/Classroom
**C:** Clinical/Field Testing
**P:** Practicum
**A:** Assessment/Mock Exam

**TEST INFORMATION**
**Test Statistics:** N/A
**Reference(s):** Norkin & White (2009)

## MUSCULOSKELETAL SYSTEM—REGION 9: WRIST AND HAND
# OSTEOKINEMATIC JOINT MOTION

| NATA EC 5th | BOC RD6 | SKILL |
|---|---|---|
| CE-21d | D2-0203 | Goniometric Assessment: Radiocarpal (Extension) |

**Supplies Needed:** Table, chairs, small or large goniometer

*This problem allows you the opportunity to demonstrate a* **goniometric assessment** *for* **radiocarpal (extension)**. *You have 2 minutes to complete this task.*

| Goniometric Assessment: Radiocarpal (Extension) | Course or Site Assessor Environment | | Test 1 | | Test 2 | | Test 3 | |
|---|---|---|---|---|---|---|---|---|
| **Tester places patient and limb in appropriate position** | | | **Y** | **N** | **Y** | **N** | **Y** | **N** |
| Seated with forearm on table, shoulder and elbow at 90 degrees | | | ○ | ○ | ○ | ○ | ○ | ○ |
| Allow hand/wrist to lie off the edge of the table, palm down | | | ○ | ○ | ○ | ○ | ○ | ○ |
| **Tester and goniometer placed in proper position** | | | **Y** | **N** | **Y** | **N** | **Y** | **N** |
| Sits or stands next to or in front of the patient | | | ○ | ○ | ○ | ○ | ○ | ○ |
| Places center of fulcrum over triquetrum on lateral aspect of wrist | | | ○ | ○ | ○ | ○ | ○ | ○ |
| Stationary arm aligned with lateral midline of ulna | | | ○ | ○ | ○ | ○ | ○ | ○ |
| Moving arm aligned with lateral midline of fifth metacarpal | | | ○ | ○ | ○ | ○ | ○ | ○ |
| **Tester performs test according to accepted guidelines** | | | **Y** | **N** | **Y** | **N** | **Y** | **N** |
| Instructs the patient to extend the wrist as far as possible | | | ○ | ○ | ○ | ○ | ○ | ○ |
| Takes proper goniometric measurement once the patient reaches end range | | | ○ | ○ | ○ | ○ | ○ | ○ |
| **Identifies implications** | | | **Y** | **N** | **Y** | **N** | **Y** | **N** |
| Identifies normal ranges (radiocarpal extension = 60 to 80 degrees) | | | ○ | ○ | ○ | ○ | ○ | ○ |
| Total | | | __/9 | | __/9 | | __/9 | |
| Must achieve >6 to pass this examination | | | ⓟ | Ⓕ | ⓟ | Ⓕ | ⓟ | Ⓕ |

| Assessor:<br>Date: | Test 1 Comments: |
|---|---|
| Assessor:<br>Date: | Test 2 Comments: |
| Assessor:<br>Date: | Test 3 Comments: |

**TEST ENVIRONMENTS**
**L:** Laboratory/Classroom
**C:** Clinical/Field Testing
**P:** Practicum
**A:** Assessment/Mock Exam

**TEST INFORMATION**
**Test Statistics:** N/A
**Reference(s):** Norkin & White (2009)

# OSTEOKINEMATIC JOINT MOTION

| NATA EC 5th | BOC RD6 | SKILL |
|---|---|---|
| CE-21d | D2-0203 | Goniometric Assessment: Radiocarpal (Radial Deviation) |

**Supplies Needed:** Table, chairs, small or large goniometer

*This problem allows you the opportunity to demonstrate a* **goniometric assessment** *for* **radiocarpal (radial deviation)**. *You have 2 minutes to complete this task.*

| Goniometric Assessment: Radiocarpal (Radial Deviation) | Course or Site Assessor Environment _____ _____ _____ | | | | | |
|---|---|---|---|---|---|---|
| | | Test 1 | | Test 2 | | Test 3 |
| **Tester places patient and limb in appropriate position** | | Y | N | Y | N | Y | N |
| Seated with forearm on table, shoulder and elbow at 90 degrees | | O | O | O | O | O | O |
| Allow hand/wrist to rest on table, palm down | | O | O | O | O | O | O |
| **Tester and goniometer placed in proper position** | | Y | N | Y | N | Y | N |
| Sits or stands next to or in front of the patient | | O | O | O | O | O | O |
| Places center of fulcrum over capitate on dorsal aspect of wrist | | O | O | O | O | O | O |
| Stationary arm aligned with dorsal midline of forearm | | O | O | O | O | O | O |
| Moving arm aligned with dorsal midline of third metacarpal | | O | O | O | O | O | O |
| **Tester performs test according to accepted guidelines** | | Y | N | Y | N | Y | N |
| Instructs the patient to radially deviate as far as possible | | O | O | O | O | O | O |
| Takes proper goniometric measurement once the patient reaches end range | | O | O | O | O | O | O |
| **Identifies implications** | | Y | N | Y | N | Y | N |
| Identifies normal ranges (radiocarpal radial deviation = 20 degrees) | | O | O | O | O | O | O |
| Total | | ___/9 | | ___/9 | | ___/9 | |
| Must achieve >6 to pass this examination | | P | F | P | F | P | F |

| Assessor: Date: | Test 1 Comments: |
|---|---|
| Assessor: Date: | Test 2 Comments: |
| Assessor: Date: | Test 3 Comments: |

**TEST ENVIRONMENTS**
**L:** Laboratory/Classroom
**C:** Clinical/Field Testing
**P:** Practicum
**A:** Assessment/Mock Exam

**TEST INFORMATION**
**Test Statistics:** N/A
**Reference(s):** Norkin & White (2009)

## MUSCULOSKELETAL SYSTEM—REGION 9: WRIST AND HAND
# OSTEOKINEMATIC JOINT MOTION

| NATA EC 5th | BOC RD6 | SKILL |
|---|---|---|
| CE-21d | D2-0203 | Goniometric Assessment: Radiocarpal (Ulnar Deviation) |

**Supplies Needed:** Table, chairs, small or large goniometer

*This problem allows you the opportunity to demonstrate a* **goniometric assessment** *for* **radiocarpal (ulnar deviation)**. *You have 2 minutes to complete this task.*

| Goniometric Assessment: Radiocarpal (Ulnar Deviation) | Course or Site Assessor Environment | | Test 1 | | Test 2 | | Test 3 | |
|---|---|---|---|---|---|---|---|---|
| **Tester places patient and limb in appropriate position** | | | **Y** | **N** | **Y** | **N** | **Y** | **N** |
| Seated with forearm on table, shoulder and elbow at 90 degrees | | | O | O | O | O | O | O |
| Allow hand/wrist to rest on table, palm down | | | O | O | O | O | O | O |
| **Tester and goniometer placed in proper position** | | | **Y** | **N** | **Y** | **N** | **Y** | **N** |
| Sits or stands next to or in front of the patient | | | O | O | O | O | O | O |
| Places center of fulcrum over capitate on dorsal aspect of wrist | | | O | O | O | O | O | O |
| Stationary arm aligned with dorsal midline of forearm | | | O | O | O | O | O | O |
| Moving arm aligned with dorsal midline of third metacarpal | | | O | O | O | O | O | O |
| **Tester performs test according to accepted guidelines** | | | **Y** | **N** | **Y** | **N** | **Y** | **N** |
| Instructs the patient to ulnarly deviate as far as possible | | | O | O | O | O | O | O |
| Takes proper goniometric measurement once the patient reaches end range | | | O | O | O | O | O | O |
| **Identifies implications** | | | **Y** | **N** | **Y** | **N** | **Y** | **N** |
| Identifies normal ranges (cervical lateral flexion right = 30 to 40 degrees) | | | O | O | O | O | O | O |
| Total | | | ___/9 | | ___/9 | | ___/9 | |
| Must achieve >6 to pass this examination | | | Ⓟ | Ⓕ | Ⓟ | Ⓕ | Ⓟ | Ⓕ |

| Assessor: Date: | Test 1 Comments: |
|---|---|
| Assessor: Date: | Test 2 Comments: |
| Assessor: Date: | Test 3 Comments: |

**TEST ENVIRONMENTS**
**L:** Laboratory/Classroom
**C:** Clinical/Field Testing
**P:** Practicum
**A:** Assessment/Mock Exam

**TEST INFORMATION**
**Test Statistics:** N/A
**Reference(s):** Norkin & White (2009)

MUSCULOSKELETAL SYSTEM—REGION 9: WRIST AND HAND
# CAPSULAR AND LIGAMENTOUS STRESS TESTING

| NATA EC 5th | BOC RD6 | SKILL |
|---|---|---|
| CE-21e | D2-0203 | Gamekeeper's Thumb Test (Ulnar Collateral Ligament Test) |

**Supplies Needed:** Table or chair

*This problem allows you the opportunity to demonstrate an* **orthopedic test** *known as the* **gamekeeper's thumb test (ulnar collateral ligament test)**. *You have 2 minutes to complete this task.*

| Gamekeeper's Thumb Test (Ulnar Collateral Ligament Test) | Course or Site Assessor Environment | | Test 1 | | Test 2 | | Test 3 | |
|---|---|---|---|---|---|---|---|---|
| **Tester places patient and limb in appropriate position** | | | Y | N | Y | N | Y | N |
| Seated or standing | | | ○ | ○ | ○ | ○ | ○ | ○ |
| **Tester placed in proper position** | | | Y | N | Y | N | Y | N |
| Stands in front of the patient | | | ○ | ○ | ○ | ○ | ○ | ○ |
| One hand stabilizes first metacarpal | | | ○ | ○ | ○ | ○ | ○ | ○ |
| Other hand stabilizes first proximal phalanx | | | ○ | ○ | ○ | ○ | ○ | ○ |
| **Tester performs test according to accepted guidelines** | | | Y | N | Y | N | Y | N |
| Applies a valgus stress to UCL with thumb slightly abducted and extended | | | ○ | ○ | ○ | ○ | ○ | ○ |
| **Identifies positive findings and implications** | | | Y | N | Y | N | Y | N |
| Ulnar side of first MCP joint gaps farther than uninjured side or the patient has pain, or both | | | ○ | ○ | ○ | ○ | ○ | ○ |
| Sprain of the UCL, avulsion fracture | | | ○ | ○ | ○ | ○ | ○ | ○ |
| Total | | | ___/7 | | ___/7 | | ___/7 | |
| Must achieve >4 to pass this examination | | | Ⓟ | Ⓕ | Ⓟ | Ⓕ | Ⓟ | Ⓕ |

| Assessor: Date: | Test 1 Comments: |
|---|---|
| Assessor: Date: | Test 2 Comments: |
| Assessor: Date: | Test 3 Comments: |

**TEST ENVIRONMENTS**
**L:** Laboratory/Classroom
**C:** Clinical/Field Testing
**P:** Practicum
**A:** Assessment/Mock Exam

**TEST INFORMATION**
**Test Statistics:** No data available
**Reference(s):**  Starkey & Brown (2015)

## MUSCULOSKELETAL SYSTEM—REGION 9: WRIST AND HAND
# CAPSULAR AND LIGAMENTOUS STRESS TESTING

| NATA EC 5th | BOC RD6 | SKILL |
|---|---|---|
| CE-21e | D2-0203 | Interphalangeal Joint Valgus Stress Test |

**Supplies Needed:** Table or chair

*This problem allows you the opportunity to demonstrate an* **orthopedic test** *known as the* **interphalangeal joint valgus stress test**. *You have 2 minutes to complete this task.*

| Interphalangeal Joint Valgus Stress Test | Course or Site _____ _____ _____<br>Assessor _____ _____ _____<br>Environment _____ _____ _____ | Test 1 | | Test 2 | | Test 3 | |
|---|---|---|---|---|---|---|---|
| **Tester places patient and limb in appropriate position** | | Y | N | Y | N | Y | N |
| Seated or standing | | ○ | ○ | ○ | ○ | ○ | ○ |
| Joint being tested is in extension | | ○ | ○ | ○ | ○ | ○ | ○ |
| **Tester placed in proper position** | | Y | N | Y | N | Y | N |
| Stands in front of the patient | | ○ | ○ | ○ | ○ | ○ | ○ |
| One hand stabilizes the phalanx proximal to the joint being tested | | ○ | ○ | ○ | ○ | ○ | ○ |
| Other hand grasps distal phalanx to the joint being tested | | ○ | ○ | ○ | ○ | ○ | ○ |
| **Tester performs test according to accepted guidelines** | | Y | N | Y | N | Y | N |
| Applies a valgus stress to joint | | ○ | ○ | ○ | ○ | ○ | ○ |
| **Identifies positive findings and implications** | | Y | N | Y | N | Y | N |
| Increased gapping compared to uninjured side and/or pain | | ○ | ○ | ○ | ○ | ○ | ○ |
| Collateral ligament sprain of IP joint, avulsion fracture | | ○ | ○ | ○ | ○ | ○ | ○ |
| Total | | ____ /8 | | ____ /8 | | ____ /8 | |
| Must achieve >5 to pass this examination | | Ⓟ | Ⓕ | Ⓟ | Ⓕ | Ⓟ | Ⓕ |

| Assessor:<br>Date: | Test 1 Comments: |
|---|---|
| Assessor:<br>Date: | Test 2 Comments: |
| Assessor:<br>Date: | Test 3 Comments: |

**TEST ENVIRONMENTS**
**L:** Laboratory/Classroom
**C:** Clinical/Field Testing
**P:** Practicum
**A:** Assessment/Mock Exam

**TEST INFORMATION**
**Test Statistics:** No data available
**Reference(s):** Starkey & Brown (2015)

# CAPSULAR AND LIGAMENTOUS STRESS TESTING

| NATA EC 5th | BOC RD6 | SKILL |
|---|---|---|
| CE-21e | D2-0203 | Interphalangeal Joint Varus Stress Test |

**Supplies Needed:** Table or chair

*This problem allows you the opportunity to demonstrate an* **orthopedic test** *known as the* **interphalangeal joint varus stress test**. *You have 2 minutes to complete this task.*

| Interphalangeal Joint Varus Stress Test | Course or Site<br>Assessor<br>Environment | | Test 1 | | Test 2 | | Test 3 |
|---|---|---|---|---|---|---|---|
| | | **Y** | **N** | **Y** | **N** | **Y** | **N** |
| **Tester places patient and limb in appropriate position** | | **Y** | **N** | **Y** | **N** | **Y** | **N** |
| Seated or standing | | O | O | O | O | O | O |
| Joint being tested is in extension | | O | O | O | O | O | O |
| **Tester placed in proper position** | | **Y** | **N** | **Y** | **N** | **Y** | **N** |
| Stands in front of the patient | | O | O | O | O | O | O |
| One hand stabilizes the phalanx proximal to the joint being tested | | O | O | O | O | O | O |
| Other hand grasps distal phalanx to the joint being tested | | O | O | O | O | O | O |
| **Tester performs test according to accepted guidelines** | | **Y** | **N** | **Y** | **N** | **Y** | **N** |
| Applies a varus stress to joint | | O | O | O | O | O | O |
| **Identifies positive findings and implications** | | **Y** | **N** | **Y** | **N** | **Y** | **N** |
| Increased gapping compared to uninjured side and/or pain | | O | O | O | O | O | O |
| Collateral ligament sprain of IP joint, avulsion fracture | | O | O | O | O | O | O |
| **Total** | | ___/8 | | ___/8 | | ___/8 | |
| **Must achieve >5 to pass this examination** | | Ⓟ | Ⓕ | Ⓟ | Ⓕ | Ⓟ | Ⓕ |

| Assessor:<br>Date: | **Test 1 Comments:** |
|---|---|
| Assessor:<br>Date: | **Test 2 Comments:** |
| Assessor:<br>Date: | **Test 3 Comments:** |

**TEST ENVIRONMENTS**
**L:** Laboratory/Classroom
**C:** Clinical/Field Testing
**P:** Practicum
**A:** Assessment/Mock Exam

**TEST INFORMATION**
**Test Statistics:** No data available
**Reference(s):** Starkey & Brown (2015)

## MUSCULOSKELETAL SYSTEM—REGION 9: WRIST AND HAND
# CAPSULAR AND LIGAMENTOUS STRESS TESTING

| NATA EC 5th | BOC RD6 | SKILL |
|---|---|---|
| CE-21e | D2-0203 | Radiocarpal Valgus Stress Test |

**Supplies Needed:** Table or chair

*This problem allows you the opportunity to demonstrate an* **orthopedic test** *known as the* **radiocarpal valgus stress test**. *You have 2 minutes to complete this task.*

| Radiocarpal Valgus Stress Test | Course or Site<br>Assessor<br>Environment | | | | | |
|---|---|---|---|---|---|---|
| | | Test 1 | | Test 2 | | Test 3 |
| **Tester places patient and limb in appropriate position** | | Y | N | Y | N | Y | N |
| Seated | | ○ | ○ | ○ | ○ | ○ | ○ |
| Elbow flexed to 90 degrees, forearm pronated, fingers relaxed in flexion | | ○ | ○ | ○ | ○ | ○ | ○ |
| **Tester placed in proper position** | | Y | N | Y | N | Y | N |
| Sits or stands lateral to wrist | | ○ | ○ | ○ | ○ | ○ | ○ |
| One hand grips distal forearm | | ○ | ○ | ○ | ○ | ○ | ○ |
| Other hand grasps hand across the metacarpals | | ○ | ○ | ○ | ○ | ○ | ○ |
| **Tester performs test according to accepted guidelines** | | Y | N | Y | N | Y | N |
| A valgus stress test is applied, radially deviating the wrist | | ○ | ○ | ○ | ○ | ○ | ○ |
| **Identifies positive findings and implications** | | Y | N | Y | N | Y | N |
| Pain or laxity (or both) compared with other wrist | | ○ | ○ | ○ | ○ | ○ | ○ |
| Stretching or tearing of ulnar collateral ligament | | ○ | ○ | ○ | ○ | ○ | ○ |
| Total | | ___/8 | | ___/8 | | ___/8 |
| Must achieve >5 to pass this examination | | Ⓟ | Ⓕ | Ⓟ | Ⓕ | Ⓟ | Ⓕ |

| Assessor:<br>Date: | Test 1 Comments: |
|---|---|
| Assessor:<br>Date: | Test 2 Comments: |
| Assessor:<br>Date: | Test 3 Comments: |

**TEST ENVIRONMENTS**
**L:** Laboratory/Classroom
**C:** Clinical/Field Testing
**P:** Practicum
**A:** Assessment/Mock Exam

**TEST INFORMATION**
**Test Statistics:** No data available
**Reference(s):** Starkey & Brown (2015)

# CAPSULAR AND LIGAMENTOUS STRESS TESTING

| NATA EC 5th | BOC RD6 | SKILL |
|---|---|---|
| CE-21e | D2-0203 | Radiocarpal Varus Stress Test |

**Supplies Needed:** Table or chair

*This problem allows you the opportunity to demonstrate an* **orthopedic test** *known as the* **radiocarpal varus stress test.** *You have 2 minutes to complete this task.*

| Radiocarpal Varus Stress Test | Course or Site Assessor Environment | | Test 1 | | Test 2 | | Test 3 | |
|---|---|---|---|---|---|---|---|---|
| **Tester places patient and limb in appropriate position** | | | Y | N | Y | N | Y | N |
| Seated | | | ○ | ○ | ○ | ○ | ○ | ○ |
| Elbow flexed to 90 degrees, forearm pronated, fingers relaxed in flexion | | | ○ | ○ | ○ | ○ | ○ | ○ |
| **Tester placed in proper position** | | | Y | N | Y | N | Y | N |
| Sits or stands lateral to wrist | | | ○ | ○ | ○ | ○ | ○ | ○ |
| One hand grips distal forearm | | | ○ | ○ | ○ | ○ | ○ | ○ |
| Other hand grasps hand across the metacarpals | | | ○ | ○ | ○ | ○ | ○ | ○ |
| **Tester performs test according to accepted guidelines** | | | Y | N | Y | N | Y | N |
| A varus stress test is applied, ulnarly deviating the wrist | | | ○ | ○ | ○ | ○ | ○ | ○ |
| **Identifies positive findings and implications** | | | Y | N | Y | N | Y | N |
| Pain or laxity (or both) compared with other wrist | | | ○ | ○ | ○ | ○ | ○ | ○ |
| Stretching or tearing of radial collateral ligament | | | ○ | ○ | ○ | ○ | ○ | ○ |
| Total | | | ___/8 | | ___/8 | | ___/8 | |
| **Must achieve >5 to pass this examination** | | | Ⓟ | Ⓕ | Ⓟ | Ⓕ | Ⓟ | Ⓕ |
| Assessor: Date: | Test 1 Comments: | | | | | | | |
| Assessor: Date: | Test 2 Comments: | | | | | | | |
| Assessor: Date: | Test 3 Comments: | | | | | | | |

**TEST ENVIRONMENTS**
**L:** Laboratory/Classroom
**C:** Clinical/Field Testing
**P:** Practicum
**A:** Assessment/Mock Exam

**TEST INFORMATION**
**Test Statistics:** No data available
**Reference(s):** Starkey & Brown (2015)

## MUSCULOSKELETAL SYSTEM—REGION 9: WRIST AND HAND
# JOINT PLAY (ARTHROKINEMATICS)

| NATA EC 5th | BOC RD6 | SKILL |
|---|---|---|
| CE-21f | D2-0203 | Intermetacarpal Glide |

**Supplies Needed:** Table or chair

*This problem allows you the opportunity to demonstrate an* **orthopedic test** *known as the* **intermetacarpal glide.** *You have 2 minutes to complete this task.*

| Intermetacarpal Glide | Course or Site<br>Assessor<br>Environment | | | | | | |
|---|---|---|---|---|---|---|---|
| | | Test 1 | | Test 2 | | Test 3 | |
| **Tester places patient and limb in appropriate position** | | Y | N | Y | N | Y | N |
| Seated | | ○ | ○ | ○ | ○ | ○ | ○ |
| Elbow flexed to 90 degrees, forearm pronated, fingers relaxed | | ○ | ○ | ○ | ○ | ○ | ○ |
| **Tester placed in proper position** | | Y | N | Y | N | Y | N |
| Sits or stands lateral to wrist | | ○ | ○ | ○ | ○ | ○ | ○ |
| One hand grasps the head of one metacarpal | | ○ | ○ | ○ | ○ | ○ | ○ |
| Other hand grasps the head of the metacarpal right next to it | | ○ | ○ | ○ | ○ | ○ | ○ |
| **Tester performs test according to accepted guidelines** | | Y | N | Y | N | Y | N |
| Applies a shear force by gliding one metacarpal in a palmar and dorsal aspect | | ○ | ○ | ○ | ○ | ○ | ○ |
| **Identifies positive findings and implications** | | Y | N | Y | N | Y | N |
| Pain or significant change in glide compared to other side | | ○ | ○ | ○ | ○ | ○ | ○ |
| Trauma to tissue between metacarpals, decreased glide may indicate adhesions | | ○ | ○ | ○ | ○ | ○ | ○ |
| Total | | ___/8 | | ___/8 | | ___/8 | |
| **Must achieve >5 to pass this examination** | | Ⓟ | Ⓕ | Ⓟ | Ⓕ | Ⓟ | Ⓕ |

| Assessor:<br>Date: | **Test 1 Comments:** |
|---|---|
| Assessor:<br>Date: | **Test 2 Comments:** |
| Assessor:<br>Date: | **Test 3 Comments:** |

**TEST ENVIRONMENTS**
**L:** Laboratory/Classroom
**C:** Clinical/Field Testing
**P:** Practicum
**A:** Assessment/Mock Exam

**TEST INFORMATION**
**Test Statistics:** No data available
**Reference(s):** Starkey & Brown (2015)

## MUSCULOSKELETAL SYSTEM—REGION 9: WRIST AND HAND
# JOINT PLAY (ARTHROKINEMATICS)

| NATA EC 5th | BOC RD6 | SKILL |
|---|---|---|
| CE-21f | D2-0203 | Carpometacarpal Glide |

**Supplies Needed:** Table or chair

*This problem allows you the opportunity to demonstrate an* **orthopedic test** *known as the* **carpometacarpal glide***. You have 2 minutes to complete this task.*

| Carpometacarpal Glide | Course or Site Assessor Environment | Test 1 | | Test 2 | | Test 3 | |
|---|---|---|---|---|---|---|---|
| | | **Y** | **N** | **Y** | **N** | **Y** | **N** |
| **Tester places patient and limb in appropriate position** | | **Y** | **N** | **Y** | **N** | **Y** | **N** |
| Seated | | ○ | ○ | ○ | ○ | ○ | ○ |
| Elbow flexed to 90 degrees, forearm pronated, fingers relaxed | | ○ | ○ | ○ | ○ | ○ | ○ |
| **Tester placed in proper position** | | **Y** | **N** | **Y** | **N** | **Y** | **N** |
| Sits or stands lateral to wrist | | ○ | ○ | ○ | ○ | ○ | ○ |
| One hand stabilizes the distal row of carpal bones | | ○ | ○ | ○ | ○ | ○ | ○ |
| Other hand grasps the base of one metacarpal being tested | | ○ | ○ | ○ | ○ | ○ | ○ |
| **Tester performs test according to accepted guidelines** | | **Y** | **N** | **Y** | **N** | **Y** | **N** |
| Applies a shear force by gliding the metacarpal in a palmar and dorsal aspect | | ○ | ○ | ○ | ○ | ○ | ○ |
| **Identifies positive findings and implications** | | **Y** | **N** | **Y** | **N** | **Y** | **N** |
| Pain or significant change in glide compared to other side | | ○ | ○ | ○ | ○ | ○ | ○ |
| Tear or stretching of carpometacarpal ligaments, decreased glide may indicate adhesions and capsular stiffness | | ○ | ○ | ○ | ○ | ○ | ○ |
| Total | | ___/8 | | ___/8 | | ___/8 | |
| **Must achieve >5 to pass this examination** | | Ⓟ | Ⓕ | Ⓟ | Ⓕ | Ⓟ | Ⓕ |

| Assessor: Date: | Test 1 Comments: |
|---|---|
| Assessor: Date: | Test 2 Comments: |
| Assessor: Date: | Test 3 Comments: |

**TEST ENVIRONMENTS**
**L:** Laboratory/Classroom
**C:** Clinical/Field Testing
**P:** Practicum
**A:** Assessment/Mock Exam

**TEST INFORMATION**
**Test Statistics:** No data available
**Reference(s):** Starkey & Brown (2015)

# JOINT PLAY (ARTHROKINEMATICS)

| NATA EC 5th | BOC RD6 | SKILL |
|---|---|---|
| CE-21f | D2-0203 | Radiocarpal Glide |

**Supplies Needed:** Table or chair

*This problem allows you the opportunity to demonstrate an* **orthopedic test** *known as the* **radiocarpal glide.**
*You have 2 minutes to complete this task.*

| Radiocarpal Glide | Course or Site Assessor Environment | | Test 1 | | Test 2 | | Test 3 |
|---|---|---|---|---|---|---|---|
| | | Y | N | Y | N | Y | N |
| **Tester places patient and limb in appropriate position** | | Y | N | Y | N | Y | N |
| Seated | | ○ | ○ | ○ | ○ | ○ | ○ |
| Elbow flexed to 90 degrees, forearm pronated, fingers relaxed | | ○ | ○ | ○ | ○ | ○ | ○ |
| **Tester placed in proper position** | | Y | N | Y | N | Y | N |
| Sits or stands lateral to wrist | | ○ | ○ | ○ | ○ | ○ | ○ |
| One hand grips the distal radius | | ○ | ○ | ○ | ○ | ○ | ○ |
| Other hand grasps the proximal carpal row | | ○ | ○ | ○ | ○ | ○ | ○ |
| **Tester performs test according to accepted guidelines** | | Y | N | Y | N | Y | N |
| Applies a shear force by gliding the distal segment in a radial and ulnar direction, then in a dorsal and palmar direction | | ○ | ○ | ○ | ○ | ○ | ○ |
| **Identifies positive findings and implications** | | Y | N | Y | N | Y | N |
| Pain or significant change in glide compared to other side | | ○ | ○ | ○ | ○ | ○ | ○ |
| Sprain of the collateral or intercarpal ligaments or trauma to the triangular fibrocartilage, decreased glide may indicate adhesions and capsular stiffness | | ○ | ○ | ○ | ○ | ○ | ○ |
| **Total** | | __/8 | | __/8 | | __/8 | |
| **Must achieve >5 to pass this examination** | | Ⓟ | Ⓕ | Ⓟ | Ⓕ | Ⓟ | Ⓕ |

| Assessor: Date: | Test 1 Comments: |
|---|---|
| Assessor: Date: | Test 2 Comments: |
| Assessor: Date: | Test 3 Comments: |

**TEST ENVIRONMENTS**
**L:** Laboratory/Classroom
**C:** Clinical/Field Testing
**P:** Practicum
**A:** Assessment/Mock Exam

**TEST INFORMATION**
**Test Statistics:** No data available
**Reference(s):** Starkey & Brown (2015)

## MUSCULOSKELETAL SYSTEM—REGION 9: WRIST AND HAND
# SPECIAL TESTS

| NATA EC 5th | BOC RD6 | SKILL |
|---|---|---|
| CE-21g, CE-20e | D2-0203 | Allen's Test |

**Supplies Needed:** Table or chair

*This problem allows you the opportunity to demonstrate a **special test** known as **Allen's test**.*
*You have 2 minutes to complete this task.*

| Allen's Test | Course or Site<br>Assessor<br>Environment | Test 1 | | Test 2 | | Test 3 | |
|---|---|---|---|---|---|---|---|
| | | **Y** | **N** | **Y** | **N** | **Y** | **N** |
| **Tester places patient and limb in appropriate position** | | | | | | | |
| Seated or standing | | ○ | ○ | ○ | ○ | ○ | ○ |
| **Tester placed in proper position** | | **Y** | **N** | **Y** | **N** | **Y** | **N** |
| Stands in front of the patient | | ○ | ○ | ○ | ○ | ○ | ○ |
| Applies pressure to the radial and ulnar arteries to compress them | | ○ | ○ | ○ | ○ | ○ | ○ |
| **Tester performs test according to accepted guidelines** | | **Y** | **N** | **Y** | **N** | **Y** | **N** |
| Instructs the patient to open and close hand rapidly and then to keep a tightly closed fist | | ○ | ○ | ○ | ○ | ○ | ○ |
| Releases pressure on one artery and observes hand | | ○ | ○ | ○ | ○ | ○ | ○ |
| **Identifies positive findings and implications** | | **Y** | **N** | **Y** | **N** | **Y** | **N** |
| Uneven filling (return of redness/color) into the hand | | ○ | ○ | ○ | ○ | ○ | ○ |
| Restriction of blood flow | | ○ | ○ | ○ | ○ | ○ | ○ |
| Total | | ___/7 | | ___/7 | | ___/7 | |
| Must achieve >4 to pass this examination | | Ⓟ | Ⓕ | Ⓟ | Ⓕ | Ⓟ | Ⓕ |

| Assessor:<br>Date: | Test 1 Comments: |
|---|---|
| Assessor:<br>Date: | Test 2 Comments: |
| Assessor:<br>Date: | Test 3 Comments: |

**TEST ENVIRONMENTS**
**L:** Laboratory/Classroom
**C:** Clinical/Field Testing
**P:** Practicum
**A:** Assessment/Mock Exam

**TEST INFORMATION**
**Test Statistics:** No data available
**Reference(s):** Starkey & Brown (2015)

## MUSCULOSKELETAL SYSTEM—REGION 9: WRIST AND HAND
# SPECIAL TESTS

| NATA EC 5th | BOC RD6 | SKILL |
|---|---|---|
| CE-21g, CE-20e | D2-0203 | Finkelstein's Test |

**Supplies Needed:** Table or chair

*This problem allows you the opportunity to demonstrate a **special test** known as **Finkelstein's test** to rule out possible **de Quervain's syndrome**. You have 2 minutes to complete this task.*

| Finkelstein's Test | Course or Site Assessor Environment | | | | | |
|---|---|---|---|---|---|---|
| | | Test 1 | | Test 2 | | Test 3 |
| **Tester places patient and limb in appropriate position** | | Y | N | Y | N | Y | N |
| Seated or standing | | ○ | ○ | ○ | ○ | ○ | ○ |
| **Tester placed in proper position** | | Y | N | Y | N | Y | N |
| Stands in front of the patient | | ○ | ○ | ○ | ○ | ○ | ○ |
| **Tester performs test according to accepted guidelines** | | Y | N | Y | N | Y | N |
| Instructs the patient to tuck the thumb under the fingers by making a fist | | ○ | ○ | ○ | ○ | ○ | ○ |
| Instructs the patient to then ulnarly deviate the wrist | | ○ | ○ | ○ | ○ | ○ | ○ |
| **Identifies positive findings and implications** | | Y | N | Y | N | Y | N |
| Increased pain in area of radial styloid process and along length of extensor pollicis brevis/abductor pollicis longus tendons | | ○ | ○ | ○ | ○ | ○ | ○ |
| De Quervain's syndrome (tenosynovitis of those tendons) | | ○ | ○ | ○ | ○ | ○ | ○ |
| **Total** | | ___/6 | | ___/6 | | ___/6 |
| **Must achieve >4 to pass this examination** | | Ⓟ | Ⓕ | Ⓟ | Ⓕ | Ⓟ | Ⓕ |

| Assessor: Date: | Test 1 Comments: |
|---|---|
| Assessor: Date: | Test 2 Comments: |
| Assessor: Date: | Test 3 Comments: |

**TEST ENVIRONMENTS**
**L:** Laboratory/Classroom
**C:** Clinical/Field Testing
**P:** Practicum
**A:** Assessment/Mock Exam

**TEST INFORMATION**
**Test Statistics:** Sensitivity .81
Specificity .5
(+) LR 1.62
(-) LR .38
**Reference(s):** Cook & Hegedus (2013)
Starkey & Brown (2015)

## MUSCULOSKELETAL SYSTEM—REGION 9: WRIST AND HAND
# SPECIAL TESTS

| NATA EC 5th | BOC RD6 | SKILL |
|---|---|---|
| CE-21g, CE-20e | D2-0203 | Phalen's Test (Wrist Flexion Test) |

**Supplies Needed:** Table or chair

*This problem allows you the opportunity to demonstrate a* **special test** *known as* **Phalen's test (wrist flexion test)** *to rule out possible* **carpal tunnel syndrome***. You have 2 minutes to complete this task.*

| Phalen's Test (Wrist Flexion Test) | Course or Site Assessor Environment | Test 1 | | Test 2 | | Test 3 | |
|---|---|---|---|---|---|---|---|
| | | Y | N | Y | N | Y | N |
| **Tester places patient and limb in appropriate position** | | Y | N | Y | N | Y | N |
| Seated or standing | | ○ | ○ | ○ | ○ | ○ | ○ |
| **Tester placed in proper position** | | Y | N | Y | N | Y | N |
| Stands in front of the patient | | ○ | ○ | ○ | ○ | ○ | ○ |
| **Tester performs test according to accepted guidelines** | | Y | N | Y | N | Y | N |
| Applies overpressure during passive wrist flexion | | ○ | ○ | ○ | ○ | ○ | ○ |
| Holds position for 1 minute | | ○ | ○ | ○ | ○ | ○ | ○ |
| **Identifies positive findings and implications** | | Y | N | Y | N | Y | N |
| Tingling into the thumb, index finger, middle finger, and radial half of the fourth finger | | ○ | ○ | ○ | ○ | ○ | ○ |
| Medial nerve compression (carpal tunnel syndrome) | | ○ | ○ | ○ | ○ | ○ | ○ |
| | Total | ___/6 | | ___/6 | | ___/6 | |
| **Must achieve >4 to pass this examination** | | Ⓟ | Ⓕ | Ⓟ | Ⓕ | Ⓟ | Ⓕ |

| Assessor: Date: | Test 1 Comments: |
|---|---|
| Assessor: Date: | Test 2 Comments: |
| Assessor: Date: | Test 3 Comments: |

**TEST ENVIRONMENTS**
**L:** Laboratory/Classroom
**C:** Clinical/Field Testing
**P:** Practicum
**A:** Assessment/Mock Exam

**TEST INFORMATION**
**Test Statistics:** Sensitivity .1–.92
Specificity .33–1
(+) LR .57–41.5
(-) LR 1–.15
**Reference(s):** Cook & Hegedus (2013)
Starkey & Brown (2015)

## MUSCULOSKELETAL SYSTEM—REGION 9: WRIST AND HAND
# SPECIAL TESTS

| NATA EC 5th | BOC RD6 | SKILL |
|---|---|---|
| CE-21g, CE-20e | D2-0203 | Reagan's Test |

**Supplies Needed:** Table or chair

*This problem allows you the opportunity to demonstrate a* **special test** *known as* **Reagan's test** *to rule out possible* **instability of the joint between lunate and triquetrum** *and/or* **dislocation/subluxation of lunate**. *You have 2 minutes to complete this task.*

| Reagan's Test | Course or Site _____ Assessor _____ Environment _____ | | Test 1 | | Test 2 | | Test 3 |
|---|---|---|---|---|---|---|---|
| | | **Y** | **N** | **Y** | **N** | **Y** | **N** |
| **Tester places patient and limb in appropriate position** | | **Y** | **N** | **Y** | **N** | **Y** | **N** |
| Seated | | O | O | O | O | O | O |
| **Tester placed in proper position** | | **Y** | **N** | **Y** | **N** | **Y** | **N** |
| Stands in front of the patient | | O | O | O | O | O | O |
| One hand grips the triquetrum with index finger and thumb | | O | O | O | O | O | O |
| Other hand grasps the lunate on anterior and posterior surfaces | | O | O | O | O | O | O |
| **Tester performs test according to accepted guidelines** | | **Y** | **N** | **Y** | **N** | **Y** | **N** |
| Moves lunate in an anterior-posterior direction | | O | O | O | O | O | O |
| **Identifies positive findings and implications** | | **Y** | **N** | **Y** | **N** | **Y** | **N** |
| Pain, laxity, and/or crepitus | | O | O | O | O | O | O |
| Instability of joint between lunate and triquetrum and/or dislocation/subluxation of lunate | | O | O | O | O | O | O |
| **Total** | | ___/7 | | ___/7 | | ___/7 | |
| **Must achieve >4 to pass this examination** | | Ⓟ | Ⓕ | Ⓟ | Ⓕ | Ⓟ | Ⓕ |

| Assessor:<br>Date: | Test 1 Comments: |
|---|---|
| Assessor:<br>Date: | Test 2 Comments: |
| Assessor:<br>Date: | Test 3 Comments: |

**TEST ENVIRONMENTS**
**L:** Laboratory/Classroom
**C:** Clinical/Field Testing
**P:** Practicum
**A:** Assessment/Mock Exam

**TEST INFORMATION**
**Test Statistics:** Sensitivity .64
Specificity .44
(+) LR 1.14
(-) LR .82
**Reference(s):** Cook & Hegedus (2013)
Starkey & Brown (2015)

## MUSCULOSKELETAL SYSTEM—REGION 9: WRIST AND HAND
# SPECIAL TESTS

| NATA EC 5th | BOC RD6 | SKILL |
|---|---|---|
| CE-21g, CE-20e | D2-0203 | Reverse Phalen's Test |

**Supplies Needed:** Table or chair

*This problem allows you the opportunity to demonstrate a **special test** known as the **reverse Phalen's test** to rule out possible **carpal tunnel syndrome**. You have 2 minutes to complete this task.*

| Reverse Phalen's Test | Course or Site Assessor Environment | | Test 1 | | Test 2 | | Test 3 | |
|---|---|---|---|---|---|---|---|---|
| **Tester places patient and limb in appropriate position** | | | Y | N | Y | N | Y | N |
| Seated or standing | | | ○ | ○ | ○ | ○ | ○ | ○ |
| **Tester placed in proper position** | | | Y | N | Y | N | Y | N |
| Stands in front of the patient | | | ○ | ○ | ○ | ○ | ○ | ○ |
| **Tester performs test according to accepted guidelines** | | | Y | N | Y | N | Y | N |
| Applies overpressure during passive wrist extension | | | ○ | ○ | ○ | ○ | ○ | ○ |
| Holds position for 1 minute | | | ○ | ○ | ○ | ○ | ○ | ○ |
| **Identifies positive findings and implications** | | | Y | N | Y | N | Y | N |
| Tingling into the thumb, index finger, middle finger, and radial half of the fourth finger | | | ○ | ○ | ○ | ○ | ○ | ○ |
| Medial nerve compression (carpal tunnel syndrome) | | | ○ | ○ | ○ | ○ | ○ | ○ |
| | | Total | __/6 | | __/6 | | __/6 | |
| | **Must achieve >4 to pass this examination** | | Ⓟ | Ⓕ | Ⓟ | Ⓕ | Ⓟ | Ⓕ |

| Assessor: Date: | Test 1 Comments: |
|---|---|
| Assessor: Date: | Test 2 Comments: |
| Assessor: Date: | Test 3 Comments: |

**TEST ENVIRONMENTS**
**L:** Laboratory/Classroom
**C:** Clinical/Field Testing
**P:** Practicum
**A:** Assessment/Mock Exam

**TEST INFORMATION**
**Test Statistics:** No data available
**Reference(s):** Starkey & Brown (2015)

## MUSCULOSKELETAL SYSTEM—REGION 9: WRIST AND HAND
# SPECIAL TESTS

| NATA EC 5th | BOC RD6 | SKILL |
|---|---|---|
| CE-21g, CE-20e | D2-0203 | Scaphoid Compression Test |

**Supplies Needed:** Table or chair

*This problem allows you the opportunity to demonstrate a* **special test** *known as the* **scaphoid compression test** *to rule out possible* **scaphoid fracture**. *You have 2 minutes to complete this task.*

| Scaphoid Compression Test | Course or Site Assessor Environment | | Test 1 | | Test 2 | | Test 3 | |
|---|---|---|---|---|---|---|---|---|
| **Tester places patient and limb in appropriate position** | | Y | N | Y | N | Y | N | |
| Seated | | O | O | O | O | O | O | |
| **Tester placed in proper position** | | Y | N | Y | N | Y | N | |
| Stands or sits in front of the patient | | O | O | O | O | O | O | |
| One hand stabilizes wrist | | O | O | O | O | O | O | |
| Other hand grasps first metacarpal shaft | | O | O | O | O | O | O | |
| **Tester performs test according to accepted guidelines** | | Y | N | Y | N | Y | N | |
| Translates first metacarpal and then applies an axial load to metacarpal, toward scaphoid | | O | O | O | O | O | O | |
| **Identifies positive findings and implications** | | Y | N | Y | N | Y | N | |
| Pain, crepitus | | O | O | O | O | O | O | |
| Scaphoid fracture, Bennett's fracture | | O | O | O | O | O | O | |
| **Total** | | ___/7 | | ___/7 | | ___/7 | | |
| **Must achieve >4 to pass this examination** | | Ⓟ | Ⓕ | Ⓟ | Ⓕ | Ⓟ | Ⓕ | |

| Assessor: Date: | Test 1 Comments: |
|---|---|
| Assessor: Date: | Test 2 Comments: |
| Assessor: Date: | Test 3 Comments: |

**TEST ENVIRONMENTS**
**L:** Laboratory/Classroom
**C:** Clinical/Field Testing
**P:** Practicum
**A:** Assessment/Mock Exam

**TEST INFORMATION**
**Test Statistics:** Sensitivity .7
Specificity .22
(+) LR 1.38
(-) LR .9
**Reference(s):** Cook & Hegedus (2013)
Starkey & Brown (2015)

## MUSCULOSKELETAL SYSTEM—REGION 9: WRIST AND HAND
# SPECIAL TESTS

| NATA EC 5th | BOC RD6 | SKILL |
|---|---|---|
| CE-21g, CE-20e | D2-0203 | Tinel's Sign (Median Nerve) |

**Supplies Needed:** Table or chair

*This problem allows you the opportunity to demonstrate a* **special test** *known as* **Tinel's sign (median nerve)** *to rule out possible* **median nerve pathology**. *You have 2 minutes to complete this task.*

| Tinel's Sign (Median Nerve) | Course or Site Assessor Environment _____ _____ _____ | | Test 1 | | Test 2 | | Test 3 | |
|---|---|---|---|---|---|---|---|---|
| **Tester places patient and limb in appropriate position** | | | Y | N | Y | N | Y | N |
| Seated or standing | | | ◯ | ◯ | ◯ | ◯ | ◯ | ◯ |
| **Tester placed in proper position** | | | Y | N | Y | N | Y | N |
| Stands in front of the patient | | | ◯ | ◯ | ◯ | ◯ | ◯ | ◯ |
| **Tester performs test according to accepted guidelines** | | | Y | N | Y | N | Y | N |
| Taps the surface over the carpal tunnel | | | ◯ | ◯ | ◯ | ◯ | ◯ | ◯ |
| **Identifies positive findings and implications** | | | Y | N | Y | N | Y | N |
| Tingling into the thumb, index finger, middle finger, and radial half of the fourth finger | | | ◯ | ◯ | ◯ | ◯ | ◯ | ◯ |
| Nerve pathology | | | ◯ | ◯ | ◯ | ◯ | ◯ | ◯ |
| Total | | | ____/5 | | ____/5 | | ____/5 | |
| Must achieve >3 to pass this examination | | | Ⓟ | Ⓕ | Ⓟ | Ⓕ | Ⓟ | Ⓕ |
| **Assessor:** **Date:** | Test 1 Comments: | | | | | | | |
| **Assessor:** **Date:** | Test 2 Comments: | | | | | | | |
| **Assessor:** **Date:** | Test 3 Comments: | | | | | | | |

**TEST ENVIRONMENTS**
**L:** Laboratory/Classroom
**C:** Clinical/Field Testing
**P:** Practicum
**A:** Assessment/Mock Exam

**TEST INFORMATION**
**Test Statistics:** Sensitivity .25–.97
Specificity .31–.99
(+) LR .7–64
(-) LR 1.1–.3
**Reference(s):** Cook & Hegedus (2013)
Starkey & Brown (2015)

## MUSCULOSKELETAL SYSTEM—REGION 9: WRIST AND HAND
# SPECIAL TESTS

| NATA EC 5th | BOC RD6 | SKILL |
|---|---|---|
| CE-21g, CE-20e | D2-0203 | Watson's Test (Scapholunate Instability) |

**Supplies Needed:** Table or chair

*This problem allows you the opportunity to demonstrate a* **special test** *known as* **Watson's test** *to rule out possible* **scapholunate instability**. *You have 2 minutes to complete this task.*

| Watson's Test (Scapholunate Instability) | Course or Site Assessor Environment _____ _____ _____ | | Test 1 | | Test 2 | | Test 3 |
|---|---|---|---|---|---|---|---|
| **Tester places patient and limb in appropriate position** | | **Y** | **N** | **Y** | **N** | **Y** | **N** |
| Seated | | ○ | ○ | ○ | ○ | ○ | ○ |
| Elbow flexed on table, forearm and hand pointing up (arm wrestling pose) | | ○ | ○ | ○ | ○ | ○ | ○ |
| **Tester placed in proper position** | | **Y** | **N** | **Y** | **N** | **Y** | **N** |
| Stands or sits in front of the patient | | ○ | ○ | ○ | ○ | ○ | ○ |
| Places thumb of one hand over dorsal pole of scaphoid | | ○ | ○ | ○ | ○ | ○ | ○ |
| Other hand grasps hand over metacarpals | | ○ | ○ | ○ | ○ | ○ | ○ |
| **Tester performs test according to accepted guidelines** | | **Y** | **N** | **Y** | **N** | **Y** | **N** |
| Moves wrist into radial and ulnar deviation while applying pressure over dorsal pole of scaphoid | | ○ | ○ | ○ | ○ | ○ | ○ |
| **Identifies positive findings and implications** | | **Y** | **N** | **Y** | **N** | **Y** | **N** |
| Pain, notable pop at scapholunate articulation | | ○ | ○ | ○ | ○ | ○ | ○ |
| Scapholunate dissociation | | ○ | ○ | ○ | ○ | ○ | ○ |
| Total | | ___/8 | | ___/8 | | ___/8 | |
| **Must achieve >5 to pass this examination** | | Ⓟ | Ⓕ | Ⓟ | Ⓕ | Ⓟ | Ⓕ |

| Assessor: Date: | Test 1 Comments: |
|---|---|
| Assessor: Date: | Test 2 Comments: |
| Assessor: Date: | Test 3 Comments: |

**TEST ENVIRONMENTS**
**L:** Laboratory/Classroom
**C:** Clinical/Field Testing
**P:** Practicum
**A:** Assessment/Mock Exam

**TEST INFORMATION**
**Test Statistics:** Sensitivity .69
Specificity .66
(+) LR 2.0
(-) LR .47
**Reference(s):** Cook & Hegedus (2013)
Starkey & Brown (2015)

MUSCULOSKELETAL SYSTEM—REGION 9: WRIST AND HAND
# NEUROLOGICAL ASSESSMENT

| NATA EC 5th | BOC RD6 | SKILL |
|---|---|---|
| CE-21h, CE-20f | D2-0203 | Median Nerve |

**Supplies Needed:** Table or chair

*This problem allows you the opportunity to demonstrate a* **neurological test** *for the* **median nerve.** *You have 2 minutes to complete this task.*

| Median Nerve | Course or Site<br>Assessor<br>Environment \_\_\_\_\_ \_\_\_\_\_ \_\_\_\_\_ | | | | | |
|---|---|---|---|---|---|---|
| | Test 1 | | Test 2 | | Test 3 | |
| **Tester places patient and limb in appropriate position** | **Y** | **N** | **Y** | **N** | **Y** | **N** |
| Seated | ○ | ○ | ○ | ○ | ○ | ○ |
| Elbow flexed to 90 degrees, forearm supinated | ○ | ○ | ○ | ○ | ○ | ○ |
| **Tester placed in proper position** | **Y** | **N** | **Y** | **N** | **Y** | **N** |
| Stands or sits diagonal from the patient | ○ | ○ | ○ | ○ | ○ | ○ |
| Instructs the patient to oppose thumb and fifth fingers | ○ | ○ | ○ | ○ | ○ | ○ |
| Places one hand over thenar eminence | ○ | ○ | ○ | ○ | ○ | ○ |
| Places other hand over hypothenar eminence | ○ | ○ | ○ | ○ | ○ | ○ |
| **Tester performs test according to accepted guidelines** | **Y** | **N** | **Y** | **N** | **Y** | **N** |
| Attempts to separate the thumb and fifth finger by applying resistance at the distal first and fifth metacarpals | ○ | ○ | ○ | ○ | ○ | ○ |
| **Identifies positive findings and implications** | **Y** | **N** | **Y** | **N** | **Y** | **N** |
| Decrease in strength as compared to the other side | ○ | ○ | ○ | ○ | ○ | ○ |
| Median nerve pathology | ○ | ○ | ○ | ○ | ○ | ○ |
| Any paresthesia over the palmar aspect of second and third metacarpals and phalanges | ○ | ○ | ○ | ○ | ○ | ○ |
| **Total** | \_\_\_\_/10 | | \_\_\_\_/10 | | \_\_\_\_/10 | |
| **Must achieve >6 to pass this examination** | Ⓟ | Ⓕ | Ⓟ | Ⓕ | Ⓟ | Ⓕ |

| Assessor:<br>Date: | **Test 1 Comments:** |
|---|---|
| Assessor:<br>Date: | **Test 2 Comments:** |
| Assessor:<br>Date: | **Test 3 Comments:** |

**TEST ENVIRONMENTS**
**L:** Laboratory/Classroom
**C:** Clinical/Field Testing
**P:** Practicum
**A:** Assessment/Mock Exam

**TEST INFORMATION**
**Test Statistics:** No data available
**Reference(s):** Starkey & Brown (2015)

## MUSCULOSKELETAL SYSTEM—REGION 9: WRIST AND HAND
# NEUROLOGICAL ASSESSMENT

| NATA EC 5th | BOC RD6 | SKILL |
|---|---|---|
| CE-21h, CE-20f | D2-0203 | Radial Nerve |

**Supplies Needed:** Table or chair

*This problem allows you the opportunity to demonstrate a* **neurological test** *for the* **radial nerve.**
*You have 2 minutes to complete this task.*

| Radial Nerve | Course or Site Assessor Environment | | Test 1 | | Test 2 | | Test 3 | |
|---|---|---|---|---|---|---|---|---|
| **Tester places patient and limb in appropriate position** | | | **Y** | **N** | **Y** | **N** | **Y** | **N** |
| Seated | | | ○ | ○ | ○ | ○ | ○ | ○ |
| Elbow flexed to 90 degrees, forearm pronated, wrist extended and radially deviated | | | ○ | ○ | ○ | ○ | ○ | ○ |
| **Tester placed in proper position** | | | **Y** | **N** | **Y** | **N** | **Y** | **N** |
| Stands or sits diagonal from the patient | | | ○ | ○ | ○ | ○ | ○ | ○ |
| One hand supports forearm | | | ○ | ○ | ○ | ○ | ○ | ○ |
| Other hand applies resistance over dorsal surface of second and third metacarpals | | | ○ | ○ | ○ | ○ | ○ | ○ |
| **Tester performs test according to accepted guidelines** | | | **Y** | **N** | **Y** | **N** | **Y** | **N** |
| Instructs the patient to extend wrist in radial deviation against resistance | | | ○ | ○ | ○ | ○ | ○ | ○ |
| Applies resistance into flexion and ulnar deviation | | | ○ | ○ | ○ | ○ | ○ | ○ |
| Resistance is held for 5 seconds | | | ○ | ○ | ○ | ○ | ○ | ○ |
| Performs bilaterally | | | ○ | ○ | ○ | ○ | ○ | ○ |
| **Identifies positive findings and implications** | | | **Y** | **N** | **Y** | **N** | **Y** | **N** |
| Decrease in strength as compared bilaterally | | | ○ | ○ | ○ | ○ | ○ | ○ |
| Radial nerve pathology, may result in drop wrist syndrome | | | ○ | ○ | ○ | ○ | ○ | ○ |
| Any paresthesia to the tunnel of Guyon | | | ○ | ○ | ○ | ○ | ○ | ○ |
| | | Total | ___/12 | | ___/12 | | ___/12 | |
| | Must achieve >8 to pass this examination | | Ⓟ | Ⓕ | Ⓟ | Ⓕ | Ⓟ | Ⓕ |

| Assessor:
Date: | Test 1 Comments: |
|---|---|
| Assessor:
Date: | Test 2 Comments: |
| Assessor:
Date: | Test 3 Comments: |

**TEST ENVIRONMENTS**
**L:** Laboratory/Classroom
**C:** Clinical/Field Testing
**P:** Practicum
**A:** Assessment/Mock Exam

**TEST INFORMATION**
**Test Statistics:** No data available
**Reference(s):** Starkey & Brown (2015)

## MUSCULOSKELETAL SYSTEM—REGION 9: WRIST AND HAND
## NEUROLOGICAL ASSESSMENT

| NATA EC 5th | BOC RD6 | SKILL |
|---|---|---|
| CE-21h, CE-20f | D2-0203 | Ulnar Nerve |

**Supplies Needed:** Table or chair

*This problem allows you the opportunity to demonstrate a* **neurological test** *for the* **ulnar nerve**. *You have 2 minutes to complete this task.*

| Ulnar Nerve | Course or Site Assessor Environment | | | | | |
|---|---|---|---|---|---|---|
| | Test 1 | | Test 2 | | Test 3 | |
| **Tester places patient and limb in appropriate position** | **Y** | **N** | **Y** | **N** | **Y** | **N** |
| Seated | ○ | ○ | ○ | ○ | ○ | ○ |
| Elbow flexed to 90 degrees, forearm pronated, hand resting on table | ○ | ○ | ○ | ○ | ○ | ○ |
| **Tester placed in proper position** | **Y** | **N** | **Y** | **N** | **Y** | **N** |
| Sits or stands in front of or next to the patient | ○ | ○ | ○ | ○ | ○ | ○ |
| One hand over the ulnar aspect of the fifth metacarpal | ○ | ○ | ○ | ○ | ○ | ○ |
| Other hand stabilizes hand | ○ | ○ | ○ | ○ | ○ | ○ |
| **Tester performs test according to accepted guidelines** | **Y** | **N** | **Y** | **N** | **Y** | **N** |
| Applies resistance over ulnar aspect of proximal fifth phalanx | ○ | ○ | ○ | ○ | ○ | ○ |
| **Identifies positive findings and implications** | **Y** | **N** | **Y** | **N** | **Y** | **N** |
| Decrease in strength as compared to other side | ○ | ○ | ○ | ○ | ○ | ○ |
| Ulnar nerve pathology | ○ | ○ | ○ | ○ | ○ | ○ |
| Any paresthesia over the fifth metacarpal and phalanges | ○ | ○ | ○ | ○ | ○ | ○ |
| **Total** | ___/9 | | ___/9 | | ___/9 | |
| **Must achieve >6 to pass this examination** | Ⓟ | Ⓕ | Ⓟ | Ⓕ | Ⓟ | Ⓕ |

| Assessor: Date: | Test 1 Comments: |
|---|---|
| Assessor: Date: | Test 2 Comments: |
| Assessor: Date: | Test 3 Comments: |

**TEST ENVIRONMENTS**
**L:** Laboratory/Classroom
**C:** Clinical/Field Testing
**P:** Practicum
**A:** Assessment/Mock Exam

**TEST INFORMATION**
**Test Statistics:** No data available
**Reference(s):** Starkey & Brown (2015)

# 13

# MUSCULOSKELETAL SYSTEM— REGION 10: HEAD AND FACE

Hauth, J. M., Gloyeske, B. M., & Amato, H. K.
*Clinical Skills Documentation Guide for Athletic Training, Third Edition* (pp. 415-451).
© 2016 SLACK Incorporated.

## MUSCULOSKELETAL SYSTEM—REGION 10: HEAD AND FACE
# KNOWLEDGE AND SKILLS

| Musculoskeletal System—Region 10: Head and Face | | | | Skill: Acquisition, Reinforcement, Proficiency | | |
|---|---|---|---|---|---|---|
| **NATA EC 5th** | **BOC RD6** | **Palpation** | **Page #** | | | |
| CE-21b, CE-20c | D2-0202 | Palpation: Head and Face – 01 | 417 | | | |
| CE-21b, CE-20c | D2-0202 | Palpation: Head and Face – 02 | 418 | | | |
| CE-21b, CE-20c | D2-0202 | Palpation: Head and Face – 03 | 419 | | | |
| **NATA EC 5th** | **BOC RD6** | **Special Tests** | **Page #** | | | |
| CE-21g, CE-20e | D2-0203 | Halo Test | 420 | | | |
| CE-21g, CE-20e | D2-0203 | Tongue Blade Test | 421 | | | |
| **NATA EC 5th** | **BOC RD6** | **Neurological Assessment** | **Page #** | | | |
| CE-21h, CE-20f | D2-0203 | Balance Error Scoring System (BESS) Test | 422 | | | |
| CE-21h, CE-20f | D2-0203 | Tandem Walking | 423 | | | |
| CE-21h, CE-20f | D2-0203 | Romberg Test | 424 | | | |
| CE-21h, CE-20f | D2-0203 | Determination of Anterograde Amnesia | 425 | | | |
| CE-21h, CE-20f | D2-0203 | Determination of Retrograde Amnesia | 426 | | | |
| CE-21h, CE-20f | D2-0203 | Maddock's Questions | 427 | | | |
| CE-21h, CE-20f | D2-0203 | Cranial Nerve I (Olfactory) | 428 | | | |
| CE-21h, CE-20f | D2-0203 | Cranial Nerve II (Optic) | 429 | | | |
| CE-21h, CE-20f | D2-0203 | Cranial Nerve III (Oculomotor) | 430 | | | |
| CE-21h, CE-20f | D2-0203 | Cranial Nerve IV (Trochlear) | 431 | | | |
| CE-21h, CE-20f | D2-0203 | Cranial Nerve V (Trigeminal) | 432 | | | |
| CE-21h, CE-20f | D2-0203 | Cranial Nerve VI (Abducens) | 433 | | | |
| CE-21h, CE-20f | D2-0203 | Cranial Nerve VII (Facial) | 434 | | | |
| CE-21h, CE-20f | D2-0203 | Cranial Nerve VIII (Vestibulocochlear) | 435 | | | |
| CE-21h, CE-20f | D2-0203 | Cranial Nerve IX (Glossopharyngeal) | 436 | | | |
| CE-21h, CE-20f | D2-0203 | Cranial Nerve X (Vagus) | 437 | | | |
| CE-21h, CE-20f | D2-0203 | Cranial Nerve XI (Spinal Accessory) | 438 | | | |
| CE-21h, CE-20f | D2-0203 | Cranial Nerve XII (Hypoglossal) | 439 | | | |
| **NATA EC 5th** | **BOC RD6** | **Clinical Assessment** | **Page #** | | | |
| CE-21m | D2-0203 | Convergence | 440 | | | |
| CE-21m | D2-0203 | Fluorescent Dye Testing | 441 | | | |
| CE-21m | D2-0203 | Gaze Stability (Horizontal Vestibulo-Ocular Reflex) | 442 | | | |
| CE-21m | D2-0203 | Gaze Stability (Vertical Vestibulo-Ocular Reflex) | 443 | | | |
| CE-21m | D2-0203 | Pupil Reaction to Light | 444 | | | |
| CE-21m | D2-0203 | Saccadic Eye Movement (Horizontal) | 445 | | | |
| CE-21m | D2-0203 | Saccadic Eye Movement (Vertical) | 446 | | | |
| CE-21m | D2-0203 | Smooth Pursuits | 447 | | | |
| CE-21m | D2-0203 | Snellen Eye Chart | 448 | | | |
| CE-21n | D2-0203 | Otoscope Use (Ear) | 449 | | | |
| CE-21n | D2-0203 | Otoscope Use (Nose) | 450 | | | |
| CE-21n | D2-0203 | Otoscope Use (Throat) | 451 | | | |

## MUSCULOSKELETAL SYSTEM—REGION 10: HEAD AND FACE
# PALPATION

| NATA EC 5th | BOC RD6 | SKILL |
|---|---|---|
| CE-21b, CE-20c | D2-0202 | Palpation: Head and Face – 01 |

**Supplies Needed:** Table

*This problem allows you the opportunity to demonstrate your ability to* **palpate** *the* **head and face.**
*You have 2 minutes to complete this task.*

| Palpation: Head and Face – 01 | Course or Site Assessor Environment | | | | | |
|---|---|---|---|---|---|---|
| | | Test 1 | | Test 2 | | Test 3 |
| | | Y | N | Y | N | Y | N |
| Mastoid process | | O | O | O | O | O | O |
| Zygomatic arch | | O | O | O | O | O | O |
| Temporal mandibular joint (external) | | O | O | O | O | O | O |
| External ear | | O | O | O | O | O | O |
| Sternocleidomastoid | | O | O | O | O | O | O |
| Lingual frenulum | | O | O | O | O | O | O |
| Masseter | | O | O | O | O | O | O |
| Total | | ___/7 | | ___/7 | | ___/7 | |
| Must achieve >4 to pass this examination | | Ⓟ | Ⓕ | Ⓟ | Ⓕ | Ⓟ | Ⓕ |

| Assessor:<br>Date: | Test 1 Comments: |
|---|---|
| Assessor:<br>Date: | Test 2 Comments: |
| Assessor:<br>Date: | Test 3 Comments: |

**TEST ENVIRONMENTS**
**L:** Laboratory/Classroom
**C:** Clinical/Field Testing
**P:** Practicum
**A:** Assessment/Mock Exam

**TEST INFORMATION**
**Test Statistics:** N/A
**Reference(s):** Starkey & Brown (2015)

MUSCULOSKELETAL SYSTEM—REGION 10: HEAD AND FACE
# PALPATION

| NATA EC 5th | BOC RD6 | SKILL |
|---|---|---|
| CE-21b, CE-20c | D2-0202 | Palpation: Head and Face – 02 |

**Supplies Needed:** Table

*This problem allows you the opportunity to demonstrate your ability to* **palpate** *the* **head and face.**
*You have 2 minutes to complete this task.*

| Palpation: Head and Face – 02 | Course or Site / Assessor / Environment | Test 1 | | Test 2 | | Test 3 | |
|---|---|---|---|---|---|---|---|
| | | Y | N | Y | N | Y | N |
| Orbital | | ○ | ○ | ○ | ○ | ○ | ○ |
| Nasal cartilage | | ○ | ○ | ○ | ○ | ○ | ○ |
| Periauricular area | | ○ | ○ | ○ | ○ | ○ | ○ |
| Mandible | | ○ | ○ | ○ | ○ | ○ | ○ |
| Hyoid | | ○ | ○ | ○ | ○ | ○ | ○ |
| Carotid artery | | ○ | ○ | ○ | ○ | ○ | ○ |
| Cricoid cartilage | | ○ | ○ | ○ | ○ | ○ | ○ |
| Total | | ___/7 | | ___/7 | | ___/7 | |
| Must achieve >4 to pass this examination | | P | F | P | F | P | F |

| Assessor: Date: | Test 1 Comments: |
|---|---|
| Assessor: Date: | Test 2 Comments: |
| Assessor: Date: | Test 3 Comments: |

**TEST ENVIRONMENTS**
**L:** Laboratory/Classroom
**C:** Clinical/Field Testing
**P:** Practicum
**A:** Assessment/Mock Exam

**TEST INFORMATION**
**Test Statistics:** N/A
**Reference(s):** Starkey & Brown (2015)

## MUSCULOSKELETAL SYSTEM—REGION 10: HEAD AND FACE
# PALPATION

| NATA EC 5th | BOC RD6 | SKILL |
|---|---|---|
| CE-21b, CE-20c | D2-0202 | Palpation: Head and Face – 03 |

**Supplies Needed:** Table

*This problem allows you the opportunity to demonstrate your ability to* **palpate** *the* **head and face**. *You have 2 minutes to complete this task.*

| Palpation: Head and Face – 03 | Course or Site Assessor Environment | | | | | |
|---|---|---|---|---|---|---|
| | | Test 1 | | Test 2 | | Test 3 |
| | | Y | N | Y | N | Y | N |
| Nasal bone | | O | O | O | O | O | O |
| Frontal bone | | O | O | O | O | O | O |
| Maxilla | | O | O | O | O | O | O |
| Temporal mandibular joint (internal) | | O | O | O | O | O | O |
| Teeth | | O | O | O | O | O | O |
| Scalene | | O | O | O | O | O | O |
| Thyroid | | O | O | O | O | O | O |
| Total | | ___/7 | | ___/7 | | ___/7 |
| Must achieve >4 to pass this examination | | P | F | P | F | P | F |

| Assessor: Date: | Test 1 Comments: |
|---|---|
| Assessor: Date: | Test 2 Comments: |
| Assessor: Date: | Test 3 Comments: |

**TEST ENVIRONMENTS**
**L:** Laboratory/Classroom
**C:** Clinical/Field Testing
**P:** Practicum
**A:** Assessment/Mock Exam

**TEST INFORMATION**
**Test Statistics:** N/A
**Reference(s):** Starkey & Brown (2015)

## MUSCULOSKELETAL SYSTEM—REGION 10: HEAD AND FACE
# SPECIAL TESTS

| NATA EC 5th | BOC RD6 | SKILL |
|---|---|---|
| CE-21g, CE-20e | D2-0203 | Halo Test |

**Supplies Needed:** Table

*This problem allows you the opportunity to demonstrate an* **orthopedic test** *known as the* **halo test** *for* **cerebrospinal fluid leakage***. You have 2 minutes to complete this task.*

| Halo Test | Course or Site Assessor Environment | | Test 1 | | Test 2 | | Test 3 | |
|---|---|---|---|---|---|---|---|---|
| **Tester places patient and limb in appropriate position** | | | **Y** | **N** | **Y** | **N** | **Y** | **N** |
| Lying down or seated | | | ○ | ○ | ○ | ○ | ○ | ○ |
| **Tester placed in proper position** | | | **Y** | **N** | **Y** | **N** | **Y** | **N** |
| Lateral to the ear being tested | | | ○ | ○ | ○ | ○ | ○ | ○ |
| **Tester performs test according to accepted guidelines** | | | **Y** | **N** | **Y** | **N** | **Y** | **N** |
| Folds a piece of sterile gauze into a triangle | | | ○ | ○ | ○ | ○ | ○ | ○ |
| Using the corner of the gauze, inserts into ear and collects a sample of fluid | | | ○ | ○ | ○ | ○ | ○ | ○ |
| Unfolds gauze and inspects fluid | | | ○ | ○ | ○ | ○ | ○ | ○ |
| **Identifies positive findings and implications** | | | **Y** | **N** | **Y** | **N** | **Y** | **N** |
| A pale yellow "halo" will form around the sample of fluid | | | ○ | ○ | ○ | ○ | ○ | ○ |
| **Total** | | | ___/6 | | ___/6 | | ___/6 | |
| **Must achieve >4 to pass this examination** | | | Ⓟ | Ⓕ | Ⓟ | Ⓕ | Ⓟ | Ⓕ |
| **Assessor:** **Date:** | **Test 1 Comments:** | | | | | | | |
| **Assessor:** **Date:** | **Test 2 Comments:** | | | | | | | |
| **Assessor:** **Date:** | **Test 3 Comments:** | | | | | | | |

**TEST ENVIRONMENTS**
**L:** Laboratory/Classroom
**C:** Clinical/Field Testing
**P:** Practicum
**A:** Assessment/Mock Exam

**TEST INFORMATION**
**Test Statistics:** No data available
**Reference(s):** Starkey & Brown (2015)

## MUSCULOSKELETAL SYSTEM—REGION 10: HEAD AND FACE
# SPECIAL TESTS

| NATA EC 5th | BOC RD6 | SKILL |
|---|---|---|
| CE-21g, CE-20e | D2-0203 | Tongue Blade Test |

**Supplies Needed:** Table or chair

*This problem allows you the opportunity to demonstrate an* **orthopedic test** *known as the* **tongue blade test** *for* **mandibular fracture**. *You have 2 minutes to complete this task.*

| Tongue Blade Test | Course or Site Assessor Environment | | Test 1 | | Test 2 | | Test 3 |
|---|---|---|---|---|---|---|---|
| | | | | | | | |
| **Tester places patient and limb in appropriate position** | | Y | N | Y | N | Y | N |
| Seated | | O | O | O | O | O | O |
| **Tester placed in proper position** | | Y | N | Y | N | Y | N |
| Stands in front of the patient | | O | O | O | O | O | O |
| **Tester performs test according to accepted guidelines** | | Y | N | Y | N | Y | N |
| Places tongue blade in the patient's mouth | | O | O | O | O | O | O |
| Instructs the patient to bite down and hold blade in place | | O | O | O | O | O | O |
| Rotates the blade while the patient attempts to hold on | | O | O | O | O | O | O |
| **Identifies positive findings and implications** | | Y | N | Y | N | Y | N |
| The patient is unable to maintain a firm bite or pain is elicited | | O | O | O | O | O | O |
| Total | | __/6 | | __/6 | | __/6 | |
| **Must achieve >4 to pass this examination** | | Ⓟ | Ⓕ | Ⓟ | Ⓕ | Ⓟ | Ⓕ |

| Assessor: Date: | Test 1 Comments: |
|---|---|
| Assessor: Date: | Test 2 Comments: |
| Assessor: Date: | Test 3 Comments: |

**TEST ENVIRONMENTS**
**L:** Laboratory/Classroom
**C:** Clinical/Field Testing
**P:** Practicum
**A:** Assessment/Mock Exam

**TEST INFORMATION**
**Test Statistics:** No data available
**Reference(s):** Starkey & Brown (2015)

## MUSCULOSKELETAL SYSTEM—REGION 10: HEAD AND FACE
# NEUROLOGICAL ASSESSMENT

| NATA EC 5th | BOC RD6 | SKILL |
|---|---|---|
| CE-21h, CE-20f | D2-0203 | Balance Error Scoring System (BESS) Test |

**Supplies Needed:** Table, stopwatch, Airex pad

*This problem allows you the opportunity to demonstrate a* **neurological assessment** *known as the* **Balance Error Scoring System (BESS) test** *for* **impaired cerebral function**. *You have 2 minutes to complete this task.*

| Balance Error Scoring System (BESS) Test | Course or Site _____ _____ _____ <br> Assessor _____ _____ _____ <br> Environment _____ _____ _____ <br> Test 1 / Test 2 / Test 3 | | | | | |
|---|---|---|---|---|---|---|
| | Test 1 Y | Test 1 N | Test 2 Y | Test 2 N | Test 3 Y | Test 3 N |
| **Tester places patient and limb in appropriate position** | Y | N | Y | N | Y | N |
| The patient is barefoot | ○ | ○ | ○ | ○ | ○ | ○ |
| The patient listens to the tester for proper instructions | ○ | ○ | ○ | ○ | ○ | ○ |
| **Tester placed in proper position** | Y | N | Y | N | Y | N |
| Stands in front of the patient | ○ | ○ | ○ | ○ | ○ | ○ |
| **Tester performs test according to accepted guidelines** | Y | N | Y | N | Y | N |
| Instructs the patient to close eyes and keep hands on iliac crest | ○ | ○ | ○ | ○ | ○ | ○ |
| Instructs the patient to perform double-leg stance (firm/foam surface) | ○ | ○ | ○ | ○ | ○ | ○ |
| Instructs the patient to perform nondominant single-leg stance (firm/foam surface) | ○ | ○ | ○ | ○ | ○ | ○ |
| Instructs the patient to perform tandem stance (firm/foam surface) | ○ | ○ | ○ | ○ | ○ | ○ |
| Times each stance for 30 seconds and records errors | ○ | ○ | ○ | ○ | ○ | ○ |
| **Identifies positive findings and implications** | Y | N | Y | N | Y | N |
| Errors are hands off iliac crest; opens eyes; steps, stumbles, or falls; lifting forefoot or heel; remaining out of test position >5 seconds | ○ | ○ | ○ | ○ | ○ | ○ |
| Decline in perform from baseline | ○ | ○ | ○ | ○ | ○ | ○ |
| **Total** | /10 | | /10 | | /10 | |
| **Must achieve >6 to pass this examination** | Ⓟ | Ⓕ | Ⓟ | Ⓕ | Ⓟ | Ⓕ |

| Assessor: Date: | Test 1 Comments: |
|---|---|
| Assessor: Date: | Test 2 Comments: |
| Assessor: Date: | Test 3 Comments: |

**TEST ENVIRONMENTS**
**L:** Laboratory/Classroom
**C:** Clinical/Field Testing
**P:** Practicum
**A:** Assessment/Mock Exam

**TEST INFORMATION**
**Test Statistics:** N/A
**Reference(s):** Starkey & Brown (2015)

**MUSCULOSKELETAL SYSTEM—REGION 10: HEAD AND FACE**
## NEUROLOGICAL ASSESSMENT

| NATA EC 5th | BOC RD6 | SKILL |
|---|---|---|
| CE-21h, CE-20f | D2-0203 | Tandem Walking |

**Supplies Needed:** Open and safe space for walking

*This problem allows you the opportunity to demonstrate a* **neurological assessment** *known as* **tandem walking** *for* **cerebral or inner ear dysfunction**. *You have 2 minutes to complete this task.*

| Tandem Walking | Course or Site Assessor Environment | | Test 1 | | Test 2 | | Test 3 | |
|---|---|---|---|---|---|---|---|---|
| **Tester places patient and limb in appropriate position** | | Y | N | Y | N | Y | N | |
| Stands with feet in a straight line | | ○ | ○ | ○ | ○ | ○ | ○ | |
| **Tester placed in proper position** | | Y | N | Y | N | Y | N | |
| Stands beside the patient ready to provide support | | ○ | ○ | ○ | ○ | ○ | ○ | |
| **Tester performs test according to accepted guidelines** | | Y | N | Y | N | Y | N | |
| Instructs the patient to walk heel to toe along a straight line for approximately 10 yards | | ○ | ○ | ○ | ○ | ○ | ○ | |
| Instructs the patient to walk backward in a straight line to the starting position | | ○ | ○ | ○ | ○ | ○ | ○ | |
| **Identifies positive findings and implications** | | Y | N | Y | N | Y | N | |
| The patient is unable to maintain balance | | ○ | ○ | ○ | ○ | ○ | ○ | |
| | Total | ___/5 | | ___/5 | | ___/5 | | |
| | Must achieve >3 to pass this examination | Ⓟ | Ⓕ | Ⓟ | Ⓕ | Ⓟ | Ⓕ | |

| Assessor: Date: | Test 1 Comments: |
|---|---|
| Assessor: Date: | Test 2 Comments: |
| Assessor: Date: | Test 3 Comments: |

**TEST ENVIRONMENTS**
**L:** Laboratory/Classroom
**C:** Clinical/Field Testing
**P:** Practicum
**A:** Assessment/Mock Exam

**TEST INFORMATION**
**Test Statistics:** N/A
**Reference(s):** Starkey & Brown (2015)

## MUSCULOSKELETAL SYSTEM—REGION 10: HEAD AND FACE
# NEUROLOGICAL ASSESSMENT

| NATA EC 5th | BOC RD6 | SKILL |
|---|---|---|
| CE-21h, CE-20f | D2-0203 | Romberg Test |

**Supplies Needed:** N/A

*This problem allows you the opportunity to demonstrate a* **neurological assessment** *known as the* **Romberg test** *to rule out a* **cerebellar or cranial nerve VIII dysfunction***. You have 2 minutes to complete this task.*

| Romberg Test | Course or Site<br>Assessor<br>Environment | | Test 1 | | Test 2 | | Test 3 | |
|---|---|---|---|---|---|---|---|---|
| **Tester places patient and limb in appropriate position** | | | Y | N | Y | N | Y | N |
| Stands with feet shoulder width apart | | | ◯ | ◯ | ◯ | ◯ | ◯ | ◯ |
| **Tester placed in proper position** | | | Y | N | Y | N | Y | N |
| Stands to the side of the patient, ready for support | | | ◯ | ◯ | ◯ | ◯ | ◯ | ◯ |
| **Tester performs test according to accepted guidelines** | | | Y | N | Y | N | Y | N |
| Instructs the patient to shut eyes and abduct arms 90 degrees with elbows extended | | | ◯ | ◯ | ◯ | ◯ | ◯ | ◯ |
| Instructs the patient to tilt the head backward and lift one foot off the ground | | | ◯ | ◯ | ◯ | ◯ | ◯ | ◯ |
| If previous portion is adequate, the tester instructs the patient to touch the index finger to the nose | | | ◯ | ◯ | ◯ | ◯ | ◯ | ◯ |
| **Identifies positive findings and implications** | | | Y | N | Y | N | Y | N |
| The patient displays gross unsteadiness | | | ◯ | ◯ | ◯ | ◯ | ◯ | ◯ |
| | | Total | ___/6 | | ___/6 | | ___/6 | |
| | Must achieve >4 to pass this examination | | Ⓟ | Ⓕ | Ⓟ | Ⓕ | Ⓟ | Ⓕ |

| Assessor:<br>Date: | Test 1 Comments: |
|---|---|
| Assessor:<br>Date: | Test 2 Comments: |
| Assessor:<br>Date: | Test 3 Comments: |

**TEST ENVIRONMENTS**
**L:** Laboratory/Classroom
**C:** Clinical/Field Testing
**P:** Practicum
**A:** Assessment/Mock Exam

**TEST INFORMATION**
**Test Statistics:** N/A
**Reference(s):** Starkey & Brown (2015)

**MUSCULOSKELETAL SYSTEM—REGION 10: HEAD AND FACE**
# NEUROLOGICAL ASSESSMENT

| NATA EC 5th | BOC RD6 | SKILL |
|---|---|---|
| CE-21h, CE-20f | D2-0203 | Determination of Anterograde Amnesia |

**Supplies Needed:** Table, clock

*This problem allows you the opportunity to demonstrate a* **neurological assessment** *to* **determine the presence of anterograde amnesia**. *You have 2 minutes to complete this task.*

| Determination of Anterograde Amnesia | Course or Site Assessor Environment | | | | | |
|---|---|---|---|---|---|---|
| | | Test 1 | | Test 2 | | Test 3 |
| **Tester places patient and limb in appropriate position** | | Y | N | Y | N | Y | N |
| Standing, seated, or lying down | | O | O | O | O | O | O |
| **Tester placed in proper position** | | Y | N | Y | N | Y | N |
| In a position to hear the patient's response | | O | O | O | O | O | O |
| **Tester performs test according to accepted guidelines** | | Y | N | Y | N | Y | N |
| Tells the patient a series of four unrelated items with instructions to memorize them | | O | O | O | O | O | O |
| Repeats the list to ensure the patient heard the items | | O | O | O | O | O | O |
| Asks the patient to repeat the list of items every 5 minutes | | O | O | O | O | O | O |
| **Identifies positive findings and implications** | | Y | N | Y | N | Y | N |
| Inability to recite the list properly | | O | O | O | O | O | O |
| Total | | ___/6 | | ___/6 | | ___/6 |
| Must achieve >4 to pass this examination | | Ⓟ | Ⓕ | Ⓟ | Ⓕ | Ⓟ | Ⓕ |

| Assessor:<br>Date: | Test 1 Comments: |
|---|---|
| Assessor:<br>Date: | Test 2 Comments: |
| Assessor:<br>Date: | Test 3 Comments: |

**TEST ENVIRONMENTS**
**L:** Laboratory/Classroom
**C:** Clinical/Field Testing
**P:** Practicum
**A:** Assessment/Mock Exam

**TEST INFORMATION**
**Test Statistics:** N/A
**Reference(s):** Starkey & Brown (2015)

## MUSCULOSKELETAL SYSTEM—REGION 10: HEAD AND FACE
## NEUROLOGICAL ASSESSMENT

| NATA EC 5th | BOC RD6 | SKILL |
|---|---|---|
| CE-21h, CE-20f | D2-0203 | Determination of Retrograde Amnesia |

**Supplies Needed:** Table

*This problem allows you the opportunity to demonstrate a* **neurological assessment** *to* **determine retrograde amnesia***. You have 2 minutes to complete this task.*

| Determination of Retrograde Amnesia | Course or Site / Assessor / Environment | | Test 1 | | Test 2 | | Test 3 | |
|---|---|---|---|---|---|---|---|---|
| | | | Y | N | Y | N | Y | N |
| **Tester places patient and limb in appropriate position** | | | Y | N | Y | N | Y | N |
| On-field: In the patient's current position | | | O | O | O | O | O | O |
| Off-field: Seated, standing, or lying down | | | O | O | O | O | O | O |
| **Tester placed in proper position** | | | Y | N | Y | N | Y | N |
| In a position to hear the patient's response | | | O | O | O | O | O | O |
| **Tester performs test according to accepted guidelines** | | | Y | N | Y | N | Y | N |
| The tester asks the patient a series of questions beginning with the time of injury | | | O | O | O | O | O | O |
| Each question progresses backward in time | | | O | O | O | O | O | O |
| **Identifies positive findings and implications** | | | Y | N | Y | N | Y | N |
| The patient has difficulty remembering or cannot remember events prior to the injury | | | O | O | O | O | O | O |
| Total | | | ___/6 | | ___/6 | | ___/6 | |
| Must achieve >4 to pass this examination | | | P | F | P | F | P | F |

| Assessor: Date: | Test 1 Comments: |
|---|---|
| Assessor: Date: | Test 2 Comments: |
| Assessor: Date: | Test 3 Comments: |

**TEST ENVIRONMENTS**
**L:** Laboratory/Classroom
**C:** Clinical/Field Testing
**P:** Practicum
**A:** Assessment/Mock Exam

**TEST INFORMATION**
**Test Statistics:** N/A
**Reference(s):** Starkey & Brown (2015)

## MUSCULOSKELETAL SYSTEM—REGION 10: HEAD AND FACE
# NEUROLOGICAL ASSESSMENT

| NATA EC 5th | BOC RD6 | SKILL |
|---|---|---|
| CE-21h, CE-20f | D2-0203 | Maddock's Questions |

**Supplies Needed:** Table

*This problem allows you the opportunity to demonstrate a* **neurological assessment** *known as* **Maddock's questions***. You have 2 minutes to complete this task.*

| Maddock's Questions | Course or Site Assessor Environment | | Test 1 | | Test 2 | | Test 3 | |
|---|---|---|---|---|---|---|---|---|
| | | | Y | N | Y | N | Y | N |
| **Tester places patient and limb in appropriate position** | | | **Y** | **N** | **Y** | **N** | **Y** | **N** |
| Seated | | | O | O | O | O | O | O |
| **Tester placed in proper position** | | | **Y** | **N** | **Y** | **N** | **Y** | **N** |
| In a position to hear the patient's response | | | O | O | O | O | O | O |
| **Tester performs test according to accepted guidelines** | | | **Y** | **N** | **Y** | **N** | **Y** | **N** |
| Tells the patient "I am going to ask you a few questions, please listen carefully and give your best effort." | | | O | O | O | O | O | O |
| Asks the patient "What venue are we at?" | | | O | O | O | O | O | O |
| Asks the patient "Which half is it now?" | | | O | O | O | O | O | O |
| Asks the patient "Who scored last in this match?" | | | O | O | O | O | O | O |
| Asks the patient "What team did you play last week/game?" | | | O | O | O | O | O | O |
| Asks the patient "Did your team win the last game?" | | | O | O | O | O | O | O |
| **Identifies positive findings and implications** | | | **Y** | **N** | **Y** | **N** | **Y** | **N** |
| Inability to answer questions | | | O | O | O | O | O | O |
| Total | | | ___/9 | | ___/9 | | ___/9 | |
| Must achieve >6 to pass this examination | | | Ⓟ | Ⓕ | Ⓟ | Ⓕ | Ⓟ | Ⓕ |

| Assessor: Date: | Test 1 Comments: |
|---|---|
| Assessor: Date: | Test 2 Comments: |
| Assessor: Date: | Test 3 Comments: |

**TEST ENVIRONMENTS**
**L:** Laboratory/Classroom
**C:** Clinical/Field Testing
**P:** Practicum
**A:** Assessment/Mock Exam

**TEST INFORMATION**
**Test Statistics:** N/A
**Reference(s):** Starkey & Brown (2015)

MUSCULOSKELETAL SYSTEM—REGION 10: HEAD AND FACE
# NEUROLOGICAL ASSESSMENT

| NATA EC 5th | BOC RD6 | SKILL |
|---|---|---|
| CE-21h, CE-20f | D2-0203 | Cranial Nerve I (Olfactory) |

**Supplies Needed:** Table or chair, scented item

*This problem allows you the opportunity to demonstrate a* **neurological assessment** *for* **cranial nerve I (olfactory)**. *You have 2 minutes to complete this task.*

| Cranial Nerve I (Olfactory) | Course or Site Assessor Environment | | Test 1 | | Test 2 | | Test 3 | |
|---|---|---|---|---|---|---|---|---|
| **Tester places patient and limb in appropriate position** | | | Y | N | Y | N | Y | N |
| Seated or standing | | | O | O | O | O | O | O |
| **Tester placed in proper position** | | | Y | N | Y | N | Y | N |
| Stands in front of the patient | | | O | O | O | O | O | O |
| **Tester performs test according to accepted guidelines** | | | Y | N | Y | N | Y | N |
| Instructs the patient close his/her eyes | | | O | O | O | O | O | O |
| The tester chooses an item with a smell that is potent and familiar (e.g., mints, citrus) | | | O | O | O | O | O | O |
| Instructs the patient to smell the item without opening his/her eyes or touching the item | | | O | O | O | O | O | O |
| Instructs the patient to identify the smell | | | O | O | O | O | O | O |
| **Identifies positive findings and implications** | | | Y | N | Y | N | Y | N |
| The patient is unable to identify the smell correctly or increased symptoms | | | O | O | O | O | O | O |
| Possible damage to cranial nerve I (olfactory) | | | O | O | O | O | O | O |
| Total | | | /8 | | /8 | | /8 | |
| Must achieve >5 to pass this examination | | | P | F | P | F | P | F |

| Assessor: Date: | Test 1 Comments: |
|---|---|
| Assessor: Date: | Test 2 Comments: |
| Assessor: Date: | Test 3 Comments: |

**TEST ENVIRONMENTS**
L: Laboratory/Classroom
C: Clinical/Field Testing
P: Practicum
A: Assessment/Mock Exam

**TEST INFORMATION**
**Test Statistics:** No data available
**Reference(s):** Starkey & Brown (2015)

## MUSCULOSKELETAL SYSTEM—REGION 10: HEAD AND FACE
# NEUROLOGICAL ASSESSMENT

| NATA EC 5th | BOC RD6 | SKILL |
|---|---|---|
| CE-21h, CE-20f | D2-0203 | Cranial Nerve II (Optic) |

**Supplies Needed:** Target with 14-point font writing

*This problem allows you the opportunity to demonstrate a* **neurological assessment** *for* **cranial nerve II (optic)**. *You have 2 minutes to complete this task.*

| Cranial Nerve II (Optic) | Course or Site<br>Assessor<br>Environment | | Test 1 | | Test 2 | | Test 3 | |
|---|---|---|---|---|---|---|---|---|
| **Tester places patient and limb in appropriate position** | | **Y** | **N** | **Y** | **N** | **Y** | **N** | |
| Standing | | ○ | ○ | ○ | ○ | ○ | ○ | |
| **Tester placed in proper position** | | **Y** | **N** | **Y** | **N** | **Y** | **N** | |
| Stands in front of the patient | | ○ | ○ | ○ | ○ | ○ | ○ | |
| **Tester performs test according to accepted guidelines** | | **Y** | **N** | **Y** | **N** | **Y** | **N** | |
| Instructs the patient to read a target with 14-point font at arm's length | | ○ | ○ | ○ | ○ | ○ | ○ | |
| **Identifies positive findings and implications** | | **Y** | **N** | **Y** | **N** | **Y** | **N** | |
| Inability to read material or increased symptoms | | ○ | ○ | ○ | ○ | ○ | ○ | |
| Possible damage to the optic nerves | | ○ | ○ | ○ | ○ | ○ | ○ | |
| **Total** | | _____ /5 | | _____ /5 | | _____ /5 | | |
| **Must achieve >3 to pass this examination** | | Ⓟ | Ⓕ | Ⓟ | Ⓕ | Ⓟ | Ⓕ | |

| Assessor:<br>Date: | Test 1 Comments: |
|---|---|
| Assessor:<br>Date: | Test 2 Comments: |
| Assessor:<br>Date: | Test 3 Comments: |

**TEST ENVIRONMENTS**
**L:** Laboratory/Classroom
**C:** Clinical/Field Testing
**P:** Practicum
**A:** Assessment/Mock Exam

**TEST INFORMATION**
**Test Statistics:** No data available
**Reference(s):** Mucha et al. (2014)
Starkey & Brown (2015)

## MUSCULOSKELETAL SYSTEM—REGION 10: HEAD AND FACE
# NEUROLOGICAL ASSESSMENT

| NATA EC 5th | BOC RD6 | SKILL |
|---|---|---|
| CE-21h, CE-20f | D2-0203 | Cranial Nerve III (Oculomotor) |

**Supplies Needed:** Table or chair, penlight

*This problem allows you the opportunity to demonstrate a* **neurological assessment** *for* **cranial nerve III (oculomotor)**. *You have 2 minutes to complete this task.*

| Cranial Nerve III (Oculomotor) | Course or Site / Assessor / Environment | | Test 1 | | Test 2 | | Test 3 | |
|---|---|---|---|---|---|---|---|---|
| | | | Y | N | Y | N | Y | N |
| **Tester places patient and limb in appropriate position** | | | Y | N | Y | N | Y | N |
| Seated or standing | | | ○ | ○ | ○ | ○ | ○ | ○ |
| **Tester placed in proper position** | | | Y | N | Y | N | Y | N |
| Stands in front of the patient | | | ○ | ○ | ○ | ○ | ○ | ○ |
| Holds penlight 18 inches from the patient's face | | | ○ | ○ | ○ | ○ | ○ | ○ |
| **Tester performs test according to accepted guidelines** | | | Y | N | Y | N | Y | N |
| Instructs the patient to open eyes | | | ○ | ○ | ○ | ○ | ○ | ○ |
| Instructs the patient to gaze over the tester's shoulder | | | ○ | ○ | ○ | ○ | ○ | ○ |
| Shines penlight into one of the patient's eyes, while watching both pupils for reaction to light | | | ○ | ○ | ○ | ○ | ○ | ○ |
| Instructs the patient to follow penlight with only eye movement while moving the penlight laterally to 30 degrees of abduction to each side | | | ○ | ○ | ○ | ○ | ○ | ○ |
| **Identifies positive findings and implications** | | | Y | N | Y | N | Y | N |
| Inability to open eyes, unequal pupil reaction, inability to perform adduction of the eyes, or increased symptoms | | | ○ | ○ | ○ | ○ | ○ | ○ |
| Possible damage to cranial nerve III (oculomotor) | | | ○ | ○ | ○ | ○ | ○ | ○ |
| | | Total | __/9 | | __/9 | | __/9 | |
| | Must achieve >6 to pass this examination | | ⓟ | Ⓕ | ⓟ | Ⓕ | ⓟ | Ⓕ |

| Assessor: Date: | Test 1 Comments: |
|---|---|
| Assessor: Date: | Test 2 Comments: |
| Assessor: Date: | Test 3 Comments: |

**TEST ENVIRONMENTS**
**L:** Laboratory/Classroom
**C:** Clinical/Field Testing
**P:** Practicum
**A:** Assessment/Mock Exam

**TEST INFORMATION**
**Test Statistics:** N/A
**Reference(s):** Starkey & Brown (2015)

MUSCULOSKELETAL SYSTEM—REGION 10: HEAD AND FACE
# NEUROLOGICAL ASSESSMENT

| NATA EC 5th | BOC RD6 | SKILL |
|---|---|---|
| CE-21h, CE-20f | D2-0203 | Cranial Nerve IV (Trochlear) |

**Supplies Needed:** Table or chair, penlight

*This problem allows you the opportunity to demonstrate a* **neurological assessment** *for* **cranial nerve IV (trochlear)**. *You have 2 minutes to complete this task.*

| Cranial Nerve IV (Trochlear) | Course or Site Assessor Environment | | Test 1 | | Test 2 | | Test 3 | |
|---|---|---|---|---|---|---|---|---|
| | | | Y | N | Y | N | Y | N |
| **Tester places patient and limb in appropriate position** | | | Y | N | Y | N | Y | N |
| Seated or standing | | | O | O | O | O | O | O |
| **Tester placed in proper position** | | | Y | N | Y | N | Y | N |
| Stands in front of the patient | | | O | O | O | O | O | O |
| Holds the penlight 18 inches from the patient's face | | | O | O | O | O | O | O |
| **Tester performs test according to accepted guidelines** | | | Y | N | Y | N | Y | N |
| Instructs the patient to focus on the penlight movements without moving the head and neck | | | O | O | O | O | O | O |
| Moves the penlight vertically from top of the patient's head to bottom of the patient's chin | | | O | O | O | O | O | O |
| Watches the patient's eyes for lagging, nystagmus, or other abnormal reactions | | | O | O | O | O | O | O |
| **Identifies positive findings and implications** | | | Y | N | Y | N | Y | N |
| Inability to follow penlight, nystagmus, or increased symptoms | | | O | O | O | O | O | O |
| Possible damage to cranial nerve IV (trochlear) | | | O | O | O | O | O | O |
| Total | | | __/8 | | __/8 | | __/8 | |
| Must achieve >5 to pass this examination | | | P | F | P | F | P | F |

| Assessor: Date: | Test 1 Comments: |
|---|---|
| Assessor: Date: | Test 2 Comments: |
| Assessor: Date: | Test 3 Comments: |

**TEST ENVIRONMENTS**
**L:** Laboratory/Classroom
**C:** Clinical/Field Testing
**P:** Practicum
**A:** Assessment/Mock Exam

**TEST INFORMATION**
**Test Statistics:** N/A
**Reference(s):** Starkey & Brown (2015)

## MUSCULOSKELETAL SYSTEM—REGION 10: HEAD AND FACE
## NEUROLOGICAL ASSESSMENT

| NATA EC 5th | BOC RD6 | SKILL |
|---|---|---|
| CE-21h, CE-20f | D2-0203 | Cranial Nerve V (Trigeminal) |

**Supplies Needed:** Table or chair, Taylor Hammer

*This problem allows you the opportunity to demonstrate a* **neurological assessment** *for* **cranial nerve V (trigeminal)**. *You have 2 minutes to complete this task.*

| Cranial Nerve V (Trigeminal) | Course or Site Assessor Environment | Test 1 | | Test 2 | | Test 3 | |
|---|---|---|---|---|---|---|---|
| | | Y | N | Y | N | Y | N |
| **Tester places patient and limb in appropriate position** | | Y | N | Y | N | Y | N |
| Seated or standing | | O | O | O | O | O | O |
| **Tester placed in proper position** | | Y | N | Y | N | Y | N |
| Stands in front of the patient | | O | O | O | O | O | O |
| **Tester performs test according to accepted guidelines** | | Y | N | Y | N | Y | N |
| Instructs the patient to clench teeth and palpates masseter muscle bilaterally | | O | O | O | O | O | O |
| Then instructs the patient to close his/her eyes | | O | O | O | O | O | O |
| Uses Taylor Hammer to test sensation of the patient's nose, forehead, temple, scalp, lips, and lower jaw | | O | O | O | O | O | O |
| **Identifies positive findings and implications** | | Y | N | Y | N | Y | N |
| Inability to clench teeth or decreased sensation to the face | | O | O | O | O | O | O |
| Possible damage to cranial nerve V (trigeminal) | | O | O | O | O | O | O |
| Total | | ___/7 | | ___/7 | | ___/7 | |
| **Must achieve >4 to pass this examination** | | P | F | P | F | P | F |

| Assessor: Date: | Test 1 Comments: |
|---|---|
| Assessor: Date: | Test 2 Comments: |
| Assessor: Date: | Test 3 Comments: |

**TEST ENVIRONMENTS**
L: Laboratory/Classroom
C: Clinical/Field Testing
P: Practicum
A: Assessment/Mock Exam

**TEST INFORMATION**
**Test Statistics:** No data available
**Reference(s):** Cook & Hegedus (2013)

## MUSCULOSKELETAL SYSTEM—REGION 10: HEAD AND FACE
# NEUROLOGICAL ASSESSMENT

| NATA EC 5th | BOC RD6 | SKILL |
|---|---|---|
| CE-21h, CE-20f | D2-0203 | Cranial Nerve VI (Abducens) |

**Supplies Needed:** Table or chair, penlight

*This problem allows you the opportunity to demonstrate a* **neurological assessment** *for* **cranial nerve VI (abducens)**. *You have 2 minutes to complete this task.*

| Cranial Nerve VI (Abducens) | Course or Site Assessor Environment | | Test 1 | | Test 2 | | Test 3 |
|---|---|---|---|---|---|---|---|
| **Tester places patient and limb in appropriate position** | | Y | N | Y | N | Y | N |
| Seated or standing | | O | O | O | O | O | O |
| **Tester placed in proper position** | | Y | N | Y | N | Y | N |
| Stands in front of the patient | | O | O | O | O | O | O |
| Places penlight 18 inches from the patient's face | | O | O | O | O | O | O |
| **Tester performs test according to accepted guidelines** | | Y | N | Y | N | Y | N |
| Instructs the patient to follow the penlight without moving the head and neck | | O | O | O | O | O | O |
| Moves penlight to 30 degrees abduction in both directions | | O | O | O | O | O | O |
| **Identifies positive findings and implications** | | Y | N | Y | N | Y | N |
| Nystagmus or lagging of eye motions or increased symptoms | | O | O | O | O | O | O |
| Possible damage to cranial nerve VI (abducens) | | O | O | O | O | O | O |
| **Total** | | ___/7 | | ___/7 | | ___/7 | |
| **Must achieve >4 to pass this examination** | | Ⓟ | Ⓕ | Ⓟ | Ⓕ | Ⓟ | Ⓕ |

| Assessor: Date: | Test 1 Comments: |
|---|---|
| Assessor: Date: | Test 2 Comments: |
| Assessor: Date: | Test 3 Comments: |

**TEST ENVIRONMENTS**
L: Laboratory/Classroom
C: Clinical/Field Testing
P: Practicum
A: Assessment/Mock Exam

**TEST INFORMATION**
**Test Statistics:** No data available
**Reference(s):** Starkey & Brown (2015)

## MUSCULOSKELETAL SYSTEM—REGION 10: HEAD AND FACE
## NEUROLOGICAL ASSESSMENT

| NATA EC 5th | BOC RD6 | SKILL |
|---|---|---|
| CE-21h, CE-20f | D2-0203 | Cranial Nerve VII (Facial) |

**Supplies Needed:** Table or chair, item to be tasted

*This problem allows you the opportunity to demonstrate a* **neurological assessment** *for* **cranial nerve VII (facial)**. *You have 2 minutes to complete this task.*

| Cranial Nerve VII (Facial) | Course or Site / Assessor / Environment | | Test 1 | | Test 2 | | Test 3 |
|---|---|---|---|---|---|---|---|
| | | Y | N | Y | N | Y | N |
| **Tester places patient and limb in appropriate position** | | Y | N | Y | N | Y | N |
| Seated or standing | | ○ | ○ | ○ | ○ | ○ | ○ |
| **Tester placed in proper position** | | Y | N | Y | N | Y | N |
| Stands in front of the patient | | ○ | ○ | ○ | ○ | ○ | ○ |
| Prepares to administer item to be tasted | | ○ | ○ | ○ | ○ | ○ | ○ |
| **Tester performs test according to accepted guidelines** | | Y | N | Y | N | Y | N |
| Instructs the patient to smile and grimace | | ○ | ○ | ○ | ○ | ○ | ○ |
| Instructs the patient to close both eyes | | ○ | ○ | ○ | ○ | ○ | ○ |
| Provides item that has potent and familiar taste | | ○ | ○ | ○ | ○ | ○ | ○ |
| The patient is instructed to identify the taste using posterior portion of the tongue without opening eyes | | ○ | ○ | ○ | ○ | ○ | ○ |
| **Identifies positive findings and implications** | | Y | N | Y | N | Y | N |
| Inability to identify tasted item, form facial expressions, or increased symptoms | | ○ | ○ | ○ | ○ | ○ | ○ |
| Possible damage to cranial nerve VII (facial) | | ○ | ○ | ○ | ○ | ○ | ○ |
| Total | | ___/9 | | ___/9 | | ___/9 | |
| Must achieve >6 to pass this examination | | Ⓟ | Ⓕ | Ⓟ | Ⓕ | Ⓟ | Ⓕ |

| Assessor: Date: | Test 1 Comments: |
|---|---|
| Assessor: Date: | Test 2 Comments: |
| Assessor: Date: | Test 3 Comments: |

**TEST ENVIRONMENTS**
**L:** Laboratory/Classroom
**C:** Clinical/Field Testing
**P:** Practicum
**A:** Assessment/Mock Exam

**TEST INFORMATION**
**Test Statistics:** No data available
**Reference(s):** Starkey & Brown (2015)

MUSCULOSKELETAL SYSTEM—REGION 10: HEAD AND FACE
# NEUROLOGICAL ASSESSMENT

| NATA EC 5th | BOC RD6 | SKILL |
|---|---|---|
| CE-21h, CE-20f | D2-0203 | Cranial Nerve VIII (Vestibulocochlear) |

**Supplies Needed:** Table or chair

*This problem allows you the opportunity to demonstrate a* **neurological assessment** *for* **cranial nerve VIII (vestibulocochlear)**. *You have 2 minutes to complete this task.*

| Cranial Nerve VIII (Vestibulocochlear) | Course or Site Assessor Environment | | Test 1 | | Test 2 | | Test 3 |
|---|---|---|---|---|---|---|---|
| | | **Y** | **N** | **Y** | **N** | **Y** | **N** |
| **Tester places patient and limb in appropriate position** | | **Y** | **N** | **Y** | **N** | **Y** | **N** |
| Seated or standing | | O | O | O | O | O | O |
| **Tester placed in proper position** | | **Y** | **N** | **Y** | **N** | **Y** | **N** |
| Stands behind the patient | | O | O | O | O | O | O |
| One hand on each side of the patient's head | | O | O | O | O | O | O |
| **Tester performs test according to accepted guidelines** | | **Y** | **N** | **Y** | **N** | **Y** | **N** |
| Instructs the patient to indicate which side a "snap" is heard | | O | O | O | O | O | O |
| Then snaps fingers at random one side at a time, allowing time between snaps for the patient to indicate which side | | O | O | O | O | O | O |
| Performs this test for _____ snaps | | O | O | O | O | O | O |
| Then moves to the side of the patient, and instructs the patient to place hands against his/her side, feet together, and close eyes | | O | O | O | O | O | O |
| The patient maintains stance for 30 seconds | | O | O | O | O | O | O |
| **Identifies positive findings and implications** | | **Y** | **N** | **Y** | **N** | **Y** | **N** |
| Inability to identify sound, unsteadiness, or increased symptoms | | O | O | O | O | O | O |
| Possible damage to cranial nerve VIII (vestibulocochlear) | | O | O | O | O | O | O |
| | Total | /10 | | /10 | | /10 | |
| | Must achieve >6 to pass this examination | Ⓟ | Ⓕ | Ⓟ | Ⓕ | Ⓟ | Ⓕ |

| Assessor: Date: | Test 1 Comments: |
|---|---|
| Assessor: Date: | Test 2 Comments: |
| Assessor: Date: | Test 3 Comments: |

**TEST ENVIRONMENTS**
**L:** Laboratory/Classroom
**C:** Clinical/Field Testing
**P:** Practicum
**A:** Assessment/Mock Exam

**TEST INFORMATION**
**Test Statistics:** No data available
**Reference(s):** Konin et al. (2016)
Starkey & Brown (2015)

## MUSCULOSKELETAL SYSTEM—REGION 10: HEAD AND FACE
# NEUROLOGICAL ASSESSMENT

| NATA EC 5th | BOC RD6 | SKILL |
|---|---|---|
| CE-21h, CE-20f | D2-0203 | Cranial Nerve IX (Glossopharyngeal) |

**Supplies Needed:** Table or chair, item to be tasted

*This problem allows you the opportunity to demonstrate a* **neurological assessment** *for* **cranial nerve IX (glossopharyngeal)**. *You have 2 minutes to complete this task.*

| Cranial Nerve IX (Glossopharyngeal) | Course or Site Assessor Environment | | | | | |
|---|---|---|---|---|---|---|
| | | Test 1 | | Test 2 | | Test 3 | |
| **Tester places patient and limb in appropriate position** | | Y | N | Y | N | Y | N |
| Seated or standing | | O | O | O | O | O | O |
| **Tester placed in proper position** | | Y | N | Y | N | Y | N |
| Stands in front of the patient | | O | O | O | O | O | O |
| **Tester performs test according to accepted guidelines** | | Y | N | Y | N | Y | N |
| Instructs the patient to swallow | | O | O | O | O | O | O |
| Instructs the patient to close both eyes | | O | O | O | O | O | O |
| Provides item that has potent and familiar taste | | O | O | O | O | O | O |
| The patient is instructed to identify the taste using posterior portion of the tongue without opening eyes | | O | O | O | O | O | O |
| **Identifies positive findings and implications** | | Y | N | Y | N | Y | N |
| Inability to swallow, identify taste, or symptoms increase | | O | O | O | O | O | O |
| Possible damage to cranial nerve IX (glossopharyngeal) | | O | O | O | O | O | O |
| Total | | __/8 | | __/8 | | __/8 | |
| Must achieve >5 to pass this examination | | Ⓟ | Ⓕ | Ⓟ | Ⓕ | Ⓟ | Ⓕ |

| Assessor: Date: | Test 1 Comments: |
|---|---|
| Assessor: Date: | Test 2 Comments: |
| Assessor: Date: | Test 3 Comments: |

**TEST ENVIRONMENTS**
**L:** Laboratory/Classroom
**C:** Clinical/Field Testing
**P:** Practicum
**A:** Assessment/Mock Exam

**TEST INFORMATION**
**Test Statistics:** No data available
**Reference(s):** Starkey & Brown (2015)

## MUSCULOSKELETAL SYSTEM—REGION 10: HEAD AND FACE
# NEUROLOGICAL ASSESSMENT

| NATA EC 5th | BOC RD6 | SKILL |
|---|---|---|
| CE-21h, CE-20f | D2-0203 | Cranial Nerve X (Vagus) |

**Supplies Needed:** Table or chair, tongue depressor

*This problem allows you the opportunity to demonstrate a* **neurological assessment** *for* **cranial nerve X (vagus)**. *You have 2 minutes to complete this task.*

| Cranial Nerve X (Vagus) | Course or Site Assessor Environment | | Test 1 | | Test 2 | | Test 3 | |
|---|---|---|---|---|---|---|---|---|
| **Tester places patient and limb in appropriate position** | | | Y | N | Y | N | Y | N |
| Seated or standing | | | O | O | O | O | O | O |
| **Tester placed in proper position** | | | Y | N | Y | N | Y | N |
| Stands in front of the patient | | | O | O | O | O | O | O |
| **Tester performs test according to accepted guidelines** | | | Y | N | Y | N | Y | N |
| Instructs the patient to say "Ahh" | | | O | O | O | O | O | O |
| Then instructs the patient to keep mouth open and induces gag reflex by placing a tongue depressor on posterior aspect of the tongue | | | O | O | O | O | O | O |
| **Identifies positive findings and implications** | | | Y | N | Y | N | Y | N |
| Inability to produce sound, reduced gag reflex, or increased symptoms | | | O | O | O | O | O | O |
| Possible damage to cranial nerve X (vagus) | | | O | O | O | O | O | O |
| **Total** | | | ___/6 | | ___/6 | | ___/6 | |
| **Must achieve >4 to pass this examination** | | | P | F | P | F | P | F |

| Assessor:<br>Date: | Test 1 Comments: |
|---|---|
| Assessor:<br>Date: | Test 2 Comments: |
| Assessor:<br>Date: | Test 3 Comments: |

**TEST ENVIRONMENTS**
**L:** Laboratory/Classroom
**C:** Clinical/Field Testing
**P:** Practicum
**A:** Assessment/Mock Exam

**TEST INFORMATION**
**Test Statistics:** No data available
**Reference(s):** Starkey & Brown (2015)

## MUSCULOSKELETAL SYSTEM—REGION 10: HEAD AND FACE
# NEUROLOGICAL ASSESSMENT

| NATA EC 5th | BOC RD6 | SKILL |
|---|---|---|
| CE-21h, CE-20f | D2-0203 | Cranial Nerve XI (Spinal Accessory) |

**Supplies Needed:** Table or chair

*This problem allows you the opportunity to demonstrate a* **neurological assessment** *for* **cranial nerve XI (spinal accessory)**. *You have 2 minutes to complete this task.*

| Cranial Nerve XI (Spinal Accessory) | Course or Site / Assessor / Environment | | | | | |
|---|---|---|---|---|---|---|
| | | Test 1 | | Test 2 | | Test 3 | |
| | | Y | N | Y | N | Y | N |
| **Tester places patient and limb in appropriate position** | | Y | N | Y | N | Y | N |
| Seated or standing | | ○ | ○ | ○ | ○ | ○ | ○ |
| **Tester placed in proper position** | | Y | N | Y | N | Y | N |
| Stands behind the patient | | ○ | ○ | ○ | ○ | ○ | ○ |
| **Tester performs test according to accepted guidelines** | | Y | N | Y | N | Y | N |
| Instructs the patient to perform a shoulder shrug | | ○ | ○ | ○ | ○ | ○ | ○ |
| The tester applies manual resistance to the shoulders into depression of the shoulder | | ○ | ○ | ○ | ○ | ○ | ○ |
| **Identifies positive findings and implications** | | Y | N | Y | N | Y | N |
| The patient is unable to elevate shoulders | | ○ | ○ | ○ | ○ | ○ | ○ |
| Possible damage to cranial nerve XI (spinal accessory) | | ○ | ○ | ○ | ○ | ○ | ○ |
| **Total** | | /6 | | /6 | | /6 | |
| **Must achieve >4 to pass this examination** | | Ⓟ | Ⓕ | Ⓟ | Ⓕ | Ⓟ | Ⓕ |

| Assessor: Date: | Test 1 Comments: |
|---|---|
| Assessor: Date: | Test 2 Comments: |
| Assessor: Date: | Test 3 Comments: |

**TEST ENVIRONMENTS**
**L:** Laboratory/Classroom
**C:** Clinical/Field Testing
**P:** Practicum
**A:** Assessment/Mock Exam

**TEST INFORMATION**
**Test Statistics:** No data available
**Reference(s):** Starkey & Brown (2015)

## MUSCULOSKELETAL SYSTEM—REGION 10: HEAD AND FACE
# NEUROLOGICAL ASSESSMENT

| NATA EC 5th | BOC RD6 | SKILL |
|---|---|---|
| CE-21h, CE-20f | D2-0203 | Cranial Nerve XII (Hypoglossal) |

**Supplies Needed:** Table or chair

*This problem allows you the opportunity to demonstrate a* **neurological assessment** *for* **cranial nerve XII (hypoglossal)**. *You have 2 minutes to complete this task.*

| Cranial Nerve XII (Hypoglossal) | Course or Site<br>Assessor<br>Environment | | | | | | |
|---|---|---|---|---|---|---|---|
| | | Test 1 | | Test 2 | | Test 3 | |
| **Tester places patient and limb in appropriate position** | | Y | N | Y | N | Y | N |
| Seated or standing | | O | O | O | O | O | O |
| **Tester placed in proper position** | | Y | N | Y | N | Y | N |
| Stands in front of the patient | | O | O | O | O | O | O |
| **Tester performs test according to accepted guidelines** | | Y | N | Y | N | Y | N |
| Instructs the patient to stick out his/her tongue | | O | O | O | O | O | O |
| **Identifies positive findings and implications** | | Y | N | Y | N | Y | N |
| Inability to stick out tongue or increased symptoms | | O | O | O | O | O | O |
| Possible damage to cranial nerve XII (hypoglossal) | | O | O | O | O | O | O |
| | Total | ___/5 | | ___/5 | | ___/5 | |
| | Must achieve >3 to pass this examination | Ⓟ | Ⓕ | Ⓟ | Ⓕ | Ⓟ | Ⓕ |

| Assessor:<br>Date: | Test 1 Comments: |
|---|---|
| Assessor:<br>Date: | Test 2 Comments: |
| Assessor:<br>Date: | Test 3 Comments: |

**TEST ENVIRONMENTS**
**L:** Laboratory/Classroom
**C:** Clinical/Field Testing
**P:** Practicum
**A:** Assessment/Mock Exam

**TEST INFORMATION**
**Test Statistics:** No data available
**Reference(s):** Starkey & Brown (2015)

## MUSCULOSKELETAL SYSTEM—REGION 10: HEAD AND FACE
# CLINICAL ASSESSMENT

| NATA EC 5th | BOC RD6 | SKILL |
|---|---|---|
| CE-21m | D2-0203 | Convergence |

**Supplies Needed:** Chair, penlight

*This problem allows you the opportunity to demonstrate a* **physical examination** *known as* **convergence**. *You have 2 minutes to complete this task.*

| Convergence | Course or Site Assessor Environment | Test 1 | | Test 2 | | Test 3 | |
|---|---|---|---|---|---|---|---|
| | | Y | N | Y | N | Y | N |
| **Tester places patient and limb in appropriate position** | | Y | N | Y | N | Y | N |
| Seated, wearing corrective lenses if needed | | ○ | ○ | ○ | ○ | ○ | ○ |
| **Tester placed in proper position** | | Y | N | Y | N | Y | N |
| Seated in front of the patient | | ○ | ○ | ○ | ○ | ○ | ○ |
| **Tester performs test according to accepted guidelines** | | Y | N | Y | N | Y | N |
| Holds penlight arm's length away from the patient | | ○ | ○ | ○ | ○ | ○ | ○ |
| Slowly moves penlight to tip of the patient's nose | | ○ | ○ | ○ | ○ | ○ | ○ |
| Instructs the patient to focus on tip of penlight and tell the tester when image becomes blurry | | ○ | ○ | ○ | ○ | ○ | ○ |
| **Identifies positive findings and implications** | | Y | N | Y | N | Y | N |
| Image becomes blurry at a distance >6 cm from tip of nose | | ○ | ○ | ○ | ○ | ○ | ○ |
| **Total** | | /6 | | /6 | | /6 | |
| **Must achieve >4 to pass this examination** | | Ⓟ | Ⓕ | Ⓟ | Ⓕ | Ⓟ | Ⓕ |

| Assessor: Date: | Test 1 Comments: |
|---|---|
| Assessor: Date: | Test 2 Comments: |
| Assessor: Date: | Test 3 Comments: |

**TEST ENVIRONMENTS**
**L:** Laboratory/Classroom
**C:** Clinical/Field Testing
**P:** Practicum
**A:** Assessment/Mock Exam

**TEST INFORMATION**
**Test Statistics:** No data available
**Reference(s):** Mucha et al. (2014)

# CLINICAL ASSESSMENT

| NATA EC 5th | BOC RD6 | SKILL |
|---|---|---|
| CE-21m | D2-0203 | Fluorescent Dye Testing |

**Supplies Needed:** Table or chair, fluorescent strips, saline solution

*This problem allows you the opportunity to demonstrate a* **physical assessment** *known as* **fluorescent dye testing** *for* **corneal abrasion**. *You have 2 minutes to complete this task.*

| Fluorescent Dye Testing | Course or Site<br>Assessor<br>Environment | | | | | |
|---|---|---|---|---|---|---|
| | | Test 1 | | Test 2 | | Test 3 |
| | | Y | N | Y | N | Y | N |
| **Tester places patient and limb in appropriate position** | | Y | N | Y | N | Y | N |
| Seated | | O | O | O | O | O | O |
| **Tester placed in proper position** | | Y | N | Y | N | Y | N |
| Stands in front of the patient | | O | O | O | O | O | O |
| **Tester performs test according to accepted guidelines** | | Y | N | Y | N | Y | N |
| Soaks the fluorescent strip with sterile saline solution | | O | O | O | O | O | O |
| Lightly touches the wet fluorescent strip to the conjunctiva of the lower eyelid | | O | O | O | O | O | O |
| Asks the patient to blink the eyes a few times | | O | O | O | O | O | O |
| **Identifies positive findings and implications** | | Y | N | Y | N | Y | N |
| When viewed with a cobalt blue light, corneal abrasions appear as bright yellowish-green pattern on the eye | | O | O | O | O | O | O |
| **Total** | | __/6 | | __/6 | | __/6 |
| **Must achieve >4 to pass this examination** | | Ⓟ | Ⓕ | Ⓟ | Ⓕ | Ⓟ | Ⓕ |

| Assessor:<br>Date: | Test 1 Comments: |
|---|---|
| Assessor:<br>Date: | Test 2 Comments: |
| Assessor:<br>Date: | Test 3 Comments: |

**TEST ENVIRONMENTS**
L: Laboratory/Classroom
C: Clinical/Field Testing
P: Practicum
A: Assessment/Mock Exam

**TEST INFORMATION**
**Test Statistics:** No data available
**Reference(s):** Starkey & Brown (2015)

## Musculoskeletal System—Region 10: Head and Face
# Clinical Assessment

| NATA EC 5th | BOC RD6 | SKILL |
|---|---|---|
| CE-21m | D2-0203 | Gaze Stability (Horizontal Vestibulo-Ocular Reflex) |

**Supplies Needed:** Table, target with 14-point font writing

*This problem allows you the opportunity to demonstrate a* **physical assessment** *known as* **horizontal gaze stability**. *You have 2 minutes to complete this task.*

| Gaze Stability (Horizontal Vestibulo-Ocular Reflex) | Course or Site Assessor Environment | | Test 1 | | Test 2 | | Test 3 | |
|---|---|---|---|---|---|---|---|---|
| **Tester places patient and limb in appropriate position** | | | Y | N | Y | N | Y | N |
| Seated | | | O | O | O | O | O | O |
| **Tester placed in proper position** | | | Y | N | Y | N | Y | N |
| Sits in front of the patient | | | O | O | O | O | O | O |
| **Tester performs test according to accepted guidelines** | | | Y | N | Y | N | Y | N |
| Holds a target of approximately 14-point font size in front of the patient | | | O | O | O | O | O | O |
| Instructs the patient to rotate head horizontally while maintaining focus on target | | | O | O | O | O | O | O |
| **Identifies positive findings and implications** | | | Y | N | Y | N | Y | N |
| Inability to perform 10 repetitions | | | O | O | O | O | O | O |
| Increase in symptoms | | | O | O | O | O | O | O |
| **Total** | | | ___/6 | | ___/6 | | ___/6 | |
| **Must achieve >4 to pass this examination** | | | Ⓟ | Ⓕ | Ⓟ | Ⓕ | Ⓟ | Ⓕ |
| Assessor: Date: | Test 1 Comments: | | | | | | | |
| Assessor: Date: | Test 2 Comments: | | | | | | | |
| Assessor: Date: | Test 3 Comments: | | | | | | | |

**TEST ENVIRONMENTS**
**L:** Laboratory/Classroom
**C:** Clinical/Field Testing
**P:** Practicum
**A:** Assessment/Mock Exam

**TEST INFORMATION**
**Test Statistics:** N/A
**Reference(s):** Mucha et al. (2014)

# CLINICAL ASSESSMENT

| NATA EC 5th | BOC RD6 | SKILL |
|---|---|---|
| CE-21m | D2-0203 | Gaze Stability (Vertical Vestibulo-Ocular Reflex) |

**Supplies Needed:** Table, target with 14-point font writing

*This problem allows you the opportunity to demonstrate a* **physical assessment** *known as* **vertical gaze stability.** *You have 2 minutes to complete this task.*

| Gaze Stability (Vertical Vestibulo-Ocular Reflex) | Course or Site Assessor Environment | | Test 1 | | Test 2 | | Test 3 | |
|---|---|---|---|---|---|---|---|---|
| **Tester places patient and limb in appropriate position** | | Y | | N | Y | N | Y | N |
| Seated | | ○ | | ○ | ○ | ○ | ○ | ○ |
| **Tester placed in proper position** | | Y | | N | Y | N | Y | N |
| Seated in front of the patient | | ○ | | ○ | ○ | ○ | ○ | ○ |
| **Tester performs test according to accepted guidelines** | | Y | | N | Y | N | Y | N |
| Holds a target of approximately 14-point font size in front of the patient | | ○ | | ○ | ○ | ○ | ○ | ○ |
| Instructs the patient to rotate head vertically while maintaining focus on target | | ○ | | ○ | ○ | ○ | ○ | ○ |
| **Identifies positive findings and implications** | | Y | | N | Y | N | Y | N |
| Inability to perform 10 repetitions | | ○ | | ○ | ○ | ○ | ○ | ○ |
| Increase in symptoms | | ○ | | ○ | ○ | ○ | ○ | ○ |
| Total | | ___/6 | | | ___/6 | | ___/6 | |
| Must achieve >4 to pass this examination | | Ⓟ | | Ⓕ | Ⓟ | Ⓕ | Ⓟ | Ⓕ |

| Assessor: Date: | Test 1 Comments: |
|---|---|
| Assessor: Date: | Test 2 Comments: |
| Assessor: Date: | Test 3 Comments: |

**TEST ENVIRONMENTS**
**L:** Laboratory/Classroom
**C:** Clinical/Field Testing
**P:** Practicum
**A:** Assessment/Mock Exam

**TEST INFORMATION**
**Test Statistics:** N/A
**Reference(s):** Starkey & Brown (2015)

## MUSCULOSKELETAL SYSTEM—REGION 10: HEAD AND FACE
# CLINICAL ASSESSMENT

| NATA EC 5th | BOC RD6 | SKILL |
|---|---|---|
| CE-21m | D2-0203 | Pupil Reaction to Light |

**Supplies Needed:** Occluder, penlight

*This problem allows you the opportunity to demonstrate a* **physical assessment** *known as* **pupil reaction to light**. *You have 2 minutes to complete this task.*

| Pupil Reaction to Light | Course or Site / Assessor / Environment | Test 1 | | Test 2 | | Test 3 | |
|---|---|---|---|---|---|---|---|
| | | Y | N | Y | N | Y | N |
| **Tester places patient and limb in appropriate position** | | Y | N | Y | N | Y | N |
| Standing | | ○ | ○ | ○ | ○ | ○ | ○ |
| **Tester placed in proper position** | | Y | N | Y | N | Y | N |
| Stands in front of the patient | | ○ | ○ | ○ | ○ | ○ | ○ |
| **Tester performs test according to accepted guidelines** | | Y | N | Y | N | Y | N |
| Places occluder in front of the eye not being tested | | ○ | ○ | ○ | ○ | ○ | ○ |
| Slowly moves penlight into the patient's eye for 1 second | | ○ | ○ | ○ | ○ | ○ | ○ |
| Observes for pupil constriction when light is applied and dilation when light is removed | | ○ | ○ | ○ | ○ | ○ | ○ |
| **Identifies positive findings and implications** | | Y | N | Y | N | Y | N |
| Pupil is unresponsive to light | | ○ | ○ | ○ | ○ | ○ | ○ |
| Total | | ___/6 | | ___/6 | | ___/6 | |
| **Must achieve >4 to pass this examination** | | Ⓟ | Ⓕ | Ⓟ | Ⓕ | Ⓟ | Ⓕ |

| Assessor: Date: | Test 1 Comments: |
|---|---|
| Assessor: Date: | Test 2 Comments: |
| Assessor: Date: | Test 3 Comments: |

**TEST ENVIRONMENTS**
**L:** Laboratory/Classroom
**C:** Clinical/Field Testing
**P:** Practicum
**A:** Assessment/Mock Exam

**TEST INFORMATION**
**Test Statistics:** N/A
**Reference(s):** Starkey & Brown (2015)

## MUSCULOSKELETAL SYSTEM—REGION 10: HEAD AND FACE
# CLINICAL ASSESSMENT

| NATA EC 5th | BOC RD6 | SKILL |
|---|---|---|
| CE-21m | D2-0203 | Saccadic Eye Movement (Horizontal) |

**Supplies Needed:** Table

*This problem allows you the opportunity to demonstrate a* **physical assessment** *known as* **horizontal saccadic eye movement**. *You have 2 minutes to complete this task.*

| Saccadic Eye Movement (Horizontal) | Course or Site Assessor Environment | | | | | |
|---|---|---|---|---|---|---|
| | | Test 1 | | Test 2 | | Test 3 |
| **Tester places patient and limb in appropriate position** | Y | N | Y | N | Y | N |
| Seated | O | O | O | O | O | O |
| **Tester placed in proper position** | Y | N | Y | N | Y | N |
| Seated in front of the patient | O | O | O | O | O | O |
| **Tester performs test according to accepted guidelines** | Y | N | Y | N | Y | N |
| Holds two single points (fingertips) horizontally at a distance of 3 feet from the patient, 1.5 feet to the left, and 1.5 feet to the right of the midline | O | O | O | O | O | O |
| Instructs the patient to move his/her eyes as quickly as possible between targets without moving the head | O | O | O | O | O | O |
| 10 repetitions are performed | O | O | O | O | O | O |
| **Identifies positive findings and implications** | Y | N | Y | N | Y | N |
| Increase in symptoms | O | O | O | O | O | O |
| Total | /6 | | /6 | | /6 | |
| Must achieve >4 to pass this examination | Ⓟ | Ⓕ | Ⓟ | Ⓕ | Ⓟ | Ⓕ |

| Assessor:<br>Date: | Test 1 Comments: |
|---|---|
| Assessor:<br>Date: | Test 2 Comments: |
| Assessor:<br>Date: | Test 3 Comments: |

**TEST ENVIRONMENTS**
**L:** Laboratory/Classroom
**C:** Clinical/Field Testing
**P:** Practicum
**A:** Assessment/Mock Exam

**TEST INFORMATION**
**Test Statistics:** N/A
**Reference(s):** Mucha et al. (2014)

# CLINICAL ASSESSMENT

| NATA EC 5th | BOC RD6 | SKILL |
|---|---|---|
| CE-21m | D2-0203 | Saccadic Eye Movement (Vertical) |

**Supplies Needed:** Table

*This problem allows you the opportunity to demonstrate a* **physical assessment** *known as* **vertical saccadic eye movement**. *You have 2 minutes to complete this task.*

| Saccadic Eye Movement (Vertical) | Course or Site Assessor Environment | Test 1 | | Test 2 | | Test 3 | |
|---|---|---|---|---|---|---|---|
| | | Y | N | Y | N | Y | N |
| **Tester places patient and limb in appropriate position** | | Y | N | Y | N | Y | N |
| Seated | | ○ | ○ | ○ | ○ | ○ | ○ |
| **Tester placed in proper position** | | Y | N | Y | N | Y | N |
| Seated in front of the patient | | ○ | ○ | ○ | ○ | ○ | ○ |
| **Tester performs test according to accepted guidelines** | | Y | N | Y | N | Y | N |
| Holds two single points (fingertips) vertically at a distance of 3 feet from the patient, 1.5 feet above and 1.5 feet below the midline | | ○ | ○ | ○ | ○ | ○ | ○ |
| Instructs the patient to move his/her eyes as quickly as possible between targets without moving the head | | ○ | ○ | ○ | ○ | ○ | ○ |
| 10 repetitions are performed | | ○ | ○ | ○ | ○ | ○ | ○ |
| **Identifies positive findings and implications** | | Y | N | Y | N | Y | N |
| Increase in symptoms | | ○ | ○ | ○ | ○ | ○ | ○ |
| **Total** | | /6 | | /6 | | /6 | |
| **Must achieve >4 to pass this examination** | | Ⓟ | Ⓕ | Ⓟ | Ⓕ | Ⓟ | Ⓕ |

| Assessor: Date: | Test 1 Comments: |
|---|---|
| Assessor: Date: | Test 2 Comments: |
| Assessor: Date: | Test 3 Comments: |

**TEST ENVIRONMENTS**
**L:** Laboratory/Classroom
**C:** Clinical/Field Testing
**P:** Practicum
**A:** Assessment/Mock Exam

**TEST INFORMATION**
**Test Statistics:** N/A
**Reference(s):** Mucha et al. (2014)

## MUSCULOSKELETAL SYSTEM—REGION 10: HEAD AND FACE
# CLINICAL ASSESSMENT

| NATA EC 5th | BOC RD6 | SKILL |
|---|---|---|
| CE-21m | D2-0203 | Smooth Pursuits |

**Supplies Needed:** Table

*This problem allows you the opportunity to demonstrate a* **physical assessment** *known as* **smooth pursuit eye movement**. *You have 2 minutes to complete this task.*

| Smooth Pursuits | Course or Site / Assessor / Environment | | Test 1 | | Test 2 | | Test 3 | |
|---|---|---|---|---|---|---|---|---|
| | | | Y | N | Y | N | Y | N |
| **Tester places patient and limb in appropriate position** | | | Y | N | Y | N | Y | N |
| Standing | | | O | O | O | O | O | O |
| **Tester placed in proper position** | | | Y | N | Y | N | Y | N |
| Stands in front of the patient | | | O | O | O | O | O | O |
| **Tester performs test according to accepted guidelines** | | | Y | N | Y | N | Y | N |
| Holds fingertip 3 feet away from the patient | | | O | O | O | O | O | O |
| Instructs the patient to maintain focus on the fingertip | | | O | O | O | O | O | O |
| Moves the fingertip in a horizontal direction to the left and right 1.5 feet | | | O | O | O | O | O | O |
| Moves fingertip at a consistent rate | | | O | O | O | O | O | O |
| **Identifies positive findings and implications** | | | Y | N | Y | N | Y | N |
| Increase in symptoms | | | O | O | O | O | O | O |
| | | Total | __/7 | | __/7 | | __/7 | |
| | Must achieve >4 to pass this examination | | Ⓟ | Ⓕ | Ⓟ | Ⓕ | Ⓟ | Ⓕ |

| Assessor: Date: | Test 1 Comments: |
|---|---|
| Assessor: Date: | Test 2 Comments: |
| Assessor: Date: | Test 3 Comments: |

**TEST ENVIRONMENTS**
**L:** Laboratory/Classroom
**C:** Clinical/Field Testing
**P:** Practicum
**A:** Assessment/Mock Exam

**TEST INFORMATION**
**Test Statistics:** N/A
**Reference(s):** Mucha et al. (2014)

## MUSCULOSKELETAL SYSTEM—REGION 10: HEAD AND FACE
# CLINICAL ASSESSMENT

| NATA EC 5th | BOC RD6 | SKILL |
|---|---|---|
| CE-21m | D2-0203 | Snellen Eye Chart |

**Supplies Needed:** Vision occluder, Snellen eye chart

*This problem allows you the opportunity to demonstrate a* **physical assessment** *known as the* **Snellen eye chart**. *You have 2 minutes to complete this task.*

| Snellen Eye Chart | Course or Site Assessor Environment | | Test 1 | | Test 2 | | Test 3 | |
|---|---|---|---|---|---|---|---|---|
| **Tester places patient and limb in appropriate position** | | **Y** | **N** | **Y** | **N** | **Y** | **N** | |
| Standing 20 feet away from chart in well-illuminated area | | ○ | ○ | ○ | ○ | ○ | ○ | |
| **Tester placed in proper position** | | **Y** | **N** | **Y** | **N** | **Y** | **N** | |
| Stands next to eye chart | | ○ | ○ | ○ | ○ | ○ | ○ | |
| **Tester performs test according to accepted guidelines** | | **Y** | **N** | **Y** | **N** | **Y** | **N** | |
| Instructs the patient to cover eye not being tested | | ○ | ○ | ○ | ○ | ○ | ○ | |
| Instructs the patient to read line 6 (20/20) from left to right | | ○ | ○ | ○ | ○ | ○ | ○ | |
| Asks the patient to repeat with opposite eye in reverse order | | ○ | ○ | ○ | ○ | ○ | ○ | |
| **Identifies positive findings and implications** | | **Y** | **N** | **Y** | **N** | **Y** | **N** | |
| The patient is unable to read line | | ○ | ○ | ○ | ○ | ○ | ○ | |
| **Total** | | ___/6 | | ___/6 | | ___/6 | | |
| **Must achieve >4 to pass this examination** | | Ⓟ | Ⓕ | Ⓟ | Ⓕ | Ⓟ | Ⓕ | |

| Assessor:<br>Date: | Test 1 Comments: |
|---|---|
| Assessor:<br>Date: | Test 2 Comments: |
| Assessor:<br>Date: | Test 3 Comments: |

**TEST ENVIRONMENTS**
**L:** Laboratory/Classroom
**C:** Clinical/Field Testing
**P:** Practicum
**A:** Assessment/Mock Exam

**TEST INFORMATION**
**Test Statistics:** N/A
**Reference(s):** Stevens (2007)

# MUSCULOSKELETAL SYSTEM—REGION 10: HEAD AND FACE
## CLINICAL ASSESSMENT

| NATA EC 5th | BOC RD6 | SKILL |
|---|---|---|
| CE-21n | D2-0203 | Otoscope Use (Ear) |

**Supplies Needed:** Table, otoscope

*This problem allows you the opportunity to demonstrate use of an* **otoscope** *to examine the* **ear***.*
*You have 2 minutes to complete this task.*

| Otoscope Use (Ear) | Course or Site Assessor Environment | | Test 1 | | Test 2 | | Test 3 | |
|---|---|---|---|---|---|---|---|---|
| | | | Y | N | Y | N | Y | N |
| **Tester places patient and limb in appropriate position** | | | Y | N | Y | N | Y | N |
| Seated | | | O | O | O | O | O | O |
| **Tester placed in proper position** | | | Y | N | Y | N | Y | N |
| Position to easily access the ear | | | O | O | O | O | O | O |
| **Tester performs test according to accepted guidelines** | | | Y | N | Y | N | Y | N |
| Fits speculum on the otoscope | | | O | O | O | O | O | O |
| Opens the auditory canal by gently pulling upward and backward on the pinna or downward on the earlobe | | | O | O | O | O | O | O |
| Inserts the otoscope gently and examines the canal | | | O | O | O | O | O | O |
| **Identifies implications** | | | Y | N | Y | N | Y | N |
| Redding or bulging tympanic membrane, fluid buildup behind the tympanic membrane, ruptured tympanic membrane | | | O | O | O | O | O | O |
| Total | | | ___/6 | | ___/6 | | ___/6 | |
| Must achieve >4 to pass this examination | | | P | F | P | F | P | F |

| Assessor: Date: | Test 1 Comments: |
|---|---|
| Assessor: Date: | Test 2 Comments: |
| Assessor: Date: | Test 3 Comments: |

**TEST ENVIRONMENTS**
**L:** Laboratory/Classroom
**C:** Clinical/Field Testing
**P:** Practicum
**A:** Assessment/Mock Exam

**TEST INFORMATION**
**Test Statistics:** N/A
**Reference(s):** Starkey & Brown (2015)

## MUSCULOSKELETAL SYSTEM—REGION 10: HEAD AND FACE
# CLINICAL ASSESSMENT

| NATA EC 5th | BOC RD6 | SKILL |
|---|---|---|
| CE-21n | D2-0203 | Otoscope Use (Nose) |

**Supplies Needed:** Table, otoscope

*This problem allows you the opportunity to demonstrate use of an* **otoscope** *to examine the* **nose**. *You have 2 minutes to complete this task.*

| Otoscope Use (Nose) | Course or Site / Assessor / Environment | | Test 1 | | Test 2 | | Test 3 | |
|---|---|---|---|---|---|---|---|---|
| **Tester places patient and limb in appropriate position** | | | Y | N | Y | N | Y | N |
| Seated | | | ○ | ○ | ○ | ○ | ○ | ○ |
| **Tester placed in proper position** | | | Y | N | Y | N | Y | N |
| Position to easily access the nose | | | ○ | ○ | ○ | ○ | ○ | ○ |
| **Tester performs test according to accepted guidelines** | | | Y | N | Y | N | Y | N |
| Fits speculum on the otoscope | | | ○ | ○ | ○ | ○ | ○ | ○ |
| Inserts the otoscope gently and examines the canal | | | ○ | ○ | ○ | ○ | ○ | ○ |
| **Identifies implications** | | | Y | N | Y | N | Y | N |
| Deviation or deformity of the nasal passage | | | ○ | ○ | ○ | ○ | ○ | ○ |
| Total | | | ___/5 | | ___/5 | | ___/5 | |
| Must achieve >3 to pass this examination | | | Ⓟ | Ⓕ | Ⓟ | Ⓕ | Ⓟ | Ⓕ |

| Assessor: Date: | Test 1 Comments: |
|---|---|
| Assessor: Date: | Test 2 Comments: |
| Assessor: Date: | Test 3 Comments: |

**TEST ENVIRONMENTS**
**L:** Laboratory/Classroom
**C:** Clinical/Field Testing
**P:** Practicum
**A:** Assessment/Mock Exam

**TEST INFORMATION**
**Test Statistics:** N/A
**Reference(s):** Starkey & Brown (2015)

## MUSCULOSKELETAL SYSTEM—REGION 10: HEAD AND FACE
# CLINICAL ASSESSMENT

| NATA EC 5th | BOC RD6 | SKILL |
|---|---|---|
| CE-21n | D2-0203 | Otoscope Use (Throat) |

**Supplies Needed:** Table, otoscope

*This problem allows you the opportunity to demonstrate use of an* **otoscope** *to examine the* **throat**. *You have 2 minutes to complete this task.*

| Otoscope Use (Throat) | Course or Site Assessor Environment | | Test 1 | | Test 2 | | Test 3 | |
|---|---|---|---|---|---|---|---|---|
| **Tester places patient and limb in appropriate position** | | | Y | N | Y | N | Y | N |
| Seated | | | O | O | O | O | O | O |
| **Tester placed in proper position** | | | Y | N | Y | N | Y | N |
| Position to easily access the throat | | | O | O | O | O | O | O |
| **Tester performs test according to accepted guidelines** | | | Y | N | Y | N | Y | N |
| Instructs the patient to open mouth and keep mouth open | | | O | O | O | O | O | O |
| Uses light on otoscope to examine the back of throat | | | O | O | O | O | O | O |
| **Identifies implications** | | | Y | N | Y | N | Y | N |
| Abnormal discoloration or swelling in throat | | | O | O | O | O | O | O |
| Total | | | _/5 | | _/5 | | _/5 | |
| Must achieve >3 to pass this examination | | | Ⓟ | Ⓕ | Ⓟ | Ⓕ | Ⓟ | Ⓕ |
| Assessor: Date: | Test 1 Comments: | | | | | | | |
| Assessor: Date: | Test 2 Comments: | | | | | | | |
| Assessor: Date: | Test 3 Comments: | | | | | | | |

**TEST ENVIRONMENTS**
**L:** Laboratory/Classroom
**C:** Clinical/Field Testing
**P:** Practicum
**A:** Assessment/Mock Exam

**TEST INFORMATION**
**Test Statistics:** N/A
**Reference(s):** Starkey & Brown (2015)

# IV

---

# ACUTE CARE OF
# INJURIES AND ILLNESSES

# 14

# ACUTE CARE OF
# INJURIES AND ILLNESSES

Hauth, J. M., Gloyeske, B. M., & Amato, H. K.
*Clinical Skills Documentation Guide for Athletic Training, Third Edition* (pp. 454-504).
© 2016 SLACK Incorporated.

## ACUTE CARE OF INJURIES AND ILLNESSES
# KNOWLEDGE AND SKILLS

| Acute Care of Injuries and Illnesses | | | | Skill: Acquisition, Reinforcement, Proficiency | | |
|---|---|---|---|---|---|---|
| **NATA EC 5th** | **BOC RD6** | **Assessment** | **Page #** | | | |
| AC-4 | D3-0302 | Primary and Secondary Surveys | 457 | | | |
| AC-6 | D3-0302 | Vital Signs (Blood Pressure) | 458 | | | |
| AC-6 | D3-0302 | Vital Signs (Core Temperature) | 459 | | | |
| AC-6 | D3-0302 | Vital Signs (Heart Rate) | 460 | | | |
| AC-6, AC-18 | D3-0302 | Vital Signs (Pulse Oximetry) | 461 | | | |
| AC-6 | D3-0302 | Vital Signs (Respiratory Rate) | 462 | | | |
| AC-7 | D3-0302, D1-0102 | Heart Auscultation | 463 | | | |
| AC-7 | D3-0302, D1-0102 | Lung Auscultation | 464 | | | |
| AC-10 | D3-0302 | Oropharyngeal Airways | 465 | | | |
| AC-10 | D3-0302 | Nasopharyngeal Airways | 466 | | | |
| AC-10 | D3-0302 | Facemask Removal (Cordless Screwdriver) | 467 | | | |
| AC-10 | D3-0302 | Facemask Removal (FM Extractor) | 468 | | | |
| AC-10 | D3-0302 | Facemask Removal (Quick Release Tool) | 469 | | | |
| AC-10 | D3-0302 | Facemask Removal (Trainer's Angel) | 470 | | | |
| AC-11 | D3-0303 | Suction for Airway Management | 471 | | | |
| AC-13 | D3-0303 | Automated External Defibrillator | 472 | | | |
| AC-14 | D3-0303 | Cardiopulmonary Resuscitation (1P Adult) | 473 | | | |
| AC-14 | D3-0303 | Cardiopulmonary Resuscitation (2P Adult) | 474 | | | |
| AC-15 | D3-0303 | Bag Valve Mask (Child and Adult Nonbreathing) | 475 | | | |
| AC-15 | D3-0303 | Pocket Mask (Child and Adult) | 476 | | | |
| AC-17 | D3-0303 | Supplemental Oxygen (Nasal Cannula) | 477 | | | |
| AC-17 | D3-0303 | Supplemental Oxygen (Reservoir Bag Valve Facemask) | 478 | | | |
| AC-20 | D4-0404 | External Hemorrhage Management | 479 | | | |
| AC-22 | D4-0404 | Wound Care (Forearm Abrasion) | 480 | | | |
| AC-23 | D3-0303 | Cervical Spine Stabilization | 481 | | | |
| AC-25 | D3-0303 | Patient Transfer Technique (Six-Person Lift) | 482 | | | |
| AC-25 | D3-0303 | Patient Transfer Technique (Prone Log Roll) | 483 | | | |
| AC-25 | D3-0303 | Patient Transfer Technique (Supine Log Roll) | 484 | | | |
| AC-29 | D3-0302 | Rectal Temperature | 485 | | | |
| AC-31 | D3-0303 | Nebulizer Treatment | 486 | | | |
| AC-33 | D3-0303 | Metered-Dose Inhaler | 487 | | | |
| AC-35 | D3-0303 | Auto-Injectable Epinephrine | 488 | | | |

*(continued on the next page)*

ACUTE CARE OF INJURIES AND ILLNESSES
# KNOWLEDGE AND SKILLS

| NATA EC 5th | BOC RD6 | Protective Device Fitting | Page # | | | |
|---|---|---|---|---|---|---|
| AC-37 | D3-0303, D4-0403 | Adjustable SAM Splint (Ladder Splint) | 489 | | | |
| AC-37 | D3-0303, D4-0403 | Immobilization (Knee Immobilizer) | 490 | | | |
| **NATA EC 5th** | **BOC RD6** | **Protective Device Construction** | **Page #** | | | |
| AC-37 | D3-0303, D4-0403 | Immobilization (Sling and Swath) | 491 | | | |
| AC-37 | D3-0303, D4-0403 | Splinting – Arm (Humerus) | 492 | | | |
| AC-37 | D3-0303, D4-0403 | Splinting – Finger (Proximal Interphalangeal Joint) | 493 | | | |
| AC-37 | D3-0303, D4-0403 | Splinting – Foot/Ankle (Tarsals/Metatarsals) | 494 | | | |
| AC-37 | D3-0303, D4-0403 | Splinting – Hand/Wrist (Carpals/Metacarpals) | 495 | | | |
| AC-37 | D3-0303, D4-0403 | Splinting – Leg (Femur) | 496 | | | |
| AC-37 | D3-0303, D4-0403 | Splinting – Lower Leg (Tibia) | 497 | | | |
| **NATA EC 5th** | **BOC RD6** | **Ambulation Assistance** | **Page #** | | | |
| AC-39 | D4-0403 | Cane Fitting | 498 | | | |
| AC-39 | D4-0403 | Crutch Fitting | 499 | | | |
| AC-39 | D4-0403 | Four-Point Gait Method | 500 | | | |
| AC-39 | D4-0403 | Nonweightbearing (Ascending/Descending Stairs) | 501 | | | |
| AC-39 | D4-0403 | Nonweightbearing (Tripod) | 502 | | | |
| **NATA EC 5th** | **BOC RD6** | **Patient Transport** | **Page #** | | | |
| AC-42 | D4-0403 | Patient Transport (Assisted Walk) | 503 | | | |
| AC-42 | D4-0403 | Patient Transport (Carry) | 504 | | | |

## ACUTE CARE OF INJURIES AND ILLNESSES
# ASSESSMENT

| NATA EC 5th | BOC RD6 | SKILL |
|---|---|---|
| AC-4 | D3-0302 | Primary and Secondary Surveys |

**Supplies Needed:** Mannequin, personal protective equipment

*This problem allows you the opportunity to demonstrate an acute care assessment known as the* **Primary and Secondary Surveys** *to rule out* **life-threatening conditions**. *You have 2 minutes to complete this task.*

| Primary and Secondary Surveys | Course or Site / Assessor / Environment | | | | | |
|---|---|---|---|---|---|---|
| | | Test 1 | | Test 2 | | Test 3 |
| **Tester performs test according to accepted guidelines** | | Y | N | Y | N | Y | N |
| Checks the scene to ensure safety | | ○ | ○ | ○ | ○ | ○ | ○ |
| Applies appropriate PPE prior to approaching the patient | | ○ | ○ | ○ | ○ | ○ | ○ |
| Scans the patient for life- or limb-threatening conditions and immediately corrects them | | ○ | ○ | ○ | ○ | ○ | ○ |
| Checks airway, breathing, circulation, neurological disability/applies defibrillator, and exposure level of the patient | | ○ | ○ | ○ | ○ | ○ | ○ |
| Activates EAP, if appropriate | | ○ | ○ | ○ | ○ | ○ | ○ |
| Performs complete head-to-toe examination to rule out non-life-threatening conditions | | ○ | ○ | ○ | ○ | ○ | ○ |
| Continues to monitor vital signs throughout survey | | ○ | ○ | ○ | ○ | ○ | ○ |
| Recognizes and corrects deterioration in vital signs quickly | | ○ | ○ | ○ | ○ | ○ | ○ |
| Communicates status clearly to EMS upon arrival | | ○ | ○ | ○ | ○ | ○ | ○ |
| **Total** | | __/9 | | __/9 | | __/9 | |
| **Must achieve >6 to pass this examination** | | ⓟ | Ⓕ | ⓟ | Ⓕ | ⓟ | Ⓕ |

| Assessor: Date: | Test 1 Comments: |
|---|---|
| Assessor: Date: | Test 2 Comments: |
| Assessor: Date: | Test 3 Comments: |

**TEST ENVIRONMENTS**
**L:** Laboratory/Classroom
**C:** Clinical/Field Testing
**P:** Practicum
**A:** Assessment/Mock Exam

**TEST INFORMATION**
**Test Statistics:** N/A
**Reference(s):** Starkey & Brown (2015)

## ACUTE CARE OF INJURIES AND ILLNESSES
# ASSESSMENT

| NATA EC 5th | BOC RD6 | SKILL |
|---|---|---|
| AC-6 | D3-0302 | Vital Signs (Blood Pressure) |

**Supplies Needed:** Chair, table, sphygmomanometer, stethoscope

*This problem allows you the opportunity to demonstrate an acute care assessment of* **vital signs (blood pressure)**. *You have 2 minutes to complete this task.*

| Vital Signs (Blood Pressure) | Course or Site / Assessor / Environment | Test 1 | | Test 2 | | Test 3 | |
|---|---|---|---|---|---|---|---|
| | | Y | N | Y | N | Y | N |
| **Tester places patient and limb in appropriate position** | | Y | N | Y | N | Y | N |
| Seated, with arm resting on a table at chest height | | ○ | ○ | ○ | ○ | ○ | ○ |
| **Tester placed in proper position** | | Y | N | Y | N | Y | N |
| Stands in front of the patient | | ○ | ○ | ○ | ○ | ○ | ○ |
| **Tester performs test according to accepted guidelines** | | Y | N | Y | N | Y | N |
| Places appropriate-sized sphygmomanometer around the patient's bare upper arm | | ○ | ○ | ○ | ○ | ○ | ○ |
| Palpates and places stethoscope over brachial artery | | ○ | ○ | ○ | ○ | ○ | ○ |
| Inflates sphygmomanometer to 15 to 20 mm Hg beyond the point where Korotkoff sounds are no longer heard | | ○ | ○ | ○ | ○ | ○ | ○ |
| Allows sphygmomanometer to deflate at a slow, controlled rate, noting systolic and diastolic blood pressures | | ○ | ○ | ○ | ○ | ○ | ○ |
| **Identifies positive findings and implications** | | Y | N | Y | N | Y | N |
| Normal blood pressure – 120/80 mm Hg | | ○ | ○ | ○ | ○ | ○ | ○ |
| **Total** | | ___/7 | | ___/7 | | ___/7 | |
| **Must achieve >4 to pass this examination** | | Ⓟ | Ⓕ | Ⓟ | Ⓕ | Ⓟ | Ⓕ |

| Assessor: Date: | Test 1 Comments: |
|---|---|
| Assessor: Date: | Test 2 Comments: |
| Assessor: Date: | Test 3 Comments: |

**TEST ENVIRONMENTS**
**L:** Laboratory/Classroom
**C:** Clinical/Field Testing
**P:** Practicum
**A:** Assessment/Mock Exam

**TEST INFORMATION**
**Test Statistics:** N/A
**Reference(s):** Gorse et al. (2010)

# ASSESSMENT

| NATA EC 5th | BOC RD6 | SKILL |
|:---:|:---:|:---:|
| AC-6 | D3-0302 | Vital Signs (Core Temperature) |

**Supplies Needed:** Thermometer, lubricating or petroleum jelly

*This problem allows you the opportunity to demonstrate an acute care assessment of* **vital signs (core temperature)**. *You have 2 minutes to complete this task.*

| Vital Signs (Core Temperature) | Course or Site Assessor Environment | | Test 1 | | Test 2 | | Test 3 |
|---|---|:---:|:---:|:---:|:---:|:---:|:---:|
| **Tester places patient and limb in appropriate position** | | **Y** | **N** | **Y** | **N** | **Y** | **N** |
| Places the patient on his/her stomach or side | | O | O | O | O | O | O |
| Places the hip into flexion and spreads the buttocks | | O | O | O | O | O | O |
| **Tester placed in proper position** | | **Y** | **N** | **Y** | **N** | **Y** | **N** |
| At the side of the patient | | O | O | O | O | O | O |
| **Tester performs test according to accepted guidelines** | | **Y** | **N** | **Y** | **N** | **Y** | **N** |
| Covers the tip of the glass thermometer or a flexible digital thermometer with lubricating or petroleum jelly | | O | O | O | O | O | O |
| Gently inserts the thermometer 8 to 10 cm into the rectum. Does not force it. Holds the buttocks together to keep the thermometer in place. | | O | O | O | O | O | O |
| Does not release his/her grip on glass thermometer | | O | O | O | O | O | O |
| Leaves the thermometer in place for 3 minutes | | O | O | O | O | O | O |
| Carefully removes and cleans the thermometer | | O | O | O | O | O | O |
| **Identifies positive findings and implications** | | **Y** | **N** | **Y** | **N** | **Y** | **N** |
| Heat stroke >104.8°F | | O | O | O | O | O | O |
| Cools the patient in a cold water tub | | O | O | O | O | O | O |
| | **Total** | \_\_\_\_/10 | | \_\_\_\_/10 | | \_\_\_\_/10 | |
| | **Must achieve >7 to pass this examination** | Ⓟ | Ⓕ | Ⓟ | Ⓕ | Ⓟ | Ⓕ |

| Assessor:<br>Date: | **Test 1 Comments:** |
|---|---|
| Assessor:<br>Date: | **Test 2 Comments:** |
| Assessor:<br>Date: | **Test 3 Comments:** |

**TEST ENVIRONMENTS**
**L:** Laboratory/Classroom
**C:** Clinical/Field Testing
**P:** Practicum
**A:** Assessment/Mock Exam

**TEST INFORMATION**
**Test Statistics:** N/A
**Reference(s):** Gorse et al. (2010)

# ASSESSMENT

| NATA EC 5th | BOC RD6 | SKILL |
|---|---|---|
| AC-6 | D3-0302 | Vital Signs (Heart Rate) |

**Supplies Needed:** Table

*This problem allows you the opportunity to demonstrate an acute care assessment of **vital signs (heart rate)**. You have 2 minutes to complete this task.*

| Vital Signs (Heart Rate) | Course or Site Assessor Environment | | Test 1 | | Test 2 | | Test 3 | |
|---|---|---|---|---|---|---|---|---|
| **Tester places patient and limb in appropriate position** | | | **Y** | **N** | **Y** | **N** | **Y** | **N** |
| Seated or standing | | | ○ | ○ | ○ | ○ | ○ | ○ |
| **Tester placed in proper position** | | | **Y** | **N** | **Y** | **N** | **Y** | **N** |
| Stands next to the patient | | | ○ | ○ | ○ | ○ | ○ | ○ |
| **Tester performs test according to accepted guidelines** | | | **Y** | **N** | **Y** | **N** | **Y** | **N** |
| Palpates the patient's radial artery for at least 30 seconds | | | ○ | ○ | ○ | ○ | ○ | ○ |
| Notes regularity and strength of the patient's pulse | | | ○ | ○ | ○ | ○ | ○ | ○ |
| **Identifies positive findings and implications** | | | **Y** | **N** | **Y** | **N** | **Y** | **N** |
| Normative values – adult: 60 to 100 bpm; child: >20 bpm | | | ○ | ○ | ○ | ○ | ○ | ○ |
| Weak pulse may indicate shock | | | ○ | ○ | ○ | ○ | ○ | ○ |
| Irregular rates require careful evaluation and should be referred | | | ○ | ○ | ○ | ○ | ○ | ○ |
| Total | | | ___/7 | | ___/7 | | ___/7 | |
| Must achieve >4 to pass this examination | | | Ⓟ | Ⓕ | Ⓟ | Ⓕ | Ⓟ | Ⓕ |
| Assessor: Date: | **Test 1 Comments:** | | | | | | | |
| Assessor: Date: | **Test 2 Comments:** | | | | | | | |
| Assessor: Date: | **Test 3 Comments:** | | | | | | | |

**TEST ENVIRONMENTS**
**L:** Laboratory/Classroom
**C:** Clinical/Field Testing
**P:** Practicum
**A:** Assessment/Mock Exam

**TEST INFORMATION**
**Test Statistics:** N/A
**Reference(s):** Gorse et al. (2010)

ACUTE CARE OF INJURIES AND ILLNESSES
# ASSESSMENT

| NATA EC 5th | BOC RD6 | SKILL |
|---|---|---|
| AC-6, AC-18 | D3-0302 | Vital Signs (Pulse Oximetry) |

**Supplies Needed:** Chair, pulse oximeter

*This problem allows you the opportunity to demonstrate an acute care assessment of* **vital signs (pulse oximetry)**. *You have 2 minutes to complete this task.*

| Vital Signs (Pulse Oximetry) | Course or Site / Assessor / Environment | | Test 1 | | Test 2 | | Test 3 | |
|---|---|---|---|---|---|---|---|---|
| **Tester places patient and limb in appropriate position** | | | Y | N | Y | N | Y | N |
| Seated in a chair | | | O | O | O | O | O | O |
| **Tester placed in proper position** | | | Y | N | Y | N | Y | N |
| Stands to the side of the patient | | | O | O | O | O | O | O |
| **Tester performs test according to accepted guidelines** | | | Y | N | Y | N | Y | N |
| Instructs the patient to hold out pointer or middle finger | | | O | O | O | O | O | O |
| Turns on and places pulse oximeter on the patient's finger | | | O | O | O | O | O | O |
| Records values from pulse oximeter | | | O | O | O | O | O | O |
| **Identifies positive findings and implications** | | | Y | N | Y | N | Y | N |
| Normative values – $SPO_2$ >95% | | | O | O | O | O | O | O |
| Values under 90% require supplemental oxygen | | | O | O | O | O | O | O |
| Abnormally high values could indicate carbon monoxide poisoning | | | O | O | O | O | O | O |
| | | Total | ___/8 | | ___/8 | | ___/8 | |
| | Must achieve >5 to pass this examination | | Ⓟ | Ⓕ | Ⓟ | Ⓕ | Ⓟ | Ⓕ |

| Assessor:<br>Date: | Test 1 Comments: |
|---|---|
| Assessor:<br>Date: | Test 2 Comments: |
| Assessor:<br>Date: | Test 3 Comments: |

**TEST ENVIRONMENTS**
**L:** Laboratory/Classroom
**C:** Clinical/Field Testing
**P:** Practicum
**A:** Assessment/Mock Exam

**TEST INFORMATION**
**Test Statistics:** N/A
**Reference(s):** Gorse et al. (2010)

## ACUTE CARE OF INJURIES AND ILLNESSES
# ASSESSMENT

| NATA EC 5th | BOC RD6 | SKILL |
|---|---|---|
| AC-6 | D3-0302 | Vital Signs (Respiratory Rate) |

**Supplies Needed:** Chair

*This problem allows you the opportunity to demonstrate an acute care assessment of* **vital signs (respiratory rate)**. *You have 2 minutes to complete this task.*

| Vital Signs (Respiratory Rate) | Course or Site Assessor Environment | Test 1 | | Test 2 | | Test 3 | |
|---|---|---|---|---|---|---|---|
| | | **Y** | **N** | **Y** | **N** | **Y** | **N** |
| **Tester places patient and limb in appropriate position** | | **Y** | **N** | **Y** | **N** | **Y** | **N** |
| Seated or standing | | ○ | ○ | ○ | ○ | ○ | ○ |
| **Tester placed in proper position** | | **Y** | **N** | **Y** | **N** | **Y** | **N** |
| Stands next to the patient, palpating radial pulse | | ○ | ○ | ○ | ○ | ○ | ○ |
| **Tester performs test according to accepted guidelines** | | **Y** | **N** | **Y** | **N** | **Y** | **N** |
| Informs the patient he/she will be assessing the patient's pulse | | ○ | ○ | ○ | ○ | ○ | ○ |
| While palpating pulse, the tester observes the patient's chest rise | | ○ | ○ | ○ | ○ | ○ | ○ |
| Counts respirations for at least 15 seconds (preferably 30 seconds) | | ○ | ○ | ○ | ○ | ○ | ○ |
| **Identifies positive findings and implications** | | **Y** | **N** | **Y** | **N** | **Y** | **N** |
| Normative values – adult: 10 to 20 bpm; child: >20 bpm | | ○ | ○ | ○ | ○ | ○ | ○ |
| **Total** | | ___/6 | | ___/6 | | ___/6 | |
| **Must achieve >3 to pass this examination** | | Ⓟ | Ⓕ | Ⓟ | Ⓕ | Ⓟ | Ⓕ |

| Assessor: Date: | **Test 1 Comments:** |
|---|---|
| Assessor: Date: | **Test 2 Comments:** |
| Assessor: Date: | **Test 3 Comments:** |

**TEST ENVIRONMENTS**
**L:** Laboratory/Classroom
**C:** Clinical/Field Testing
**P:** Practicum
**A:** Assessment/Mock Exam

**TEST INFORMATION**
**Test Statistics:** N/A
**Reference(s):** Gorse et al. (2010)

## ACUTE CARE OF INJURIES AND ILLNESSES
# ASSESSMENT

| NATA EC 5th | BOC RD6 | SKILL |
|---|---|---|
| AC-7 | D3-0302, D1-0102 | Heart Auscultation |

**Supplies Needed:** Table or chair, stethoscope

*This problem allows you the opportunity to demonstrate an acute care assessment known as* **heart auscultation.** *You have 2 minutes to complete this task.*

| Heart Auscultation | Course or Site Assessor Environment | | Test 1 | | Test 2 | | Test 3 | |
|---|---|---|---|---|---|---|---|---|
| | | | Y | N | Y | N | Y | N |
| **Tester places patient and limb in appropriate position** | | | Y | N | Y | N | Y | N |
| Seated or supine | | | O | O | O | O | O | O |
| The patient should have minimal clothing on thorax | | | O | O | O | O | O | O |
| **Tester placed in proper position** | | | Y | N | Y | N | Y | N |
| Stands to the right of the patient | | | O | O | O | O | O | O |
| Stethoscope set to auscultate with diaphragm | | | O | O | O | O | O | O |
| **Tester performs test according to accepted guidelines** | | | Y | N | Y | N | Y | N |
| Auscultates over aortic valve (right sternum, ribs 2-3) | | | O | O | O | O | O | O |
| Auscultates over pulmonic valve (left sternum, ribs 2-3) | | | O | O | O | O | O | O |
| Auscultates over tricuspid valve (left sternum, ribs 5-6) | | | O | O | O | O | O | O |
| Auscultates over mitral valve (mid-clavicular line, ribs 5-6) | | | O | O | O | O | O | O |
| Repeats procedure auscultating with stethoscope bell | | | O | O | O | O | O | O |
| **Identifies positive findings and implications** | | | Y | N | Y | N | Y | N |
| Identifies sounds as normal or abnormal | | | O | O | O | O | O | O |
| | Total | | ___/10 | | ___/10 | | ___/10 | |
| | Must achieve >7 to pass this examination | | (P) | (F) | (P) | (F) | (P) | (F) |

| Assessor: Date: | Test 1 Comments: |
|---|---|
| Assessor: Date: | Test 2 Comments: |
| Assessor: Date: | Test 3 Comments: |

**TEST ENVIRONMENTS**
**L:** Laboratory/Classroom
**C:** Clinical/Field Testing
**P:** Practicum
**A:** Assessment/Mock Exam

**TEST INFORMATION**
**Test Statistics:** N/A
**Reference(s):** McChesney & McChesney (2001)

## ACUTE CARE OF INJURIES AND ILLNESSES
# ASSESSMENT

| NATA EC 5th | BOC RD6 | SKILL |
|---|---|---|
| AC-7 | D3-0302, D1-0102 | Lung Auscultation |

**Supplies Needed:** Table, stethoscope

*This problem allows you the opportunity to demonstrate an acute care assessment known as* **lung auscultation***. You have 2 minutes to complete this task.*

| Lung Auscultation | Course or Site / Assessor / Environment | | Test 1 | | Test 2 | | Test 3 | |
|---|---|---|---|---|---|---|---|---|
| | | | Y | N | Y | N | Y | N |
| **Tester places patient and limb in appropriate position** | | | Y | N | Y | N | Y | N |
| Seated | | | ○ | ○ | ○ | ○ | ○ | ○ |
| **Tester placed in proper position** | | | Y | N | Y | N | Y | N |
| Stands to the right of the patient | | | ○ | ○ | ○ | ○ | ○ | ○ |
| Stethoscope set to auscultate with diaphragm | | | ○ | ○ | ○ | ○ | ○ | ○ |
| **Tester performs test according to accepted guidelines** | | | Y | N | Y | N | Y | N |
| Auscultates bilaterally at superior angle of the scapulae | | | ○ | ○ | ○ | ○ | ○ | ○ |
| Auscultates bilaterally at medial spine of the scapulae | | | ○ | ○ | ○ | ○ | ○ | ○ |
| Auscultates bilaterally at inferior angle of the scapulae | | | ○ | ○ | ○ | ○ | ○ | ○ |
| Auscultates bilaterally at posterior mid-axillary region | | | ○ | ○ | ○ | ○ | ○ | ○ |
| Auscultates bilaterally just inferior to the clavicle | | | ○ | ○ | ○ | ○ | ○ | ○ |
| Auscultates bilaterally at mid-sternum height | | | ○ | ○ | ○ | ○ | ○ | ○ |
| Auscultates bilaterally at ribs 3-4 | | | ○ | ○ | ○ | ○ | ○ | ○ |
| Auscultates bilaterally at ribs 5-6 | | | ○ | ○ | ○ | ○ | ○ | ○ |
| Auscultates bilaterally at anterior mid-axillary region | | | ○ | ○ | ○ | ○ | ○ | ○ |
| **Identifies positive findings and implications** | | | Y | N | Y | N | Y | N |
| Identifies sounds as normal or abnormal | | | ○ | ○ | ○ | ○ | ○ | ○ |
| | | Total | ___/13 | | ___/13 | | ___/13 | |
| | Must achieve >9 to pass this examination | | Ⓟ | Ⓕ | Ⓟ | Ⓕ | Ⓟ | Ⓕ |
| **Assessor:** **Date:** | **Test 1 Comments:** | | | | | | | |
| **Assessor:** **Date:** | **Test 2 Comments:** | | | | | | | |
| **Assessor:** **Date:** | **Test 3 Comments:** | | | | | | | |

**TEST ENVIRONMENTS**
**L:** Laboratory/Classroom
**C:** Clinical/Field Testing
**P:** Practicum
**A:** Assessment/Mock Exam

**TEST INFORMATION**
**Test Statistics:** N/A
**Reference(s):** McChesney & McChesney (2001)

# ASSESSMENT

| NATA EC 5th | BOC RD6 | SKILL |
|---|---|---|
| AC-10 | D3-0302 | Oropharyngeal Airways |

**Supplies Needed:** Oropharyngeal airway, mannequin

*This problem allows you the opportunity to demonstrate an acute care technique using* **oropharyngeal airways**. *You have 2 minutes to complete this task.*

| Oropharyngeal Airways | Course or Site / Assessor / Environment | | Test 1 | | Test 2 | | Test 3 |
|---|---|---|---|---|---|---|---|
| **Tester places patient and limb in appropriate position** | | Y | N | Y | N | Y | N |
| Uses head-tilt, chin-lift, or jaw-thrust to establish airway | | ○ | ○ | ○ | ○ | ○ | ○ |
| **Tester placed in proper position** | | Y | N | Y | N | Y | N |
| Kneels to the side of the patient | | ○ | ○ | ○ | ○ | ○ | ○ |
| **Tester performs test according to accepted guidelines** | | Y | N | Y | N | Y | N |
| Measures from the corner of the mouth to the tip of the ear | | ○ | ○ | ○ | ○ | ○ | ○ |
| Uses a cross-finger technique to open the patient's mouth | | ○ | ○ | ○ | ○ | ○ | ○ |
| Using correctly sized OPA, the tester inserts OPA "upside-down" until resistance is felt against the soft palate | | ○ | ○ | ○ | ○ | ○ | ○ |
| Rotates OPA 180 degrees so that the tip is pointed down the patient's throat | | ○ | ○ | ○ | ○ | ○ | ○ |
| Removes OPA by pulling it out without rotating the OPA | | ○ | ○ | ○ | ○ | ○ | ○ |
| **Total** | | __/7 | | __/7 | | __/7 | |
| **Must achieve >4 to pass this examination** | | Ⓟ | Ⓕ | Ⓟ | Ⓕ | Ⓟ | Ⓕ |

| Assessor: Date: | Test 1 Comments: |
|---|---|
| Assessor: Date: | Test 2 Comments: |
| Assessor: Date: | Test 3 Comments: |

**TEST ENVIRONMENTS**
**L:** Laboratory/Classroom
**C:** Clinical/Field Testing
**P:** Practicum
**A:** Assessment/Mock Exam

**TEST INFORMATION**
**Test Statistics:** N/A
**Reference(s):** Gorse et al. (2010)

## ACUTE CARE OF INJURIES AND ILLNESSES
# ASSESSMENT

| NATA EC 5th | BOC RD6 | SKILL |
|---|---|---|
| AC-10 | D3-0302 | Nasopharyngeal Airways |

**Supplies Needed:** Nasopharyngeal airway, water-based lubricant, mannequin

*This problem allows you the opportunity to demonstrate an acute care technique using* **nasopharyngeal airways***. You have 2 minutes to complete this task.*

| Nasopharyngeal Airways | Course or Site Assessor Environment | | Test 1 | | Test 2 | | Test 3 | |
|---|---|---|---|---|---|---|---|---|
| | | | Y | N | Y | N | Y | N |
| **Tester places patient and limb in appropriate position** | | | Y | N | Y | N | Y | N |
| Uses head-tilt, chin-lift, or jaw-thrust to establish airway | | | O | O | O | O | O | O |
| **Tester placed in proper position** | | | Y | N | Y | N | Y | N |
| Kneels to the side of the patient | | | O | O | O | O | O | O |
| **Tester performs test according to accepted guidelines** | | | Y | N | Y | N | Y | N |
| Measures from the end of the nose to the tip of the ear | | | O | O | O | O | O | O |
| Coats the NPA with water-based lubricant | | | O | O | O | O | O | O |
| Flares the nares by pressing the tip of the nose toward the forehead | | | O | O | O | O | O | O |
| Places NPA's bevel edge against the right septal wall | | | O | O | O | O | O | O |
| Gently inserts the NPA parallel to the nasal floor following the contour of the nasal passage and the device | | | O | O | O | O | O | O |
| Inserts NPA until the flange rests on the nare | | | O | O | O | O | O | O |
| Removes NPA by pulling gently | | | O | O | O | O | O | O |
| Total | | | _____ /9 | | _____ /9 | | _____ /9 | |
| Must achieve >5 to pass this examination | | | Ⓟ | Ⓕ | Ⓟ | Ⓕ | Ⓟ | Ⓕ |

| Assessor: Date: | Test 1 Comments: |
|---|---|
| Assessor: Date: | Test 2 Comments: |
| Assessor: Date: | Test 3 Comments: |

**TEST ENVIRONMENTS**
**L:** Laboratory/Classroom
**C:** Clinical/Field Testing
**P:** Practicum
**A:** Assessment/Mock Exam

**TEST INFORMATION**
**Test Statistics:** N/A
**Reference(s):** Gorse et al. (2010)

## ACUTE CARE OF INJURIES AND ILLNESSES
# ASSESSMENT

| NATA EC 5th | BOC RD6 | SKILL |
|---|---|---|
| AC-10 | D3-0302 | Facemask Removal (Cordless Screwdriver) |

**Supplies Needed:** Football helmet, mannequin, cordless screwdriver

*This problem allows you the opportunity to demonstrate an acute care technique known as* **facemask removal (cordless screwdriver)**. *You have 2 minutes to complete this task.*

| Facemask Removal (Cordless Screwdriver) | Course or Site Assessor Environment | | Test 1 | | Test 2 | | Test 3 | |
|---|---|---|---|---|---|---|---|---|
| **Tester places patient and limb in appropriate position** | | **Y** | **N** | **Y** | **N** | **Y** | **N** | |
| Supine | | O | O | O | O | O | O | |
| **Tester placed in proper position** | | **Y** | **N** | **Y** | **N** | **Y** | **N** | |
| Kneels beside the patient | | O | O | O | O | O | O | |
| Helmet and cervical spine stabilized | | O | O | O | O | O | O | |
| **Tester performs test according to accepted guidelines** | | **Y** | **N** | **Y** | **N** | **Y** | **N** | |
| Uses cordless screwdriver to extract screws from facemask | | O | O | O | O | O | O | |
| Removes facemask from helmet | | O | O | O | O | O | O | |
| Completes procedure within 2 minutes | | O | O | O | O | O | O | |
| Maintains cervical alignment throughout the motion | | O | O | O | O | O | O | |
| **Total** | | ___/7 | | ___/7 | | ___/7 | | |
| **Must achieve >4 to pass this examination** | | Ⓟ | Ⓕ | Ⓟ | Ⓕ | Ⓟ | Ⓕ | |

| Assessor: Date: | Test 1 Comments: |
|---|---|
| Assessor: Date: | Test 2 Comments: |
| Assessor: Date: | Test 3 Comments: |

**TEST ENVIRONMENTS**
**L:** Laboratory/Classroom
**C:** Clinical/Field Testing
**P:** Practicum
**A:** Assessment/Mock Exam

**TEST INFORMATION**
**Test Statistics:** N/A
**Reference(s):** Prentice (2014)

## Acute Care of Injuries and Illnesses
# Assessment

| NATA EC 5th | BOC RD6 | SKILL |
|---|---|---|
| AC-10 | D3-0302 | Facemask Removal (FM Extractor) |

**Supplies Needed:** Football helmet, mannequin, FM Extractor

*This problem allows you the opportunity to demonstrate an acute care technique known as* **facemask removal (FM Extractor [Sports Medicine Concepts])**. *You have 2 minutes to complete this task.*

| Facemask Removal (FM Extractor) | Course or Site<br>Assessor<br>Environment | | | | | |
|---|---|---|---|---|---|---|
| | | Test 1 | | Test 2 | | Test 3 |
| **Tester places patient and limb in appropriate position** | | Y | N | Y | N | Y | N |
| Supine | | O | O | O | O | O | O |
| **Tester placed in proper position** | | Y | N | Y | N | Y | N |
| Kneels beside the patient | | O | O | O | O | O | O |
| Helmet and cervical spine stabilized | | O | O | O | O | O | O |
| **Tester performs test according to accepted guidelines** | | Y | N | Y | N | Y | N |
| Uses FM Extractor to cut through clips on facemask | | O | O | O | O | O | O |
| Removes facemask from helmet | | O | O | O | O | O | O |
| Completes the motion within 2 minutes | | O | O | O | O | O | O |
| Maintains cervical alignment throughout the motion | | O | O | O | O | O | O |
| Total | | __/7 | | __/7 | | __/7 |
| Must achieve >4 to pass this examination | | P | F | P | F | P | F |

| Assessor:<br>Date: | Test 1 Comments: |
|---|---|
| Assessor:<br>Date: | Test 2 Comments: |
| Assessor:<br>Date: | Test 3 Comments: |

**TEST ENVIRONMENTS**
**L:** Laboratory/Classroom
**C:** Clinical/Field Testing
**P:** Practicum
**A:** Assessment/Mock Exam

**TEST INFORMATION**
**Test Statistics:** N/A
**Reference(s):** Prentice (2014)

ACUTE CARE OF INJURIES AND ILLNESSES
# ASSESSMENT

| NATA EC 5th | BOC RD6 | SKILL |
|---|---|---|
| AC-10 | D3-0302 | Facemask Removal (Quick Release Tool) |

**Supplies Needed:** Football helmet, mannequin, Quick Release Tool

*This problem allows you the opportunity to demonstrate an acute care technique known as* **facemask removal (Quick Release Tool [Riddell]).** *You have 2 minutes to complete this task.*

| Facemask Removal (Quick Release Tool) | Course or Site Assessor Environment | | Test 1 | | Test 2 | | Test 3 |
|---|---|---|---|---|---|---|---|
| **Tester places patient and limb in appropriate position** | | Y | N | Y | N | Y | N |
| Supine | | ○ | ○ | ○ | ○ | ○ | ○ |
| **Tester placed in proper position** | | Y | N | Y | N | Y | N |
| Kneels beside the patient | | ○ | ○ | ○ | ○ | ○ | ○ |
| Helmet and cervical spine stabilized | | ○ | ○ | ○ | ○ | ○ | ○ |
| **Tester performs test according to accepted guidelines** | | Y | N | Y | N | Y | N |
| Uses Quick Release Tool to release clips on facemask | | ○ | ○ | ○ | ○ | ○ | ○ |
| Removes facemask from helmet | | ○ | ○ | ○ | ○ | ○ | ○ |
| Completes the motion within 2 minutes | | ○ | ○ | ○ | ○ | ○ | ○ |
| Maintains cervical alignment throughout the motion | | ○ | ○ | ○ | ○ | ○ | ○ |
| | Total | ___/7 | | ___/7 | | ___/7 | |
| | Must achieve >4 to pass this examination | Ⓟ | Ⓕ | Ⓟ | Ⓕ | Ⓟ | Ⓕ |

| Assessor: Date: | Test 1 Comments: |
|---|---|
| Assessor: Date: | Test 2 Comments: |
| Assessor: Date: | Test 3 Comments: |

**TEST ENVIRONMENTS**
**L:** Laboratory/Classroom
**C:** Clinical/Field Testing
**P:** Practicum
**A:** Assessment/Mock Exam

**TEST INFORMATION**
**Test Statistics:** N/A
**Reference(s):** Prentice (2014)

## ACUTE CARE OF INJURIES AND ILLNESSES
# ASSESSMENT

| NATA EC 5th | BOC RD6 | SKILL |
|---|---|---|
| AC-10 | D3-0302 | Facemask Removal (Trainer's Angel) |

**Supplies Needed:** Football helmet, mannequin, Trainer's Angel

*This problem allows you the opportunity to demonstrate an acute care technique known as* **facemask removal (Trainer's Angel)**. *You have 2 minutes to complete this task.*

| Facemask Removal (Trainer's Angel) | Course or Site<br>Assessor<br>Environment | | Test 1 | | Test 2 | | Test 3 | |
|---|---|---|---|---|---|---|---|---|
| | | | Y | N | Y | N | Y | N |
| **Tester places patient and limb in appropriate position** | | | Y | N | Y | N | Y | N |
| Supine | | | ○ | ○ | ○ | ○ | ○ | ○ |
| **Tester placed in proper position** | | | Y | N | Y | N | Y | N |
| Kneels beside the patient | | | ○ | ○ | ○ | ○ | ○ | ○ |
| Helmet and cervical spine stabilized | | | ○ | ○ | ○ | ○ | ○ | ○ |
| **Tester performs test according to accepted guidelines** | | | Y | N | Y | N | Y | N |
| Uses Trainer's Angel to cut through clips on facemask | | | ○ | ○ | ○ | ○ | ○ | ○ |
| Removes facemask from helmet | | | ○ | ○ | ○ | ○ | ○ | ○ |
| Completes the motion within 2 minutes | | | ○ | ○ | ○ | ○ | ○ | ○ |
| Maintains cervical alignment throughout the motion | | | ○ | ○ | ○ | ○ | ○ | ○ |
| **Total** | | | __/7 | | __/7 | | __/7 | |
| **Must achieve >4 to pass this examination** | | | Ⓟ | Ⓕ | Ⓟ | Ⓕ | Ⓟ | Ⓕ |
| **Assessor:**<br>**Date:** | **Test 1 Comments:** | | | | | | | |
| **Assessor:**<br>**Date:** | **Test 2 Comments:** | | | | | | | |
| **Assessor:**<br>**Date:** | **Test 3 Comments:** | | | | | | | |

**TEST ENVIRONMENTS**
**L:** Laboratory/Classroom
**C:** Clinical/Field Testing
**P:** Practicum
**A:** Assessment/Mock Exam

**TEST INFORMATION**
**Test Statistics:** N/A
**Reference(s):** Prentice (2014)

ACUTE CARE OF INJURIES AND ILLNESSES
# ASSESSMENT

| NATA EC 5th | BOC RD6 | SKILL |
|---|---|---|
| AC-11 | D3-0303 | Suction for Airway Management |

**Supplies Needed:** Manual suction device

*This problem allows you the opportunity to demonstrate* **suction for airway management** *to maintain a patent airway. You have 2 minutes to complete this task.*

| Suction for Airway Management | Course or Site Assessor Environment | Test 1 | | Test 2 | | Test 3 | |
|---|---|---|---|---|---|---|---|
| | | Y | N | Y | N | Y | N |
| **Tester places patient and limb in appropriate position** | | Y | N | Y | N | Y | N |
| Supine | | ○ | ○ | ○ | ○ | ○ | ○ |
| **Tester placed in proper position** | | Y | N | Y | N | Y | N |
| Kneels beside the patient | | ○ | ○ | ○ | ○ | ○ | ○ |
| Applies appropriate PPE | | ○ | ○ | ○ | ○ | ○ | ○ |
| **Tester performs test according to accepted guidelines** | | Y | N | Y | N | Y | N |
| Turns the patient's head to one side (if cervical injury is suspected, a log roll is performed, keeping cervical alignment) | | ○ | ○ | ○ | ○ | ○ | ○ |
| Opens the patient's mouth and wipes away large debris with two gloved fingers, performing a circular motion toward the ground | | ○ | ○ | ○ | ○ | ○ | ○ |
| Measures the suction catheter from the corner of the patient's mouth to the earlobe | | ○ | ○ | ○ | ○ | ○ | ○ |
| Inserts suction tip and slowly draws it from the mouth while suctioning | | ○ | ○ | ○ | ○ | ○ | ○ |
| Suctions for no longer than 15 seconds (adult) or 10 seconds (child) | | ○ | ○ | ○ | ○ | ○ | ○ |
| Total | | ___/8 | | ___/8 | | ___/8 | |
| **Must achieve >5 to pass this examination** | | Ⓟ | Ⓕ | Ⓟ | Ⓕ | Ⓟ | Ⓕ |

| Assessor: Date: | Test 1 Comments: |
|---|---|
| Assessor: Date: | Test 2 Comments: |
| Assessor: Date: | Test 3 Comments: |

**TEST ENVIRONMENTS**
**L:** Laboratory/Classroom
**C:** Clinical/Field Testing
**P:** Practicum
**A:** Assessment/Mock Exam

**TEST INFORMATION**
**Test Statistics:** N/A
**Reference(s):** Gorse et al. (2010)

## ACUTE CARE OF INJURIES AND ILLNESSES
# ASSESSMENT

| NATA EC 5th | BOC RD6 | SKILL |
|---|---|---|
| AC-13 | D3-0303 | Automated External Defibrillator |

**Supplies Needed:** Automated external defibrillator, mannequin

*This problem allows you the opportunity to demonstrate an acute care technique using an* **automated external defibrillator**. *You have 2 minutes to complete this task.*

| Automated External Defibrillator | Course or Site / Assessor / Environment | | Test 1 | | Test 2 | | Test 3 | |
|---|---|---|---|---|---|---|---|---|
| **Tester places patient and limb in appropriate position** | | | Y | N | Y | N | Y | N |
| Supine | | | ○ | ○ | ○ | ○ | ○ | ○ |
| **Tester placed in proper position** | | | Y | N | Y | N | Y | N |
| Kneels beside the patient | | | ○ | ○ | ○ | ○ | ○ | ○ |
| **Tester performs test according to accepted guidelines** | | | Y | N | Y | N | Y | N |
| Assesses vital signs and determines there is no pulse | | | ○ | ○ | ○ | ○ | ○ | ○ |
| Activates EMS, and grabs AED | | | ○ | ○ | ○ | ○ | ○ | ○ |
| Turns on the AED and places it near the patient's head | | | ○ | ○ | ○ | ○ | ○ | ○ |
| Exposes the patient's chest and ensures it is clean and dry | | | ○ | ○ | ○ | ○ | ○ | ○ |
| Removes adhesive backing and applies AED pads on the patient's upper right border of the sternum and left lower ribs | | | ○ | ○ | ○ | ○ | ○ | ○ |
| Ensures electrodes are plugged in | | | ○ | ○ | ○ | ○ | ○ | ○ |
| Removes hands from the patient and pushes "analyze" on AED | | | ○ | ○ | ○ | ○ | ○ | ○ |
| If defibrillation is needed, the tester continues CPR as AED charges | | | ○ | ○ | ○ | ○ | ○ | ○ |
| When AED is ready to administer a shock, the tester stops CPR and removes hands from the patient, then presses "shock" button | | | ○ | ○ | ○ | ○ | ○ | ○ |
| Resumes CPR for 5 cycles and reanalyzes | | | ○ | ○ | ○ | ○ | ○ | ○ |
| **Total** | | | ___/12 | | ___/12 | | ___/12 | |
| **Must achieve >9 to pass this examination** | | | Ⓟ | Ⓕ | Ⓟ | Ⓕ | Ⓟ | Ⓕ |

| Assessor: Date: | Test 1 Comments: |
|---|---|
| Assessor: Date: | Test 2 Comments: |
| Assessor: Date: | Test 3 Comments: |

**TEST ENVIRONMENTS**
**L:** Laboratory/Classroom
**C:** Clinical/Field Testing
**P:** Practicum
**A:** Assessment/Mock Exam

**TEST INFORMATION**
**Test Statistics:** No data available
**Reference(s):** Gorse et al. (2010)

| NATA EC 5th | BOC RD6 | SKILL |
|---|---|---|
| AC-14 | D3-0303 | Cardiopulmonary Resuscitation (1P Adult) |

**Supplies Needed:** Mannequin

*This problem allows you the opportunity to demonstrate an acute care technique on an unresponsive patient called* **cardiopulmonary resuscitation (1P adult)**. *You have 2 minutes to complete this task.*

| Cardiopulmonary Resuscitation (1P Adult) | Course or Site / Assessor / Environment | | Test 1 | | Test 2 | | Test 3 | |
|---|---|---|---|---|---|---|---|---|
| | | | Y | N | Y | N | Y | N |
| **Tester places patient and limb in appropriate position** | | | Y | N | Y | N | Y | N |
| Supine | | | O | O | O | O | O | O |
| **Tester placed in proper position** | | | Y | N | Y | N | Y | N |
| Kneels next to the patient | | | O | O | O | O | O | O |
| **Tester performs test according to accepted guidelines** | | | Y | N | Y | N | Y | N |
| Provides verbal and physical stimulation to determine responsiveness | | | O | O | O | O | O | O |
| Simultaneously checks pulse and performs head-tilt, chin-lift, or jaw-thrust maneuver (if trauma is suspected) to open airway and checks breathing using the "look, listen, feel" method | | | O | O | O | O | O | O |
| If no pulse/breathing is found, the tester begins EMS | | | O | O | O | O | O | O |
| Begins chest compressions, with hands laced and the heel of the dominant hand lined up with the patient's nipple line | | | O | O | O | O | O | O |
| Performs 30 compressions at 100 bpm with arms straight, then provides 2 breaths, watching the chest rise to ensure open airway | | | O | O | O | O | O | O |
| Performs 5 cycles (approximately 2 minutes) and rechecks vitals | | | O | O | O | O | O | O |
| If the patient resumes consciousness, the tester places the patient in the recovery position and monitors vitals until EMS arrival | | | O | O | O | O | O | O |
| Total | | | __/9 | | __/9 | | __/9 | |
| Must achieve >6 to pass this examination | | | P | F | P | F | P | F |

| Assessor: Date: | Test 1 Comments: |
|---|---|
| Assessor: Date: | Test 2 Comments: |
| Assessor: Date: | Test 3 Comments: |

**TEST ENVIRONMENTS**
**L:** Laboratory/Classroom
**C:** Clinical/Field Testing
**P:** Practicum
**A:** Assessment/Mock Exam

**TEST INFORMATION**
**Test Statistics:** No data available
**Reference(s):** Starkey & Brown (2015)

ACUTE CARE OF INJURIES AND ILLNESSES
# ASSESSMENT

| NATA EC 5th | BOC RD6 | SKILL |
|---|---|---|
| AC-14 | D3-0303 | Cardiopulmonary Resuscitation (2P Adult) |

**Supplies Needed:** Mannequin

*This problem allows you the opportunity to demonstrate an acute care technique on an unresponsive patient called* **cardiopulmonary resuscitation (2P adult)**. *You have 2 minutes to complete this task.*

| Cardiopulmonary Resuscitation (2P Adult) | Course or Site Assessor Environment | | | | | |
|---|---|---|---|---|---|---|
| | | Test 1 | | Test 2 | | Test 3 |
| **Tester places patient and limb in appropriate position** | | Y | N | Y | N | Y | N |
| Supine | | ○ | ○ | ○ | ○ | ○ | ○ |
| **Tester placed in proper position** | | Y | N | Y | N | Y | N |
| Kneels on opposite sides of the patient | | ○ | ○ | ○ | ○ | ○ | ○ |
| **Tester performs test according to accepted guidelines** | | Y | N | Y | N | Y | N |
| Tester 1 provides verbal and physical stimulation to determine responsiveness | | ○ | ○ | ○ | ○ | ○ | ○ |
| Tester 1 simultaneously checks pulse and performs head-tilt, chin-lift, or jaw-thrust maneuver (if trauma is suspected) to open airway and checks breathing using the "look, listen, feel" method | | ○ | ○ | ○ | ○ | ○ | ○ |
| If no pulse/breathing is found, tester 2 begins EMS | | ○ | ○ | ○ | ○ | ○ | ○ |
| Tester 1 begins chest compressions, with hands laced and the heel of the dominant hand lined up with the patient's nipple line | | ○ | ○ | ○ | ○ | ○ | ○ |
| Tester 1 performs 30 compressions at 100 bpm with arms straight, then tester 2 provides two breaths, watching the chest rise to ensure an open airway | | ○ | ○ | ○ | ○ | ○ | ○ |
| The testers perform two cycles, then switch places | | ○ | ○ | ○ | ○ | ○ | ○ |
| If the patient resumes consciousness, the testers place the patient in the recovery position and monitor vitals until EMS arrival | | ○ | ○ | ○ | ○ | ○ | ○ |
| Total | | ___/9 | | ___/9 | | ___/9 | |
| Must achieve >6 to pass this examination | | Ⓟ | Ⓕ | Ⓟ | Ⓕ | Ⓟ | Ⓕ |
| Assessor: Date: | Test 1 Comments: | | | | | | |
| Assessor: Date: | Test 2 Comments: | | | | | | |
| Assessor: Date: | Test 3 Comments: | | | | | | |

**TEST ENVIRONMENTS**
L: Laboratory/Classroom
C: Clinical/Field Testing
P: Practicum
A: Assessment/Mock Exam

**TEST INFORMATION**
**Test Statistics:** No data available
**Reference(s):** Starkey & Brown (2015)

# ASSESSMENT

| NATA EC 5th | BOC RD6 | SKILL |
|---|---|---|
| AC-15 | D3-0303 | Bag Valve Mask (Child and Adult Nonbreathing) |

**Supplies Needed:** Table, bag valve mask

*This problem allows you the opportunity to demonstrate an acute care technique on a nonbreathing patient called rescue breathing with a* **bag valve mask**. *You have 2 minutes to complete this task.*

| Bag Valve Mask (Child and Adult Nonbreathing) | Course or Site<br>Assessor<br>Environment | Test 1 | | Test 2 | | Test 3 | |
|---|---|---|---|---|---|---|---|
| | | Y | N | Y | N | Y | N |
| **Tester places patient and limb in appropriate position** | | Y | N | Y | N | Y | N |
| Supine | | O | O | O | O | O | O |
| **Tester placed in proper position** | | Y | N | Y | N | Y | N |
| Kneels behind the patient's head | | O | O | O | O | O | O |
| Hands on the patient's jaw | | O | O | O | O | O | O |
| **Tester performs test according to accepted guidelines** | | Y | N | Y | N | Y | N |
| Performs a head-tilt, chin-lift, or jaw-thrust maneuver to open the airway | | O | O | O | O | O | O |
| Places mask over the mouth and nose of the patient | | O | O | O | O | O | O |
| Forms a tight seal by forming "C" with the thumb and index finger | | O | O | O | O | O | O |
| Forms an "F" with the middle, ring, and pinky fingers to help assist in maintaining an airway | | O | O | O | O | O | O |
| Uses other hand to squeeze bag to deliver oxygen saturated air to the nonbreathing patient | | O | O | O | O | O | O |
| **Total** | | ___/8 | | ___/8 | | ___/8 | |
| **Must achieve >5 to pass this examination** | | Ⓟ | Ⓕ | Ⓟ | Ⓕ | Ⓟ | Ⓕ |

| Assessor:<br>Date: | Test 1 Comments: |
|---|---|
| Assessor:<br>Date: | Test 2 Comments: |
| Assessor:<br>Date: | Test 3 Comments: |

**TEST ENVIRONMENTS**
**L:** Laboratory/Classroom
**C:** Clinical/Field Testing
**P:** Practicum
**A:** Assessment/Mock Exam

**TEST INFORMATION**
**Test Statistics:** No data available
**Reference(s):** Gulli et al. (2012)

## ACUTE CARE OF INJURIES AND ILLNESSES
# ASSESSMENT

| NATA EC 5th | BOC RD6 | SKILL |
|---|---|---|
| AC-15 | D3-0303 | Pocket Mask (Child and Adult) |

**Supplies Needed:** Table, pocket mask

*This problem allows you the opportunity to demonstrate an acute care technique on a nonbreathing patient called rescue breathing with a* **pocket mask.** *You have 2 minutes to complete this task.*

| Pocket Mask (Child and Adult) | Course or Site Assessor Environment | | Test 1 | | Test 2 | | Test 3 | |
|---|---|---|---|---|---|---|---|---|
| | | | **Y** | **N** | **Y** | **N** | **Y** | **N** |
| **Tester places patient and limb in appropriate position** | | | **Y** | **N** | **Y** | **N** | **Y** | **N** |
| Supine | | | ○ | ○ | ○ | ○ | ○ | ○ |
| **Tester placed in proper position** | | | **Y** | **N** | **Y** | **N** | **Y** | **N** |
| Kneels behind the patient's head | | | ○ | ○ | ○ | ○ | ○ | ○ |
| Hands on both sides of the patient's face | | | ○ | ○ | ○ | ○ | ○ | ○ |
| **Tester performs test according to accepted guidelines** | | | **Y** | **N** | **Y** | **N** | **Y** | **N** |
| Performs a head-tilt, chin-lift, or jaw-thrust maneuver to open the airway | | | ○ | ○ | ○ | ○ | ○ | ○ |
| Places mask over the mouth and nose of the patient | | | ○ | ○ | ○ | ○ | ○ | ○ |
| Forms a tight seal by forming a "C" with the thumb and index finger | | | ○ | ○ | ○ | ○ | ○ | ○ |
| Forms an "F" with the middle, ring, and pinky fingers to help assist in maintaining an airway | | | ○ | ○ | ○ | ○ | ○ | ○ |
| **Total** | | | ___/7 | | ___/7 | | ___/7 | |
| **Must achieve >4 to pass this examination** | | | Ⓟ | Ⓕ | Ⓟ | Ⓕ | Ⓟ | Ⓕ |
| **Assessor:** **Date:** | **Test 1 Comments:** | | | | | | | |
| **Assessor:** **Date:** | **Test 2 Comments:** | | | | | | | |
| **Assessor:** **Date:** | **Test 3 Comments:** | | | | | | | |

**TEST ENVIRONMENTS**
**L:** Laboratory/Classroom
**C:** Clinical/Field Testing
**P:** Practicum
**A:** Assessment/Mock Exam

**TEST INFORMATION**
**Test Statistics:** No data available
**Reference(s):** Starkey & Brown (2015)

## ACUTE CARE OF INJURIES AND ILLNESSES
# ASSESSMENT

| NATA EC 5th | BOC RD6 | SKILL |
|---|---|---|
| AC-17 | D3-0303 | Supplemental Oxygen (Nasal Cannula) |

**Supplies Needed:** Table, oxygen tank, nasal cannula

*This problem allows you the opportunity to demonstrate an acute care technique called oxygen administration with a **nasal cannula**. You have 2 minutes to complete this task.*

| Supplemental Oxygen (Nasal Cannula) | Course or Site Assessor Environment | | Test 1 | | Test 2 | | Test 3 |
|---|---|---|---|---|---|---|---|
| | | Y | N | Y | N | Y | N |
| **Tester places patient and limb in appropriate position** | | Y | N | Y | N | Y | N |
| Supine or seated | | O | O | O | O | O | O |
| **Tester placed in proper position** | | Y | N | Y | N | Y | N |
| Stands in front of the patient | | O | O | O | O | O | O |
| **Tester performs test according to accepted guidelines** | | Y | N | Y | N | Y | N |
| Applies appropriate PPE | | O | O | O | O | O | O |
| Assembles the regulator to tank and opens the tank | | O | O | O | O | O | O |
| Checks for leaks and tank pressure, adjusts flow to 6 liters per minute or less | | O | O | O | O | O | O |
| Attaches nasal cannula to the patient's nasal passages and wraps around the ears | | O | O | O | O | O | O |
| Total | | ___/6 | | ___/6 | | ___/6 | |
| Must achieve >3 to pass this examination | | P | F | P | F | P | F |

| Assessor: Date: | Test 1 Comments: |
|---|---|
| Assessor: Date: | Test 2 Comments: |
| Assessor: Date: | Test 3 Comments: |

**TEST ENVIRONMENTS**
**L:** Laboratory/Classroom
**C:** Clinical/Field Testing
**P:** Practicum
**A:** Assessment/Mock Exam

**TEST INFORMATION**
**Test Statistics:** No data available
**Reference(s):** Gorse et al. (2010)

## ACUTE CARE OF INJURIES AND ILLNESSES
# ASSESSMENT

| NATA EC 5th | BOC RD6 | SKILL |
|---|---|---|
| AC-17 | D3-0303 | Supplemental Oxygen<br>(Reservoir Bag Valve Facemask) |

**Supplies Needed:** Table, oxygen tank, reservoir bag valve facemask

*This problem allows you the opportunity to demonstrate an acute care technique called oxygen administration with a* **reservoir bag valve facemask.** *You have 2 minutes to complete this task.*

| Supplemental Oxygen<br>(Reservoir Bag Valve Facemask) | Course or Site<br>Assessor<br>Environment | Test 1 | | Test 2 | | Test 3 | |
|---|---|---|---|---|---|---|---|
| | | Y | N | Y | N | Y | N |
| **Tester places patient and limb in appropriate position** | | Y | N | Y | N | Y | N |
| Supine or seated | | ○ | ○ | ○ | ○ | ○ | ○ |
| **Tester placed in proper position** | | Y | N | Y | N | Y | N |
| Stands in front of the patient | | ○ | ○ | ○ | ○ | ○ | ○ |
| **Tester performs test according to accepted guidelines** | | Y | N | Y | N | Y | N |
| Applies appropriate PPE | | ○ | ○ | ○ | ○ | ○ | ○ |
| Assembles the regulator to tank and opens the tank | | ○ | ○ | ○ | ○ | ○ | ○ |
| Checks for leaks and tank pressure, adjusts flow to 6 liters per minute or less | | ○ | ○ | ○ | ○ | ○ | ○ |
| Attaches mask to oxygen and prefills the reservoir | | ○ | ○ | ○ | ○ | ○ | ○ |
| Adjusts liter flow to 12 liters per minute, applies and adjusts facemask | | ○ | ○ | ○ | ○ | ○ | ○ |
| Total | | __/7 | | __/7 | | __/7 | |
| Must achieve >3 to pass this examination | | Ⓟ | Ⓕ | Ⓟ | Ⓕ | Ⓟ | Ⓕ |

| Assessor:<br>Date: | Test 1 Comments: |
|---|---|
| Assessor:<br>Date: | Test 2 Comments: |
| Assessor:<br>Date: | Test 3 Comments: |

**TEST ENVIRONMENTS**
**L:** Laboratory/Classroom
**C:** Clinical/Field Testing
**P:** Practicum
**A:** Assessment/Mock Exam

**TEST INFORMATION**
**Test Statistics:** No data available
**Reference(s):** Gorse et al. (2010)

# ASSESSMENT

| NATA EC 5th | BOC RD6 | SKILL |
|---|---|---|
| AC-20 | D4-0404 | External Hemorrhage Management |

**Supplies Needed:** Table or chair, saline spray or faucet, gloves, syringe, antibiotic ointment, dressings

*This problem allows you the opportunity to demonstrate an acute care technique for* **external hemorrhage management**. *You have 2 minutes to complete this task.*

| External Hemorrhage Management | Course or Site Assessor Environment _____ _____ _____ | | Test 1 | | Test 2 | | Test 3 |
|---|---|---|---|---|---|---|---|
| **Tester places patient and limb in appropriate position** | | **Y** | **N** | **Y** | **N** | **Y** | **N** |
| Seated or standing | | O | O | O | O | O | O |
| **Tester placed in proper position** | | **Y** | **N** | **Y** | **N** | **Y** | **N** |
| Stands in front of the patient | | O | O | O | O | O | O |
| **Tester performs test according to accepted guidelines** | | **Y** | **N** | **Y** | **N** | **Y** | **N** |
| Applies PPE | | O | O | O | O | O | O |
| Washes the wound with soap and water | | O | O | O | O | O | O |
| Flushes the wound under running water or with saline spray | | O | O | O | O | O | O |
| Applies antibiotic ointment | | O | O | O | O | O | O |
| Covers the wound with sterile external dressings | | O | O | O | O | O | O |
| **Total** | | ____/7 | | ____/7 | | ____/7 | |
| **Must achieve >5 to pass this examination** | | Ⓟ | Ⓕ | Ⓟ | Ⓕ | Ⓟ | Ⓕ |

| Assessor: Date: | Test 1 Comments: |
|---|---|
| Assessor: Date: | Test 2 Comments: |
| Assessor: Date: | Test 3 Comments: |

**TEST ENVIRONMENTS**
**L:** Laboratory/Classroom
**C:** Clinical/Field Testing
**P:** Practicum
**A:** Assessment/Mock Exam

**TEST INFORMATION**
**Test Statistics:** No data available
**Reference(s):** Thygerson et al. (2012)

## ACUTE CARE OF INJURIES AND ILLNESSES
# ASSESSMENT

| NATA EC 5th | BOC RD6 | SKILL |
|:---:|:---:|:---:|
| AC-22 | D4-0404 | Wound Care (Forearm Abrasion) |

**Supplies Needed:** Table or chair, saline spray or faucet, gloves, syringe, antibiotic ointment, dressings

*This problem allows you the opportunity to demonstrate an acute care technique called* **wound care** *for a* **forearm abrasion**. *You have 2 minutes to complete this task.*

| Wound Care (Forearm Abrasion) | Course or Site<br>Assessor<br>Environment | | Test 1 | | Test 2 | | Test 3 | |
|---|---|---|:---:|:---:|:---:|:---:|:---:|:---:|
| **Tester places patient and limb in appropriate position** | | | **Y** | **N** | **Y** | **N** | **Y** | **N** |
| Seated or standing | | | ○ | ○ | ○ | ○ | ○ | ○ |
| **Tester placed in proper position** | | | **Y** | **N** | **Y** | **N** | **Y** | **N** |
| Stands in front of the patient | | | ○ | ○ | ○ | ○ | ○ | ○ |
| **Tester performs test according to accepted guidelines** | | | **Y** | **N** | **Y** | **N** | **Y** | **N** |
| Applies PPE | | | ○ | ○ | ○ | ○ | ○ | ○ |
| Washes the wound with soap and water | | | ○ | ○ | ○ | ○ | ○ | ○ |
| Flushes the wound under running water or with saline spray | | | ○ | ○ | ○ | ○ | ○ | ○ |
| Covers the wound with sterile external dressings | | | ○ | ○ | ○ | ○ | ○ | ○ |
| **Total** | | | \_\_\_\_/6 | | \_\_\_\_/6 | | \_\_\_\_/6 | |
| **Must achieve >3 to pass this examination** | | | Ⓟ | Ⓕ | Ⓟ | Ⓕ | Ⓟ | Ⓕ |
| Assessor:<br>Date: | **Test 1 Comments:** | | | | | | | |
| Assessor:<br>Date: | **Test 2 Comments:** | | | | | | | |
| Assessor:<br>Date: | **Test 3 Comments:** | | | | | | | |

**TEST ENVIRONMENTS**
**L:** Laboratory/Classroom
**C:** Clinical/Field Testing
**P:** Practicum
**A:** Assessment/Mock Exam

**TEST INFORMATION**
**Test Statistics:** No data available
**Reference(s):** Thygerson et al. (2012)

| NATA EC 5th | BOC RD6 | SKILL |
|---|---|---|
| AC-23 | D3-0303 | Cervical Spine Stabilization |

**Supplies Needed:** N/A

*This problem allows you the opportunity to demonstrate an acute care technique called* **cervical spine stabilization***. You have 2 minutes to complete this task.*

| Cervical Spine Stabilization | Course or Site<br>Assessor<br>Environment | Test 1 | | Test 2 | | Test 3 | |
|---|---|---|---|---|---|---|---|
| | | **Y** | **N** | **Y** | **N** | **Y** | **N** |
| **Tester places patient and limb in appropriate position** | | **Y** | **N** | **Y** | **N** | **Y** | **N** |
| Supine | | ○ | ○ | ○ | ○ | ○ | ○ |
| **Tester placed in proper position** | | **Y** | **N** | **Y** | **N** | **Y** | **N** |
| Kneels behind the patient's head | | ○ | ○ | ○ | ○ | ○ | ○ |
| **Tester performs test according to accepted guidelines** | | **Y** | **N** | **Y** | **N** | **Y** | **N** |
| Places both hands on the patient's upper trapezius region | | ○ | ○ | ○ | ○ | ○ | ○ |
| Firmly holds on the trapezius while firmly grasping the head between the tester's forearms | | ○ | ○ | ○ | ○ | ○ | ○ |
| Total | | ___/4 | | ___/4 | | ___/4 | |
| Must achieve >2 to pass this examination | | Ⓟ | Ⓕ | Ⓟ | Ⓕ | Ⓟ | Ⓕ |

| Assessor:<br>Date: | Test 1 Comments: |
|---|---|
| Assessor:<br>Date: | Test 2 Comments: |
| Assessor:<br>Date: | Test 3 Comments: |

**TEST ENVIRONMENTS**
**L:** Laboratory/Classroom
**C:** Clinical/Field Testing
**P:** Practicum
**A:** Assessment/Mock Exam

**TEST INFORMATION**
**Test Statistics:** No data available
**Reference(s):** Gorse et al. (2010)

## ACUTE CARE OF INJURIES AND ILLNESSES
# ASSESSMENT

| NATA EC 5th | BOC RD6 | SKILL |
|:---:|:---:|:---:|
| AC-25 | D3-0303 | Patient Transfer Technique (Six-Person Lift) |

**Supplies Needed:** Spine board and straps

*This problem allows you the opportunity to demonstrate an acute care technique for* **patient transfer** *called the* **six-person lift**. *You have 2 minutes to complete this task.*

| Patient Transfer Technique (Six-Person Lift) | Course or Site / Assessor / Environment | | Test 1 | | Test 2 | | Test 3 | |
|---|---|---|:---:|:---:|:---:|:---:|:---:|:---:|
| **Tester places patient and limb in appropriate position** | | | Y | N | Y | N | Y | N |
| Supine | | | ○ | ○ | ○ | ○ | ○ | ○ |
| **Tester placed in proper position** | | | Y | N | Y | N | Y | N |
| One tester is positioned behind the head of the patient, maintaining in-line stabilization | | | ○ | ○ | ○ | ○ | ○ | ○ |
| Two testers are positioned on each side of the patient's torso | | | ○ | ○ | ○ | ○ | ○ | ○ |
| Two testers are positioned on each side of the patient's lower extremity | | | ○ | ○ | ○ | ○ | ○ | ○ |
| One tester stands on the side of the patient with the spine board | | | ○ | ○ | ○ | ○ | ○ | ○ |
| **Tester performs test according to accepted guidelines** | | | Y | N | Y | N | Y | N |
| The testers at the torso and lower extremity cross hands over each other | | | ○ | ○ | ○ | ○ | ○ | ○ |
| Once all testers have a firm grasp of the patient, a verbal cue is given by the tester at the head: "On the count of 3, we will lift the patient, 1, 2, 3" | | | ○ | ○ | ○ | ○ | ○ | ○ |
| As the patient is lifted, the tester with the spine board slides it under the suspended patient | | | ○ | ○ | ○ | ○ | ○ | ○ |
| Once the spine board is in place, the patient is slowly lowered and strapped on | | | ○ | ○ | ○ | ○ | ○ | ○ |
| Total | | | ___/9 | | ___/9 | | ___/9 | |
| Must achieve >6 to pass this examination | | | Ⓟ | Ⓕ | Ⓟ | Ⓕ | Ⓟ | Ⓕ |

| Assessor: Date: | Test 1 Comments: |
|---|---|
| Assessor: Date: | Test 2 Comments: |
| Assessor: Date: | Test 3 Comments: |

**TEST ENVIRONMENTS**
**L:** Laboratory/Classroom
**C:** Clinical/Field Testing
**P:** Practicum
**A:** Assessment/Mock Exam

**TEST INFORMATION**
**Test Statistics:** No data available
**Reference(s):** Rehberg (2013)

ACUTE CARE OF INJURIES AND ILLNESSES
# ASSESSMENT

| NATA EC 5th | BOC RD6 | SKILL |
|---|---|---|
| AC-25 | D3-0303 | Patient Transfer Technique (Prone Log Roll) |

**Supplies Needed:** Spine board and straps

*This problem allows you the opportunity to demonstrate an acute care technique for* **patient transfer** *called the* **prone log roll.** *You have 2 minutes to complete this task.*

| Patient Transfer Technique (Prone Log Roll) | Course or Site Assessor Environment | | Test 1 | | Test 2 | | Test 3 | |
|---|---|---|---|---|---|---|---|---|
| | | **Y** | **N** | **Y** | **N** | **Y** | **N** | |
| **Tester places patient and limb in appropriate position** | | **Y** | **N** | **Y** | **N** | **Y** | **N** |
| Prone | | ○ | ○ | ○ | ○ | ○ | ○ |
| **Tester placed in proper position** | | **Y** | **N** | **Y** | **N** | **Y** | **N** |
| One tester is positioned behind the head of the patient, maintaining in-line stabilization | | ○ | ○ | ○ | ○ | ○ | ○ |
| Four testers are positioned on the side of the patient from torso to lower legs | | ○ | ○ | ○ | ○ | ○ | ○ |
| One tester stands on the side of the patient with the spine board | | ○ | ○ | ○ | ○ | ○ | ○ |
| **Tester performs test according to accepted guidelines** | | **Y** | **N** | **Y** | **N** | **Y** | **N** |
| The testers at the torso and lower extremity cross hands over each other | | ○ | ○ | ○ | ○ | ○ | ○ |
| Once all testers have a firm grasp of the patient, a verbal cue is given by the tester at the head: "On the count of 3, we will roll the patient, 1, 2, 3" | | ○ | ○ | ○ | ○ | ○ | ○ |
| As the patient is rolled over, the tester with the spine board slides it under the patient | | ○ | ○ | ○ | ○ | ○ | ○ |
| Once the spine board is in place, the patient is slowly lowered and strapped on | | ○ | ○ | ○ | ○ | ○ | ○ |
| **Total** | | ___/8 | | ___/8 | | ___/8 | |
| **Must achieve >5 to pass this examination** | | Ⓟ | Ⓕ | Ⓟ | Ⓕ | Ⓟ | Ⓕ |

| Assessor: Date: | Test 1 Comments: |
|---|---|
| Assessor: Date: | Test 2 Comments: |
| Assessor: Date: | Test 3 Comments: |

**TEST ENVIRONMENTS**
**L:** Laboratory/Classroom
**C:** Clinical/Field Testing
**P:** Practicum
**A:** Assessment/Mock Exam

**TEST INFORMATION**
**Test Statistics:** No data available
**Reference(s):** Rehberg (2013)

## ACUTE CARE OF INJURIES AND ILLNESSES
# ASSESSMENT

| NATA EC 5th | BOC RD6 | SKILL |
|---|---|---|
| AC-25 | D3-0303 | Patient Transfer Technique (Supine Log Roll) |

**Supplies Needed:** Spine board and straps

*This problem allows you the opportunity to demonstrate an acute care technique for* **patient transfer** *called the* **supine log roll.** *You have 2 minutes to complete this task.*

| Patient Transfer Technique (Supine Log Roll) | Course or Site Assessor Environment | | Test 1 | | Test 2 | | Test 3 | |
|---|---|---|---|---|---|---|---|---|
| **Tester places patient and limb in appropriate position** | | | Y | N | Y | N | Y | N |
| Supine | | | ○ | ○ | ○ | ○ | ○ | ○ |
| **Tester placed in proper position** | | | Y | N | Y | N | Y | N |
| One tester is positioned behind the head of the patient, maintaining in-line stabilization | | | ○ | ○ | ○ | ○ | ○ | ○ |
| Four testers are positioned on the side of the patient from torso to lower legs | | | ○ | ○ | ○ | ○ | ○ | ○ |
| One tester stands on the side of the patient with the spine board | | | ○ | ○ | ○ | ○ | ○ | ○ |
| **Tester performs test according to accepted guidelines** | | | Y | N | Y | N | Y | N |
| The testers at the torso and lower extremity cross hands over each other | | | ○ | ○ | ○ | ○ | ○ | ○ |
| Once all testers have a firm grasp of the patient, a verbal cue is given by the tester at the head: "On the count of 3, we will roll the patient, 1, 2, 3" | | | ○ | ○ | ○ | ○ | ○ | ○ |
| As the patient is rolled over, the tester with the spine board slides it under the patient | | | ○ | ○ | ○ | ○ | ○ | ○ |
| Once the spine board is in place, the patient is slowly lowered and strapped on | | | ○ | ○ | ○ | ○ | ○ | ○ |
| **Total** | | | ___/8 | | ___/8 | | ___/8 | |
| **Must achieve >5 to pass this examination** | | | Ⓟ | Ⓕ | Ⓟ | Ⓕ | Ⓟ | Ⓕ |
| **Assessor: Date:** | **Test 1 Comments:** | | | | | | | |
| **Assessor: Date:** | **Test 2 Comments:** | | | | | | | |
| **Assessor: Date:** | **Test 3 Comments:** | | | | | | | |

**TEST ENVIRONMENTS**
**L:** Laboratory/Classroom
**C:** Clinical/Field Testing
**P:** Practicum
**A:** Assessment/Mock Exam

**TEST INFORMATION**
**Test Statistics:** No data available
**Reference(s):** Rehberg (2013)

| NATA EC 5th | BOC RD6 | SKILL |
|---|---|---|
| AC-29 | D3-0302 | Rectal Temperature |

**Supplies Needed:** Table, rectal thermometer, lubricating or petroleum jelly

*This problem allows you the opportunity to demonstrate an acute care technique for core body temperature called* **rectal temperature**. *You have 2 minutes to complete this task.*

| Rectal Temperature | Course or Site Assessor Environment | | | | | | |
|---|---|---|---|---|---|---|---|
| | | Test 1 | | Test 2 | | Test 3 | |
| **Tester places patient and limb in appropriate position** | | Y | N | Y | N | Y | N |
| Side lying | | ○ | ○ | ○ | ○ | ○ | ○ |
| **Tester placed in proper position** | | Y | N | Y | N | Y | N |
| Kneels at the side of the patient | | ○ | ○ | ○ | ○ | ○ | ○ |
| If using a glass thermometer shake down to below 97.8°F | | ○ | ○ | ○ | ○ | ○ | ○ |
| Cover the tip of the thermometer with lubricating or petroleum jelly | | ○ | ○ | ○ | ○ | ○ | ○ |
| **Tester performs test according to accepted guidelines** | | Y | N | Y | N | Y | N |
| Spreads the buttocks and gently inserts the thermometer 8 to 10 cm (never force it) and keeps the thermometer in place | | ○ | ○ | ○ | ○ | ○ | ○ |
| Leaves thermometer in place for 3 minutes | | ○ | ○ | ○ | ○ | ○ | ○ |
| Washes the thermometer once done | | ○ | ○ | ○ | ○ | ○ | ○ |
| Total | | __/7 | | __/7 | | __/7 | |
| Must achieve >5 to pass this examination | | Ⓟ | Ⓕ | Ⓟ | Ⓕ | Ⓟ | Ⓕ |

| Assessor: Date: | Test 1 Comments: |
|---|---|
| Assessor: Date: | Test 2 Comments: |
| Assessor: Date: | Test 3 Comments: |

**TEST ENVIRONMENTS**
**L:** Laboratory/Classroom
**C:** Clinical/Field Testing
**P:** Practicum
**A:** Assessment/Mock Exam

**TEST INFORMATION**
**Test Statistics:** No data available
**Reference(s):** Rehberg (2013)

## ACUTE CARE OF INJURIES AND ILLNESSES
# ASSESSMENT

| NATA EC 5th | BOC RD6 | SKILL |
|---|---|---|
| AC-31 | D3-0303 | Nebulizer Treatment |

**Supplies Needed:** Table, nebulizer

*This problem allows you the opportunity to demonstrate an acute care technique for administration of a breathing treatment called a* **nebulizer treatment**. *You have 2 minutes to complete this task.*

| Nebulizer Treatment | Course or Site Assessor Environment | | Test 1 | | Test 2 | | Test 3 | |
|---|---|---|---|---|---|---|---|---|
| | | | Y | N | Y | N | Y | N |
| **Tester places patient and limb in appropriate position** | | | Y | N | Y | N | Y | N |
| Seated | | | ○ | ○ | ○ | ○ | ○ | ○ |
| **Tester placed in proper position** | | | Y | N | Y | N | Y | N |
| Stands next to the patient | | | ○ | ○ | ○ | ○ | ○ | ○ |
| Assembles nebulizer | | | ○ | ○ | ○ | ○ | ○ | ○ |
| **Tester performs test according to accepted guidelines** | | | Y | N | Y | N | Y | N |
| The tester places appropriate amount of medication into cup | | | ○ | ○ | ○ | ○ | ○ | ○ |
| Turns on power source | | | ○ | ○ | ○ | ○ | ○ | ○ |
| Instructs the patient to breath normally for duration of treatment | | | ○ | ○ | ○ | ○ | ○ | ○ |
| Total | | | ___/6 | | ___/6 | | ___/6 | |
| Must achieve >3 to pass this examination | | | Ⓟ | Ⓕ | Ⓟ | Ⓕ | Ⓟ | Ⓕ |
| Assessor:<br>Date: | Test 1 Comments: | | | | | | | |
| Assessor:<br>Date: | Test 2 Comments: | | | | | | | |
| Assessor:<br>Date: | Test 3 Comments: | | | | | | | |

**TEST ENVIRONMENTS**
**L:** Laboratory/Classroom
**C:** Clinical/Field Testing
**P:** Practicum
**A:** Assessment/Mock Exam

**TEST INFORMATION**
**Test Statistics:** No data available
**Reference(s):** Rehberg (2013)

## ACUTE CARE OF INJURIES AND ILLNESSES
# ASSESSMENT

| NATA EC 5th | BOC RD6 | SKILL |
|:---:|:---:|:---:|
| AC-33 | D3-0303 | Metered-Dose Inhaler |

**Supplies Needed:** Table, metered-dose inhaler

*This problem allows you the opportunity to demonstrate an acute care technique for asthma treatment called a* **metered-dose inhaler.** *You have 2 minutes to complete this task.*

| Metered-Dose Inhaler | Course or Site Assessor Environment | | Test 1 | | Test 2 | | Test 3 | |
|---|---|---|:---:|:---:|:---:|:---:|:---:|:---:|
| | | | Y | N | Y | N | Y | N |
| **Tester places patient and limb in appropriate position** | | | Y | N | Y | N | Y | N |
| Seated | | | O | O | O | O | O | O |
| **Tester placed in proper position** | | | Y | N | Y | N | Y | N |
| Stands at the side of the patient | | | O | O | O | O | O | O |
| Places a spacer on the MDI | | | O | O | O | O | O | O |
| MDI must be primed if not used for 14 days | | | O | O | O | O | O | O |
| **Tester performs test according to accepted guidelines** | | | Y | N | Y | N | Y | N |
| The patient is instructed to take two deep breaths and to hold each breath for 10 seconds to practice | | | O | O | O | O | O | O |
| Once ready, the patient takes a deep breath and simultaneously depresses the MDI | | | O | O | O | O | O | O |
| The patient inhales medication and holds inhalation for 10 seconds; the patient can take second dose after 1 minute if needed | | | O | O | O | O | O | O |
| Total | | | ___/7 | | ___/7 | | ___/7 | |
| **Must achieve >5 to pass this examination** | | | (P) | (F) | (P) | (F) | (P) | (F) |

| Assessor: Date: | Test 1 Comments: |
|---|---|
| Assessor: Date: | Test 2 Comments: |
| Assessor: Date: | Test 3 Comments: |

**TEST ENVIRONMENTS**
**L:** Laboratory/Classroom
**C:** Clinical/Field Testing
**P:** Practicum
**A:** Assessment/Mock Exam

**TEST INFORMATION**
**Test Statistics:** No data available
**Reference(s):** Rehberg (2013)

## ACUTE CARE OF INJURIES AND ILLNESSES
# ASSESSMENT

| NATA EC 5th | BOC RD6 | SKILL |
|---|---|---|
| AC-35 | D3-0303 | Auto-Injectable Epinephrine |

**Supplies Needed:** Table, epinephrine

*This problem allows you the opportunity to demonstrate an acute care technique for anaphylaxis treatment called* **auto-injectable epinephrine**. *You have 2 minutes to complete this task.*

| Auto-Injectable Epinephrine | Course or Site / Assessor / Environment | | Test 1 | | Test 2 | | Test 3 | |
|---|---|---|---|---|---|---|---|---|
| | | | Y | N | Y | N | Y | N |
| **Tester places patient and limb in appropriate position** | | | Y | N | Y | N | Y | N |
| Seated | | | ○ | ○ | ○ | ○ | ○ | ○ |
| **Tester placed in proper position** | | | Y | N | Y | N | Y | N |
| Stands at the side of the patient | | | ○ | ○ | ○ | ○ | ○ | ○ |
| **Tester performs test according to accepted guidelines** | | | Y | N | Y | N | Y | N |
| Pulls off blue safety cap | | | ○ | ○ | ○ | ○ | ○ | ○ |
| Firmly grasps the pen and firmly pushes the orange tip into the vastus lateralis and holds for 10 seconds | | | ○ | ○ | ○ | ○ | ○ | ○ |
| Gently rubs the area to increase absorption | | | ○ | ○ | ○ | ○ | ○ | ○ |
| Total | | | ___/5 | | ___/5 | | ___/5 | |
| Must achieve >3 to pass this examination | | | Ⓟ | Ⓕ | Ⓟ | Ⓕ | Ⓟ | Ⓕ |

| Assessor: Date: | Test 1 Comments: |
|---|---|
| Assessor: Date: | Test 2 Comments: |
| Assessor: Date: | Test 3 Comments: |

**TEST ENVIRONMENTS**
**L:** Laboratory/Classroom
**C:** Clinical/Field Testing
**P:** Practicum
**A:** Assessment/Mock Exam

**TEST INFORMATION**
**Test Statistics:** No data available
**Reference(s):** Rehberg (2013)

# PROTECTIVE DEVICE FITTING

| NATA EC 5th | BOC RD6 | SKILL |
|---|---|---|
| AC-37 | D3-0303, D4-0403 | Adjustable SAM Splint (Ladder Splint) |

**Supplies Needed:** SAM splint (ladder splint), white tape, compression wrap

*This problem allows you the opportunity to demonstrate how to appropriately apply an* **adjustable SAM splint ([SAM Medical Products] ladder splint)**. *You have 4 minutes to complete this task.*

| Adjustable SAM Splint (Ladder Splint) | Course or Site Assessor Environment | Test 1 Y | Test 1 N | Test 2 Y | Test 2 N | Test 3 Y | Test 3 N |
|---|---|---|---|---|---|---|---|
| **Tester places patient and limb in appropriate position** | | Y | N | Y | N | Y | N |
| Maintains injured body part in position it was found | | ○ | ○ | ○ | ○ | ○ | ○ |
| Limits movement of injured area as much as possible | | ○ | ○ | ○ | ○ | ○ | ○ |
| **Selects appropriate device and applies to injured area** | | Y | N | Y | N | Y | N |
| Positions splint in horseshoe shape around the foot and ankle (forms around deformity and does not relocate) | | ○ | ○ | ○ | ○ | ○ | ○ |
| Applies compression wrap distal to proximal | | ○ | ○ | ○ | ○ | ○ | ○ |
| Secures splint, stabilizing the bones above and below the ankle joint | | ○ | ○ | ○ | ○ | ○ | ○ |
| **Tester evaluates injured area after device application** | | Y | N | Y | N | Y | N |
| Checks distal pulse | | ○ | ○ | ○ | ○ | ○ | ○ |
| Checks distal sensation and capillary refill | | ○ | ○ | ○ | ○ | ○ | ○ |
| Total | | /7 | | /7 | | /7 | |
| **Must achieve >5 to pass this examination** | | Ⓟ | Ⓕ | Ⓟ | Ⓕ | Ⓟ | Ⓕ |

| Assessor: Date: | Test 1 Comments: |
|---|---|
| Assessor: Date: | Test 2 Comments: |
| Assessor: Date: | Test 3 Comments: |

**TEST ENVIRONMENTS**
**L:** Laboratory/Classroom
**C:** Clinical/Field Testing
**P:** Practicum
**A:** Assessment/Mock Exam

**TEST INFORMATION**
**Test Statistics:** N/A
**Reference(s):** Manufacturer's recommendation

ACUTE CARE OF INJURIES AND ILLNESSES
# PROTECTIVE DEVICE FITTING

| NATA EC 5th | BOC RD6 | SKILL |
|---|---|---|
| AC-37 | D3-0303, D4-0403 | Immobilization (Knee Immobilizer) |

**Supplies Needed:** Knee immobilizers of various sizes

*This problem allows you the opportunity to demonstrate how to appropriately* **fit a knee immobilizer.**
*You have 4 minutes to complete this task.*

| Immobilization (Knee Immobilizer) | Course or Site Assessor Environment | | Test 1 | | Test 2 | | Test 3 | |
|---|---|---|---|---|---|---|---|---|
| | | | Y | N | Y | N | Y | N |
| **Tester places patient and limb in appropriate position** | | | **Y** | **N** | **Y** | **N** | **Y** | **N** |
| Knee extended | | | ○ | ○ | ○ | ○ | ○ | ○ |
| Limits movement of injured area as much as possible | | | ○ | ○ | ○ | ○ | ○ | ○ |
| **Selects appropriate device and applies to injured area** | | | **Y** | **N** | **Y** | **N** | **Y** | **N** |
| Obtains appropriate-sized immobilizer | | | ○ | ○ | ○ | ○ | ○ | ○ |
| Slides immobilizer under affected limb | | | ○ | ○ | ○ | ○ | ○ | ○ |
| Secures straps near joint first | | | ○ | ○ | ○ | ○ | ○ | ○ |
| Follows by securing proximal and distal straps | | | ○ | ○ | ○ | ○ | ○ | ○ |
| Verifies that device is snug but comfortable | | | ○ | ○ | ○ | ○ | ○ | ○ |
| **Tester evaluates injured area after device application** | | | **Y** | **N** | **Y** | **N** | **Y** | **N** |
| Checks distal pulse | | | ○ | ○ | ○ | ○ | ○ | ○ |
| Checks distal sensation and capillary refill | | | ○ | ○ | ○ | ○ | ○ | ○ |
| **Total** | | | ___/9 | | ___/9 | | ___/9 | |
| **Must achieve >7 to pass this examination** | | | Ⓟ | Ⓕ | Ⓟ | Ⓕ | Ⓟ | Ⓕ |

| Assessor: Date: | Test 1 Comments: |
|---|---|
| Assessor: Date: | Test 2 Comments: |
| Assessor: Date: | Test 3 Comments: |

**TEST ENVIRONMENTS**
**L:** Laboratory/Classroom
**C:** Clinical/Field Testing
**P:** Practicum
**A:** Assessment/Mock Exam

**TEST INFORMATION**
**Test Statistics:** N/A
**Reference(s):** Starkey & Brown (2015)

# PROTECTIVE DEVICE CONSTRUCTION

| NATA EC 5th | BOC RD6 | SKILL |
|:---:|:---:|:---:|
| AC-37 | D3-0303, D4-0403 | Immobilization (Sling and Swath) |

**Supplies Needed:** Triangular bandage, swath, safety pin

*This problem allows you the opportunity to demonstrate how to appropriately apply a* **cervical arm sling and swath** *to immobilize the* **upper extremity.** *You have 3 minutes to complete this task.*

| Immobilization (Sling and Swath) | Course or Site Assessor Environment | | | | | |
|---|---|:---:|:---:|:---:|:---:|:---:|
| | | \_\_\_\_ Test 1 | | \_\_\_\_ Test 2 | | \_\_\_\_ Test 3 |
| **Tester places patient and limb in appropriate position** | | **Y** | **N** | **Y** | **N** | **Y** | **N** |
| Standing | | ○ | ○ | ○ | ○ | ○ | ○ |
| Elbow flexed to approximately 70 degrees | | ○ | ○ | ○ | ○ | ○ | ○ |
| **Applies protective device to injured area** | | **Y** | **N** | **Y** | **N** | **Y** | **N** |
| Slides sling underneath injured extremity with apex facing elbow | | ○ | ○ | ○ | ○ | ○ | ○ |
| Drapes end of bandage closest to body over the injured shoulder | | ○ | ○ | ○ | ○ | ○ | ○ |
| Pulls other end of bandage over the opposite shoulder | | ○ | ○ | ○ | ○ | ○ | ○ |
| Secures sling with square knot behind the neck | | ○ | ○ | ○ | ○ | ○ | ○ |
| Fastens apex of the bandage at the elbow using a safety pin | | ○ | ○ | ○ | ○ | ○ | ○ |
| Secures sling to body by applying swath around the trunk | | ○ | ○ | ○ | ○ | ○ | ○ |
| **Tester evaluates injured area after device application** | | **Y** | **N** | **Y** | **N** | **Y** | **N** |
| Checks distal pulse | | ○ | ○ | ○ | ○ | ○ | ○ |
| Checks distal sensation and capillary refill | | ○ | ○ | ○ | ○ | ○ | ○ |
| Total | | \_\_\_\_/10 | | \_\_\_\_/10 | | \_\_\_\_/10 | |
| Must achieve >7 to pass this examination | | Ⓟ | Ⓕ | Ⓟ | Ⓕ | Ⓟ | Ⓕ |

| Assessor: Date: | Test 1 Comments: |
|---|---|
| Assessor: Date: | Test 2 Comments: |
| Assessor: Date: | Test 3 Comments: |

**TEST ENVIRONMENTS**
**L:** Laboratory/Classroom
**C:** Clinical/Field Testing
**P:** Practicum
**A:** Assessment/Mock Exam

**TEST INFORMATION**
**Test Statistics:** N/A
**Reference(s):** Prentice (2014)

ACUTE CARE OF INJURIES AND ILLNESSES
# PROTECTIVE DEVICE CONSTRUCTION

| NATA EC 5th | BOC RD6 | SKILL |
|---|---|---|
| AC-37 | D3-0303, D4-0403 | Splinting – Arm (Humerus) |

**Supplies Needed:** Table, vacuum splint (small or medium – to fit whole length of arm), vacuum pump

*This problem allows you the opportunity to demonstrate how to appropriately apply a* **splint to the humerus** *to immobilize the* **arm***. You have 3 minutes to complete this task.*

| Splinting – Arm (Humerus) | Course or Site Assessor Environment | Test 1 | | Test 2 | | Test 3 | |
|---|---|---|---|---|---|---|---|
| | | Y | N | Y | N | Y | N |
| **Tester places patient and limb in appropriate position** | | Y | N | Y | N | Y | N |
| Seated, lying down, or standing (whatever is most comfortable) | | O | O | O | O | O | O |
| Splints arm in position found with elbow extended (straight arm) | | O | O | O | O | O | O |
| Moves injured area as little as possible | | O | O | O | O | O | O |
| **Applies protective device to injured area** | | Y | N | Y | N | Y | N |
| The tester has another person carefully lift and hold the injured arm below and above the injury | | O | O | O | O | O | O |
| Carefully slides the vacuum splint under the injured arm and carefully wraps it around | | O | O | O | O | O | O |
| Adjusts splint to immobilize shoulder and elbow and secures the straps | | O | O | O | O | O | O |
| Sucks the air out of the splint with pump until it firmly supports limb (but not tight enough to hurt or cut off circulation) | | O | O | O | O | O | O |
| **Tester evaluates injured area after device application** | | Y | N | Y | N | Y | N |
| Splint properly immobilizes joints proximal and distal to injury | | O | O | O | O | O | O |
| Checks distal pulse | | O | O | O | O | O | O |
| Checks distal sensation and capillary refill | | O | O | O | O | O | O |
| Total | | __/10 | | __/10 | | __/10 | |
| Must achieve >7 to pass this examination | | Ⓟ | Ⓕ | Ⓟ | Ⓕ | Ⓟ | Ⓕ |

| Assessor: Date: | Test 1 Comments: |
|---|---|
| Assessor: Date: | Test 2 Comments: |
| Assessor: Date: | Test 3 Comments: |

**TEST ENVIRONMENTS**
**L:** Laboratory/Classroom
**C:** Clinical/Field Testing
**P:** Practicum
**A:** Assessment/Mock Exam

**TEST INFORMATION**
**Test Statistics:** N/A
**Reference(s):** Prentice (2014)

# PROTECTIVE DEVICE CONSTRUCTION

| NATA EC 5th | BOC RD6 | SKILL |
|---|---|---|
| AC-37 | D3-0303, D4-0403 | Splinting – Finger (Proximal Interphalangeal Joint) |

**Supplies Needed:** Table, finger splint, 1-inch white tape

*This problem allows you the opportunity to demonstrate how to appropriately apply a* **finger splint** *to immobilize the* **PIP joint** *of a finger. You have 3 minutes to complete this task.*

| Splinting – Finger (Proximal Interphalangeal Joint) | Course or Site / Assessor / Environment | | | | | |
|---|---|---|---|---|---|---|
| | | Test 1 | | Test 2 | | Test 3 |
| | | Y | N | Y | N | Y | N |
| **Tester places patient and limb in appropriate position** | | Y | N | Y | N | Y | N |
| Seated | | O | O | O | O | O | O |
| Places hand in appropriate position | | O | O | O | O | O | O |
| Moves injured area as little as possible | | O | O | O | O | O | O |
| **Applies protective device to injured area** | | Y | N | Y | N | Y | N |
| Slides splint under the affected finger | | O | O | O | O | O | O |
| Adjusts splint to cover one joint above and below the fracture site | | O | O | O | O | O | O |
| Secures splint to affected finger with white tape | | O | O | O | O | O | O |
| **Tester evaluates injured area after device application** | | Y | N | Y | N | Y | N |
| Checks distal pulse | | O | O | O | O | O | O |
| Checks distal sensation and capillary refill | | O | O | O | O | O | O |
| Total | | /8 | | /8 | | /8 |
| Must achieve >6 to pass this examination | | P | F | P | F | P | F |

| Assessor: Date: | Test 1 Comments: |
|---|---|
| Assessor: Date: | Test 2 Comments: |
| Assessor: Date: | Test 3 Comments: |

**TEST ENVIRONMENTS**
L: Laboratory/Classroom
C: Clinical/Field Testing
P: Practicum
A: Assessment/Mock Exam

**TEST INFORMATION**
**Test Statistics:** N/A
**Reference(s):** Prentice (2014)

ACUTE CARE OF INJURIES AND ILLNESSES
# PROTECTIVE DEVICE CONSTRUCTION

| NATA EC 5th | BOC RD6 | SKILL |
|---|---|---|
| AC-37 | D3-0303, D4-0403 | Splinting – Foot/Ankle (Tarsals/Metatarsals) |

**Supplies Needed:** Table, SAM splint, elastic wrap, white tape

*This problem allows you the opportunity to demonstrate how to appropriately* **splint the foot/ankle.** *You have 3 minutes to complete this task.*

| Splinting – Foot/Ankle (Tarsals/Metatarsals) | Course or Site Assessor Environment _____ _____ _____ | | | | | |
|---|---|---|---|---|---|---|
| | | Test 1 | | Test 2 | | Test 3 |
| **Tester places patient and limb in appropriate position** | | **Y** | **N** | **Y** | **N** | **Y** | **N** |
| Seated or lying down | | ○ | ○ | ○ | ○ | ○ | ○ |
| Splints foot/ankle in position found | | ○ | ○ | ○ | ○ | ○ | ○ |
| Moves injured area as little as possible | | ○ | ○ | ○ | ○ | ○ | ○ |
| **Applies protective device to injured area** | | **Y** | **N** | **Y** | **N** | **Y** | **N** |
| Molds a SAM splint or another hard splint to the length and shape of the patient's foot/ankle (must support knee as well) | | ○ | ○ | ○ | ○ | ○ | ○ |
| Instructs another person to carefully lift and hold the injured foot/ankle by gently lifting from the lower leg while supporting the distal foot | | ○ | ○ | ○ | ○ | ○ | ○ |
| Slides splint under foot/ankle and carefully forms splint to the patient (should have most of this done before placing on the patient) | | ○ | ○ | ○ | ○ | ○ | ○ |
| Secures splint with an elastic wrap and white tape, but not too tight | | ○ | ○ | ○ | ○ | ○ | ○ |
| **Tester evaluates injured area after device application** | | **Y** | **N** | **Y** | **N** | **Y** | **N** |
| Splint properly immobilizes the joints proximal and distal to injury | | ○ | ○ | ○ | ○ | ○ | ○ |
| Checks distal pulse | | ○ | ○ | ○ | ○ | ○ | ○ |
| Checks distal sensation and capillary refill | | ○ | ○ | ○ | ○ | ○ | ○ |
| | Total | ___/10 | | ___/10 | | ___/10 | |
| | Must achieve >7 to pass this examination | Ⓟ | Ⓕ | Ⓟ | Ⓕ | Ⓟ | Ⓕ |
| **Assessor: Date:** | Test 1 Comments: | | | | | | |
| **Assessor: Date:** | Test 2 Comments: | | | | | | |
| **Assessor: Date:** | Test 3 Comments: | | | | | | |

**TEST ENVIRONMENTS**
**L:** Laboratory/Classroom
**C:** Clinical/Field Testing
**P:** Practicum
**A:** Assessment/Mock Exam

**TEST INFORMATION**
**Test Statistics:** N/A
**Reference(s):** Prentice (2014)

## ACUTE CARE OF INJURIES AND ILLNESSES
# PROTECTIVE DEVICE CONSTRUCTION

| NATA EC 5th | BOC RD6 | SKILL |
|---|---|---|
| AC-37 | D3-0303, D4-0403 | Splinting – Hand/Wrist (Carpals/Metacarpals) |

**Supplies Needed:** Table, SAM splint, elastic wrap, white tape

*This problem allows you the opportunity to demonstrate how to appropriately* **splint the hand/wrist**. *You have 3 minutes to complete this task.*

| Splinting – Hand/Wrist (Carpals/Metacarpals) | Course or Site Assessor Environment | Test 1 | | Test 2 | | Test 3 | |
|---|---|---|---|---|---|---|---|
| | | Y | N | Y | N | Y | N |
| **Tester places patient and limb in appropriate position** | | **Y** | **N** | **Y** | **N** | **Y** | **N** |
| Seated | | ○ | ○ | ○ | ○ | ○ | ○ |
| Splints hand/wrist in position found | | ○ | ○ | ○ | ○ | ○ | ○ |
| Moves injured area as little as possible | | ○ | ○ | ○ | ○ | ○ | ○ |
| **Applies protective device to injured area** | | **Y** | **N** | **Y** | **N** | **Y** | **N** |
| Instructs the patient to support wrist | | ○ | ○ | ○ | ○ | ○ | ○ |
| Molds a SAM splint for the patient with wrist in a relaxed position (slightly flexed), made with "handle" for the patient's hand to rest on | | ○ | ○ | ○ | ○ | ○ | ○ |
| Applies splint to the patient carefully – should support the elbow as well | | ○ | ○ | ○ | ○ | ○ | ○ |
| Secures splint to the patient with elastic wrap and tape | | ○ | ○ | ○ | ○ | ○ | ○ |
| **Tester evaluates injured area after device application** | | **Y** | **N** | **Y** | **N** | **Y** | **N** |
| Splint properly immobilizes the joints proximal and distal to injury | | ○ | ○ | ○ | ○ | ○ | ○ |
| Checks distal pulse | | ○ | ○ | ○ | ○ | ○ | ○ |
| Checks distal sensation and capillary refill | | ○ | ○ | ○ | ○ | ○ | ○ |
| Total | | ___/10 | | ___/10 | | ___/10 | |
| Must achieve >7 to pass this examination | | Ⓟ | Ⓕ | Ⓟ | Ⓕ | Ⓟ | Ⓕ |

| Assessor: Date: | Test 1 Comments: |
|---|---|
| Assessor: Date: | Test 2 Comments: |
| Assessor: Date: | Test 3 Comments: |

**TEST ENVIRONMENTS**
**L:** Laboratory/Classroom
**C:** Clinical/Field Testing
**P:** Practicum
**A:** Assessment/Mock Exam

**TEST INFORMATION**
**Test Statistics:** N/A
**Reference(s):** Prentice (2014)

## ACUTE CARE OF INJURIES AND ILLNESSES
# PROTECTIVE DEVICE CONSTRUCTION

| NATA EC 5th | BOC RD6 | SKILL |
|---|---|---|
| AC-37 | D3-0303, D4-0403 | Splinting – Leg (Femur) |

**Supplies Needed:** Table, vacuum splint (medium to large – needs to immobilize the knee and hip), vacuum pump

*This problem allows you the opportunity to demonstrate how to appropriately **splint the femur** to immobilize the **leg**. You have 3 minutes to complete this task.*

| Splinting – Leg (Femur) | Course or Site Assessor Environment | | Test 1 | | Test 2 | | Test 3 |
|---|---|---|---|---|---|---|---|
| | | Y | N | Y | N | Y | N |
| **Tester places patient and limb in appropriate position** | | Y | N | Y | N | Y | N |
| Lying down | | ○ | ○ | ○ | ○ | ○ | ○ |
| Splints leg in position found | | ○ | ○ | ○ | ○ | ○ | ○ |
| Moves injured area as little as possible | | ○ | ○ | ○ | ○ | ○ | ○ |
| **Applies protective device to injured area** | | Y | N | Y | N | Y | N |
| Instructs another person to carefully lift leg distal and proximal to injury | | ○ | ○ | ○ | ○ | ○ | ○ |
| Slides vacuum splint under leg and wraps it around | | ○ | ○ | ○ | ○ | ○ | ○ |
| Adjusts splint to support the hip, knee, and ankle joints, and then secures straps | | ○ | ○ | ○ | ○ | ○ | ○ |
| Sucks the air out of the splint with the pump | | ○ | ○ | ○ | ○ | ○ | ○ |
| **Tester evaluates injured area after device application** | | Y | N | Y | N | Y | N |
| Splint properly immobilizes the joints proximal and distal to injury | | ○ | ○ | ○ | ○ | ○ | ○ |
| Checks distal pulse | | ○ | ○ | ○ | ○ | ○ | ○ |
| Checks distal sensation and capillary refill | | ○ | ○ | ○ | ○ | ○ | ○ |
| **Total** | | /10 | | /10 | | /10 | |
| **Must achieve >7 to pass this examination** | | Ⓟ | Ⓕ | Ⓟ | Ⓕ | Ⓟ | Ⓕ |

| Assessor: Date: | Test 1 Comments: |
|---|---|
| Assessor: Date: | Test 2 Comments: |
| Assessor: Date: | Test 3 Comments: |

**TEST ENVIRONMENTS**
L: Laboratory/Classroom
C: Clinical/Field Testing
P: Practicum
A: Assessment/Mock Exam

**TEST INFORMATION**
**Test Statistics:** N/A
**Reference(s):** Prentice (2014)

## ACUTE CARE OF INJURIES AND ILLNESSES
# PROTECTIVE DEVICE CONSTRUCTION

| NATA EC 5th | BOC RD6 | SKILL |
|---|---|---|
| AC-37 | D3-0303, D4-0403 | Splinting – Lower Leg (Tibia) |

**Supplies Needed:** Table, vacuum splint (medium to large – needs to immobilize the ankle and knee), vacuum pump

*This problem allows you the opportunity to demonstrate how to appropriately* **splint the tibia** *to immobilize the* **lower leg**. *You have 3 minutes to complete this task.*

| Splinting – Lower Leg (Tibia) | Course or Site Assessor Environment | Test 1 Y | Test 1 N | Test 2 Y | Test 2 N | Test 3 Y | Test 3 N |
|---|---|---|---|---|---|---|---|
| **Tester places patient and limb in appropriate position** | | **Y** | **N** | **Y** | **N** | **Y** | **N** |
| Lying down | | O | O | O | O | O | O |
| Splints leg in position found | | O | O | O | O | O | O |
| Moves injured area as little as possible | | O | O | O | O | O | O |
| **Applies protective device to injured area** | | **Y** | **N** | **Y** | **N** | **Y** | **N** |
| Instructs another person to carefully lift leg distal and proximal to injury | | O | O | O | O | O | O |
| Slides vacuum splint under leg and wraps it around | | O | O | O | O | O | O |
| Adjusts splint to support the knee and ankle joints, and then secures straps | | O | O | O | O | O | O |
| Sucks the air out of the splint with the pump | | O | O | O | O | O | O |
| **Tester evaluates injured area after device application** | | **Y** | **N** | **Y** | **N** | **Y** | **N** |
| Splint properly immobilizes the joints proximal and distal to injury | | O | O | O | O | O | O |
| Checks distal pulse | | O | O | O | O | O | O |
| Checks distal sensation and capillary refill | | O | O | O | O | O | O |
| Total | | __ /10 | | __ /10 | | __ /10 | |
| Must achieve >7 to pass this examination | | ⓟ | Ⓕ | ⓟ | Ⓕ | ⓟ | Ⓕ |

| Assessor: Date: | Test 1 Comments: |
|---|---|
| Assessor: Date: | Test 2 Comments: |
| Assessor: Date: | Test 3 Comments: |

**TEST ENVIRONMENTS**
**L:** Laboratory/Classroom
**C:** Clinical/Field Testing
**P:** Practicum
**A:** Assessment/Mock Exam

**TEST INFORMATION**
**Test Statistics:** N/A
**Reference(s):** Prentice (2014)

## Acute Care of Injuries and Illnesses
# Ambulation Assistance

| NATA EC 5th | BOC RD6 | SKILL |
|---|---|---|
| AC-39 | D4-0403 | Cane Fitting |

**Supplies Needed:** Canes of various sizes

*This problem allows you the opportunity to demonstrate how to appropriately* **fit a cane.**
*You have 3 minutes to complete this task.*

| Cane Fitting | Course or Site Assessor Environment | Test 1 | | Test 2 | | Test 3 | |
|---|---|---|---|---|---|---|---|
| | | Y | N | Y | N | Y | N |
| **Tester places patient and limb in appropriate position** | | Y | N | Y | N | Y | N |
| Standing with good posture | | ○ | ○ | ○ | ○ | ○ | ○ |
| Feet shoulder width apart | | ○ | ○ | ○ | ○ | ○ | ○ |
| Wearing low-heeled/flat shoes | | ○ | ○ | ○ | ○ | ○ | ○ |
| **Measures patient for ambulation device** | | Y | N | Y | N | Y | N |
| Measures from greater trochanter of femur to the floor | | ○ | ○ | ○ | ○ | ○ | ○ |
| Adjusts cane to the measured length | | ○ | ○ | ○ | ○ | ○ | ○ |
| **Instructs patient in walking with ambulatory device** | | Y | N | Y | N | Y | N |
| Cane is placed on uninjured side | | ○ | ○ | ○ | ○ | ○ | ○ |
| The patient steps forward with cane and injured leg | | ○ | ○ | ○ | ○ | ○ | ○ |
| The patient follows with uninjured leg | | ○ | ○ | ○ | ○ | ○ | ○ |
| **Total** | | __/8 | | __/8 | | __/8 | |
| **Must achieve >6 to pass this examination** | | Ⓟ | Ⓕ | Ⓟ | Ⓕ | Ⓟ | Ⓕ |

| Assessor: Date: | Test 1 Comments: |
|---|---|
| Assessor: Date: | Test 2 Comments: |
| Assessor: Date: | Test 3 Comments: |

**TEST ENVIRONMENTS**
**L:** Laboratory/Classroom
**C:** Clinical/Field Testing
**P:** Practicum
**A:** Assessment/Mock Exam

**TEST INFORMATION**
**Test Statistics:** N/A
**Reference(s):** Prentice (2014)

## ACUTE CARE OF INJURIES AND ILLNESSES
# AMBULATION ASSISTANCE

| NATA EC 5th | BOC RD6 | SKILL |
|---|---|---|
| AC-39 | D4-0403 | Crutch Fitting |

**Supplies Needed:** Crutches of various sizes

*This problem allows you the opportunity to demonstrate how to appropriately **fit crutches**. You have 3 minutes to complete this task.*

| Crutch Fitting | Course or Site Assessor Environment | | Test 1 | | Test 2 | | Test 3 | |
|---|---|---|---|---|---|---|---|---|
| | | | Y | N | Y | N | Y | N |
| **Tester places patient and limb in appropriate position** | | | Y | N | Y | N | Y | N |
| Standing with good posture | | | ○ | ○ | ○ | ○ | ○ | ○ |
| Feet shoulder width apart | | | ○ | ○ | ○ | ○ | ○ | ○ |
| Wearing low-heeled/flat shoes | | | ○ | ○ | ○ | ○ | ○ | ○ |
| **Measures patient for ambulation device** | | | Y | N | Y | N | Y | N |
| Places crutch slightly in front of the involved limb (2 to 4 inches) | | | ○ | ○ | ○ | ○ | ○ | ○ |
| Places crutch slightly to the side of the involved limb (4 to 6 inches) | | | ○ | ○ | ○ | ○ | ○ | ○ |
| Places axillary pas approximately 1 to 1.5 inches below axilla | | | ○ | ○ | ○ | ○ | ○ | ○ |
| Places elbow in approximately 30 degrees flexion | | | ○ | ○ | ○ | ○ | ○ | ○ |
| **Instructs patient in walking with ambulatory device** | | | Y | N | Y | N | Y | N |
| Tightens all fasteners | | | ○ | ○ | ○ | ○ | ○ | ○ |
| Verifies axilla and hand grips are well-padded | | | ○ | ○ | ○ | ○ | ○ | ○ |
| Verifies that rubberized tips are not damaged | | | ○ | ○ | ○ | ○ | ○ | ○ |
| Instructs the patient to bear weight on hands not axilla | | | ○ | ○ | ○ | ○ | ○ | ○ |
| | Total | | ___/11 | | ___/11 | | ___/11 | |
| Must achieve >8 to pass this examination | | | Ⓟ | Ⓕ | Ⓟ | Ⓕ | Ⓟ | Ⓕ |
| Assessor: Date: | Test 1 Comments: | | | | | | | |
| Assessor: Date: | Test 2 Comments: | | | | | | | |
| Assessor: Date: | Test 3 Comments: | | | | | | | |

**TEST ENVIRONMENTS**
**L:** Laboratory/Classroom
**C:** Clinical/Field Testing
**P:** Practicum
**A:** Assessment/Mock Exam

**TEST INFORMATION**
**Test Statistics:** N/A
**Reference(s):** Prentice (2014)

## ACUTE CARE OF INJURIES AND ILLNESSES
# AMBULATION ASSISTANCE

| NATA EC 5th | BOC RD6 | SKILL |
|---|---|---|
| AC-39 | D4-0403 | Four-Point Gait Method |

**Supplies Needed:** Crutches of various sizes

*This problem allows you the opportunity to instruct a patient in the **four-point gait method**.*
*You have 3 minutes to complete this task.*

| Four-Point Gait Method | Course or Site Assessor Environment | | | | | |
|---|---|---|---|---|---|---|
| | Test 1 | | Test 2 | | Test 3 | |
| | Y | N | Y | N | Y | N |
| **Tester places patient and limb in appropriate position** | Y | N | Y | N | Y | N |
| Standing with good posture | ○ | ○ | ○ | ○ | ○ | ○ |
| Feet shoulder width apart | ○ | ○ | ○ | ○ | ○ | ○ |
| Wearing low-heeled/flat shoes | ○ | ○ | ○ | ○ | ○ | ○ |
| **Measures patient for ambulation device** | Y | N | Y | N | Y | N |
| Places crutch slightly in front of the involved limb (2 to 4 inches) | ○ | ○ | ○ | ○ | ○ | ○ |
| Places crutch slightly to the side of the involved limb (4 to 6 inches) | ○ | ○ | ○ | ○ | ○ | ○ |
| Places axillary pas approximately 1 to 1.5 inches below axilla | ○ | ○ | ○ | ○ | ○ | ○ |
| Places elbow in approximately 30 degrees flexion | ○ | ○ | ○ | ○ | ○ | ○ |
| **Instructs patient in walking with ambulatory device** | Y | N | Y | N | Y | N |
| Weight evenly distributed on crutches | ○ | ○ | ○ | ○ | ○ | ○ |
| The patient places one crutch tip forward | ○ | ○ | ○ | ○ | ○ | ○ |
| The patient steps forward with opposite foot | ○ | ○ | ○ | ○ | ○ | ○ |
| The patient places other crutch tip forward | ○ | ○ | ○ | ○ | ○ | ○ |
| The patient steps forward with other foot | ○ | ○ | ○ | ○ | ○ | ○ |
| Total | ___/12 | | ___/12 | | ___/12 | |
| **Must achieve >9 to pass this examination** | Ⓟ | Ⓕ | Ⓟ | Ⓕ | Ⓟ | Ⓕ |

| Assessor: Date: | Test 1 Comments: |
|---|---|
| Assessor: Date: | Test 2 Comments: |
| Assessor: Date: | Test 3 Comments: |

**TEST ENVIRONMENTS**
**L:** Laboratory/Classroom
**C:** Clinical/Field Testing
**P:** Practicum
**A:** Assessment/Mock Exam

**TEST INFORMATION**
**Test Statistics:** N/A
**Reference(s):**  Prentice (2014)

## ACUTE CARE OF INJURIES AND ILLNESSES
# AMBULATION ASSISTANCE

| NATA EC 5th | BOC RD6 | SKILL |
|---|---|---|
| AC-39 | D4-0403 | Nonweightbearing (Ascending/Descending Stairs) |

**Supplies Needed:** Crutches of various sizes

*This problem allows you the opportunity to instruct a patient in* **nonweightbearing (ascending/descending stairs).** *You have 4 minutes to complete this task.*

| Nonweightbearing (Ascending/Descending Stairs) | Course or Site Assessor Environment | | Test 1 | | Test 2 | | Test 3 | |
|---|---|---|---|---|---|---|---|---|
| **Tester places patient and limb in appropriate position** | | | **Y** | **N** | **Y** | **N** | **Y** | **N** |
| Standing with good posture | | | ○ | ○ | ○ | ○ | ○ | ○ |
| Feet shoulder width apart | | | ○ | ○ | ○ | ○ | ○ | ○ |
| Wearing low-heeled/flat shoes | | | ○ | ○ | ○ | ○ | ○ | ○ |
| **Measures patient for ambulation device** | | | **Y** | **N** | **Y** | **N** | **Y** | **N** |
| Places crutch slightly in front of the involved limb (2 to 4 inches) | | | ○ | ○ | ○ | ○ | ○ | ○ |
| Places crutch slightly to the side of the involved limb (4 to 6 inches) | | | ○ | ○ | ○ | ○ | ○ | ○ |
| Places axillary pas approximately 1 to 1.5 inches below axilla | | | ○ | ○ | ○ | ○ | ○ | ○ |
| Places elbow in approximately 30 degrees flexion | | | ○ | ○ | ○ | ○ | ○ | ○ |
| **Instructs patient in walking with ambulatory device** | | | **Y** | **N** | **Y** | **N** | **Y** | **N** |
| Weight evenly distributed on crutches | | | ○ | ○ | ○ | ○ | ○ | ○ |
| The patient steps up with uninjured leg | | | ○ | ○ | ○ | ○ | ○ | ○ |
| The patient follows with injured leg and crutches | | | ○ | ○ | ○ | ○ | ○ | ○ |
| Instructs the patient in descending stairs | | | ○ | ○ | ○ | ○ | ○ | ○ |
| Weight evenly distributed on crutches | | | ○ | ○ | ○ | ○ | ○ | ○ |
| The patient steps down with injured leg and crutches | | | ○ | ○ | ○ | ○ | ○ | ○ |
| The patient follows with uninjured leg | | | ○ | ○ | ○ | ○ | ○ | ○ |
| | | Total | ___/14 | | ___/14 | | ___/14 | |
| | Must achieve >10 to pass this examination | | Ⓟ | Ⓕ | Ⓟ | Ⓕ | Ⓟ | Ⓕ |

| Assessor: Date: | **Test 1 Comments:** |
|---|---|
| Assessor: Date: | **Test 2 Comments:** |
| Assessor: Date: | **Test 3 Comments:** |

**TEST ENVIRONMENTS**
**L:** Laboratory/Classroom
**C:** Clinical/Field Testing
**P:** Practicum
**A:** Assessment/Mock Exam

**TEST INFORMATION**
**Test Statistics:** N/A
**Reference(s):** Prentice (2014)

ACUTE CARE OF INJURIES AND ILLNESSES
# AMBULATION ASSISTANCE

| NATA EC 5th | BOC RD6 | SKILL |
|---|---|---|
| AC-39 | D4-0403 | Nonweightbearing (Tripod) |

**Supplies Needed:** Crutches of various sizes

*This problem allows you the opportunity to instruct a patient in* **nonweightbearing (tripod)**. *You have 4 minutes to complete this task.*

| Nonweightbearing (Tripod) | Course or Site / Assessor / Environment | | | | | |
|---|---|---|---|---|---|---|
| | | Test 1 | | Test 2 | | Test 3 |
| **Tester places patient and limb in appropriate position** | | Y | N | Y | N | Y | N |
| Standing with good posture | | O | O | O | O | O | O |
| Feet shoulder width apart | | O | O | O | O | O | O |
| Wearing low-heeled/flat shoes | | O | O | O | O | O | O |
| **Measures patient for ambulation device** | | Y | N | Y | N | Y | N |
| Places crutch slightly in front of the involved limb (2 to 4 inches) | | O | O | O | O | O | O |
| Places crutch slightly to the side of the involved limb (4 to 6 inches) | | O | O | O | O | O | O |
| Places axillary pas approximately 1 to 1.5 inches below axilla | | O | O | O | O | O | O |
| Places elbow in approximately 30 degrees flexion | | O | O | O | O | O | O |
| **Instructs patient in walking with ambulatory device** | | Y | N | Y | N | Y | N |
| Weight evenly distributed on crutches | | O | O | O | O | O | O |
| Instructs the patient not to put weight on axilla | | O | O | O | O | O | O |
| Involved limb is off the floor (flexed position) | | O | O | O | O | O | O |
| The patient moves both crutches forward (6 to 8 inches) | | O | O | O | O | O | O |
| The patient swings the noninjured limb forward (swing-to) or (swing-through) | | O | O | O | O | O | O |
| Repeat the above two steps | | O | O | O | O | O | O |
| Total | | ___/13 | | ___/13 | | ___/13 | |
| Must achieve >10 to pass this examination | | P | F | P | F | P | F |

| Assessor: Date: | Test 1 Comments: |
|---|---|
| Assessor: Date: | Test 2 Comments: |
| Assessor: Date: | Test 3 Comments: |

**TEST ENVIRONMENTS**
**L:** Laboratory/Classroom
**C:** Clinical/Field Testing
**P:** Practicum
**A:** Assessment/Mock Exam

**TEST INFORMATION**
**Test Statistics:** N/A
**Reference(s):** Prentice (2014)

## ACUTE CARE OF INJURIES AND ILLNESSES
# PATIENT TRANSPORT

| NATA EC 5th | BOC RD6 | SKILL |
|---|---|---|
| AC-42 | D4-0403 | Patient Transport (Assisted Walk) |

**Supplies Needed:** N/A

*This problem allows you the opportunity to demonstrate how to appropriately perform a* **patient transport (assisted walk)**. *You have 4 minutes to complete this task.*

| Patient Transport (Assisted Walk) | Course or Site / Assessor / Environment | | Test 1 | | Test 2 | | Test 3 |
|---|---|---|---|---|---|---|---|
| **Appropriately prepares patient** | | Y | N | Y | N | Y | N |
| Makes sure the injury is minor (walking should be prohibited in patients with major injuries) | | ○ | ○ | ○ | ○ | ○ | ○ |
| Has the patient go from prone to supine, side lying to sitting, and should sit for 30 seconds prior to standing | | ○ | ○ | ○ | ○ | ○ | ○ |
| Instructs the patient what is going to happen before it is performed | | ○ | ○ | ○ | ○ | ○ | ○ |
| **Appropriately performs transport** | | Y | N | Y | N | Y | N |
| Instructs the patient to keep all weight on uninvolved leg, bend uninvolved knee, and grasp the tester's hand | | ○ | ○ | ○ | ○ | ○ | ○ |
| Holds the patient's hand and supports the patient's torso by grasping around the shoulder/back (on injured side) | | ○ | ○ | ○ | ○ | ○ | ○ |
| Instructs the patient to stand up with uninvolved leg | | ○ | ○ | ○ | ○ | ○ | ○ |
| Two people who are about the same height as the patient should provide complete support on both sides of the patient | | ○ | ○ | ○ | ○ | ○ | ○ |
| The patient's arms are draped over the assistants' shoulders, and their arms encircle his/her back | | ○ | ○ | ○ | ○ | ○ | ○ |
| **Total** | | ___/8 | | ___/8 | | ___/8 | |
| **Must achieve >6 to pass this examination** | | Ⓟ | Ⓕ | Ⓟ | Ⓕ | Ⓟ | Ⓕ |

| Assessor: Date: | Test 1 Comments: |
|---|---|
| Assessor: Date: | Test 2 Comments: |
| Assessor: Date: | Test 3 Comments: |

**TEST ENVIRONMENTS**
**L:** Laboratory/Classroom
**C:** Clinical/Field Testing
**P:** Practicum
**A:** Assessment/Mock Exam

**TEST INFORMATION**
**Test Statistics:** N/A
**Reference(s):** Prentice (2014)

## ACUTE CARE OF INJURIES AND ILLNESSES
# PATIENT TRANSPORT

| NATA EC 5th | BOC RD6 | SKILL |
|---|---|---|
| AC-42 | D4-0403 | Patient Transport (Carry) |

**Supplies Needed:** N/A

*This problem allows you the opportunity to demonstrate how to appropriately perform a* **patient transport (carry)***. You have 4 minutes to complete this task.*

| Patient Transport (Carry) | Course or Site<br>Assessor<br>Environment | | Test 1 | | Test 2 | | Test 3 |
|---|---|---|---|---|---|---|---|
| **Appropriately prepares patient** | | **Y** | **N** | **Y** | **N** | **Y** | **N** |
| Makes sure the injury is minor/mild (carrying is used to move a patient with mild injury a greater distance than comfortable to walk) | | ○ | ○ | ○ | ○ | ○ | ○ |
| The tester has the patient go from prone to supine, side lying to sitting, and should sit for 30 seconds prior to standing | | ○ | ○ | ○ | ○ | ○ | ○ |
| Instruct the patient what is going to happen before it is performed | | ○ | ○ | ○ | ○ | ○ | ○ |
| **Appropriately performs carry** | | **Y** | **N** | **Y** | **N** | **Y** | **N** |
| Instructs the patient to keep all weight on uninvolved leg, bend uninvolved knee, and grasps the tester's hand | | ○ | ○ | ○ | ○ | ○ | ○ |
| Should hold the patient's hand and also support the patient's torso by grasping around the shoulder/back (on injured side) | | ○ | ○ | ○ | ○ | ○ | ○ |
| Instructs the patient to stand up with uninvolved leg | | ○ | ○ | ○ | ○ | ○ | ○ |
| Two people who are about the same height should provide complete support on both sides of the patient | | ○ | ○ | ○ | ○ | ○ | ○ |
| The patient's arms are draped over the assistants' shoulders, and their arms encircle his/her back | | ○ | ○ | ○ | ○ | ○ | ○ |
| Instructs assistants to lock arms (grasp each other's wrists), behind the patient's knees | | ○ | ○ | ○ | ○ | ○ | ○ |
| Instructs the patient to slowly sit back onto their arms | | ○ | ○ | ○ | ○ | ○ | ○ |
| Assistants carry the patient, without causing any more harm to the patient | | ○ | ○ | ○ | ○ | ○ | ○ |
| **Total** | | __/11 | | __/11 | | __/11 | |
| **Must achieve >8 to pass this examination** | | Ⓟ | Ⓕ | Ⓟ | Ⓕ | Ⓟ | Ⓕ |
| Assessor:<br>Date: | Test 1 Comments: | | | | | | |
| Assessor:<br>Date: | Test 2 Comments: | | | | | | |
| Assessor:<br>Date: | Test 3 Comments: | | | | | | |

**TEST ENVIRONMENTS**
**L:** Laboratory/Classroom
**C:** Clinical/Field Testing
**P:** Practicum
**A:** Assessment/Mock Exam

**TEST INFORMATION**
**Test Statistics:** N/A
**Reference(s):** Prentice (2014)

# V

---

**THERAPEUTIC INTERVENTIONS**

# 15

# THERAPEUTIC INTERVENTIONS

Hauth, J. M., Gloyeske, B. M., & Amato, H. K.
*Clinical Skills Documentation Guide for Athletic Training, Third Edition* (pp. 506-633).
© 2016 SLACK Incorporated.

## THERAPEUTIC INTERVENTIONS
# KNOWLEDGE AND SKILLS

| *Therapeutic Interventions* | | | | *Skill: Acquisition, Reinforcement, Proficiency* | | |
|---|---|---|---|---|---|---|
| **NATA EC 5th** | **BOC RD6** | **Therapeutic Modalities—Self-Treatment** | **Page #** | | | |
| TI-10 | D4-0401 | Self-Stretching | 510 | | | |
| **NATA EC 5th** | **BOC RD6** | **Therapeutic Modalities—Acoustic Energy** | **Page #** | | | |
| TI-11a/b/c/e/f | D4-0402 | Phonophoresis | 512 | | | |
| TI-11a/b/c/e/f | D4-0402 | Therapeutic Ultrasound 1 MHz | 514 | | | |
| TI-11a/b/c/e/f | D4-0402 | Therapeutic Ultrasound 3 MHz | 516 | | | |
| TI-11a/b/c/e/f | D4-0402 | Therapeutic Ultrasound Immersion | 518 | | | |
| **NATA EC 5th** | **BOC RD6** | **Therapeutic Modalities—Cryotherapy** | **Page #** | | | |
| TI-11a/b/c/e/f | D4-0402 | Contrast Bath | 520 | | | |
| TI-11a/b/c/e/f | D4-0402 | Cold Whirlpool | 522 | | | |
| TI-11a/b/c/e/f | D4-0402 | Ice Bag | 524 | | | |
| TI-11a/b/c/e/f | D4-0402 | Ice Massage | 525 | | | |
| TI-11a/b/c/e/f | D4-0402 | Vapo-Coolant Spray | 527 | | | |
| **NATA EC 5th** | **BOC RD6** | **Therapeutic Modalities—Electrical Energy** | **Page #** | | | |
| TI-11a/b/c/e/f | D4-0402 | Electrical Stimulation (Interferential) | 528 | | | |
| TI-11a/b/c/e/f | D4-0402 | Electrical Stimulation (Low-Intensity Microcurrent) | 530 | | | |
| TI-11a/b/c/e/f | D4-0402 | Electrical Stimulation (Iontophoresis) | 532 | | | |
| **NATA EC 5th** | **BOC RD6** | **Therapeutic Modalities—Manual Therapy** | **Page #** | | | |
| TI-11a/b/c/e/f | D4-0402 | Intermittent Compression | 534 | | | |
| TI-11a/b/c/e/f | D4-0402 | Cross-Fiber Friction Massage | 536 | | | |
| TI-11a/b/c/e/f | D4-0402 | Effleurage Massage | 538 | | | |
| TI-11a/b/c/e/f | D4-0402 | Fine Vibration Massage | 540 | | | |
| TI-11a/b/c/e/f | D4-0402 | Petrissage Massage | 542 | | | |
| TI-11a/b/c/e/f | D4-0402 | Tapotement Massage | 544 | | | |
| **NATA EC 5th** | **BOC RD6** | **Therapeutic Modalities—Thermotherapy** | **Page #** | | | |
| TI-11a/b/c/e/f | D4-0402 | Hot Whirlpool | 546 | | | |
| TI-11a/b/c/e/f | D4-0402 | Moist Heat Pack | 548 | | | |
| TI-11a/b/c/e/f | D4-0402 | Paraffin Bath | 550 | | | |
| **NATA EC 5th** | **BOC RD6** | **Therapeutic Exercise—Lower Extremity** | **Page #** | | | |
| TI-11a/b/d | D4-0401 | Lower Extremity Endurance (Ankle) | 552 | | | |
| TI-11a/b/d | D4-0401 | Lower Extremity Endurance (Hip) | 553 | | | |
| TI-11a/b/d | D4-0401 | Lower Extremity Endurance (Knee) | 554 | | | |
| TI-11a/b/d | D4-0401 | Lower Extremity Isometrics (Ankle) | 555 | | | |
| TI-11a/b/d | D4-0401 | Lower Extremity Isometrics (Hip) | 556 | | | |
| TI-11a/b/d | D4-0401 | Lower Extremity Isometrics (Knee) | 557 | | | |
| TI-11a/b/d | D4-0401 | Lower Extremity Proprioception (Static) | 558 | | | |
| TI-11a/b/d | D4-0401 | Lower Extremity Proprioception (Dynamic) | 559 | | | |
| TI-11a/b/d | D4-0401 | Lower Extremity Strength (Ankle) | 560 | | | |
| TI-11a/b/d | D4-0401 | Lower Extremity Strength (Hip) | 561 | | | |
| TI-11a/b/d | D4-0401 | Lower Extremity Strength (Knee) | 562 | | | |

*(continued on the next page)*

## THERAPEUTIC INTERVENTIONS
# KNOWLEDGE AND SKILLS

| NATA EC 5th | BOC RD6 | Therapeutic Exercise—Upper Extremity | Page # | | | |
|---|---|---|---|---|---|---|
| TI-11a/b/d | D4-0401 | Upper Extremity Endurance (Shoulder) | 563 | | | |
| TI-11a/b/d | D4-0401 | Upper Extremity Isometrics (Elbow) | 564 | | | |
| TI-11a/b/d | D4-0401 | Upper Extremity Isometrics (Shoulder) | 565 | | | |
| TI-11a/b/d | D4-0401 | Upper Extremity Proprioception (Static) | 566 | | | |
| TI-11a/b/d | D4-0401 | Upper Extremity Proprioception (Dynamic) | 567 | | | |
| TI-11a/b/d | D4-0401 | Upper Extremity Strength (Elbow) | 568 | | | |
| TI-11a/b/d | D4-0401 | Upper Extremity Strength (Hand) | 569 | | | |
| TI-11a/b/d | D4-0401 | Upper Extremity Strength (Shoulder) | 570 | | | |
| TI-11a/b/d | D4-0401 | Upper Extremity Strength (Wrist) | 571 | | | |
| **NATA EC 5th** | **BOC RD6** | **Proprioceptive Neuromuscular Facilitation—Stretching** | **Page #** | | | |
| TI-11a/b/d | D4-0401 | PNF: Contract/Relax (Wrist Flexors) | 572 | | | |
| TI-11a/b/d | D4-0401 | PNF: Contract/Relax (Hip Extensors/Hamstrings) | 574 | | | |
| TI-11a/b/d | D4-0401 | PNF: Hold/Relax (Wrist Flexors) | 576 | | | |
| TI-11a/b/d | D4-0401 | PNF: Hold/Relax (Hip Extensors/Hamstrings) | 578 | | | |
| TI-11a/b/d | D4-0401 | PNF: Slow-Reversal-Hold-Relax (Wrist Flexors) | 580 | | | |
| TI-11a/b/d | D4-0401 | PNF: Slow-Reversal-Hold-Relax (Hip Extensors/Hamstrings) | 582 | | | |
| **NATA EC 5th** | **BOC RD6** | **Proprioceptive Neuromuscular Facilitation—Strengthening** | **Page #** | | | |
| TI-11a/b/d | D4-0401 | PNF: Rhythmic Initiation (Elbow Flexors) | 584 | | | |
| TI-11a/b/d | D4-0401 | PNF: Rhythmic Initiation (Ankle Dorsiflexors) | 586 | | | |
| TI-11a/b/d | D4-0401 | PNF: Repeated Contraction (Ankle Dorsiflexors) | 588 | | | |
| TI-11a/b/d | D4-0401 | PNF: Slow Reversal (Lower Extremity D1 Flexion) | 590 | | | |
| TI-11a/b/d | D4-0401 | PNF: Slow Reversal (Lower Extremity D1 Extension) | 592 | | | |
| TI-11a/b/d | D4-0401 | PNF: Slow Reversal (Lower Extremity D2 Flexion) | 594 | | | |
| TI-11a/b/d | D4-0401 | PNF: Slow Reversal (Lower Extremity D2 Extension) | 596 | | | |
| TI-11a/b/d | D4-0401 | PNF: Slow Reversal (Upper Extremity D1 Flexion) | 598 | | | |
| TI-11a/b/d | D4-0401 | PNF: Slow Reversal (Upper Extremity D1 Extension) | 600 | | | |
| TI-11a/b/d | D4-0401 | PNF: Slow Reversal (Upper Extremity D2 Flexion) | 602 | | | |
| TI-11a/b/d | D4-0401 | PNF: Slow Reversal (Upper Extremity D2 Extension) | 604 | | | |
| **NATA EC 5th** | **BOC RD6** | **Joint Mobilizations—Oscillatory** | **Page #** | | | |
| TI-15 | D4-0401 | Joint Mobs: Grade 1 Oscillatory (Tibiofemoral Extension) | 606 | | | |
| TI-15 | D4-0401 | Joint Mobs: Grade 2 Oscillatory (Tibiofemoral Extension) | 608 | | | |
| TI-15 | D4-0401 | Joint Mobs: Grade 3 Oscillatory (Tibiofemoral Extension) | 610 | | | |
| TI-15 | D4-0401 | Joint Mobs: Grade 4 Oscillatory (Tibiofemoral Extension) | 612 | | | |
| TI-15 | D4-0401 | Joint Mobs: Grade 1 Oscillatory (Glenohumeral Abduction) | 614 | | | |
| TI-15 | D4-0401 | Joint Mobs: Grade 2 Oscillatory (Glenohumeral Abduction) | 616 | | | |
| TI-15 | D4-0401 | Joint Mobs: Grade 3 Oscillatory (Glenohumeral Abduction) | 618 | | | |
| TI-15 | D4-0401 | Joint Mobs: Grade 4 Oscillatory (Glenohumeral Abduction) | 620 | | | |

*(continued on the next page)*

## THERAPEUTIC INTERVENTIONS
# KNOWLEDGE AND SKILLS

| NATA EC 5th | BOC RD6 | Joint Mobilizations—Sustained | Page # | | | |
|---|---|---|---|---|---|---|
| TI-15 | D4-0401 | Joint Mobs: Grade 1 Sustained (Tibiofemoral Flexion) | 622 | | | |
| TI-15 | D4-0401 | Joint Mobs: Grade 2 Sustained (Tibiofemoral Flexion) | 624 | | | |
| TI-15 | D4-0401 | Joint Mobs: Grade 3 Sustained (Tibiofemoral Flexion) | 626 | | | |
| TI-15 | D4-0401 | Joint Mobs: Grade 1 Sustained (Glenohumeral Joint) | 628 | | | |
| TI-15 | D4-0401 | Joint Mobs: Grade 2 Sustained (Glenohumeral Joint) | 630 | | | |
| TI-15 | D4-0401 | Joint Mobs: Grade 3 Sustained (Glenohumcral Joint) | 632 | | | |

THERAPEUTIC INTERVENTIONS
# THERAPEUTIC MODALITIES—SELF-TREATMENT

| NATA EC 5th | BOC RD6 | SKILL |
|---|---|---|
| TI-10 | D4-0401 | Self-Stretching |

**Supplies Needed:** Table, towel

*This problem allows you the opportunity to instruct a patient to* **self-stretch** *the* **gastrocnemius muscle***. You have 3 minutes to complete this task.*

| Self-Stretching | Course or Site Assessor Environment | | Test 1 | | Test 2 | | Test 3 | |
|---|---|---|---|---|---|---|---|---|
| | | | Y | N | Y | N | Y | N |
| **Purpose of treatment** | | | Y | N | Y | N | Y | N |
| Increase flexibility | | | O | O | O | O | O | O |
| **Patient education/safety** | | | Y | N | Y | N | Y | N |
| Explains to the patient why this modality is appropriate | | | O | O | O | O | O | O |
| Explains to the patient what the expected treatment goals and outcomes are | | | O | O | O | O | O | O |
| Explains to the patient what he/she should or should not feel | | | O | O | O | O | O | O |
| Reviews precautions/contraindications with the patient | | | O | O | O | O | O | O |
| **Tester places patient in appropriate position** | | | Y | N | Y | N | Y | N |
| Supine | | | O | O | O | O | O | O |
| Wraps towel around ankle | | | O | O | O | O | O | O |
| **Tester administers the therapeutic modality according to accepted guidelines** | | | Y | N | Y | N | Y | N |
| Instructs the patient to hold both ends of towel firmly | | | O | O | O | O | O | O |
| The patient pulls both ends of the towel, moving the ankle into dorsiflexion, and stops once a stretch is felt | | | O | O | O | O | O | O |
| Holds for 30 seconds | | | O | O | O | O | O | O |
| Repeats three times | | | O | O | O | O | O | O |
| **Termination of treatment** | | | Y | N | Y | N | Y | N |
| Inspects treatment area | | | O | O | O | O | O | O |
| Provides the patient with feedback | | | O | O | O | O | O | O |
| Documents the treatment | | | O | O | O | O | O | O |
| **Total** | | | ___/14 | | ___/14 | | ___/14 | |

*(continued on the next page)*

| Must achieve >9 to pass this examination | Ⓟ | Ⓕ | Ⓟ | Ⓕ | Ⓟ | Ⓕ |
|---|---|---|---|---|---|---|
| **Assessor:**<br>**Date:** | **Test 1 Comments:** | | | | | |
| **Assessor:**<br>**Date:** | **Test 2 Comments:** | | | | | |
| **Assessor:**<br>**Date:** | **Test 3 Comments:** | | | | | |

## TEST ENVIRONMENTS
**L:** Laboratory/Classroom
**C:** Clinical/Field Testing
**P:** Practicum
**A:** Assessment/Mock Exam

## TEST INFORMATION
**Test Statistics:** N/A
**Reference(s):**   Starkey & Brown (2015)

# THERAPEUTIC MODALITIES—ACOUSTIC ENERGY

| NATA EC 5th | BOC RD6 | SKILL |
|---|---|---|
| TI-11a/b/c/e/f | D4-0402 | Phonophoresis |

**Supplies Needed:** Table, medication, ultrasound unit, gel

*This problem allows you the opportunity to use a* **phonophoresis treatment** *for the* **lateral epicondyle.**
*You have 3 minutes to complete this task.*

| Phonophoresis | Course or Site Assessor Environment | | Test 1 | | Test 2 | | Test 3 | |
|---|---|---|---|---|---|---|---|---|
| **Purpose of treatment** | | **Y** | **N** | **Y** | **N** | **Y** | **N** | |
| Allows medication to be absorbed into the involved area | | ○ | ○ | ○ | ○ | ○ | ○ | |
| **Patient education/safety** | | **Y** | **N** | **Y** | **N** | **Y** | **N** | |
| Explains to the patient why this modality is appropriate | | ○ | ○ | ○ | ○ | ○ | ○ | |
| Explains to the patient what the expected treatment goals and outcomes are | | ○ | ○ | ○ | ○ | ○ | ○ | |
| Explains to the patient what he/she should or should not feel | | ○ | ○ | ○ | ○ | ○ | ○ | |
| Reviews precautions/contraindications with the patient | | ○ | ○ | ○ | ○ | ○ | ○ | |
| Identifies the beam nonuniformity ratio and effective radiating area | | ○ | ○ | ○ | ○ | ○ | ○ | |
| **Tester places patient in appropriate position** | | **Y** | **N** | **Y** | **N** | **Y** | **N** | |
| Seated | | ○ | ○ | ○ | ○ | ○ | ○ | |
| **Tester administers the therapeutic modality according to accepted guidelines** | | **Y** | **N** | **Y** | **N** | **Y** | **N** | |
| Applies the appropriate amount of medication to the skin | | ○ | ○ | ○ | ○ | ○ | ○ | |
| Using the transducer, applies firm overlapping circular strokes with constant pressure | | ○ | ○ | ○ | ○ | ○ | ○ | |
| Treatment is consistent with the intended goals | | ○ | ○ | ○ | ○ | ○ | ○ | |
| Intensity | | ○ | ○ | ○ | ○ | ○ | ○ | |
| Frequency | | ○ | ○ | ○ | ○ | ○ | ○ | |
| Treatment duration | | ○ | ○ | ○ | ○ | ○ | ○ | |
| Duty cycle | | ○ | ○ | ○ | ○ | ○ | ○ | |
| **Termination of treatment** | | **Y** | **N** | **Y** | **N** | **Y** | **N** | |
| Inspects treatment area | | ○ | ○ | ○ | ○ | ○ | ○ | |
| Provides the patient with feedback | | ○ | ○ | ○ | ○ | ○ | ○ | |
| Documents the treatment | | ○ | ○ | ○ | ○ | ○ | ○ | |
| **Total** | | \_\_\_\_/17 | | \_\_\_\_/17 | | \_\_\_\_/17 | | |

*(continued on the next page)*

| | Must achieve >11 to pass this examination | Ⓟ | Ⓕ | Ⓟ | Ⓕ | Ⓟ | Ⓕ |
|---|---|---|---|---|---|---|---|
| **Assessor:**<br>**Date:** | **Test 1 Comments:** | | | | | | |
| **Assessor:**<br>**Date:** | **Test 2 Comments:** | | | | | | |
| **Assessor:**<br>**Date:** | **Test 3 Comments:** | | | | | | |

**TEST ENVIRONMENTS**
**L:** Laboratory/Classroom
**C:** Clinical/Field Testing
**P:** Practicum
**A:** Assessment/Mock Exam

**TEST INFORMATION**
**Test Statistics:** N/A
**Reference(s):**   Starkey & Brown (2015)

## THERAPEUTIC INTERVENTIONS
# THERAPEUTIC MODALITIES—ACOUSTIC ENERGY

| NATA EC 5th | BOC RD6 | SKILL |
|---|---|---|
| TI-11a/b/c/e/f | D4-0402 | Therapeutic Ultrasound 1 MHz |

**Supplies Needed:** Table, bolster, drape, ultrasound unit, gel

*This problem allows you the opportunity to use* **therapeutic ultrasound** *to heat the* **tibialis posterior tendon 1°C to 2°C.** *You have 3 minutes to complete this task.*

| Therapeutic Ultrasound 1 MHz | Course or Site / Assessor / Environment | | Test 1 | | Test 2 | | Test 3 | |
|---|---|---|---|---|---|---|---|---|
| **Purpose of treatment** | | Y | N | Y | N | Y | N |
| Increase the temperature of the skin | | O | O | O | O | O | O |
| **Patient education/safety** | | Y | N | Y | N | Y | N |
| Explains to the patient why this modality is appropriate | | O | O | O | O | O | O |
| Explains to the patient what the expected treatment goals and outcomes are | | O | O | O | O | O | O |
| Explains to the patient what he/she should or should not feel | | O | O | O | O | O | O |
| Reviews precautions/contraindications with the patient | | O | O | O | O | O | O |
| Explains the beam nonuniformity ratio and effective radiating area | | O | O | O | O | O | O |
| **Tester places patient in appropriate position** | | Y | N | Y | N | Y | N |
| Supine | | O | O | O | O | O | O |
| Places bolster under the patient's knees | | O | O | O | O | O | O |
| Drapes the patient for modesty and exposes the area | | O | O | O | O | O | O |
| **Tester administers the therapeutic modality according to accepted guidelines** | | Y | N | Y | N | Y | N |
| Applies appropriate transmission gel | | O | O | O | O | O | O |
| Applies the appropriate-sized transducer head firmly over the area | | O | O | O | O | O | O |
| Moves in circulating strokes | | O | O | O | O | O | O |
| Treatment parameters are consistent with the intended goals | | O | O | O | O | O | O |
| Intensity | | O | O | O | O | O | O |
| Frequency | | O | O | O | O | O | O |
| Treatment duration | | O | O | O | O | O | O |
| Duty cycle | | O | O | O | O | O | O |
| **Termination of treatment** | | Y | N | Y | N | Y | N |
| Inspects treatment area | | O | O | O | O | O | O |
| Provides the patient with feedback | | O | O | O | O | O | O |
| Documents the treatment | | O | O | O | O | O | O |
| **Total** | | /20 | | /20 | | /20 | |

(continued on the next page)

| Must achieve >13 to pass this examination | P | F | P | F | P | F |
|---|---|---|---|---|---|---|
| **Assessor:**<br>**Date:** | **Test 1 Comments:** | | | | | |
| **Assessor:**<br>**Date:** | **Test 2 Comments:** | | | | | |
| **Assessor:**<br>**Date:** | **Test 3 Comments:** | | | | | |

**TEST ENVIRONMENTS**
**L:** Laboratory/Classroom
**C:** Clinical/Field Testing
**P:** Practicum
**A:** Assessment/Mock Exam

**TEST INFORMATION**
**Test Statistics:** N/A
**Reference(s):**  Amato et al. (2006)
Starkey & Brown (2015)

# THERAPEUTIC MODALITIES—ACOUSTIC ENERGY

| NATA EC 5th | BOC RD6 | SKILL |
|---|---|---|
| TI-11a/b/c/e/f | D4-0402 | Therapeutic Ultrasound 3 MHz |

**Supplies Needed:** Table, bolster, drape, ultrasound unit, gel

*This problem allows you the opportunity to use* **therapeutic ultrasound** *to heat the* **patellar tendon 3°C to 4°C**. *You have 3 minutes to initiate this task.*

| Therapeutic Ultrasound 3 MHz | Course or Site Assessor Environment | | Test 1 | | Test 2 | | Test 3 | |
|---|---|---|---|---|---|---|---|---|
| **Purpose of treatment** | | **Y** | **N** | **Y** | **N** | **Y** | **N** | |
| Increase the temperature of the skin | | O | O | O | O | O | O | |
| **Patient education/safety** | | **Y** | **N** | **Y** | **N** | **Y** | **N** | |
| Explains to the patient why this modality is appropriate | | O | O | O | O | O | O | |
| Explains to the patient what the expected treatment goals and outcomes are | | O | O | O | O | O | O | |
| Explains to the patient what he/she should or should not feel | | O | O | O | O | O | O | |
| Reviews precautions/contraindications with the patient | | O | O | O | O | O | O | |
| Explains the beam nonuniformity ratio and effective radiating area | | O | O | O | O | O | O | |
| **Tester places patient in appropriate position** | | **Y** | **N** | **Y** | **N** | **Y** | **N** | |
| Supine | | O | O | O | O | O | O | |
| Places bolster under the patient's knees | | O | O | O | O | O | O | |
| Drapes the patient for modesty and exposes the area | | O | O | O | O | O | O | |
| **Tester administers the therapeutic modality according to accepted guidelines** | | **Y** | **N** | **Y** | **N** | **Y** | **N** | |
| Applies appropriate transmission gel | | O | O | O | O | O | O | |
| Applies the transducer head firmly over the area | | O | O | O | O | O | O | |
| Moves in circulating strokes | | O | O | O | O | O | O | |
| Treatment parameters are consistent with the intended goals | | O | O | O | O | O | O | |
| Intensity | | O | O | O | O | O | O | |
| Frequency | | O | O | O | O | O | O | |
| Treatment duration | | O | O | O | O | O | O | |
| Duty cycle | | O | O | O | O | O | O | |
| **Termination of treatment** | | **Y** | **N** | **Y** | **N** | **Y** | **N** | |
| Inspects treatment area | | O | O | O | O | O | O | |
| Provides the patient with feedback | | O | O | O | O | O | O | |
| Documents the treatment | | O | O | O | O | O | O | |
| **Total** | | ___/20 | | ___/20 | | ___/20 | | |

*(continued on the next page)*

| Must achieve >13 to pass this examination | Ⓟ | Ⓕ | Ⓟ | Ⓕ | Ⓟ | Ⓕ |
|---|---|---|---|---|---|---|
| **Assessor:**<br>**Date:** | **Test 1 Comments:** | | | | | |
| **Assessor:**<br>**Date:** | **Test 2 Comments:** | | | | | |
| **Assessor:**<br>**Date:** | **Test 3 Comments:** | | | | | |

**TEST ENVIRONMENTS**
**L:**  Laboratory/Classroom
**C:**  Clinical/Field Testing
**P:**  Practicum
**A:**  Assessment/Mock Exam

**TEST INFORMATION**
**Test Statistics:**  N/A
**Reference(s):**    Amato et al. (2006)
                     Starkey & Brown (2015)

## THERAPEUTIC INTERVENTIONS
# THERAPEUTIC MODALITIES—ACOUSTIC ENERGY

| NATA EC 5th | BOC RD6 | SKILL |
|---|---|---|
| TI-11a/b/c/e/f | D4-0402 | Therapeutic Ultrasound Immersion |

**Supplies Needed:** Table, immersion tub, ultrasound unit

*This problem allows you the opportunity to use* **therapeutic ultrasound immersion** *technique to* **decrease swelling** *in a* **lateral ankle sprain**. *You have 3 minutes to initiate this task.*

| Therapeutic Ultrasound Immersion | Course or Site Assessor Environment | Test 1 Y | Test 1 N | Test 2 Y | Test 2 N | Test 3 Y | Test 3 N |
|---|---|---|---|---|---|---|---|
| **Purpose of treatment** | | **Y** | **N** | **Y** | **N** | **Y** | **N** |
| Treat chronic inflammation and pain | | O | O | O | O | O | O |
| **Patient education/safety** | | **Y** | **N** | **Y** | **N** | **Y** | **N** |
| Explains to the patient why this modality is appropriate | | O | O | O | O | O | O |
| Explains to the patient what the expected treatment goals and outcomes are | | O | O | O | O | O | O |
| Explains to the patient what he/she should or should not feel | | O | O | O | O | O | O |
| Reviews precautions/contraindications with the patient | | O | O | O | O | O | O |
| Explains the beam nonuniformity ratio and effective radiating area | | O | O | O | O | O | O |
| **Tester places patient in appropriate position** | | **Y** | **N** | **Y** | **N** | **Y** | **N** |
| Seated | | O | O | O | O | O | O |
| Places ankle in a ceramic or metal tub filled with warm water | | O | O | O | O | O | O |
| **Tester administers the therapeutic modality according to accepted guidelines** | | **Y** | **N** | **Y** | **N** | **Y** | **N** |
| Places transducer in water | | O | O | O | O | O | O |
| Places transducer head 1 inch away from the ankle | | O | O | O | O | O | O |
| Does not submerge hand in water | | O | O | O | O | O | O |
| Treatment parameters are consistent with the intended goals | | O | O | O | O | O | O |
| Intensity | | O | O | O | O | O | O |
| Frequency | | O | O | O | O | O | O |
| Treatment duration | | O | O | O | O | O | O |
| **Termination of treatment** | | **Y** | **N** | **Y** | **N** | **Y** | **N** |
| Inspects treatment area | | O | O | O | O | O | O |
| Provides the patient with feedback | | O | O | O | O | O | O |
| Documents the treatment | | O | O | O | O | O | O |
| **Total** | | /18 | | /18 | | /18 | |

*(continued on the next page)*

| Must achieve >12 to pass this examination | Ⓟ | Ⓕ | Ⓟ | Ⓕ | Ⓟ | Ⓕ |
|---|---|---|---|---|---|---|
| **Assessor:**<br>**Date:** | **Test 1 Comments:** | | | | | |
| **Assessor:**<br>**Date:** | **Test 2 Comments:** | | | | | |
| **Assessor:**<br>**Date:** | **Test 3 Comments:** | | | | | |

**TEST ENVIRONMENTS**
**L:** Laboratory/Classroom
**C:** Clinical/Field Testing
**P:** Practicum
**A:** Assessment/Mock Exam

**TEST INFORMATION**
**Test Statistics:** N/A
**Reference(s):** Starkey & Brown (2015)

# THERAPEUTIC MODALITIES—CRYOTHERAPY

| NATA EC 5th | BOC RD6 | SKILL |
|---|---|---|
| TI-11a/b/c/e/f | D4-0402 | Contrast Bath |

**Supplies Needed:** Whirlpool

*This problem allows you the opportunity to use a **contrast bath** for **a subacute injury**. Your scenario is a sport-related subacute injury to the lower leg. You have 3 minutes to initiate this task.*

| Contrast Bath | Course or Site Assessor Environment | | Test 1 | | Test 2 | | Test 3 |
|---|---|---|---|---|---|---|---|
| **Purpose of treatment** | | Y | N | Y | N | Y | N |
| Decrease ecchymosis and pain | | O | O | O | O | O | O |
| **Patient education/safety** | | Y | N | Y | N | Y | N |
| Explains to the patient why this modality is appropriate | | O | O | O | O | O | O |
| Explains to the patient what the expected treatment goals and outcomes are | | O | O | O | O | O | O |
| Explains to the patient what he/she should or should not feel | | O | O | O | O | O | O |
| Reviews precautions/contraindications with the patient | | O | O | O | O | O | O |
| Prior to set up of the modality, checks all aspects for safety | | O | O | O | O | O | O |
| **Tester places patient in appropriate position** | | Y | N | Y | N | Y | N |
| Seated | | O | O | O | O | O | O |
| Contrast tubs are as close to each other as possible | | O | O | O | O | O | O |
| **Tester administers the therapeutic modality according to accepted guidelines** | | Y | N | Y | N | Y | N |
| Begins with immersing the involved limb into the hot whirlpool for 3 to 4 minutes | | O | O | O | O | O | O |
| Immediately follows by placing the involved limb into the cold whirlpool for 1 minute | | O | O | O | O | O | O |
| Repeats the cycle four times | | O | O | O | O | O | O |
| Turns turbines on prior to the patient getting into whirlpool | | O | O | O | O | O | O |
| Turns off turbines once the patient is out of the water | | O | O | O | O | O | O |
| **Termination of treatment** | | Y | N | Y | N | Y | N |
| Inspects treatment area | | O | O | O | O | O | O |
| Provides the patient with feedback | | O | O | O | O | O | O |
| Documents the treatment | | O | O | O | O | O | O |
| **Total** | | \_\_\_\_/16 | | \_\_\_\_/16 | | \_\_\_\_/16 | |

*(continued on the next page)*

| Must achieve >11 to pass this examination | Ⓟ | Ⓕ | Ⓟ | Ⓕ | Ⓟ | Ⓕ |
|---|---|---|---|---|---|---|
| **Assessor:**<br>**Date:** | **Test 1 Comments:** | | | | | |
| **Assessor:**<br>**Date:** | **Test 2 Comments:** | | | | | |
| **Assessor:**<br>**Date:** | **Test 3 Comments:** | | | | | |

## TEST ENVIRONMENTS
**L:** Laboratory/Classroom
**C:** Clinical/Field Testing
**P:** Practicum
**A:** Assessment/Mock Exam

## TEST INFORMATION
**Test Statistics:** N/A
**Reference(s):** Starkey & Brown (2015)

## THERAPEUTIC INTERVENTIONS
# THERAPEUTIC MODALITIES—CRYOTHERAPY

| NATA EC 5th | BOC RD6 | SKILL |
|---|---|---|
| TI-11a/b/c/e/f | D4-0402 | Cold Whirlpool |

**Supplies Needed:** Whirlpool

*This problem allows you the opportunity to use a **cold whirlpool** for an **acute ankle injury**.
Your scenario is a sport-related acute injury to the ankle/lower leg. You have 3 minutes to initiate this task.*

| Cold Whirlpool | Course or Site Assessor Environment | | Test 1 | | Test 2 | | Test 3 | |
|---|---|---|---|---|---|---|---|---|
| **Purpose of treatment** | | **Y** | **N** | **Y** | **N** | **Y** | **N** | |
| Application of cold to irregularly shaped body parts | | O | O | O | O | O | O | |
| **Patient education/safety** | | **Y** | **N** | **Y** | **N** | **Y** | **N** | |
| Explains to the patient why the modality is appropriate | | O | O | O | O | O | O | |
| Explains to the patient what the expected treatment goals and outcomes are | | O | O | O | O | O | O | |
| Explains to the patient what he/she should or should not feel | | O | O | O | O | O | O | |
| Reviews precautions/contraindications with the patient | | O | O | O | O | O | O | |
| Prior to set up of the modality, checks all aspects for safety | | O | O | O | O | O | O | |
| **Tester places patient in appropriate position** | | **Y** | **N** | **Y** | **N** | **Y** | **N** | |
| Seated safely with the involved limb immersed in whirlpool | | O | O | O | O | O | O | |
| **Tester administers the therapeutic modality according to accepted guidelines** | | **Y** | **N** | **Y** | **N** | **Y** | **N** | |
| Water depth is enough to cover the involved limb | | O | O | O | O | O | O | |
| Water temperature is appropriate for the nature of the injury | | O | O | O | O | O | O | |
| Turns turbines on prior to the patient getting into whirlpool | | O | O | O | O | O | O | |
| Checks the patient throughout treatment | | O | O | O | O | O | O | |
| Turns off turbines once the patient is out of the water | | O | O | O | O | O | O | |
| **Termination of treatment** | | **Y** | **N** | **Y** | **N** | **Y** | **N** | |
| Inspects treatment area | | O | O | O | O | O | O | |
| Provides the patient with feedback | | O | O | O | O | O | O | |
| Documents the treatment | | O | O | O | O | O | O | |
| **Total** | | ___/15 | | ___/15 | | ___/15 | | |

*(continued on the next page)*

| Must achieve >10 to pass this examination | Ⓟ | Ⓕ | Ⓟ | Ⓕ | Ⓟ | Ⓕ |
|---|---|---|---|---|---|---|
| **Assessor:**<br>**Date:** | **Test 1 Comments:** | | | | | |
| **Assessor:**<br>**Date:** | **Test 2 Comments:** | | | | | |
| **Assessor:**<br>**Date:** | **Test 3 Comments:** | | | | | |

**TEST ENVIRONMENTS**
**L:** Laboratory/Classroom
**C:** Clinical/Field Testing
**P:** Practicum
**A:** Assessment/Mock Exam

**TEST INFORMATION**
**Test Statistics:** N/A
**Reference(s):**   Amato et al. (2006)
Starkey & Brown (2015)

THERAPEUTIC INTERVENTIONS
# THERAPEUTIC MODALITIES—CRYOTHERAPY

| NATA EC 5th | BOC RD6 | SKILL |
|---|---|---|
| TI-11a/b/c/e/f | D4-0402 | Ice Bag |

**Supplies Needed:** Table, bag of ice, plastic or elastic wrap

*This problem allows you the opportunity to use an* **ice bag** *to* **limit inflammation** *in an* **acute lateral ankle sprain**. *You have 3 minutes to complete this task.*

| Ice Bag | Course or Site<br>Assessor<br>Environment | | Test 1 | | Test 2 | | Test 3 | |
|---|---|---|---|---|---|---|---|---|
| | | | Y | N | Y | N | Y | N |
| **Purpose of treatment** | | | Y | N | Y | N | Y | N |
| Limit inflammation and swelling | | | O | O | O | O | O | O |
| **Patient education/safety** | | | Y | N | Y | N | Y | N |
| Explains to the patient why this modality is appropriate | | | O | O | O | O | O | O |
| Explains to the patient what the expected treatment goals and outcomes are | | | O | O | O | O | O | O |
| Explains to the patient what he/she should or should not feel | | | O | O | O | O | O | O |
| Reviews precautions/contraindications with the patient | | | O | O | O | O | O | O |
| **Tester places patient in appropriate position** | | | Y | N | Y | N | Y | N |
| Supine | | | O | O | O | O | O | O |
| Ankle elevated above the level of the heart | | | O | O | O | O | O | O |
| **Tester administers the therapeutic modality according to accepted guidelines** | | | Y | N | Y | N | Y | N |
| Places appropriate amount of ice in the bag | | | O | O | O | O | O | O |
| Places the ice bag directly over the injured area | | | O | O | O | O | O | O |
| Secures the ice bag in place with a plastic or elastic wrap | | | O | O | O | O | O | O |
| Checks on the patient throughout treatment | | | O | O | O | O | O | O |
| **Termination of treatment** | | | Y | N | Y | N | Y | N |
| Treatment is terminated within an appropriate timeframe | | | O | O | O | O | O | O |
| Inspects treatment area | | | O | O | O | O | O | O |
| Provides the patient with feedback | | | O | O | O | O | O | O |
| Documents the treatment | | | O | O | O | O | O | O |
| Total | | | ___ /15 | | ___ /15 | | ___ /15 | |
| Must achieve >10 to pass this examination | | | (P) | (F) | (P) | (F) | (P) | (F) |

| Assessor:<br>Date: | Test 1 Comments: |
|---|---|
| Assessor:<br>Date: | Test 2 Comments: |
| Assessor:<br>Date: | Test 3 Comments: |

**TEST ENVIRONMENTS**
**L:** Laboratory/Classroom
**C:** Clinical/Field Testing
**P:** Practicum
**A:** Assessment/Mock Exam

**TEST INFORMATION**
**Test Statistics:** N/A
**Reference(s):**   Amato et al. (2006)
                    Starkey & Brown (2015)

# THERAPEUTIC MODALITIES—CRYOTHERAPY

| NATA EC 5th | BOC RD6 | SKILL |
|---|---|---|
| TI-11a/b/c/e/f | D4-0402 | Ice Massage |

**Supplies Needed:** Table, towels, ice cup

*This problem allows you the opportunity to use* **ice massage** *to treat* **chronic inflammation** *of the* **anterior lower leg**. *You have 3 minutes to complete this task.*

| Ice Massage | Course or Site Assessor Environment | | Test 1 | | Test 2 | | Test 3 | |
|---|---|---|---|---|---|---|---|---|
| **Purpose of treatment** | | Y | N | Y | N | Y | N |
| Decrease pain and inflammation | | ○ | ○ | ○ | ○ | ○ | ○ |
| **Patient education/safety** | | Y | N | Y | N | Y | N |
| Explains to the patient why this modality is appropriate | | ○ | ○ | ○ | ○ | ○ | ○ |
| Explains to the patient what the expected treatment goals and outcomes are | | ○ | ○ | ○ | ○ | ○ | ○ |
| Explains to the patient what he/she should or should not feel | | ○ | ○ | ○ | ○ | ○ | ○ |
| Reviews precautions/contraindications with the patient | | ○ | ○ | ○ | ○ | ○ | ○ |
| Prior to set up of the modality, checks all aspects for safety | | ○ | ○ | ○ | ○ | ○ | ○ |
| **Tester places patient in appropriate position** | | Y | N | Y | N | Y | N |
| Seated | | ○ | ○ | ○ | ○ | ○ | ○ |
| Surrounds area with towels | | ○ | ○ | ○ | ○ | ○ | ○ |
| **Tester administers the therapeutic modality according to accepted guidelines** | | Y | N | Y | N | Y | N |
| Slowly moves ice over the treatment area | | ○ | ○ | ○ | ○ | ○ | ○ |
| Uses overlapping strokes | | ○ | ○ | ○ | ○ | ○ | ○ |
| Gradually increases the pressure of the strokes | | ○ | ○ | ○ | ○ | ○ | ○ |
| Removes paper from the cup as the ice melts | | ○ | ○ | ○ | ○ | ○ | ○ |
| **Termination of treatment** | | Y | N | Y | N | Y | N |
| Inspects treatment area | | ○ | ○ | ○ | ○ | ○ | ○ |
| Provides the patient with feedback | | ○ | ○ | ○ | ○ | ○ | ○ |
| Documents the treatment | | ○ | ○ | ○ | ○ | ○ | ○ |
| Total | | /15 | | /15 | | /15 | |

*(continued on the next page)*

| Must achieve >10 to pass this examination | Ⓟ | Ⓕ | Ⓟ | Ⓕ | Ⓟ | Ⓕ |
|---|---|---|---|---|---|---|
| **Assessor:** <br> **Date:** | **Test 1 Comments:** | | | | | |
| **Assessor:** <br> **Date:** | **Test 2 Comments:** | | | | | |
| **Assessor:** <br> **Date:** | **Test 3 Comments:** | | | | | |

**TEST ENVIRONMENTS**
**L:** Laboratory/Classroom
**C:** Clinical/Field Testing
**P:** Practicum
**A:** Assessment/Mock Exam

**TEST INFORMATION**
**Test Statistics:** N/A
**Reference(s):**   Amato et al. (2006)
                    Starkey & Brown (2015)

**THERAPEUTIC INTERVENTIONS**
# THERAPEUTIC MODALITIES—CRYOTHERAPY

| NATA EC 5th | BOC RD6 | SKILL |
|---|---|---|
| TI-11a/b/c/e/f | D4-0402 | Vapo-Coolant Spray |

**Supplies Needed:** Table, vapo-coolant

*This problem allows you the opportunity to use* **vapo-coolant spray** *to* **decrease a hamstring spasm.** *You have 3 minutes to complete this task.*

| Vapo-Coolant Spray | Course or Site Assessor Environment | | Test 1 | | Test 2 | | Test 3 | |
|---|---|---|---|---|---|---|---|---|
| **Purpose of treatment** | | Y | N | Y | N | Y | N |
| Decrease muscle spasm | | ○ | ○ | ○ | ○ | ○ | ○ |
| **Patient education/safety** | | Y | N | Y | N | Y | N |
| Explains to the patient why this modality is appropriate | | ○ | ○ | ○ | ○ | ○ | ○ |
| Explains to the patient what the expected treatment goals and outcomes are | | ○ | ○ | ○ | ○ | ○ | ○ |
| Explains to the patient what he/she should or should not feel | | ○ | ○ | ○ | ○ | ○ | ○ |
| Reviews precautions/contraindications with the patient | | ○ | ○ | ○ | ○ | ○ | ○ |
| **Tester places patient in appropriate position** | | Y | N | Y | N | Y | N |
| Prone | | ○ | ○ | ○ | ○ | ○ | ○ |
| **Tester administers the therapeutic modality according to accepted guidelines** | | Y | N | Y | N | Y | N |
| Holds the container about 1 foot from the involved skin | | ○ | ○ | ○ | ○ | ○ | ○ |
| Delivers a mist of spray to the skin in a sweeping motion at about 4 inches per second | | ○ | ○ | ○ | ○ | ○ | ○ |
| Covers the treatment area | | ○ | ○ | ○ | ○ | ○ | ○ |
| **Termination of treatment** | | Y | N | Y | N | Y | N |
| Inspects treatment area | | ○ | ○ | ○ | ○ | ○ | ○ |
| Provides the patient with feedback | | ○ | ○ | ○ | ○ | ○ | ○ |
| Documents the treatment | | ○ | ○ | ○ | ○ | ○ | ○ |
| Total | | __/12 | | __/12 | | __/12 | |
| Must achieve >8 to pass this examination | | ℗ | Ⓕ | ℗ | Ⓕ | ℗ | Ⓕ |

| Assessor: Date: | Test 1 Comments: |
|---|---|
| Assessor: Date: | Test 2 Comments: |
| Assessor: Date: | Test 3 Comments: |

**TEST ENVIRONMENTS**
**L:** Laboratory/Classroom
**C:** Clinical/Field Testing
**P:** Practicum
**A:** Assessment/Mock Exam

**TEST INFORMATION**
**Test Statistics:** N/A
**Reference(s):** Amato et al. (2006)
Starkey & Brown (2015)

# THERAPEUTIC MODALITIES—ELECTRICAL ENERGY

| NATA EC 5th | BOC RD6 | SKILL |
|---|---|---|
| TI-11a/b/c/e/f | D4-0402 | Electrical Stimulation (Interferential) |

**Supplies Needed:** Table, bolster, drape, electrical stimulation unit

*This problem allows you the opportunity to use* **interferential electrical stimulation** *for* **pain modulation to the knee joint**. *You have 3 minutes to complete this task.*

| Electrical Stimulation (Inferential) | Course or Site Assessor Environment | Test 1 Y | Test 1 N | Test 2 Y | Test 2 N | Test 3 Y | Test 3 N |
|---|---|---|---|---|---|---|---|
| **Purpose of treatment** | | **Y** | **N** | **Y** | **N** | **Y** | **N** |
| Modulate pain | | O | O | O | O | O | O |
| **Patient education/safety** | | **Y** | **N** | **Y** | **N** | **Y** | **N** |
| Explains to the patient why this modality is appropriate | | O | O | O | O | O | O |
| Explains to the patient what the expected treatment goals and outcomes are | | O | O | O | O | O | O |
| Explains to the patient what he/she should or should not feel | | O | O | O | O | O | O |
| Reviews precautions/contraindications with the patient | | O | O | O | O | O | O |
| Prior to set up of the modality, checks all aspects for safety | | O | O | O | O | O | O |
| **Tester places patient in appropriate position** | | **Y** | **N** | **Y** | **N** | **Y** | **N** |
| Supine | | O | O | O | O | O | O |
| Places bolster under knee to provide a slight amount of flexion | | O | O | O | O | O | O |
| Drapes the patient modestly and exposes area to be treated | | O | O | O | O | O | O |
| **Tester administers the therapeutic modality according to accepted guidelines** | | **Y** | **N** | **Y** | **N** | **Y** | **N** |
| Places the electrodes appropriately around the painful area | | O | O | O | O | O | O |
| Turns the power on to start electrical stimulation unit | | O | O | O | O | O | O |
| Treatment parameters are consistent with intended goals | | O | O | O | O | O | O |
| Selects the proper application mode | | O | O | O | O | O | O |
| Adjusts the frequency | | O | O | O | O | O | O |
| Adjusts the sweep frequency | | O | O | O | O | O | O |
| Adjusts the duration of treatment | | O | O | O | O | O | O |
| Adjusts the intensity to the appropriate current level | | O | O | O | O | O | O |
| Presses start button once parameters are set | | O | O | O | O | O | O |
| **Termination of treatment** | | **Y** | **N** | **Y** | **N** | **Y** | **N** |
| Inspects treatment area | | O | O | O | O | O | O |
| Provides the patient with feedback | | O | O | O | O | O | O |
| Documents the treatment | | O | O | O | O | O | O |
| **Total** | | \_\_\_/21 | | \_\_\_/21 | | \_\_\_/21 | |

*(continued on the next page)*

| Must achieve >14 to pass this examination | Ⓟ | Ⓕ | Ⓟ | Ⓕ | Ⓟ | Ⓕ |
|---|---|---|---|---|---|---|
| **Assessor:**<br>**Date:** | **Test 1 Comments:** | | | | | |
| **Assessor:**<br>**Date:** | **Test 2 Comments:** | | | | | |
| **Assessor:**<br>**Date:** | **Test 3 Comments:** | | | | | |

**TEST ENVIRONMENTS**
**L:** Laboratory/Classroom
**C:** Clinical/Field Testing
**P:** Practicum
**A:** Assessment/Mock Exam

**TEST INFORMATION**
**Test Statistics:** N/A
**Reference(s):** Amato et al. (2006)
Starkey & Brown (2015)

THERAPEUTIC INTERVENTIONS
# THERAPEUTIC MODALITIES—ELECTRICAL ENERGY

| NATA EC 5th | BOC RD6 | SKILL |
|---|---|---|
| TI-11a/b/c/e/f | D4-0402 | Electrical Stimulation (Low-Intensity Microcurrent) |

**Supplies Needed:** Table, bolster, pillow, electrical stimulation unit, saline solution

*This problem allows you the opportunity to use* **microcurrent electrical stimulation** *for pain modulation of an* **acute sacroiliac joint** *injury. You have 3 minutes to complete this task.*

| Electrical Stimulation (Low-Intensity Microcurrent) | Course or Site Assessor Environment | | Test 1 | | Test 2 | | Test 3 | |
|---|---|---|---|---|---|---|---|---|
| | | **Y** | **N** | **Y** | **N** | **Y** | **N** | |
| **Purpose of treatment** | | **Y** | **N** | **Y** | **N** | **Y** | **N** |
| Treat acute inflammation | | O | O | O | O | O | O |
| **Patient education/safety** | | **Y** | **N** | **Y** | **N** | **Y** | **N** |
| Explains to the patient why this modality is appropriate | | O | O | O | O | O | O |
| Explains to the patient what the expected treatment goals and outcomes are | | O | O | O | O | O | O |
| Explains to the patient what he/she should or should not feel | | O | O | O | O | O | O |
| Reviews precautions/contraindications with the patient | | O | O | O | O | O | O |
| Prior to set up of the modality, checks all aspects for safety | | O | O | O | O | O | O |
| **Tester places patient in appropriate position** | | **Y** | **N** | **Y** | **N** | **Y** | **N** |
| Prone | | O | O | O | O | O | O |
| Places bolster under the ankles, pillow under the abdomen, and face cradle under the head | | O | O | O | O | O | O |
| **Tester administers the therapeutic modality according to accepted guidelines** | | **Y** | **N** | **Y** | **N** | **Y** | **N** |
| Selects and wets the appropriate electrodes with saline solution | | O | O | O | O | O | O |
| Places the electrodes appropriately in the painful area | | O | O | O | O | O | O |
| Treatment parameters are consistent with intended goals | | O | O | O | O | O | O |
| Selects the proper application mode | | O | O | O | O | O | O |
| Increases the output frequency | | O | O | O | O | O | O |
| Repositions the electrodes every 10 minutes (removes, rewets, repositions) | | O | O | O | O | O | O |
| **Termination of treatment** | | **Y** | **N** | **Y** | **N** | **Y** | **N** |
| Inspects treatment area | | O | O | O | O | O | O |
| Provides the patient with feedback | | O | O | O | O | O | O |
| Documents the treatment | | O | O | O | O | O | O |
| **Total** | | ___/17 | | ___/17 | | ___/17 | |

*(continued on the next page)*

| Must achieve >12 to pass this examination | P | F | P | F | P | F |
|---|---|---|---|---|---|---|
| **Assessor:**<br>**Date:** | **Test 1 Comments:** | | | | | |
| **Assessor:**<br>**Date:** | **Test 2 Comments:** | | | | | |
| **Assessor:**<br>**Date:** | **Test 3 Comments:** | | | | | |

## TEST ENVIRONMENTS
**L:** Laboratory/Classroom
**C:** Clinical/Field Testing
**P:** Practicum
**A:** Assessment/Mock Exam

## TEST INFORMATION
**Test Statistics:** N/A
**Reference(s):**     Amato et al. (2006)
                              Starkey & Brown (2015)

THERAPEUTIC INTERVENTIONS
# THERAPEUTIC MODALITIES—ELECTRICAL ENERGY

| NATA EC 5th | BOC RD6 | SKILL |
|---|---|---|
| TI-11a/b/c/e/f | D4-0402 | Electrical Stimulation (Iontophoresis) |

**Supplies Needed:** Table, iontophoresis unit, medication

*This problem allows you the opportunity to use* **iontophoresis to treat chronic inflammation** *of the* **subacromial bursa***. You have 3 minutes to initiate this task.*

| Electrical Stimulation (Iontophoresis) | Course or Site Assessor Environment | | Test 1 | | Test 2 | | Test 3 | |
|---|---|---|---|---|---|---|---|---|
| **Purpose of treatment** | | | **Y** | **N** | **Y** | **N** | **Y** | **N** |
| Treat chronic inflammation | | | O | O | O | O | O | O |
| **Patient education/safety** | | | **Y** | **N** | **Y** | **N** | **Y** | **N** |
| Explains to the patient why this modality is appropriate | | | O | O | O | O | O | O |
| Explains to the patient what the expected treatment goals and outcomes are | | | O | O | O | O | O | O |
| Explains to the patient what he/she should or should not feel | | | O | O | O | O | O | O |
| Reviews precautions/contraindications with the patient | | | O | O | O | O | O | O |
| Prior to set up of the modality, checks all aspects for safety | | | O | O | O | O | O | O |
| **Tester places patient in appropriate position** | | | **Y** | **N** | **Y** | **N** | **Y** | **N** |
| Seated | | | O | O | O | O | O | O |
| **Tester administers the therapeutic modality according to accepted guidelines** | | | **Y** | **N** | **Y** | **N** | **Y** | **N** |
| Cleans treatment area with alcohol wipes, shave area | | | O | O | O | O | O | O |
| Places the electrodes appropriately in the painful area | | | O | O | O | O | O | O |
| Fills the active electrode with the appropriate medication | | | O | O | O | O | O | O |
| Uses buffering solution to wet the return electrode | | | O | O | O | O | O | O |
| Places active electrode over the target area | | | O | O | O | O | O | O |
| Places the return electrode 4 to 6 inches away from target site | | | O | O | O | O | O | O |
| Turns the power on | | | O | O | O | O | O | O |
| Treatment parameters are consistent with intended goals | | | O | O | O | O | O | O |
| Sets the treatment duration | | | O | O | O | O | O | O |
| Selects the electrode polarity | | | O | O | O | O | O | O |
| Sets the treatment dosage (physician recommendation) | | | O | O | O | O | O | O |
| Adjusts the intensity to the appropriate level | | | O | O | O | O | O | O |
| **Termination of treatment** | | | **Y** | **N** | **Y** | **N** | **Y** | **N** |
| Inspects treatment area | | | O | O | O | O | O | O |
| Provides the patient with feedback | | | O | O | O | O | O | O |
| Documents the treatment | | | O | O | O | O | O | O |
| | **Total** | | ___/22 | | ___/22 | | ___/22 | |

*(continued on the next page)*

| Must achieve >15 to pass this examination | Ⓟ | Ⓕ | Ⓟ | Ⓕ | Ⓟ | Ⓕ |
|---|---|---|---|---|---|---|
| **Assessor:**<br>**Date:** | **Test 1 Comments:** | | | | | |
| **Assessor:**<br>**Date:** | **Test 2 Comments:** | | | | | |
| **Assessor:**<br>**Date:** | **Test 3 Comments:** | | | | | |

## TEST ENVIRONMENTS
**L:**  Laboratory/Classroom
**C:**  Clinical/Field Testing
**P:**  Practicum
**A:**  Assessment/Mock Exam

## TEST INFORMATION
**Test Statistics:** N/A
**Reference(s):**  Amato et al. (2006)
Starkey & Brown (2015)

THERAPEUTIC INTERVENTIONS
# THERAPEUTIC MODALITIES—MANUAL THERAPY

| NATA EC 5th | BOC RD6 | SKILL |
|---|---|---|
| TI-11a/b/c/e/f | D4-0402 | Intermittent Compression |

**Supplies Needed:** Table, compression unit, tape measure

*This problem allows you the opportunity to use* **intermittent compression** *to encourage* **venous return of swelling surrounding the knee**. *You have 3 minutes to initiate this task.*

| Intermittent Compression | Course or Site Assessor Environment | | Test 1 | | Test 2 | | Test 3 | |
|---|---|---|---|---|---|---|---|---|
| **Purpose of treatment** | | **Y** | **N** | **Y** | **N** | **Y** | **N** | |
| Encourage lymphatic/venous return | | ○ | ○ | ○ | ○ | ○ | ○ | |
| **Patient education/safety** | | **Y** | **N** | **Y** | **N** | **Y** | **N** | |
| Explains to the patient why this modality is appropriate | | ○ | ○ | ○ | ○ | ○ | ○ | |
| Explains to the patient what the expected treatment goals and outcomes are | | ○ | ○ | ○ | ○ | ○ | ○ | |
| Explains to the patient what he/she should or should not feel | | ○ | ○ | ○ | ○ | ○ | ○ | |
| Reviews precautions/contraindications with the patient | | ○ | ○ | ○ | ○ | ○ | ○ | |
| **Tester places patient in appropriate position** | | **Y** | **N** | **Y** | **N** | **Y** | **N** | |
| Supine | | ○ | ○ | ○ | ○ | ○ | ○ | |
| Elevates the involved limb | | ○ | ○ | ○ | ○ | ○ | ○ | |
| **Tester administers the therapeutic modality according to accepted guidelines** | | **Y** | **N** | **Y** | **N** | **Y** | **N** | |
| Measures and records limb girth | | ○ | ○ | ○ | ○ | ○ | ○ | |
| Selects the appropriate-sized compression sleeve for the unit | | ○ | ○ | ○ | ○ | ○ | ○ | |
| Selects the proper settings | | ○ | ○ | ○ | ○ | ○ | ○ | |
| Sets temperature (if applicable) | | ○ | ○ | ○ | ○ | ○ | ○ | |
| Maximum pressure | | ○ | ○ | ○ | ○ | ○ | ○ | |
| Sets on/off times | | ○ | ○ | ○ | ○ | ○ | ○ | |
| Sets treatment duration | | ○ | ○ | ○ | ○ | ○ | ○ | |
| **Termination of treatment** | | **Y** | **N** | **Y** | **N** | **Y** | **N** | |
| Inspects treatment area | | ○ | ○ | ○ | ○ | ○ | ○ | |
| Provides the patient with feedback | | ○ | ○ | ○ | ○ | ○ | ○ | |
| Documents the treatment | | ○ | ○ | ○ | ○ | ○ | ○ | |
| **Total** | | \_\_\_\_/17 | | \_\_\_\_/17 | | \_\_\_\_/17 | | |

*(continued on the next page)*

| Must achieve >11 to pass this examination | Ⓟ | Ⓕ | Ⓟ | Ⓕ | Ⓟ | Ⓕ |
|---|---|---|---|---|---|---|
| **Assessor:** **Date:** | **Test 1 Comments:** | | | | | |
| **Assessor:** **Date:** | **Test 2 Comments:** | | | | | |
| **Assessor:** **Date:** | **Test 3 Comments:** | | | | | |

**TEST ENVIRONMENTS**
**L:** Laboratory/Classroom
**C:** Clinical/Field Testing
**P:** Practicum
**A:** Assessment/Mock Exam

**TEST INFORMATION**
**Test Statistics:** N/A
**Reference(s):** Amato et al. (2006)
Starkey & Brown (2015)

THERAPEUTIC INTERVENTIONS
# THERAPEUTIC MODALITIES—MANUAL THERAPY

| NATA EC 5th | BOC RD6 | SKILL |
|---|---|---|
| TI-11a/b/c/e/f | D4-0402 | Cross-Fiber Friction Massage |

**Supplies Needed:** Table, bolster, drape

*This problem allows you the opportunity to use* **cross-fiber friction massage** *on a* **post-surgical scar**. *You have 3 minutes to complete this task.*

| Cross-Fiber Friction Massage | Course or Site / Assessor / Environment | | Test 1 | | Test 2 | | Test 3 | |
|---|---|---|---|---|---|---|---|---|
| | | | Y | N | Y | N | Y | N |
| **Purpose of treatment** | | | Y | N | Y | N | Y | N |
| Break down adhesions and scar tissue | | | ○ | ○ | ○ | ○ | ○ | ○ |
| **Patient education/safety** | | | Y | N | Y | N | Y | N |
| Explains to the patient why this modality is appropriate | | | ○ | ○ | ○ | ○ | ○ | ○ |
| Explains to the patient what the expected treatment goals and outcomes are | | | ○ | ○ | ○ | ○ | ○ | ○ |
| Explains to the patient what he/she should or should not feel | | | ○ | ○ | ○ | ○ | ○ | ○ |
| Reviews precautions/contraindications with the patient | | | ○ | ○ | ○ | ○ | ○ | ○ |
| **Tester places patient in appropriate position** | | | Y | N | Y | N | Y | N |
| Supine | | | ○ | ○ | ○ | ○ | ○ | ○ |
| Places bolster under the knees | | | ○ | ○ | ○ | ○ | ○ | ○ |
| Drapes the patient modestly and exposes area to be massaged | | | ○ | ○ | ○ | ○ | ○ | ○ |
| **Tester administers the therapeutic modality according to accepted guidelines** | | | Y | N | Y | N | Y | N |
| Preheats the tissue prior to massage (ultrasound, moist heat pack, basic massage strokes) | | | ○ | ○ | ○ | ○ | ○ | ○ |
| Thumb or fingertip strokes are performed in opposite directions | | | ○ | ○ | ○ | ○ | ○ | ○ |
| Performs strokes perpendicular to muscle fiber | | | ○ | ○ | ○ | ○ | ○ | ○ |
| Begins with light strokes; progresses to firmer strokes | | | ○ | ○ | ○ | ○ | ○ | ○ |
| **Termination of treatment** | | | Y | N | Y | N | Y | N |
| Inspects treatment area | | | ○ | ○ | ○ | ○ | ○ | ○ |
| Provides the patient with feedback | | | ○ | ○ | ○ | ○ | ○ | ○ |
| Documents the treatment | | | ○ | ○ | ○ | ○ | ○ | ○ |
| **Total** | | | ___/15 | | ___/15 | | ___/15 | |

*(continued on the next page)*

| Must achieve >10 to pass this examination | Ⓟ | Ⓕ | Ⓟ | Ⓕ | Ⓟ | Ⓕ |
|---|---|---|---|---|---|---|
| **Assessor:** <br> **Date:** | **Test 1 Comments:** | | | | | |
| **Assessor:** <br> **Date:** | **Test 2 Comments:** | | | | | |
| **Assessor:** <br> **Date:** | **Test 3 Comments:** | | | | | |

**TEST ENVIRONMENTS**
**L:** Laboratory/Classroom
**C:** Clinical/Field Testing
**P:** Practicum
**A:** Assessment/Mock Exam

**TEST INFORMATION**
**Test Statistics:** N/A
**Reference(s):**   Amato et al. (2006)
                  Starkey & Brown (2015)

# THERAPEUTIC MODALITIES—MANUAL THERAPY

| NATA EC 5th | BOC RD6 | SKILL |
|---|---|---|
| TI-11a/b/c/e/f | D4-0402 | Effleurage Massage |

**Supplies Needed:** Table, bolster, pillow, drape, lotion, towel

*This problem allows you the opportunity to use* **effleurage massage** *for a* **paraspinal spasm in the lower back***. You have 3 minutes to complete this task.*

| Effleurage Massage | Course or Site Assessor Environment | | Test 1 | | Test 2 | | Test 3 |
|---|---|---|---|---|---|---|---|
| **Purpose of treatment** | | Y | N | Y | N | Y | N |
| Interrupt the pain/spasm cycle | | O | O | O | O | O | O |
| **Patient education/safety** | | Y | N | Y | N | Y | N |
| Explains to the patient why this modality is appropriate | | O | O | O | O | O | O |
| Explains to the patient what the expected treatment goals and outcomes are | | O | O | O | O | O | O |
| Explains to the patient what he/she should or should not feel | | O | O | O | O | O | O |
| Reviews precautions/contraindications with the patient | | O | O | O | O | O | O |
| **Tester places patient in appropriate position** | | Y | N | Y | N | Y | N |
| Prone | | O | O | O | O | O | O |
| Places bolster under the ankles, pillow under the abdomen, and face cradle under head | | O | O | O | O | O | O |
| Drapes the patient modestly and exposes area to be massaged | | O | O | O | O | O | O |
| **Tester administers the therapeutic modality according to accepted guidelines** | | Y | N | Y | N | Y | N |
| Applies massage lotion, if applicable | | O | O | O | O | O | O |
| Stands to the side and slightly behind the patient | | O | O | O | O | O | O |
| Begins with light effleurage and builds up to deeper effleurage | | O | O | O | O | O | O |
| Using both hands, performs strokes with light pressure distal to proximal running parallel with the muscle fibers | | O | O | O | O | O | O |
| Glides hands back to starting position | | O | O | O | O | O | O |
| Maintains contact throughout | | O | O | O | O | O | O |
| **Termination of treatment** | | Y | N | Y | N | Y | N |
| Inspects treatment area | | O | O | O | O | O | O |
| Removes lubricant with towel | | O | O | O | O | O | O |
| Provides the patient with feedback | | O | O | O | O | O | O |
| Documents the treatment | | O | O | O | O | O | O |
| **Total** | | | /18 | | /18 | | /18 |

*(continued on the next page)*

| Must achieve >12 to pass this examination | Ⓟ | Ⓕ | Ⓟ | Ⓕ | Ⓟ | Ⓕ |
|---|---|---|---|---|---|---|
| **Assessor:** <br> **Date:** | **Test 1 Comments:** | | | | | |
| **Assessor:** <br> **Date:** | **Test 2 Comments:** | | | | | |
| **Assessor:** <br> **Date:** | **Test 3 Comments:** | | | | | |

## TEST ENVIRONMENTS
**L:** Laboratory/Classroom
**C:** Clinical/Field Testing
**P:** Practicum
**A:** Assessment/Mock Exam

## TEST INFORMATION
**Test Statistics:** N/A
**Reference(s):**   Amato et al. (2006)
                    Starkey & Brown (2015)

## THERAPEUTIC INTERVENTIONS
# THERAPEUTIC MODALITIES—MANUAL THERAPY

| NATA EC 5th | BOC RD6 | SKILL |
|---|---|---|
| TI-11a/b/c/e/f | D4-0402 | Fine Vibration Massage |

**Supplies Needed:** Table, bolster, pillow, drape

*This problem allows you the opportunity to use* **fine vibration massage** *to* **decrease minor pain and increase circulation to the hamstrings**. *You have 3 minutes to complete this task.*

| Fine Vibration Massage | Course or Site Assessor Environment | | Test 1 | | Test 2 | | Test 3 |
|---|---|---|---|---|---|---|---|
| | | Y | N | Y | N | Y | N |
| **Purpose of treatment** | | Y | N | Y | N | Y | N |
| Promote muscular relaxation, decrease pain, increase circulation | | ○ | ○ | ○ | ○ | ○ | ○ |
| **Patient education/safety** | | Y | N | Y | N | Y | N |
| Explains to the patient why this modality is appropriate | | ○ | ○ | ○ | ○ | ○ | ○ |
| Explains to the patient what the expected treatment goals and outcomes are | | ○ | ○ | ○ | ○ | ○ | ○ |
| Explains to the patient what he/she should or should not feel | | ○ | ○ | ○ | ○ | ○ | ○ |
| Reviews precautions/contraindications with the patient | | ○ | ○ | ○ | ○ | ○ | ○ |
| Prior to set up of the modality, checks all aspects for safety | | ○ | ○ | ○ | ○ | ○ | ○ |
| **Tester places patient in appropriate position** | | Y | N | Y | N | Y | N |
| Prone | | ○ | ○ | ○ | ○ | ○ | ○ |
| Places bolster under the ankles, pillow under the abdomen, and face cradle under head | | ○ | ○ | ○ | ○ | ○ | ○ |
| Drapes the patient for modesty and exposes area to be massaged | | ○ | ○ | ○ | ○ | ○ | ○ |
| **Tester administers the therapeutic modality according to accepted guidelines** | | Y | N | Y | N | Y | N |
| Stands to the side of the patient | | ○ | ○ | ○ | ○ | ○ | ○ |
| Places fingers firmly against the skin | | ○ | ○ | ○ | ○ | ○ | ○ |
| Keeps the wrist and forearm in a locked position, moves the fingers up and down rapidly | | ○ | ○ | ○ | ○ | ○ | ○ |
| The fingers should remain in contact with the skin | | ○ | ○ | ○ | ○ | ○ | ○ |
| **Termination of treatment** | | Y | N | Y | N | Y | N |
| Inspects treatment area | | ○ | ○ | ○ | ○ | ○ | ○ |
| Provides the patient with feedback | | ○ | ○ | ○ | ○ | ○ | ○ |
| Documents the treatment | | ○ | ○ | ○ | ○ | ○ | ○ |
| **Total** | | __/16 | | __/16 | | __/16 | |

*(continued on the next page)*

| Must achieve >11 to pass this examination | Ⓟ | Ⓕ | Ⓟ | Ⓕ | Ⓟ | Ⓕ |
|---|---|---|---|---|---|---|
| **Assessor:**<br>**Date:** | **Test 1 Comments:** | | | | | |
| **Assessor:**<br>**Date:** | **Test 2 Comments:** | | | | | |
| **Assessor:**<br>**Date:** | **Test 3 Comments:** | | | | | |

## TEST ENVIRONMENTS

**L:** Laboratory/Classroom
**C:** Clinical/Field Testing
**P:** Practicum
**A:** Assessment/Mock Exam

## TEST INFORMATION

**Test Statistics:** N/A
**Reference(s):**  Amato et al. (2006)
Starkey & Brown (2015)

THERAPEUTIC INTERVENTIONS
# THERAPEUTIC MODALITIES—MANUAL THERAPY

| NATA EC 5th | BOC RD6 | SKILL |
|---|---|---|
| TI-11a/b/c/e/f | D4-0402 | Petrissage Massage |

**Supplies Needed:** Table, bolster, pillow, drape

*This problem allows you the opportunity to use* **petrissage massage** *to free adhesions and promote muscle relaxation in the* **upper trapezium muscles***. You have 3 minutes to complete this task.*

| Petrissage Massage | Course or Site Assessor Environment | | Test 1 | | Test 2 | | Test 3 | |
|---|---|---|---|---|---|---|---|---|
| | | | **Y** | **N** | **Y** | **N** | **Y** | **N** |
| **Purpose of treatment** | | | **Y** | **N** | **Y** | **N** | **Y** | **N** |
| Free adhesions, muscular relaxation, and assist in venous return | | | ○ | ○ | ○ | ○ | ○ | ○ |
| **Patient education/safety** | | | **Y** | **N** | **Y** | **N** | **Y** | **N** |
| Explains to the patient why this modality is appropriate | | | ○ | ○ | ○ | ○ | ○ | ○ |
| Explains to the patient what the expected treatment goals and outcomes are | | | ○ | ○ | ○ | ○ | ○ | ○ |
| Explains to the patient what he/she should or should not feel | | | ○ | ○ | ○ | ○ | ○ | ○ |
| Reviews precautions/contraindications with the patient | | | ○ | ○ | ○ | ○ | ○ | ○ |
| **Tester places patient in appropriate position** | | | **Y** | **N** | **Y** | **N** | **Y** | **N** |
| Prone | | | ○ | ○ | ○ | ○ | ○ | ○ |
| Places bolster under the ankles, pillow under the abdomen, and face cradle under head | | | ○ | ○ | ○ | ○ | ○ | ○ |
| Drapes the patient for modesty and exposes the area to be massaged | | | ○ | ○ | ○ | ○ | ○ | ○ |
| **Tester administers the therapeutic modality according to accepted guidelines** | | | **Y** | **N** | **Y** | **N** | **Y** | **N** |
| Standing to the side of the patient | | | ○ | ○ | ○ | ○ | ○ | ○ |
| Using a "C" shape, grasps and folds the skin | | | ○ | ○ | ○ | ○ | ○ | ○ |
| Lifts, kneads, and rolls the skin | | | ○ | ○ | ○ | ○ | ○ | ○ |
| Uses both hands intermittently | | | ○ | ○ | ○ | ○ | ○ | ○ |
| Repeats several times and moves to a new area | | | ○ | ○ | ○ | ○ | ○ | ○ |
| **Termination of treatment** | | | **Y** | **N** | **Y** | **N** | **Y** | **N** |
| Inspects treatment area | | | ○ | ○ | ○ | ○ | ○ | ○ |
| Provides the patient with feedback | | | ○ | ○ | ○ | ○ | ○ | ○ |
| Documents the treatment | | | ○ | ○ | ○ | ○ | ○ | ○ |
| | Total | | ____/16 | | ____/16 | | ____/16 | |

*(continued on the next page)*

| Must achieve >11 to pass this examination | Ⓟ | Ⓕ | Ⓟ | Ⓕ | Ⓟ | Ⓕ |
|---|---|---|---|---|---|---|
| **Assessor:** **Date:** | **Test 1 Comments:** | | | | | |
| **Assessor:** **Date:** | **Test 2 Comments:** | | | | | |
| **Assessor:** **Date:** | **Test 3 Comments:** | | | | | |

**TEST ENVIRONMENTS**
**L:** Laboratory/Classroom
**C:** Clinical/Field Testing
**P:** Practicum
**A:** Assessment/Mock Exam

**TEST INFORMATION**
**Test Statistics:** N/A
**Reference(s):** Amato et al. (2006)
Starkey & Brown (2015)

# THERAPEUTIC MODALITIES—MANUAL THERAPY

| NATA EC 5th | BOC RD6 | SKILL |
|---|---|---|
| TI-11a/b/c/e/f | D4-0402 | Tapotement Massage |

**Supplies Needed:** Table, bolster, drape

*This problem allows you the opportunity to use* **tapotement massage** *to* **increase blood flow** *in the* **upper arm**. *You have 3 minutes to complete this task.*

| Tapotement Massage | Course or Site Assessor Environment | | Test 1 | | Test 2 | | Test 3 | |
|---|---|---|---|---|---|---|---|---|
| **Purpose of treatment** | | **Y** | **N** | **Y** | **N** | **Y** | **N** | |
| Increase blood flow, stimulate nerve endings, decrease pain | | ○ | ○ | ○ | ○ | ○ | ○ | |
| **Patient education/safety** | | **Y** | **N** | **Y** | **N** | **Y** | **N** | |
| Explains to the patient why this modality is appropriate | | ○ | ○ | ○ | ○ | ○ | ○ | |
| Explains to the patient what the expected treatment goals and outcomes are | | ○ | ○ | ○ | ○ | ○ | ○ | |
| Explains to the patient what he/she should or should not feel | | ○ | ○ | ○ | ○ | ○ | ○ | |
| Reviews precautions/contraindications with the patient | | ○ | ○ | ○ | ○ | ○ | ○ | |
| **Tester places patient in appropriate position** | | **Y** | **N** | **Y** | **N** | **Y** | **N** | |
| Supine | | ○ | ○ | ○ | ○ | ○ | ○ | |
| Places bolster under the patient's knees | | ○ | ○ | ○ | ○ | ○ | ○ | |
| Drapes the patient for modesty and exposes the area to be massaged | | ○ | ○ | ○ | ○ | ○ | ○ | |
| **Tester administers the therapeutic modality according to accepted guidelines** | | **Y** | **N** | **Y** | **N** | **Y** | **N** | |
| Gently taps the skin using one of the following techniques: | | | | | | | | |
|   Hacking: Contact with the skin is made using the lateral aspect of the hand and finger | | ○ | ○ | ○ | ○ | ○ | ○ | |
|   Cupping: The hands are cupped striking the skin with the heel and fingers | | ○ | ○ | ○ | ○ | ○ | ○ | |
|   Pincement: The skin is pinched using the fingertips | | ○ | ○ | ○ | ○ | ○ | ○ | |
|   Rapping: The hand is held in a loose fist striking the skin with the distal phalanges | | ○ | ○ | ○ | ○ | ○ | ○ | |
|   Tapping: The fingertips lightly drum the skin | | ○ | ○ | ○ | ○ | ○ | ○ | |
| Executes the skill softly and slowly | | ○ | ○ | ○ | ○ | ○ | ○ | |
| **Termination of treatment** | | **Y** | **N** | **Y** | **N** | **Y** | **N** | |
| Inspects treatment area | | ○ | ○ | ○ | ○ | ○ | ○ | |
| Provides the patient with feedback | | ○ | ○ | ○ | ○ | ○ | ○ | |
| Documents the treatment | | ○ | ○ | ○ | ○ | ○ | ○ | |
| **Total** | | ___/17 | | ___/17 | | ___/17 | | |

*(continued on the next page)*

| Must achieve >11 to pass this examination | P | F | P | F | P | F |
|---|---|---|---|---|---|---|
| **Assessor:** <br> **Date:** | **Test 1 Comments:** | | | | | |
| **Assessor:** <br> **Date:** | **Test 2 Comments:** | | | | | |
| **Assessor:** <br> **Date:** | **Test 3 Comments:** | | | | | |

## TEST ENVIRONMENTS
**L:** Laboratory/Classroom
**C:** Clinical/Field Testing
**P:** Practicum
**A:** Assessment/Mock Exam

## TEST INFORMATION
**Test Statistics:** N/A
**Reference(s):**   Amato et al. (2006)
Starkey & Brown (2015)

THERAPEUTIC INTERVENTIONS
# THERAPEUTIC MODALITIES—THERMOTHERAPY

| NATA EC 5th | BOC RD6 | SKILL |
|---|---|---|
| TI-11a/b/c/e/f | D4-0402 | Hot Whirlpool |

**Supplies Needed:** Table or chair, whirlpool

*This problem allows you the opportunity to use a **hot whirlpool** for a **subacute injury**. Your scenario is a sport-related subacute injury to the ankle. You have 3 minutes to complete this task.*

| Hot Whirlpool | Course or Site Assessor Environment | | Test 1 | | Test 2 | | Test 3 |
|---|---|---|---|---|---|---|---|
| **Purpose of treatment** | | Y | N | Y | N | Y | N |
| Application of heat to irregularly shaped body parts | | O | O | O | O | O | O |
| **Patient education/safety** | | Y | N | Y | N | Y | N |
| Explains to the patient why the modality is appropriate | | O | O | O | O | O | O |
| Explains to the patient what the expected treatment goals and outcomes are | | O | O | O | O | O | O |
| Explains to the patient what he/she should or should not feel | | O | O | O | O | O | O |
| Reviews precautions/contraindications with the patient | | O | O | O | O | O | O |
| Prior to set up of the modality, checks all aspects for safety | | O | O | O | O | O | O |
| **Tester places patient in appropriate position** | | Y | N | Y | N | Y | N |
| Seated with the involved limb immersed in whirlpool | | O | O | O | O | O | O |
| **Tester administers the therapeutic modality according to accepted guidelines** | | Y | N | Y | N | Y | N |
| Water depth is enough to cover the involved limb | | O | O | O | O | O | O |
| Water temperature is appropriate for the nature of the injury | | O | O | O | O | O | O |
| Turns turbines on prior to the patient getting into whirlpool | | O | O | O | O | O | O |
| Turns off turbines once the patient is out of the water | | O | O | O | O | O | O |
| **Termination of treatment** | | Y | N | Y | N | Y | N |
| Inspects treatment area | | O | O | O | O | O | O |
| Provides the patient with feedback | | O | O | O | O | O | O |
| Documents the treatment | | O | O | O | O | O | O |
| | Total | ___/14 | | ___/14 | | ___/14 | |

*(continued on the next page)*

| Must achieve >9 to pass this examination | Ⓟ | Ⓕ | Ⓟ | Ⓕ | Ⓟ | Ⓕ |
|---|---|---|---|---|---|---|
| **Assessor:** <br> **Date:** | **Test 1 Comments:** | | | | | |
| **Assessor:** <br> **Date:** | **Test 2 Comments:** | | | | | |
| **Assessor:** <br> **Date:** | **Test 3 Comments:** | | | | | |

## TEST ENVIRONMENTS
**L:** Laboratory/Classroom
**C:** Clinical/Field Testing
**P:** Practicum
**A:** Assessment/Mock Exam

## TEST INFORMATION
**Test Statistics:** N/A
**Reference(s):** Amato et al. (2006)
Starkey & Brown (2015)

THERAPEUTIC INTERVENTIONS
# THERAPEUTIC MODALITIES—THERMOTHERAPY

| NATA EC 5th | BOC RD6 | SKILL |
|---|---|---|
| TI-11a/b/c/e/f | D4-0402 | Moist Heat Pack |

**Supplies Needed:** Table, bolster, pillow, hydrocollator, moist heat pack, hot pack cover, towels

*This problem allows you the opportunity to use a **moist heat pack** to heat the **lower back**.*
*You have 3 minutes to complete this task.*

| Moist Heat Pack | Course or Site Assessor Environment | | | | | |
|---|---|---|---|---|---|---|
| | | Test 1 | | Test 2 | | Test 3 |
| **Purpose of treatment** | | Y | N | Y | N | Y | N |
| Relieve subacute or chronic muscle spasm and pain | | O | O | O | O | O | O |
| **Patient education/safety** | | Y | N | Y | N | Y | N |
| Explains to the patient why this modality is appropriate | | O | O | O | O | O | O |
| Explains to the patient what the expected treatment goals and outcomes are | | O | O | O | O | O | O |
| Explains to the patient what he/she should or should not feel | | O | O | O | O | O | O |
| Reviews precautions/contraindications with the patient | | O | O | O | O | O | O |
| **Tester places patient in appropriate position** | | Y | N | Y | N | Y | N |
| Prone | | O | O | O | O | O | O |
| Places bolster under the ankles, pillow under the abdomen, and face cradle under head | | O | O | O | O | O | O |
| **Tester administers the therapeutic modality according to accepted guidelines** | | Y | N | Y | N | Y | N |
| Places heat pack into terrycloth cover | | O | O | O | O | O | O |
| Surrounds terrycloth cover in five layers of toweling | | O | O | O | O | O | O |
| Places heat pack in appropriate area | | O | O | O | O | O | O |
| Checks the patient every 5 minutes | | O | O | O | O | O | O |
| **Termination of treatment** | | Y | N | Y | N | Y | N |
| Inspects treatment area | | O | O | O | O | O | O |
| Provides the patient with feedback | | O | O | O | O | O | O |
| Documents the treatment | | O | O | O | O | O | O |
| Total | | __/14 | | __/14 | | __/14 |

*(continued on the next page)*

| Must achieve >9 to pass this examination | Ⓟ | Ⓕ | Ⓟ | Ⓕ | Ⓟ | Ⓕ |
|---|---|---|---|---|---|---|
| **Assessor:** <br> **Date:** | **Test 1 Comments:** | | | | | |
| **Assessor:** <br> **Date:** | **Test 2 Comments:** | | | | | |
| **Assessor:** <br> **Date:** | **Test 3 Comments:** | | | | | |

## TEST ENVIRONMENTS
**L:** Laboratory/Classroom
**C:** Clinical/Field Testing
**P:** Practicum
**A:** Assessment/Mock Exam

## TEST INFORMATION
**Test Statistics:** N/A
**Reference(s):**   Amato et al. (2006)
                    Starkey & Brown (2015)

THERAPEUTIC INTERVENTIONS

# THERAPEUTIC MODALITIES—THERMOTHERAPY

| NATA EC 5th | BOC RD6 | SKILL |
|---|---|---|
| TI-11a/b/c/e/f | D4-0402 | Paraffin Bath |

**Supplies Needed:** Table, paraffin bath, plastic bag, towel

*This problem allows you the opportunity to use a* **paraffin bath** *to heat the* **hand**. *You have 3 minutes to complete this task.*

| Paraffin Bath | Course or Site Assessor Environment | | Test 1 | | Test 2 | | Test 3 | |
|---|---|---|---|---|---|---|---|---|
| | | | **Y** | **N** | **Y** | **N** | **Y** | **N** |
| **Purpose of treatment** | | | **Y** | **N** | **Y** | **N** | **Y** | **N** |
| Superficially heating small body parts | | | O | O | O | O | O | O |
| **Patient education/safety** | | | **Y** | **N** | **Y** | **N** | **Y** | **N** |
| Explains to the patient why this modality is appropriate | | | O | O | O | O | O | O |
| Explains to the patient what the expected treatment goals and outcomes are | | | O | O | O | O | O | O |
| Explains to the patient what he/she should or should not feel | | | O | O | O | O | O | O |
| Reviews precautions/contraindications with the patient | | | O | O | O | O | O | O |
| Removes all jewelry | | | O | O | O | O | O | O |
| **Tester places patient in appropriate position** | | | **Y** | **N** | **Y** | **N** | **Y** | **N** |
| Seated | | | O | O | O | O | O | O |
| **Tester administers the therapeutic modality according to accepted guidelines** | | | **Y** | **N** | **Y** | **N** | **Y** | **N** |
| Instructs the patient to dip hand into the paraffin | | | O | O | O | O | O | O |
| Removes hand from paraffin | | | O | O | O | O | O | O |
| Allows paraffin to dry before reapplying | | | O | O | O | O | O | O |
| Repeats procedure six times | | | O | O | O | O | O | O |
| Wraps the hand in a plastic bag and then a towel | | | O | O | O | O | O | O |
| **Termination of treatment** | | | **Y** | **N** | **Y** | **N** | **Y** | **N** |
| Inspects treatment area | | | O | O | O | O | O | O |
| Provides the patient with feedback | | | O | O | O | O | O | O |
| Documents the treatment | | | O | O | O | O | O | O |
| | Total | | ___/15 | | ___/15 | | ___/15 | |

*(continued on the next page)*

| Must achieve >10 to pass this examination | P | F | P | F | P | F |
|---|---|---|---|---|---|---|
| **Assessor:**<br>**Date:** | **Test 1 Comments:** | | | | | |
| **Assessor:**<br>**Date:** | **Test 2 Comments:** | | | | | |
| **Assessor:**<br>**Date:** | **Test 3 Comments:** | | | | | |

## TEST ENVIRONMENTS
**L:** Laboratory/Classroom
**C:** Clinical/Field Testing
**P:** Practicum
**A:** Assessment/Mock Exam

## TEST INFORMATION
**Test Statistics:** N/A
**Reference(s):**   Amato et al. (2006)
Starkey & Brown (2015)

THERAPEUTIC INTERVENTIONS
# THERAPEUTIC EXERCISE—LOWER EXTREMITY

| NATA EC 5th | BOC RD6 | SKILL |
|---|---|---|
| TI-11a/b/d | D4-0401 | Lower Extremity Endurance (Ankle) |

**Supplies Needed:** Table, box

*This problem allows you the opportunity to instruct a* **lower extremity endurance exercise** *for the* **ankle**. *You have 3 minutes to complete this task.*

| Lower Extremity Endurance (Ankle) | Course or Site / Assessor / Environment | | Test 1 | | Test 2 | | Test 3 | |
|---|---|---|---|---|---|---|---|---|
| | | Y | N | Y | N | Y | N | |
| **Purpose of treatment** | | Y | N | Y | N | Y | N |
| Strength development | | ○ | ○ | ○ | ○ | ○ | ○ |
| **Tester places patient in appropriate position** | | Y | N | Y | N | Y | N |
| Seated | | ○ | ○ | ○ | ○ | ○ | ○ |
| Knee in 90 degrees flexion | | ○ | ○ | ○ | ○ | ○ | ○ |
| The patient places forefoot on the edge of a box | | ○ | ○ | ○ | ○ | ○ | ○ |
| The patient allows heel to hang off the edge of the box | | ○ | ○ | ○ | ○ | ○ | ○ |
| **Tester performs the test according to accepted guidelines** | | Y | N | Y | N | Y | N |
| The patient is instructed to plantar flex the ankle, pushing the toes into the box | | ○ | ○ | ○ | ○ | ○ | ○ |
| The patient slowly lowers the ankle back to the starting position | | ○ | ○ | ○ | ○ | ○ | ○ |
| Sequence is repeated for two sets of 20 repetitions | | ○ | ○ | ○ | ○ | ○ | ○ |
| **Total** | | ___/8 | | ___/8 | | ___/8 | |
| **Must achieve >5 to pass this examination** | | Ⓟ | Ⓕ | Ⓟ | Ⓕ | Ⓟ | Ⓕ |

| Assessor: Date: | Test 1 Comments: |
|---|---|
| Assessor: Date: | Test 2 Comments: |
| Assessor: Date: | Test 3 Comments: |

**TEST ENVIRONMENTS**
**L:** Laboratory/Classroom
**C:** Clinical/Field Testing
**P:** Practicum
**A:** Assessment/Mock Exam

**TEST INFORMATION**
**Test Statistics:** N/A
**Reference(s):** Amato et al. (2006)
Starkey & Brown (2015)

# THERAPEUTIC EXERCISE—LOWER EXTREMITY

| NATA EC 5th | BOC RD6 | SKILL |
|---|---|---|
| TI-11a/b/d | D4-0401 | Lower Extremity Endurance (Hip) |

**Supplies Needed:** Table, cuff weight

*This problem allows you the opportunity to administer a* **lower extremity endurance exercise** *for* **hip extension**. *You have 3 minutes to complete this task.*

| Lower Extremity Endurance (Hip) | Course or Site Assessor Environment | | Test 1 | | Test 2 | | Test 3 | |
|---|---|---|---|---|---|---|---|---|
| | | | Y | N | Y | N | Y | N |
| **Purpose of treatment** | | | **Y** | **N** | **Y** | **N** | **Y** | **N** |
| Strength development | | | O | O | O | O | O | O |
| **Tester places patient in appropriate position** | | | **Y** | **N** | **Y** | **N** | **Y** | **N** |
| Prone | | | O | O | O | O | O | O |
| Attaches cuff weight securely to the lower leg | | | O | O | O | O | O | O |
| **Tester performs the test according to accepted guidelines** | | | **Y** | **N** | **Y** | **N** | **Y** | **N** |
| The patient tightens gluteus maximus and hamstring muscles | | | O | O | O | O | O | O |
| The patient slowly extends leg 6 inches off the table | | | O | O | O | O | O | O |
| The patient avoids hip and trunk rotation | | | O | O | O | O | O | O |
| The patient slowly lowers limb back to starting position | | | O | O | O | O | O | O |
| The patient repeats for two sets of 20 repetitions | | | O | O | O | O | O | O |
| **Total** | | | ____/8 | | ____/8 | | ____/8 | |
| **Must achieve >5 to pass this examination** | | | Ⓟ | Ⓕ | Ⓟ | Ⓕ | Ⓟ | Ⓕ |

| Assessor: Date: | Test 1 Comments: |
|---|---|
| Assessor: Date: | Test 2 Comments: |
| Assessor: Date: | Test 3 Comments: |

**TEST ENVIRONMENTS**
**L:** Laboratory/Classroom
**C:** Clinical/Field Testing
**P:** Practicum
**A:** Assessment/Mock Exam

**TEST INFORMATION**
**Test Statistics:** N/A
**Reference(s):** Amato et al. (2006)
Starkey & Brown (2015)

THERAPEUTIC INTERVENTIONS
# THERAPEUTIC EXERCISE—LOWER EXTREMITY

| NATA EC 5th | BOC RD6 | SKILL |
|---|---|---|
| TI-11a/b/d | D4-0401 | Lower Extremity Endurance (Knee) |

**Supplies Needed:** Table, cuff weight

*This problem allows you the opportunity to demonstrate a* **lower extremity endurance exercise** *for the* **knee extensors**. *You have 3 minutes to complete this task.*

| Lower Extremity Endurance (Knee) | Course or Site<br>Assessor<br>Environment | Test 1 | | Test 2 | | Test 3 | |
|---|---|---|---|---|---|---|---|
| **Purpose of treatment** | | **Y** | **N** | **Y** | **N** | **Y** | **N** |
| Strength development | | ○ | ○ | ○ | ○ | ○ | ○ |
| **Tester places patient in appropriate position** | | **Y** | **N** | **Y** | **N** | **Y** | **N** |
| Seated | | ○ | ○ | ○ | ○ | ○ | ○ |
| Cuff weight is attached to lower leg | | ○ | ○ | ○ | ○ | ○ | ○ |
| **Tester performs the test according to accepted guidelines** | | **Y** | **N** | **Y** | **N** | **Y** | **N** |
| Instructs the patient to contract the quadriceps | | ○ | ○ | ○ | ○ | ○ | ○ |
| The patient slowly extends the knee until the lower leg is parallel to the ground | | ○ | ○ | ○ | ○ | ○ | ○ |
| The patient slowly lowers leg back to starting position | | ○ | ○ | ○ | ○ | ○ | ○ |
| The patient performs two sets of 20 repetitions | | ○ | ○ | ○ | ○ | ○ | ○ |
| Total | | ___/7 | | ___/7 | | ___/7 | |
| Must achieve >4 to pass this examination | | Ⓟ | Ⓕ | Ⓟ | Ⓕ | Ⓟ | Ⓕ |
| Assessor:<br>Date: | Test 1 Comments: | | | | | | |
| Assessor:<br>Date: | Test 2 Comments: | | | | | | |
| Assessor:<br>Date: | Test 3 Comments: | | | | | | |

**TEST ENVIRONMENTS**
**L:** Laboratory/Classroom
**C:** Clinical/Field Testing
**P:** Practicum
**A:** Assessment/Mock Exam

**TEST INFORMATION**
**Test Statistics:** N/A
**Reference(s):**   Amato et al. (2006)
                    Starkey & Brown (2015)

# THERAPEUTIC EXERCISE—LOWER EXTREMITY

| NATA EC 5th | BOC RD6 | SKILL |
|---|---|---|
| TI-11a/b/d | D4-0401 | Lower Extremity Isometrics (Ankle) |

**Supplies Needed:** Table, bolster

*This problem allows you the opportunity to administer a* **lower extremity isometric exercise** *for the* **ankle.**
*You have 3 minutes to complete this task.*

| Lower Extremity Isometrics (Ankle) | Course or Site Assessor Environment | | Test 1 | | Test 2 | | Test 3 | |
|---|---|---|---|---|---|---|---|---|
| | | | **Test 1** | | **Test 2** | | **Test 3** | |
| **Purpose of treatment** | | | **Y** | **N** | **Y** | **N** | **Y** | **N** |
| Develop strength | | | ○ | ○ | ○ | ○ | ○ | ○ |
| **Tester places patient in appropriate position** | | | **Y** | **N** | **Y** | **N** | **Y** | **N** |
| Supine | | | ○ | ○ | ○ | ○ | ○ | ○ |
| Places bolster under the knee | | | ○ | ○ | ○ | ○ | ○ | ○ |
| **Tester performs the test according to accepted guidelines** | | | **Y** | **N** | **Y** | **N** | **Y** | **N** |
| Places on hand on the forefoot | | | ○ | ○ | ○ | ○ | ○ | ○ |
| Places other hand on the distal tibiofemoral syndesmotic joint | | | ○ | ○ | ○ | ○ | ○ | ○ |
| Instructs the patient to perform an isometric ankle contraction as tester applies manual resistance | | | ○ | ○ | ○ | ○ | ○ | ○ |
| | | Total | ___/6 | | ___/6 | | ___/6 | |
| | Must achieve >3 to pass this examination | | Ⓟ | Ⓕ | Ⓟ | Ⓕ | Ⓟ | Ⓕ |
| **Assessor:** **Date:** | **Test 1 Comments:** | | | | | | | |
| **Assessor:** **Date:** | **Test 2 Comments:** | | | | | | | |
| **Assessor:** **Date:** | **Test 3 Comments:** | | | | | | | |

**TEST ENVIRONMENTS**
**L:** Laboratory/Classroom
**C:** Clinical/Field Testing
**P:** Practicum
**A:** Assessment/Mock Exam

**TEST INFORMATION**
**Test Statistics:** N/A
**Reference(s):** Amato et al. (2006)
Starkey & Brown (2015)

THERAPEUTIC INTERVENTIONS
# THERAPEUTIC EXERCISE—LOWER EXTREMITY

| NATA EC 5th | BOC RD6 | SKILL |
|---|---|---|
| TI-11a/b/d | D4-0401 | Lower Extremity Isometrics (Hip) |

**Supplies Needed:** Table

*This problem allows you the opportunity to administer a* **lower extremity isometric test** *for the* **hip abductors.**
*You have 3 minutes to complete this task.*

| Lower Extremity Isometrics (Hip) | Course or Site Assessor Environment | Test 1 | | Test 2 | | Test 3 | |
|---|---|---|---|---|---|---|---|
| | | Y | N | Y | N | Y | N |
| **Purpose of treatment** | | Y | N | Y | N | Y | N |
| Develop strength | | ○ | ○ | ○ | ○ | ○ | ○ |
| **Tester places patient in appropriate position** | | Y | N | Y | N | Y | N |
| Side lying on uninvolved side | | ○ | ○ | ○ | ○ | ○ | ○ |
| The patient's hips are in neutral | | ○ | ○ | ○ | ○ | ○ | ○ |
| The patient's knees are in full extension | | ○ | ○ | ○ | ○ | ○ | ○ |
| **Tester performs the test according to accepted guidelines** | | Y | N | Y | N | Y | N |
| Places one hand on the distal portion of the femur | | ○ | ○ | ○ | ○ | ○ | ○ |
| Places the opposite hand on the lower leg | | ○ | ○ | ○ | ○ | ○ | ○ |
| Instructs the patient to perform an isometric hip abduction contraction as the tester applies manual resistance | | ○ | ○ | ○ | ○ | ○ | ○ |
| Total | | /7 | | /7 | | /7 | |
| **Must achieve >4 to pass this examination** | | Ⓟ | Ⓕ | Ⓟ | Ⓕ | Ⓟ | Ⓕ |

| Assessor: Date: | **Test 1 Comments:** |
|---|---|
| Assessor: Date: | **Test 2 Comments:** |
| Assessor: Date: | **Test 3 Comments:** |

**TEST ENVIRONMENTS**
**L:** Laboratory/Classroom
**C:** Clinical/Field Testing
**P:** Practicum
**A:** Assessment/Mock Exam

**TEST INFORMATION**
**Test Statistics:** N/A
**Reference(s):**    Amato et al. (2006)
                        Starkey & Brown (2015)

**THERAPEUTIC INTERVENTIONS**
# THERAPEUTIC EXERCISE—LOWER EXTREMITY

| NATA EC 5th | BOC RD6 | SKILL |
|---|---|---|
| TI-11a/b/d | D4-0401 | Lower Extremity Isometrics (Knee) |

**Supplies Needed:** Table

*This problem allows you the opportunity to administer a* **lower extremity isometric test** *for the* **knee**. *You have 3 minutes to complete this task.*

| Lower Extremity Isometrics (Knee) | Course or Site Assessor Environment | | Test 1 | | Test 2 | | Test 3 | |
|---|---|---|---|---|---|---|---|---|
| | | | Y | N | Y | N | Y | N |
| **Purpose of treatment** | | | Y | N | Y | N | Y | N |
| Strength development | | | O | O | O | O | O | O |
| **Tester places patient in appropriate position** | | | Y | N | Y | N | Y | N |
| Supine | | | O | O | O | O | O | O |
| Knees extended | | | O | O | O | O | O | O |
| **Tester performs the test according to accepted guidelines** | | | Y | N | Y | N | Y | N |
| Educates the patient on how to perform a isometric quadriceps contraction | | | O | O | O | O | O | O |
| The patient attempts to contract the quadriceps muscle and holds for 10 seconds | | | O | O | O | O | O | O |
| Provides biofeedback while the patient performs isometric contraction | | | O | O | O | O | O | O |
| Total | | | _/6 | | _/6 | | _/6 | |
| Must achieve >3 to pass this examination | | | P | F | P | F | P | F |
| Assessor: Date: | Test 1 Comments: | | | | | | | |
| Assessor: Date: | Test 2 Comments: | | | | | | | |
| Assessor: Date: | Test 3 Comments: | | | | | | | |

**TEST ENVIRONMENTS**
**L:** Laboratory/Classroom
**C:** Clinical/Field Testing
**P:** Practicum
**A:** Assessment/Mock Exam

**TEST INFORMATION**
**Test Statistics:** N/A
**Reference(s):** Amato et al. (2006)
Starkey & Brown (2015)

THERAPEUTIC INTERVENTIONS
## THERAPEUTIC EXERCISE—LOWER EXTREMITY

| NATA EC 5th | BOC RD6 | SKILL |
|---|---|---|
| TI-11a/b/d | D4-0401 | Lower Extremity Proprioception (Static) |

**Supplies Needed:** Table

*This problem allows you the opportunity to administer* **lower extremity proprioception (static)**.
*You have 3 minutes to complete this task.*

| Lower Extremity Propriception (Static) | Course or Site Assessor Environment | | Test 1 | | Test 2 | | Test 3 |
|---|---|---|---|---|---|---|---|
| | | Y | N | Y | N | Y | N |
| **Purpose of treatment** | | Y | N | Y | N | Y | N |
| Increase proprioception of the lower extremity | | ◯ | ◯ | ◯ | ◯ | ◯ | ◯ |
| **Tester places patient in appropriate position** | | Y | N | Y | N | Y | N |
| Standing | | ◯ | ◯ | ◯ | ◯ | ◯ | ◯ |
| **Tester performs the test according to accepted guidelines** | | Y | N | Y | N | Y | N |
| Educates the patient on proprioception exercise | | ◯ | ◯ | ◯ | ◯ | ◯ | ◯ |
| Instructs the patient to stand on the involved limb and flex uninvolved limb to 90 degrees | | ◯ | ◯ | ◯ | ◯ | ◯ | ◯ |
| Instructs the patient to hold position for 30 seconds with eyes open | | ◯ | ◯ | ◯ | ◯ | ◯ | ◯ |
| **Total** | | ___/5 | | ___/5 | | ___/5 | |
| **Must achieve >2 to pass this examination** | | Ⓟ | Ⓕ | Ⓟ | Ⓕ | Ⓟ | Ⓕ |

| Assessor: Date: | Test 1 Comments: |
|---|---|
| Assessor: Date: | Test 2 Comments: |
| Assessor: Date: | Test 3 Comments: |

**TEST ENVIRONMENTS**
**L:** Laboratory/Classroom
**C:** Clinical/Field Testing
**P:** Practicum
**A:** Assessment/Mock Exam

**TEST INFORMATION**
**Test Statistics:** N/A
**Reference(s):**  Amato et al. (2006)
                   Starkey & Brown (2015)

THERAPEUTIC INTERVENTIONS
# THERAPEUTIC EXERCISE—LOWER EXTREMITY

| NATA EC 5th | BOC RD6 | SKILL |
|---|---|---|
| TI-11a/b/d | D4-0401 | Lower Extremity Proprioception (Dynamic) |

**Supplies Needed:** Table, grid taped on floor

*This problem allows you the opportunity to administer the* **Star Excursion Balance Test for lower extremity dynamic proprioception.** *You have 3 minutes to complete this task.*

| Lower Extremity Proprioception (Dynamic) | Course or Site / Assessor / Environment | Test 1 | | Test 2 | | Test 3 | |
|---|---|---|---|---|---|---|---|
| **Purpose of treatment** | | **Y** | **N** | **Y** | **N** | **Y** | **N** |
| Increase proprioception of the lower extremity | | ○ | ○ | ○ | ○ | ○ | ○ |
| **Tester places patient in appropriate position** | | **Y** | **N** | **Y** | **N** | **Y** | **N** |
| The patient stands with the midline of stance foot in middle of the grid with hands on hips | | ○ | ○ | ○ | ○ | ○ | ○ |
| Stands in front of the patient providing support | | ○ | ○ | ○ | ○ | ○ | ○ |
| **Tester performs the test according to accepted guidelines** | | **Y** | **N** | **Y** | **N** | **Y** | **N** |
| While standing on a single limb, the patient reaches as far as possible along each line | | ○ | ○ | ○ | ○ | ○ | ○ |
| The patient lightly touches the line with the most distal portion of the reaching foot without shifting weight | | ○ | ○ | ○ | ○ | ○ | ○ |
| The patient slowly returns foot to the starting position in the center of the grid and assumes bilateral stance | | ○ | ○ | ○ | ○ | ○ | ○ |
| **Total** | | ___ /6 | | ___ /6 | | ___ /6 | |
| **Must achieve >3 to pass this examination** | | Ⓟ | Ⓕ | Ⓟ | Ⓕ | Ⓟ | Ⓕ |
| **Assessor:** **Date:** | **Test 1 Comments:** | | | | | | |
| **Assessor:** **Date:** | **Test 2 Comments:** | | | | | | |
| **Assessor:** **Date:** | **Test 3 Comments:** | | | | | | |

**TEST ENVIRONMENTS**
**L:** Laboratory/Classroom
**C:** Clinical/Field Testing
**P:** Practicum
**A:** Assessment/Mock Exam

**TEST INFORMATION**
**Test Statistics:** N/A
**Reference(s):** Gribble et al. (2012)

THERAPEUTIC INTERVENTIONS
# THERAPEUTIC EXERCISE—LOWER EXTREMITY

| NATA EC 5th | BOC RD6 | SKILL |
|---|---|---|
| TI-11a/b/d | D4-0401 | Lower Extremity Strength (Ankle) |

**Supplies Needed:** Table, elastic tubing

*This problem allows you the opportunity to administer a* **lower extremity strength exercise** *for the* **ankle**. *You have 3 minutes to complete this task.*

| Lower Extremity Strength (Ankle) | Course or Site Assessor Environment | | Test 1 | | Test 2 | | Test 3 |
|---|---|---|---|---|---|---|---|
| **Purpose of treatment** | | Y | N | Y | N | Y | N |
| Strength development | | ○ | ○ | ○ | ○ | ○ | ○ |
| **Tester places patient in appropriate position** | | Y | N | Y | N | Y | N |
| Seated with involved limb hanging over the table | | ○ | ○ | ○ | ○ | ○ | ○ |
| **Tester performs the test according to accepted guidelines** | | Y | N | Y | N | Y | N |
| Wraps resistance tubing around the patient's forefoot | | ○ | ○ | ○ | ○ | ○ | ○ |
| Holds resistance tubing below the plantar surface of the patient's foot | | ○ | ○ | ○ | ○ | ○ | ○ |
| Instructs the patient to dorsiflex the ankle against resistance | | ○ | ○ | ○ | ○ | ○ | ○ |
| Total | | ___ /5 | | ___ /5 | | ___ /5 | |
| Must achieve >2 to pass this examination | | Ⓟ | Ⓕ | Ⓟ | Ⓕ | Ⓟ | Ⓕ |

| Assessor: Date: | Test 1 Comments: |
|---|---|
| Assessor: Date: | Test 2 Comments: |
| Assessor: Date: | Test 3 Comments: |

**TEST ENVIRONMENTS**
**L:** Laboratory/Classroom
**C:** Clinical/Field Testing
**P:** Practicum
**A:** Assessment/Mock Exam

**TEST INFORMATION**
**Test Statistics:** N/A
**Reference(s):** Starkey & Brown (2015)

**THERAPEUTIC INTERVENTIONS**
# THERAPEUTIC EXERCISE—LOWER EXTREMITY

| NATA EC 5th | BOC RD6 | SKILL |
|---|---|---|
| TI-11a/b/d | D4-0401 | Lower Extremity Strength (Hip) |

**Supplies Needed:** Table, cuff weight

*This problem allows you the opportunity to administer a* **lower extremity strength exercise** *for the* **hip**. *You have 3 minutes to complete this task.*

| Lower Extremity Strength (Hip) | Course or Site<br>Assessor<br>Environment | | | | | | |
|---|---|---|---|---|---|---|---|
| | | Test 1 | | Test 2 | | Test 3 | |
| **Purpose of treatment** | | **Y** | **N** | **Y** | **N** | **Y** | **N** |
| Strength development | | ○ | ○ | ○ | ○ | ○ | ○ |
| **Tester places patient in appropriate position** | | **Y** | **N** | **Y** | **N** | **Y** | **N** |
| Seated | | ○ | ○ | ○ | ○ | ○ | ○ |
| Knees flexed to approximately 90 degrees flexion | | ○ | ○ | ○ | ○ | ○ | ○ |
| Pelvis in neutral | | ○ | ○ | ○ | ○ | ○ | ○ |
| Attaches cuff weight to distal femur | | ○ | ○ | ○ | ○ | ○ | ○ |
| **Tester performs the test according to accepted guidelines** | | **Y** | **N** | **Y** | **N** | **Y** | **N** |
| The patient tightens quadriceps and slowly lifts femur off table, maintaining good posture | | ○ | ○ | ○ | ○ | ○ | ○ |
| The patient slowly brings femur back to starting position flush on the table | | ○ | ○ | ○ | ○ | ○ | ○ |
| **Total** | | ___/7 | | ___/7 | | ___/7 | |
| **Must achieve >4 to pass this examination** | | Ⓟ | Ⓕ | Ⓟ | Ⓕ | Ⓟ | Ⓕ |
| **Assessor:**<br>**Date:** | **Test 1 Comments:** | | | | | | |
| **Assessor:**<br>**Date:** | **Test 2 Comments:** | | | | | | |
| **Assessor:**<br>**Date:** | **Test 3 Comments:** | | | | | | |

**TEST ENVIRONMENTS**
**L:** Laboratory/Classroom
**C:** Clinical/Field Testing
**P:** Practicum
**A:** Assessment/Mock Exam

**TEST INFORMATION**
**Test Statistics:** N/A
**Reference(s):** Starkey & Brown (2015)

## THERAPEUTIC INTERVENTIONS
# THERAPEUTIC EXERCISE—LOWER EXTREMITY

| NATA EC 5th | BOC RD6 | SKILL |
|---|---|---|
| TI-11a/b/d | D4-0401 | Lower Extremity Strength (Knee) |

**Supplies Needed:** Table, elastic tubing

*This problem allows you the opportunity to administer a* **lower extremity strength exercise** *for the* **knee**. *You have 3 minutes to complete this task.*

| Lower Extremity Strength (Knee) | Course or Site / Assessor / Environment | Test 1 Y | Test 1 N | Test 2 Y | Test 2 N | Test 3 Y | Test 3 N |
|---|---|---|---|---|---|---|---|
| **Purpose of treatment** | | Y | N | Y | N | Y | N |
| Strength development | | ○ | ○ | ○ | ○ | ○ | ○ |
| **Tester places patient in appropriate position** | | Y | N | Y | N | Y | N |
| The patient is standing | | ○ | ○ | ○ | ○ | ○ | ○ |
| The tester is seated in front of the patient | | ○ | ○ | ○ | ○ | ○ | ○ |
| **Tester performs the test according to accepted guidelines** | | Y | N | Y | N | Y | N |
| Places resistance tubing around the distal portion of the femur, just proximal to the popliteal fossa | | ○ | ○ | ○ | ○ | ○ | ○ |
| Instructs the patient to start with involved limb in slight flexion | | ○ | ○ | ○ | ○ | ○ | ○ |
| Instructs the patient to actively straighten involved limb by contracting quadriceps while the tester applies resistance with tubing | | ○ | ○ | ○ | ○ | ○ | ○ |
| Total | | __/6 | | __/6 | | __/6 | |
| Must achieve >3 to pass this examination | | Ⓟ | Ⓕ | Ⓟ | Ⓕ | Ⓟ | Ⓕ |

| Assessor: Date: | Test 1 Comments: |
|---|---|
| Assessor: Date: | Test 2 Comments: |
| Assessor: Date: | Test 3 Comments: |

**TEST ENVIRONMENTS**
**L:** Laboratory/Classroom
**C:** Clinical/Field Testing
**P:** Practicum
**A:** Assessment/Mock Exam

**TEST INFORMATION**
**Test Statistics:** N/A
**Reference(s):** Starkey & Brown (2015)

## THERAPEUTIC INTERVENTIONS
# THERAPEUTIC EXERCISE—UPPER EXTREMITY

| NATA EC 5th | BOC RD6 | SKILL |
|---|---|---|
| TI-11a/b/d | D4-0401 | Upper Extremity Endurance (Shoulder) |

**Supplies Needed:** Table, elastic tubing

*This problem allows you the opportunity to demonstrate an* **upper extremity endurance exercise** *for the* **subscapularis muscle***. You have 3 minutes to complete this task.*

| Upper Extremity Endurance (Shoulder) | Course or Site / Assessor / Environment | | Test 1 | | Test 2 | | Test 3 |
|---|---|---|---|---|---|---|---|
| **Purpose of treatment** | | Y | N | Y | N | Y | N |
| Strength development | | O | O | O | O | O | O |
| **Tester places patient in appropriate position** | | Y | N | Y | N | Y | N |
| Standing facing away from a wall | | O | O | O | O | O | O |
| Attaches resistance tubing to a wall mounted rack | | O | O | O | O | O | O |
| Places resistance tubing in the patient's hand and instructs the patient to move arm to 90 degrees abduction and 90 degrees elbow extension | | O | O | O | O | O | O |
| **Tester performs the test according to accepted guidelines** | | Y | N | Y | N | Y | N |
| Instructs the patient to firmly grasp the resistance band | | O | O | O | O | O | O |
| Instructs the patient to perform shoulder internal rotation until humerus is parallel with the ground | | O | O | O | O | O | O |
| Instructs the patient to slowly return to starting position | | O | O | O | O | O | O |
| Perform two sets of 25 repetitions | | O | O | O | O | O | O |
| **Total** | | /8 | | /8 | | /8 | |
| **Must achieve >5 to pass this examination** | | P | F | P | F | P | F |

| Assessor: Date: | Test 1 Comments: |
|---|---|
| Assessor: Date: | Test 2 Comments: |
| Assessor: Date: | Test 3 Comments: |

**TEST ENVIRONMENTS**
**L:** Laboratory/Classroom
**C:** Clinical/Field Testing
**P:** Practicum
**A:** Assessment/Mock Exam

**TEST INFORMATION**
**Test Statistics:** N/A
**Reference(s):** Starkey & Brown (2015)

THERAPEUTIC INTERVENTIONS
# THERAPEUTIC EXERCISE—UPPER EXTREMITY

| NATA EC 5th | BOC RD6 | SKILL |
|---|---|---|
| TI-11a/b/d | D4-0401 | Upper Extremity Isometrics (Elbow) |

**Supplies Needed:** Table

*This problem allows you the opportunity to administer an* **upper extremity isometric exercise** *for* **elbow flexion**. *You have 3 minutes to complete this task.*

| Upper Extremity Isometrics (Elbow) | Course or Site Assessor Environment | | Test 1 | | Test 2 | | Test 3 |
|---|---|---|---|---|---|---|---|
| | | **Y** | **N** | **Y** | **N** | **Y** | **N** |
| **Purpose of treatment** | | Y | N | Y | N | Y | N |
| Strength development | | O | O | O | O | O | O |
| **Tester places patient in appropriate position** | | Y | N | Y | N | Y | N |
| The patient is seated | | O | O | O | O | O | O |
| The tester is seated next to the patient's involved limb | | O | O | O | O | O | O |
| **Tester performs the test according to accepted guidelines** | | Y | N | Y | N | Y | N |
| Places one hand on the proximal radioulnar joint and the other hand on the humerus for stabilization | | O | O | O | O | O | O |
| Instructs the patient to perform an isometric contraction for elbow flexion as manual resistance is applied | | O | O | O | O | O | O |
| Total | | __/5 | | __/5 | | __/5 | |
| Must achieve >3 to pass this examination | | P | F | P | F | P | F |

| Assessor: Date: | Test 1 Comments: |
|---|---|
| Assessor: Date: | Test 2 Comments: |
| Assessor: Date: | Test 3 Comments: |

**TEST ENVIRONMENTS**
L: Laboratory/Classroom
C: Clinical/Field Testing
P: Practicum
A: Assessment/Mock Exam

**TEST INFORMATION**
**Test Statistics:** N/A
**Reference(s):** Starkey & Brown (2015)

**THERAPEUTIC INTERVENTIONS**
# THERAPEUTIC EXERCISE—UPPER EXTREMITY

| NATA EC 5th | BOC RD6 | SKILL |
|---|---|---|
| TI-11a/b/d | D4-0401 | Upper Extremity Isometrics (Shoulder) |

**Supplies Needed:** Table

*This problem allows you the opportunity to administer an* **upper extremity isometric exercise** *for* **shoulder abduction**. *You have 3 minutes to complete this task.*

| Upper Extremity Isometrics (Shoulder) | Course or Site Assessor Environment | Test 1 | | Test 2 | | Test 3 | |
|---|---|---|---|---|---|---|---|
| **Purpose of treatment** | | Y | N | Y | N | Y | N |
| Strength development | | ○ | ○ | ○ | ○ | ○ | ○ |
| **Tester places patient in appropriate position** | | Y | N | Y | N | Y | N |
| The patient is standing | | ○ | ○ | ○ | ○ | ○ | ○ |
| The tester is seated in front of the patient | | ○ | ○ | ○ | ○ | ○ | ○ |
| **Tester performs the test according to accepted guidelines** | | Y | N | Y | N | Y | N |
| The tester places on hand on the lateral aspect of the elbow and the other hand on the AC joint for stabilization | | ○ | ○ | ○ | ○ | ○ | ○ |
| Instructs the patient to perform an isometric contraction for shoulder abduction as manual resistance is applied | | ○ | ○ | ○ | ○ | ○ | ○ |
| Total | | _/5 | | _/5 | | _/5 | |
| Must achieve >3 to pass this examination | | Ⓟ | Ⓕ | Ⓟ | Ⓕ | Ⓟ | Ⓕ |

| Assessor: Date: | Test 1 Comments: |
|---|---|
| Assessor: Date: | Test 2 Comments: |
| Assessor: Date: | Test 3 Comments: |

**TEST ENVIRONMENTS**
**L:** Laboratory/Classroom
**C:** Clinical/Field Testing
**P:** Practicum
**A:** Assessment/Mock Exam

**TEST INFORMATION**
**Test Statistics:** N/A
**Reference(s):** Starkey & Brown (2015)

# THERAPEUTIC EXERCISE—UPPER EXTREMITY

| NATA EC 5th | BOC RD6 | SKILL |
|---|---|---|
| TI-11a/b/d | D4-0401 | Upper Extremity Proprioception (Static) |

**Supplies Needed:** Table, Swiss or balance ball

*This problem allows you the opportunity to administer* **upper extremity proprioception (static)**. *You have 3 minutes to complete this task.*

| Upper Extremity Proprioception (Static) | Course or Site<br>Assessor<br>Environment | | Test 1 | | Test 2 | | Test 3 |
|---|---|---|---|---|---|---|---|
| **Purpose of treatment** | | **Y** | **N** | **Y** | **N** | **Y** | **N** |
| Increase upper extremity proprioception | | ○ | ○ | ○ | ○ | ○ | ○ |
| **Tester places patient in appropriate position** | | **Y** | **N** | **Y** | **N** | **Y** | **N** |
| Prone on a Swiss ball with feet off the floor and hands placed on the floor in front of the physio ball so that the patient assumes a planking position | | ○ | ○ | ○ | ○ | ○ | ○ |
| **Tester performs the test according to accepted guidelines** | | **Y** | **N** | **Y** | **N** | **Y** | **N** |
| Instructs the patient to contract core musculature | | ○ | ○ | ○ | ○ | ○ | ○ |
| Instructs the patient to raise uninvolved limb until it is parallel with the floor and hold for 30 seconds | | ○ | ○ | ○ | ○ | ○ | ○ |
| Instructs the patient to slowly lower arm back to starting position | | ○ | ○ | ○ | ○ | ○ | ○ |
| Total | | ___/5 | | ___/5 | | ___/5 | |
| Must achieve >3 to pass this examination | | Ⓟ | Ⓕ | Ⓟ | Ⓕ | Ⓟ | Ⓕ |

| Assessor:<br>Date: | Test 1 Comments: |
|---|---|
| Assessor:<br>Date: | Test 2 Comments: |
| Assessor:<br>Date: | Test 3 Comments: |

**TEST ENVIRONMENTS**
**L:** Laboratory/Classroom
**C:** Clinical/Field Testing
**P:** Practicum
**A:** Assessment/Mock Exam

**TEST INFORMATION**
**Test Statistics:** N/A
**Reference(s):** Houglum (2005)

# THERAPEUTIC EXERCISE—UPPER EXTREMITY

| NATA EC 5th | BOC RD6 | SKILL |
|---|---|---|
| TI-11a/b/d | D4-0401 | Upper Extremity Proprioception (Dynamic) |

**Supplies Needed:** Table, tape or Y-Balance Test Kit (Functional Movement Systems)

*This problem allows you the opportunity to administer the* **Y-balance upper quarter test for upper extremity dynamic proprioception**. *You have 3 minutes to complete this task.*

| Upper Extremity Proprioception (Dynamic) | Course or Site Assessor Environment | | Test 1 | | Test 2 | | Test 3 | |
|---|---|---|---|---|---|---|---|---|
| **Purpose of treatment** | | **Y** | **N** | **Y** | **N** | **Y** | **N** | |
| Increase upper extremity proprioception | | ○ | ○ | ○ | ○ | ○ | ○ | |
| **Tester places patient in appropriate position** | | **Y** | **N** | **Y** | **N** | **Y** | **N** | |
| The patient is in the quadruped position | | ○ | ○ | ○ | ○ | ○ | ○ | |
| The patient places testing hand on platform with thumb adducted while being aligned behind the starting red line | | ○ | ○ | ○ | ○ | ○ | ○ | |
| **Tester performs the test according to accepted guidelines** | | **Y** | **N** | **Y** | **N** | **Y** | **N** | |
| Instructs the patient to perform medial reach | | ○ | ○ | ○ | ○ | ○ | ○ | |
| Instructs the patient to perform inferolateral reach | | ○ | ○ | ○ | ○ | ○ | ○ | |
| Instructs the patient to perform superolateral reach | | ○ | ○ | ○ | ○ | ○ | ○ | |
| The patient should reach as far as possible but should not push the blocks when performing the reach | | ○ | ○ | ○ | ○ | ○ | ○ | |
| **Total** | | ___/7 | | ___/7 | | ___/7 | | |
| **Must achieve >4 to pass this examination** | | Ⓟ | Ⓕ | Ⓟ | Ⓕ | Ⓟ | Ⓕ | |

| Assessor: Date: | Test 1 Comments: |
|---|---|
| Assessor: Date: | Test 2 Comments: |
| Assessor: Date: | Test 3 Comments: |

**TEST ENVIRONMENTS**
**L:** Laboratory/Classroom
**C:** Clinical/Field Testing
**P:** Practicum
**A:** Assessment/Mock Exam

**TEST INFORMATION**
**Test Statistics:** N/A
**Reference(s):** Gorman et al. (2012)

THERAPEUTIC INTERVENTIONS

# THERAPEUTIC EXERCISE—UPPER EXTREMITY

| NATA EC 5th | BOC RD6 | SKILL |
|---|---|---|
| TI-11a/b/d | D4-0401 | Upper Extremity Strength (Elbow) |

**Supplies Needed:** Table, elastic tubing

*This problem allows you the opportunity to administer an* **upper extremity strength exercise** *for the* **elbow**. *You have 3 minutes to complete this task.*

| Upper Extremity Strength (Elbow) | Course or Site Assessor Environment | | Test 1 | | Test 2 | | Test 3 | |
|---|---|---|---|---|---|---|---|---|
| | | | Y | N | Y | N | Y | N |
| **Purpose of treatment** | | | Y | N | Y | N | Y | N |
| Strength development | | | ○ | ○ | ○ | ○ | ○ | ○ |
| **Tester places patient in appropriate position** | | | Y | N | Y | N | Y | N |
| Seated | | | ○ | ○ | ○ | ○ | ○ | ○ |
| Elbow fully supinated | | | ○ | ○ | ○ | ○ | ○ | ○ |
| Attaches resistance tubing to the wall on the same side as the limb being treated | | | ○ | ○ | ○ | ○ | ○ | ○ |
| The patient grasps the tubing | | | ○ | ○ | ○ | ○ | ○ | ○ |
| **Tester performs the test according to accepted guidelines** | | | Y | N | Y | N | Y | N |
| Instructs the patient to move the limb from full supination to full pronation | | | ○ | ○ | ○ | ○ | ○ | ○ |
| The patient slowly returns back to the starting position | | | ○ | ○ | ○ | ○ | ○ | ○ |
| Total | | | ___/7 | | ___/7 | | ___/7 | |
| Must achieve >4 to pass this examination | | | Ⓟ | Ⓕ | Ⓟ | Ⓕ | Ⓟ | Ⓕ |

| Assessor: Date: | Test 1 Comments: |
|---|---|
| Assessor: Date: | Test 2 Comments: |
| Assessor: Date: | Test 3 Comments: |

**TEST ENVIRONMENTS**
**L:** Laboratory/Classroom
**C:** Clinical/Field Testing
**P:** Practicum
**A:** Assessment/Mock Exam

**TEST INFORMATION**
**Test Statistics:** N/A
**Reference(s):** Starkey & Brown (2015)

THERAPEUTIC INTERVENTIONS
# THERAPEUTIC EXERCISE—UPPER EXTREMITY

| NATA EC 5th | BOC RD6 | SKILL |
|---|---|---|
| TI-11a/b/d | D4-0401 | Upper Extremity Strength (Hand) |

**Supplies Needed:** Table, 5-pound weight

*This problem allows you the opportunity to administer an* **upper extremity strength exercise** *for the* **hand.** *You have 3 minutes to complete this task.*

| Upper Extremity Strength (Hand) | Course or Site Assessor Environment | | | | | |
|---|---|---|---|---|---|---|
| | | Test 1 | | Test 2 | | Test 3 |
| **Purpose of treatment** | | Y | N | Y | N | Y | N |
| Strength development | | ○ | ○ | ○ | ○ | ○ | ○ |
| **Tester places patient in appropriate position** | | Y | N | Y | N | Y | N |
| Seated | | ○ | ○ | ○ | ○ | ○ | ○ |
| The patient firmly holds a 5-pound weight in hand | | ○ | ○ | ○ | ○ | ○ | ○ |
| Elbow and forearm are supported by the table | | ○ | ○ | ○ | ○ | ○ | ○ |
| Wrist is placed in full ulnar deviation | | ○ | ○ | ○ | ○ | ○ | ○ |
| **Tester performs the test according to accepted guidelines** | | Y | N | Y | N | Y | N |
| The patient moves from full ulnar deviation to radial deviation | | ○ | ○ | ○ | ○ | ○ | ○ |
| The patient slowly returns to starting position | | ○ | ○ | ○ | ○ | ○ | ○ |
| Total | | ___/7 | | ___/7 | | ___/7 |
| **Must achieve >4 to pass this examination** | | Ⓟ | Ⓕ | Ⓟ | Ⓕ | Ⓟ | Ⓕ |

| Assessor: Date: | Test 1 Comments: |
|---|---|
| Assessor: Date: | Test 2 Comments: |
| Assessor: Date: | Test 3 Comments: |

**TEST ENVIRONMENTS**
L: Laboratory/Classroom
C: Clinical/Field Testing
P: Practicum
A: Assessment/Mock Exam

**TEST INFORMATION**
**Test Statistics:** N/A
**Reference(s):** Starkey & Brown (2015)

THERAPEUTIC INTERVENTIONS
# THERAPEUTIC EXERCISE—UPPER EXTREMITY

| NATA EC 5th | BOC RD6 | SKILL |
|---|---|---|
| TI-11a/b/d | D4-0401 | Upper Extremity Strength (Shoulder) |

**Supplies Needed:** Table, 5-pound weight

*This problem allows you the opportunity to administer an* **upper extremity strength exercise** *for the* **shoulder.** *You have 3 minutes to complete this task.*

| Upper Extremity Strength (Shoulder) | Course or Site Assessor Environment | Test 1 | | Test 2 | | Test 3 | |
|---|---|---|---|---|---|---|---|
| **Purpose of treatment** | | Y | N | Y | N | Y | N |
| Strength development | | O | O | O | O | O | O |
| **Tester places patient in appropriate position** | | Y | N | Y | N | Y | N |
| Standing | | O | O | O | O | O | O |
| Elbow in neutral | | O | O | O | O | O | O |
| Shoulder is internally rotated | | O | O | O | O | O | O |
| Shoulder is in the plane of the scapula | | O | O | O | O | O | O |
| The patient firmly grasps a 5-pound weight in the involved hand | | O | O | O | O | O | O |
| **Tester performs the test according to accepted guidelines** | | Y | N | Y | N | Y | N |
| The patient moves the arm through the plane of the scapula (forearm should be in neutral) | | O | O | O | O | O | O |
| The patient performs external rotation while raising arm through plane of the scapula | | O | O | O | O | O | O |
| The patient raises arm until it is parallel to the floor | | O | O | O | O | O | O |
| The patient slowly returns to the starting position | | O | O | O | O | O | O |
| Total | | /10 | | /10 | | /10 | |
| Must achieve >7 to pass this examination | | P | F | P | F | P | F |

| Assessor: Date: | Test 1 Comments: |
|---|---|
| Assessor: Date: | Test 2 Comments: |
| Assessor: Date: | Test 3 Comments: |

**TEST ENVIRONMENTS**
**L:** Laboratory/Classroom
**C:** Clinical/Field Testing
**P:** Practicum
**A:** Assessment/Mock Exam

**TEST INFORMATION**
**Test Statistics:** N/A
**Reference(s):** Starkey & Brown (2015)

**THERAPEUTIC INTERVENTIONS**
# THERAPEUTIC EXERCISE—UPPER EXTREMITY

| NATA EC 5th | BOC RD6 | SKILL |
|---|---|---|
| TI-11a/b/d | D4-0401 | Upper Extremity Strength (Wrist) |

**Supplies Needed:** Table

*This problem allows you the opportunity to administer an* **upper extremity strength exercise** *for the* **wrist**. *You have 3 minutes to complete this task.*

| Upper Extremity Strength (Wrist) | Course or Site Assessor Environment | Test 1 | | Test 2 | | Test 3 | |
|---|---|---|---|---|---|---|---|
| **Purpose of treatment** | | **Y** | **N** | **Y** | **N** | **Y** | **N** |
| Strength development | | ○ | ○ | ○ | ○ | ○ | ○ |
| **Tester places patient in appropriate position** | | **Y** | **N** | **Y** | **N** | **Y** | **N** |
| Seated | | ○ | ○ | ○ | ○ | ○ | ○ |
| Wrist/lower arm hanging over the edge of the table | | ○ | ○ | ○ | ○ | ○ | ○ |
| Wrist in full extension | | ○ | ○ | ○ | ○ | ○ | ○ |
| Places one hand on the palmar surface of the hand and other hand on the distal radioulnar joint | | ○ | ○ | ○ | ○ | ○ | ○ |
| **Tester performs the test according to accepted guidelines** | | **Y** | **N** | **Y** | **N** | **Y** | **N** |
| The patient is instructed to concentrically contract the wrist flexors | | ○ | ○ | ○ | ○ | ○ | ○ |
| The tester applies manual resistance against wrist flexion | | ○ | ○ | ○ | ○ | ○ | ○ |
| **Total** | | ___/7 | | ___/7 | | ___/7 | |
| **Must achieve >4 to pass this examination** | | Ⓟ | Ⓕ | Ⓟ | Ⓕ | Ⓟ | Ⓕ |
| **Assessor:** **Date:** | Test 1 Comments: | | | | | | |
| **Assessor:** **Date:** | Test 2 Comments: | | | | | | |
| **Assessor:** **Date:** | Test 3 Comments: | | | | | | |

**TEST ENVIRONMENTS**
**L:** Laboratory/Classroom
**C:** Clinical/Field Testing
**P:** Practicum
**A:** Assessment/Mock Exam

**TEST INFORMATION**
**Test Statistics:** N/A
**Reference(s):** Starkey & Brown (2015)

# PROPRIOCEPTIVE NEUROMUSCULAR FACILITATION—STRETCHING

| NATA EC 5th | BOC RD6 | SKILL |
|---|---|---|
| TI-11a/b/d | D4-0401 | PNF: Contract/Relax (Wrist Flexors) |

**Supplies Needed:** Table, chair

*This problem allows you the opportunity to demonstrate the PNF technique known as* **contract/relax** *to restore flexibility and coordination of the* **wrist**. *You have 2 minutes to complete this task.*

| PNF: Contract/Relax (Wrist Flexors) | Course or Site Assessor Environment | | Test 1 | | Test 2 | | Test 3 | |
|---|---|---|---|---|---|---|---|---|
| | | | Y | N | Y | N | Y | N |
| **Purpose of treatment** | | | Y | N | Y | N | Y | N |
| Restore flexibility and coordination of the wrist | | | O | O | O | O | O | O |
| **Patient education/safety** | | | Y | N | Y | N | Y | N |
| Explains to the patient why the exercise is appropriate | | | O | O | O | O | O | O |
| Explains to the patient what the expected treatment goals and outcomes are | | | O | O | O | O | O | O |
| Explains to the patient what he/she should or should not feel | | | O | O | O | O | O | O |
| Reviews precautions/contraindications with the patient | | | O | O | O | O | O | O |
| **Tester places patient in appropriate position** | | | Y | N | Y | N | Y | N |
| Seated with the wrist in full extension and forearm supinated | | | O | O | O | O | O | O |
| **Tester administers the therapeutic exercise according to accepted guidelines** | | | Y | N | Y | N | Y | N |
| Stabilizes the radius and ulna | | | O | O | O | O | O | O |
| Passively stretches the wrist flexors to end range (instructs "relax") and holds position for 6 to 10 seconds | | | O | O | O | O | O | O |
| The patient is instructed to "contract" the wrist flexors isotonically against moderate resistance over the palmar aspect of the patient's hand for 10 seconds or until fatigue | | | O | O | O | O | O | O |
| Instructs "relax" and again applies a passive stretch to the wrist flexors, increasing the end range | | | O | O | O | O | O | O |
| **Termination of treatment** | | | Y | N | Y | N | Y | N |
| Repeats treatment to accepted guidelines (three times) | | | O | O | O | O | O | O |
| Provides the patient with feedback | | | O | O | O | O | O | O |
| Documents the treatment | | | O | O | O | O | O | O |
| | Total | | ___/13 | | ___/13 | | ___/13 | |

*(continued on the next page)*

| Must achieve >9 to pass this examination | Ⓟ | Ⓕ | Ⓟ | Ⓕ | Ⓟ | Ⓕ |
|---|---|---|---|---|---|---|
| **Assessor:**<br>**Date:** | **Test 1 Comments:** | | | | | |
| **Assessor:**<br>**Date:** | **Test 2 Comments:** | | | | | |
| **Assessor:**<br>**Date:** | **Test 3 Comments:** | | | | | |

**TEST ENVIRONMENTS**
**L:** Laboratory/Classroom
**C:** Clinical/Field Testing
**P:** Practicum
**A:** Assessment/Mock Exam

**TEST INFORMATION**
**Test Statistics:** N/A
**Reference(s):**  Houglum (2005)
Prentice (2014)

# PROPRIOCEPTIVE NEUROMUSCULAR FACILITATION—STRETCHING

| NATA EC 5th | BOC RD6 | SKILL |
|---|---|---|
| TI-11a/b/d | D4-0401 | PNF: Contract/Relax (Hip Extensors/Hamstrings) |

**Supplies Needed:** Table

*This problem allows you the opportunity to demonstrate the PNF technique known as* **contract/relax** *to restore flexibility and coordination of the* **hip**. *You have 2 minutes to complete this task.*

| PNF: Contract/Relax (Hip Extensors/Hamstrings) — Course or Site / Assessor / Environment | Test 1 | | Test 2 | | Test 3 | |
|---|---|---|---|---|---|---|
| **Purpose of treatment** | Y | N | Y | N | Y | N |
| Restore flexibility and coordination of the hip | O | O | O | O | O | O |
| **Patient education/safety** | Y | N | Y | N | Y | N |
| Explains to the patient why the exercise is appropriate | O | O | O | O | O | O |
| Explains to the patient what the expected treatment goals and outcomes are | O | O | O | O | O | O |
| Explains to the patient what he/she should or should not feel | O | O | O | O | O | O |
| Reviews precautions/contraindications with the patient | O | O | O | O | O | O |
| **Tester places patient in appropriate position** | Y | N | Y | N | Y | N |
| Supine with knees in extension | O | O | O | O | O | O |
| **Tester administers the therapeutic exercise according to accepted guidelines** | Y | N | Y | N | Y | N |
| Places stabilizing hand on anterior thigh (superior to patella) | O | O | O | O | O | O |
| Places force hand on distal posterior ankle | O | O | O | O | O | O |
| Passively flexes the hip while maintaining knee extension to end range | O | O | O | O | O | O |
| Instructs "relax" and holds stretch for 6 to 10 seconds | O | O | O | O | O | O |
| The patient is instructed to "contract" the hip extensors isotonically against moderate resistance over the posterior aspect of the patient's ankle for 10 seconds or until fatigue | O | O | O | O | O | O |
| Instructs "relax" and again applies a passive stretch to the hip extensors, increasing the end range | O | O | O | O | O | O |
| **Termination of treatment** | Y | N | Y | N | Y | N |
| Repeats treatment to accepted guidelines (three times) | O | O | O | O | O | O |
| Provides the patient with feedback | O | O | O | O | O | O |
| Documents the treatment | O | O | O | O | O | O |
| **Total** | __/15 | | __/15 | | __/15 | |

*(continued on the next page)*

| Must achieve >9 to pass this examination | Ⓟ | Ⓕ | Ⓟ | Ⓕ | Ⓟ | Ⓕ |
|---|---|---|---|---|---|---|
| **Assessor:** **Date:** | **Test 1 Comments:** | | | | | |
| **Assessor:** **Date:** | **Test 2 Comments:** | | | | | |
| **Assessor:** **Date:** | **Test 3 Comments:** | | | | | |

**TEST ENVIRONMENTS**
**L:** Laboratory/Classroom
**C:** Clinical/Field Testing
**P:** Practicum
**A:** Assessment/Mock Exam

**TEST INFORMATION**
**Test Statistics:** N/A
**Reference(s):**   Houglum (2005)
                    Prentice (2014)

# PROPRIOCEPTIVE NEUROMUSCULAR FACILITATION—STRETCHING

| NATA EC 5th | BOC RD6 | SKILL |
|---|---|---|
| TI-11a/b/d | D4-0401 | PNF: Hold/Relax (Wrist Flexors) |

**Supplies Needed:** Table, chair

*This problem allows you the opportunity to demonstrate the PNF technique known as* **hold/relax** *to restore flexibility and coordination of the* **wrist**. *You have 2 minutes to complete this task.*

| PNF: Hold/Relax (Wrist Flexors) | Course or Site Assessor Environment | | Test 1 | | Test 2 | | Test 3 | |
|---|---|---|---|---|---|---|---|---|
| **Purpose of treatment** | | | **Y** | **N** | **Y** | **N** | **Y** | **N** |
| Restore flexibility and coordination of the wrist | | | O | O | O | O | O | O |
| **Patient education/safety** | | | **Y** | **N** | **Y** | **N** | **Y** | **N** |
| Explains to the patient why the exercise is appropriate | | | O | O | O | O | O | O |
| Explains to the patient what the expected treatment goals and outcomes are | | | O | O | O | O | O | O |
| Explains to the patient what he/she should or should not feel | | | O | O | O | O | O | O |
| Reviews precautions/contraindications with the patient | | | O | O | O | O | O | O |
| **Tester places patient in appropriate position** | | | **Y** | **N** | **Y** | **N** | **Y** | **N** |
| Seated with the wrist in full extension and forearm supinated | | | O | O | O | O | O | O |
| **Tester administers the therapeutic exercise according to accepted guidelines** | | | **Y** | **N** | **Y** | **N** | **Y** | **N** |
| Stabilizes the radius and ulna | | | O | O | O | O | O | O |
| Passively stretches the wrist flexors to end range (instructs "relax") and holds position for 6 to 10 seconds | | | O | O | O | O | O | O |
| The patient is instructed to "contract" the wrist flexors isometrically against moderate resistance over the palmar aspect of the patient's hand for 10 seconds or until fatigue | | | O | O | O | O | O | O |
| Instructs "relax" and again applies a passive stretch to the wrist flexors, increasing the end range | | | O | O | O | O | O | O |
| **Termination of treatment** | | | **Y** | **N** | **Y** | **N** | **Y** | **N** |
| Repeats treatment to accepted guidelines (three times) | | | O | O | O | O | O | O |
| Provides the patient with feedback | | | O | O | O | O | O | O |
| Documents the treatment | | | O | O | O | O | O | O |
| | Total | | ___/13 | | ___/13 | | ___/13 | |

*(continued on the next page)*

| Must achieve >9 to pass this examination | Ⓟ | Ⓕ | Ⓟ | Ⓕ | Ⓟ | Ⓕ |
|---|---|---|---|---|---|---|
| **Assessor:**<br>**Date:** | **Test 1 Comments:** | | | | | |
| **Assessor:**<br>**Date:** | **Test 2 Comments:** | | | | | |
| **Assessor:**<br>**Date:** | **Test 3 Comments:** | | | | | |

## TEST ENVIRONMENTS
**L:** Laboratory/Classroom
**C:** Clinical/Field Testing
**P:** Practicum
**A:** Assessment/Mock Exam

## TEST INFORMATION
**Test Statistics:** N/A
**Reference(s):**  Houglum (2005)
                   Prentice (2014)

# PROPRIOCEPTIVE NEUROMUSCULAR FACILITATION—STRETCHING

| NATA EC 5th | BOC RD6 | SKILL |
|---|---|---|
| TI-11a/b/d | D4-0401 | PNF: Hold/Relax (Hip Extensors/Hamstrings) |

**Supplies Needed:** Table

*This problem allows you the opportunity to demonstrate the PNF technique known as* **hold/relax** *to restore flexibility, strength, and coordination of the* **hip**. *You have 2 minutes to complete this task.*

| PNF: Hold/Relax (Hip Extensors/Hamstrings) | Course or Site Assessor Environment | | Test 1 | | Test 2 | | Test 3 | |
|---|---|---|---|---|---|---|---|---|
| | | | Y | N | Y | N | Y | N |
| **Purpose of treatment** | | | Y | N | Y | N | Y | N |
| Restore flexibility, strength, and coordination of the hip | | | O | O | O | O | O | O |
| **Patient education/safety** | | | Y | N | Y | N | Y | N |
| Explains to the patient why the exercise is appropriate | | | O | O | O | O | O | O |
| Explains to the patient what the expected treatment goals and outcomes are | | | O | O | O | O | O | O |
| Explains to the patient what he/she should or should not feel | | | O | O | O | O | O | O |
| Reviews precautions/contraindications with the patient | | | O | O | O | O | O | O |
| **Tester places patient in appropriate position** | | | Y | N | Y | N | Y | N |
| Supine with knees in extension | | | O | O | O | O | O | O |
| **Tester administers the therapeutic exercise according to accepted guidelines** | | | Y | N | Y | N | Y | N |
| Places stabilizing hand on anterior thigh (superior to patella) | | | O | O | O | O | O | O |
| Places force hand on distal posterior ankle | | | O | O | O | O | O | O |
| Passively flexes the hip while maintaining knee extension to end range | | | O | O | O | O | O | O |
| Instructs "relax" and holds stretch for 6 to 10 seconds | | | O | O | O | O | O | O |
| The patient is instructed to "contract" the hip extensors isometrically against moderate resistance over the posterior aspect of the patient's ankle for 10 seconds or until fatigue | | | O | O | O | O | O | O |
| Instructs "relax" and again applies a passive stretch to hip extensors, increasing the end range | | | O | O | O | O | O | O |
| **Termination of treatment** | | | Y | N | Y | N | Y | N |
| Repeats treatment to accepted guidelines (three times) | | | O | O | O | O | O | O |
| Provides the patient with feedback | | | O | O | O | O | O | O |
| Documents the treatment | | | O | O | O | O | O | O |
| **Total** | | | __/15 | | __/15 | | __/15 | |

(continued on the next page)

| Must achieve >9 to pass this examination | Ⓟ | Ⓕ | Ⓟ | Ⓕ | Ⓟ | Ⓕ |
|---|---|---|---|---|---|---|
| **Assessor:** **Date:** | **Test 1 Comments:** | | | | | |
| **Assessor:** **Date:** | **Test 2 Comments:** | | | | | |
| **Assessor:** **Date:** | **Test 3 Comments:** | | | | | |

## TEST ENVIRONMENTS
**L:** Laboratory/Classroom
**C:** Clinical/Field Testing
**P:** Practicum
**A:** Assessment/Mock Exam

## TEST INFORMATION
**Test Statistics:** N/A
**Reference(s):**  Houglum (2005)
             Prentice (2014)

THERAPEUTIC INTERVENTIONS
# PROPRIOCEPTIVE NEUROMUSCULAR FACILITATION—STRETCHING

| NATA EC 5th | BOC RD6 | SKILL |
|---|---|---|
| TI-11a/b/d | D4-0401 | PNF: Slow-Reversal-Hold-Relax (Wrist Flexors) |

**Supplies Needed:** Table, chair

*This problem allows you the opportunity to demonstrate the PNF technique known as* **slow-reversal-hold-relax** *to restore flexibility and coordination of the* **wrist***. You have 2 minutes to complete this task.*

| PNF: Slow-Reversal-Hold-Relax (Wrist Flexors) | Course or Site Assessor Environment | Test 1 | | Test 2 | | Test 3 | |
|---|---|---|---|---|---|---|---|
| **Purpose of treatment** | | **Y** | **N** | **Y** | **N** | **Y** | **N** |
| Restore flexibility and coordination of the wrist | | O | O | O | O | O | O |
| **Patient education/safety** | | **Y** | **N** | **Y** | **N** | **Y** | **N** |
| Explains to the patient why the exercise is appropriate | | O | O | O | O | O | O |
| Explains to the patient what the expected treatment goals and outcomes are | | O | O | O | O | O | O |
| Explains to the patient what he/she should or should not feel | | O | O | O | O | O | O |
| Reviews precautions/contraindications with the patient | | O | O | O | O | O | O |
| **Tester places patient in appropriate position** | | **Y** | **N** | **Y** | **N** | **Y** | **N** |
| Seated with the wrist in full extension and forearm supinated | | O | O | O | O | O | O |
| **Tester administers the therapeutic exercise according to accepted guidelines** | | **Y** | **N** | **Y** | **N** | **Y** | **N** |
| Stabilizes the radius and ulna | | O | O | O | O | O | O |
| Instructs the patient to concentrically contract the wrist extensors to the end range of extension | | O | O | O | O | O | O |
| The patient is instructed to "contract" the wrist flexors isometrically against moderate resistance over the palmar aspect of the patient's hand for 10 seconds or until fatigue | | O | O | O | O | O | O |
| The patient is again instructed to concentrically contract the wrist extensors to the new end range of extension | | O | O | O | O | O | O |
| **Termination of treatment** | | **Y** | **N** | **Y** | **N** | **Y** | **N** |
| Repeats treatment to accepted guidelines (three times) | | O | O | O | O | O | O |
| Provides the patient with feedback | | O | O | O | O | O | O |
| Documents the treatment | | O | O | O | O | O | O |
| **Total** | | ___/13 | | ___/13 | | ___/13 | |

*(continued on the next page)*

| Must achieve >9 to pass this examination | P | F | P | F | P | F |
|---|---|---|---|---|---|---|
| **Assessor:**<br>**Date:** | **Test 1 Comments:** | | | | | |
| **Assessor:**<br>**Date:** | **Test 2 Comments:** | | | | | |
| **Assessor:**<br>**Date:** | **Test 3 Comments:** | | | | | |

### TEST ENVIRONMENTS
**L:** Laboratory/Classroom
**C:** Clinical/Field Testing
**P:** Practicum
**A:** Assessment/Mock Exam

### TEST INFORMATION
**Test Statistics:** N/A
**Reference(s):** Houglum (2005)
Prentice (2014)

# PROPRIOCEPTIVE NEUROMUSCULAR FACILITATION—STRETCHING

| NATA EC 5th | BOC RD6 | SKILL |
|---|---|---|
| TI-11a/b/d | D4-0401 | PNF: Slow-Reversal-Hold-Relax (Hip Extensors/Hamstrings) |

**Supplies Needed:** Table

*This problem allows you the opportunity to demonstrate the PNF technique known as* **slow-reversal-hold-relax** *to restore flexibility, strength, and coordination of the* **hip**. *You have 2 minutes to complete this task.*

| PNF: Slow-Reversal-Hold-Relax (Hip Extensors/Hamstrings) | Course or Site Assessor Environment | | Test 1 | | Test 2 | | Test 3 |
|---|---|---|---|---|---|---|---|
| **Purpose of treatment** | | Y | N | Y | N | Y | N |
| Restore flexibility, strength, and coordination of the hip | | O | O | O | O | O | O |
| **Patient education/safety** | | Y | N | Y | N | Y | N |
| Explains to the patient why the exercise is appropriate | | O | O | O | O | O | O |
| Explains to the patient what the expected treatment goals and outcomes are | | O | O | O | O | O | O |
| Explains to the patient what he/she should or should not feel | | O | O | O | O | O | O |
| Reviews precautions/contraindications with the patient | | O | O | O | O | O | O |
| **Tester places patient in appropriate position** | | Y | N | Y | N | Y | N |
| Supine with knees in extension | | O | O | O | O | O | O |
| **Tester administers the therapeutic exercise according to accepted guidelines** | | Y | N | Y | N | Y | N |
| Places stabilizing hand on anterior thigh (superior to patella) | | O | O | O | O | O | O |
| Places force hand on distal posterior ankle | | O | O | O | O | O | O |
| Passively flexes the hip while maintaining knee extension to end range | | O | O | O | O | O | O |
| Instructs the patient to concentrically contract the hip flexors to the end range of flexion | | O | O | O | O | O | O |
| The patient is instructed to "contract" the hip extensors isometrically against moderate resistance over the posterior aspect of the patient's ankle for 10 seconds or until fatigue | | O | O | O | O | O | O |
| Again instructs the patient to concentrically contract the hip flexors to the new end range of flexion | | O | O | O | O | O | O |
| **Termination of treatment** | | Y | N | Y | N | Y | N |
| Repeats treatment to accepted guidelines (three times) | | O | O | O | O | O | O |
| Provides the patient with feedback | | O | O | O | O | O | O |
| Documents the treatment | | O | O | O | O | O | O |
| **Total** | | ___/15 | | ___/15 | | ___/15 | |

*(continued on the next page)*

| Must achieve >9 to pass this examination | P | F | P | F | P | F |
|---|---|---|---|---|---|---|
| **Assessor:** <br> **Date:** | **Test 1 Comments:** | | | | | |
| **Assessor:** <br> **Date:** | **Test 2 Comments:** | | | | | |
| **Assessor:** <br> **Date:** | **Test 3 Comments:** | | | | | |

**TEST ENVIRONMENTS**
**L:** Laboratory/Classroom
**C:** Clinical/Field Testing
**P:** Practicum
**A:** Assessment/Mock Exam

**TEST INFORMATION**
**Test Statistics:** N/A
**Reference(s):** Houglum (2005)
Prentice (2014)

# PROPRIOCEPTIVE NEUROMUSCULAR FACILITATION—STRENGTHENING

| NATA EC 5th | BOC RD6 | SKILL |
|---|---|---|
| TI-11a/b/d | D4-0401 | PNF: Rhythmic Initiation (Elbow Flexors) |

**Supplies Needed:** Table, bolster

*This problem allows you the opportunity to demonstrate the PNF technique known as **rhythmic initiation** to restore flexibility, strength, and coordination of the **elbow**. You have 2 minutes to complete this task.*

| PNF: Rhythmic Initiation (Elbow Flexors) | Course or Site _____ Assessor _____ Environment _____ | | Test 1 | | Test 2 | | Test 3 | |
|---|---|---|---|---|---|---|---|---|
| **Purpose of treatment** | | **Y** | **N** | **Y** | **N** | **Y** | **N** | |
| Increase a muscle's ability to initiate movement and stabilize | | ○ | ○ | ○ | ○ | ○ | ○ | |
| **Patient education/safety** | | **Y** | **N** | **Y** | **N** | **Y** | **N** | |
| Explains to the patient why the exercise is appropriate | | ○ | ○ | ○ | ○ | ○ | ○ | |
| Explains to the patient what the expected treatment goals and outcomes are | | ○ | ○ | ○ | ○ | ○ | ○ | |
| Explains to the patient what he/she should or should not feel | | ○ | ○ | ○ | ○ | ○ | ○ | |
| Reviews precautions/contraindications with the patient | | ○ | ○ | ○ | ○ | ○ | ○ | |
| **Tester places patient in appropriate position** | | **Y** | **N** | **Y** | **N** | **Y** | **N** | |
| Supine on table with bolster under knee | | ○ | ○ | ○ | ○ | ○ | ○ | |
| **Tester administers the therapeutic exercise according to accepted guidelines** | | **Y** | **N** | **Y** | **N** | **Y** | **N** | |
| Passively and repeatedly moves the elbow into flexion and supination while instructing the patient in the movement pattern until movement is learned | | ○ | ○ | ○ | ○ | ○ | ○ | |
| Instructs the patient to actively flex the elbow, repeating the previous movement pattern | | ○ | ○ | ○ | ○ | ○ | ○ | |
| Adds resistance against the movement pattern | | ○ | ○ | ○ | ○ | ○ | ○ | |
| **Termination of treatment** | | **Y** | **N** | **Y** | **N** | **Y** | **N** | |
| Repeats treatment to accepted guidelines | | ○ | ○ | ○ | ○ | ○ | ○ | |
| Provides the patient with feedback | | ○ | ○ | ○ | ○ | ○ | ○ | |
| Documents the treatment | | ○ | ○ | ○ | ○ | ○ | ○ | |
| **Total** | | ___/12 | | ___/12 | | ___/12 | | |

*(continued on the next page)*

| Must achieve >9 to pass this examination | (P) | (F) | (P) | (F) | (P) | (F) |
|---|---|---|---|---|---|---|

| **Assessor:** **Date:** | **Test 1 Comments:** |
|---|---|
| **Assessor:** **Date:** | **Test 2 Comments:** |
| **Assessor:** **Date:** | **Test 3 Comments:** |

**TEST ENVIRONMENTS**
**L:** Laboratory/Classroom
**C:** Clinical/Field Testing
**P:** Practicum
**A:** Assessment/Mock Exam

**TEST INFORMATION**
**Test Statistics:** N/A
**Reference(s):** Houglum (2005)
Prentice (2014)

## THERAPEUTIC INTERVENTIONS
# PROPRIOCEPTIVE NEUROMUSCULAR FACILITATION—STRENGTHENING

| NATA EC 5th | BOC RD6 | SKILL |
|---|---|---|
| TI-11a/b/d | D4-0401 | PNF: Rhythmic Initiation (Ankle Dorsiflexors) |

**Supplies Needed:** Table

*This problem allows you the opportunity to demonstrate the PNF technique known as* **rhythmic initiation** *to restore flexibility, strength, and coordination of the* **ankle**. *You have 2 minutes to complete this task.*

| PNF: Rhythmic Initiation (Ankle Dorsiflexors) | Course or Site Assessor Environment | | Test 1 | | Test 2 | | Test 3 | |
|---|---|---|---|---|---|---|---|---|
| **Purpose of treatment** | | **Y** | **N** | **Y** | **N** | **Y** | **N** | |
| Increase a muscle's ability to initiate movement and stabilize | | ○ | ○ | ○ | ○ | ○ | ○ | |
| **Patient education/safety** | | **Y** | **N** | **Y** | **N** | **Y** | **N** | |
| Explains to the patient why the exercise is appropriate | | ○ | ○ | ○ | ○ | ○ | ○ | |
| Explains to the patient what the expected treatment goals and outcomes are | | ○ | ○ | ○ | ○ | ○ | ○ | |
| Explains to the patient what he/she should or should not feel | | ○ | ○ | ○ | ○ | ○ | ○ | |
| Reviews precautions/contraindications with the patient | | ○ | ○ | ○ | ○ | ○ | ○ | |
| **Tester places patient in appropriate position** | | **Y** | **N** | **Y** | **N** | **Y** | **N** | |
| Supine with knees in extension | | ○ | ○ | ○ | ○ | ○ | ○ | |
| **Tester administers the therapeutic exercise according to accepted guidelines** | | **Y** | **N** | **Y** | **N** | **Y** | **N** | |
| Passively and repeatedly moves the ankle into dorsiflexion while instructing the patient in the movement pattern until movement is learned | | ○ | ○ | ○ | ○ | ○ | ○ | |
| Instructs the patient to actively dorsiflex the ankle, repeating the previous movement pattern | | ○ | ○ | ○ | ○ | ○ | ○ | |
| Adds resistance against the movement pattern | | ○ | ○ | ○ | ○ | ○ | ○ | |
| **Termination of treatment** | | **Y** | **N** | **Y** | **N** | **Y** | **N** | |
| Repeats treatment to accepted guidelines | | ○ | ○ | ○ | ○ | ○ | ○ | |
| Provides the patient with feedback | | ○ | ○ | ○ | ○ | ○ | ○ | |
| Documents the treatment | | ○ | ○ | ○ | ○ | ○ | ○ | |
| **Total** | | ___/12 | | ___/12 | | ___/12 | | |

*(continued on the next page)*

| Must achieve >8 to pass this examination | Ⓟ | Ⓕ | Ⓟ | Ⓕ | Ⓟ | Ⓕ |
|---|---|---|---|---|---|---|
| **Assessor:** **Date:** | **Test 1 Comments:** | | | | | |
| **Assessor:** **Date:** | **Test 2 Comments:** | | | | | |
| **Assessor:** **Date:** | **Test 3 Comments:** | | | | | |

## TEST ENVIRONMENTS
**L:** Laboratory/Classroom
**C:** Clinical/Field Testing
**P:** Practicum
**A:** Assessment/Mock Exam

## TEST INFORMATION
**Test Statistics:** N/A
**Reference(s):**   Houglum (2005)
                    Prentice (2014)

# PROPRIOCEPTIVE NEUROMUSCULAR FACILITATION—STRENGTHENING

| NATA EC 5th | BOC RD6 | SKILL |
|---|---|---|
| TI-11a/b/d | D4-0401 | PNF: Repeated Contraction (Ankle Dorsiflexors) |

**Supplies Needed:** Table

*This problem allows you the opportunity to demonstrate the PNF technique known as* **repeated contraction** *to restore flexibility, strength, and coordination of the* **ankle***. You have 2 minutes to complete this task.*

| PNF: Repeated Contraction (Ankle Dorsiflexors) | Course or Site Assessor Environment | | Test 1 | | Test 2 | | Test 3 | |
|---|---|---|---|---|---|---|---|---|
| **Purpose of treatment** | | **Y** | **N** | **Y** | **N** | **Y** | **N** | |
| Increase a muscle's ability to initiate movement and stabilize | | O | O | O | O | O | O | |
| **Patient education/safety** | | **Y** | **N** | **Y** | **N** | **Y** | **N** | |
| Explains to the patient why the exercise is appropriate | | O | O | O | O | O | O | |
| Explains to the patient what the expected treatment goals and outcomes are | | O | O | O | O | O | O | |
| Explains to the patient what he/she should or should not feel | | O | O | O | O | O | O | |
| Reviews precautions/contraindications with the patient | | O | O | O | O | O | O | |
| **Tester places patient in appropriate position** | | **Y** | **N** | **Y** | **N** | **Y** | **N** | |
| Supine with knees in extension | | O | O | O | O | O | O | |
| **Tester administers the therapeutic exercise according to accepted guidelines** | | **Y** | **N** | **Y** | **N** | **Y** | **N** | |
| Instructs the patient to actively dorsiflex the ankle while providing resistance until fatigue | | O | O | O | O | O | O | |
| Once fatigue is felt, the tester places a stretch on the muscle to facilitate more strength production | | O | O | O | O | O | O | |
| **Termination of treatment** | | **Y** | **N** | **Y** | **N** | **Y** | **N** | |
| Repeats treatment to accepted guidelines | | O | O | O | O | O | O | |
| Provides the patient with feedback | | O | O | O | O | O | O | |
| Documents the treatment | | O | O | O | O | O | O | |
| **Total** | | ___/11 | | ___/11 | | ___/11 | | |

*(continued on the next page)*

| Must achieve >8 to pass this examination | (P) | (F) | (P) | (F) | (P) | (F) |
|---|---|---|---|---|---|---|
| **Assessor:** **Date:** | **Test 1 Comments:** | | | | | |
| **Assessor:** **Date:** | **Test 2 Comments:** | | | | | |
| **Assessor:** **Date:** | **Test 3 Comments:** | | | | | |

**TEST ENVIRONMENTS**
**L:** Laboratory/Classroom
**C:** Clinical/Field Testing
**P:** Practicum
**A:** Assessment/Mock Exam

**TEST INFORMATION**
**Test Statistics:** N/A
**Reference(s):**  Houglum (2005)
Prentice (2014)

## THERAPEUTIC INTERVENTIONS
# PROPRIOCEPTIVE NEUROMUSCULAR FACILITATION—STRENGTHENING

| NATA EC 5th | BOC RD6 | SKILL |
|---|---|---|
| TI-11a/b/d | D4-0401 | PNF: Slow Reversal (Lower Extremity D1 Flexion) |

**Supplies Needed:** Table

*This problem allows you the opportunity to demonstrate the PNF technique known as **slow reversal** to restore flexibility, strength, and coordination in **lower extremity D1 flexion**. You have 2 minutes to complete this task.*

| PNF: Slow Reversal (Lower Extremity D1 Flexion) | Course or Site / Assessor / Environment | | Test 1 | | Test 2 | | Test 3 |
|---|---|---|---|---|---|---|---|
| **Purpose of treatment** | | Y | N | Y | N | Y | N |
| Increase a muscle's ability to initiate movement and stabilize | | O | O | O | O | O | O |
| **Patient education/safety** | | Y | N | Y | N | Y | N |
| Explains to the patient why the exercise is appropriate | | O | O | O | O | O | O |
| Explains to the patient what the expected treatment goals and outcomes are | | O | O | O | O | O | O |
| Explains to the patient what he/she should or should not feel | | O | O | O | O | O | O |
| Reviews precautions/contraindications with the patient | | O | O | O | O | O | O |
| **Tester places patient in appropriate position** | | Y | N | Y | N | Y | N |
| Places the patient in following: hip: extension, internal rotation, abduction; ankle: plantar flexed, everted; toes: flexed | | O | O | O | O | O | O |
| **Tester administers the therapeutic exercise according to accepted guidelines** | | Y | N | Y | N | Y | N |
| Places hands on the medial foot and medial knee for resistance | | O | O | O | O | O | O |
| Resists and gives the following verbal cues as the patient completes the movement: "Pull your toes and foot up, heel in, pull up and across" | | O | O | O | O | O | O |
| Stays in appropriate diagonal throughout test | | O | O | O | O | O | O |
| **Termination of treatment** | | Y | N | Y | N | Y | N |
| Ending position: hip: flexed, externally rotated, adducted; ankle: dorsiflexed, inverted; toes: extended | | O | O | O | O | O | O |
| Provides the patient with feedback | | O | O | O | O | O | O |
| Documents the treatment | | O | O | O | O | O | O |
| **Total** | | __/12 | | __/12 | | __/12 | |

*(continued on the next page)*

| Must achieve >8 to pass this examination | Ⓟ | Ⓕ | Ⓟ | Ⓕ | Ⓟ | Ⓕ |
|---|---|---|---|---|---|---|
| **Assessor:** **Date:** | **Test 1 Comments:** | | | | | |
| **Assessor:** **Date:** | **Test 2 Comments:** | | | | | |
| **Assessor:** **Date:** | **Test 3 Comments:** | | | | | |

**TEST ENVIRONMENTS**
**L:** Laboratory/Classroom
**C:** Clinical/Field Testing
**P:** Practicum
**A:** Assessment/Mock Exam

**TEST INFORMATION**
**Test Statistics:** N/A
**Reference(s):** Houglum (2005)
Prentice (2014)

# PROPRIOCEPTIVE NEUROMUSCULAR FACILITATION—STRENGTHENING

| NATA EC 5th | BOC RD6 | SKILL |
|---|---|---|
| TI-11a/b/d | D4-0401 | PNF: Slow Reversal (Lower Extremity D1 Extension) |

**Supplies Needed:** Table

*This problem allows you the opportunity to demonstrate the PNF technique known as* **slow reversal** *to restore flexibility, strength, and coordination in* **lower extremity D1 extension**. *You have 2 minutes to complete this task.*

| PNF: Slow Reversal (Lower Extremity D1 Extension) | Course or Site Assessor Environment | Test 1 | | Test 2 | | Test 3 | |
|---|---|---|---|---|---|---|---|
| | | Y | N | Y | N | Y | N |
| **Purpose of treatment** | | Y | N | Y | N | Y | N |
| Increase a muscle's ability to initiate movement and stabilize | | O | O | O | O | O | O |
| **Patient education/safety** | | Y | N | Y | N | Y | N |
| Explains to the patient why the exercise is appropriate | | O | O | O | O | O | O |
| Explains to the patient what the expected treatment goals and outcomes are | | O | O | O | O | O | O |
| Explains to the patient what he/she should or should not feel | | O | O | O | O | O | O |
| Reviews precautions/contraindications with the patient | | O | O | O | O | O | O |
| **Tester places patient in appropriate position** | | Y | N | Y | N | Y | N |
| Places the patient in following: hip: flexed, externally rotated, adducted; ankle: dorsiflexed, inverted; toes: extended | | O | O | O | O | O | O |
| **Tester administers the therapeutic exercise according to accepted guidelines** | | Y | N | Y | N | Y | N |
| Places hands on lateral foot and lateral knee for resistance | | O | O | O | O | O | O |
| Resists and gives the following verbal cues as the patient completes the movement: "Curl toes, push foot down, heel out, push out and down" | | O | O | O | O | O | O |
| Stays in appropriate diagonal throughout test | | O | O | O | O | O | O |
| **Termination of treatment** | | Y | N | Y | N | Y | N |
| Ending position: hip: extension, internal rotation, abduction; ankle: plantar flexed, everted, toes: flexed | | O | O | O | O | O | O |
| Provides the patient with feedback | | O | O | O | O | O | O |
| Documents the treatment | | O | O | O | O | O | O |
| Total | | ___/12 | | ___/12 | | ___/12 | |

*(continued on the next page)*

| Must achieve >8 to pass this examination | Ⓟ | Ⓕ | Ⓟ | Ⓕ | Ⓟ | Ⓕ |
|---|---|---|---|---|---|---|
| **Assessor:**<br>**Date:** | **Test 1 Comments:** | | | | | |
| **Assessor:**<br>**Date:** | **Test 2 Comments:** | | | | | |
| **Assessor:**<br>**Date:** | **Test 3 Comments:** | | | | | |

**TEST ENVIRONMENTS**
**L:** Laboratory/Classroom
**C:** Clinical/Field Testing
**P:** Practicum
**A:** Assessment/Mock Exam

**TEST INFORMATION**
**Test Statistics:** N/A
**Reference(s):**   Houglum (2005)
                    Prentice (2014)

# PROPRIOCEPTIVE NEUROMUSCULAR FACILITATION—STRENGTHENING

| NATA EC 5th | BOC RD6 | SKILL |
|---|---|---|
| TI-11a/b/d | D4-0401 | PNF: Slow Reversal (Lower Extremity D2 Flexion) |

**Supplies Needed:** Table

*This problem allows you the opportunity to demonstrate the PNF technique known as* **slow reversal** *to restore flexibility, strength, and coordination in* **lower extremity D2 flexion**. *You have 2 minutes to complete this task.*

| PNF: Slow Reversal (Lower Extremity D2 Flexion) — Course or Site / Assessor / Environment | Test 1 Y | Test 1 N | Test 2 Y | Test 2 N | Test 3 Y | Test 3 N |
|---|---|---|---|---|---|---|
| **Purpose of treatment** | Y | N | Y | N | Y | N |
| Increase a muscle's ability to initiate movement and stabilize | ○ | ○ | ○ | ○ | ○ | ○ |
| **Patient education/safety** | Y | N | Y | N | Y | N |
| Explains to the patient why the exercise is appropriate | ○ | ○ | ○ | ○ | ○ | ○ |
| Explains to the patient what the expected treatment goals and outcomes are | ○ | ○ | ○ | ○ | ○ | ○ |
| Explains to the patient what he/she should or should not feel | ○ | ○ | ○ | ○ | ○ | ○ |
| Reviews precautions/contraindications with the patient | ○ | ○ | ○ | ○ | ○ | ○ |
| **Tester places patient in appropriate position** | Y | N | Y | N | Y | N |
| Places the patient in following: hip: extended, externally rotated, adducted; ankle: plantar flexed, inverted; toes: flexed | ○ | ○ | ○ | ○ | ○ | ○ |
| **Tester administers the therapeutic exercise according to accepted guidelines** | Y | N | Y | N | Y | N |
| Places hands on lateral foot and lateral knee for resistance | ○ | ○ | ○ | ○ | ○ | ○ |
| Resists and gives the following verbal cues as the patient completes the movement: "Toes and foot up, heel out, pull up and out" | ○ | ○ | ○ | ○ | ○ | ○ |
| Stays in appropriate diagonal throughout test | ○ | ○ | ○ | ○ | ○ | ○ |
| **Termination of treatment** | Y | N | Y | N | Y | N |
| Ending position: hip: flexed, internally rotated, abducted; ankle: dorsiflexed, everted; toes: extended | ○ | ○ | ○ | ○ | ○ | ○ |
| Provides the patient with feedback | ○ | ○ | ○ | ○ | ○ | ○ |
| Documents the treatment | ○ | ○ | ○ | ○ | ○ | ○ |
| **Total** | _/12 | | _/12 | | _/12 | |

*(continued on the next page)*

| Must achieve >8 to pass this examination | Ⓟ | Ⓕ | Ⓟ | Ⓕ | Ⓟ | Ⓕ |
|---|---|---|---|---|---|---|
| **Assessor:** <br> **Date:** | **Test 1 Comments:** | | | | | |
| **Assessor:** <br> **Date:** | **Test 2 Comments:** | | | | | |
| **Assessor:** <br> **Date:** | **Test 3 Comments:** | | | | | |

## TEST ENVIRONMENTS
**L:** Laboratory/Classroom
**C:** Clinical/Field Testing
**P:** Practicum
**A:** Assessment/Mock Exam

## TEST INFORMATION
**Test Statistics:** N/A
**Reference(s):**  Houglum (2005)
Prentice (2014)

## THERAPEUTIC INTERVENTIONS
# PROPRIOCEPTIVE NEUROMUSCULAR FACILITATION—STRENGTHENING

| NATA EC 5th | BOC RD6 | SKILL |
|---|---|---|
| TI-11a/b/d | D4-0401 | PNF: Slow Reversal (Lower Extremity D2 Extension) |

**Supplies Needed:** Table

*This problem allows you the opportunity to demonstrate the PNF technique known as* **slow reversal** *to restore flexibility, strength, and coordination in* **lower extremity D2 extension***. You have 2 minutes to complete this task.*

| PNF: Slow Reversal (Lower Extremity D2 Extension) | Course or Site Assessor Environment | | Test 1 | | Test 2 | | Test 3 |
|---|---|---|---|---|---|---|---|
| **Purpose of treatment** | | Y | N | Y | N | Y | N |
| Increase a muscle's ability to initiate movement and stabilize | | O | O | O | O | O | O |
| **Patient education/safety** | | Y | N | Y | N | Y | N |
| Explains to the patient why the exercise is appropriate | | O | O | O | O | O | O |
| Explains to the patient what the expected treatment goals and outcomes are | | O | O | O | O | O | O |
| Explains to the patient what he/she should or should not feel | | O | O | O | O | O | O |
| Reviews precautions/contraindications with the patient | | O | O | O | O | O | O |
| **Tester places patient in appropriate position** | | Y | N | Y | N | Y | N |
| Places the patient in following: hip: flexed, internally rotated, abducted; ankle: dorsiflexed, everted; toes: extended | | O | O | O | O | O | O |
| **Tester administers the therapeutic exercise according to accepted guidelines** | | Y | N | Y | N | Y | N |
| Places hands on medial foot and medial knee for resistance | | O | O | O | O | O | O |
| Resists and gives the following verbal cues as the patient completes the movement: "Toes and foot down, heel in, push down and across" | | O | O | O | O | O | O |
| Stays in appropriate diagonal throughout test | | O | O | O | O | O | O |
| **Termination of treatment** | | Y | N | Y | N | Y | N |
| Ending position: hip: extended, externally rotated, adducted; ankle: plantar flexed, inverted; toes: flexed | | O | O | O | O | O | O |
| Provides the patient with feedback | | O | O | O | O | O | O |
| Documents the treatment | | O | O | O | O | O | O |
| **Total** | | ___/12 | | ___/12 | | ___/12 | |

*(continued on the next page)*

| Must achieve >8 to pass this examination | P | F | P | F | P | F |
|---|---|---|---|---|---|---|
| **Assessor:**<br>**Date:** | **Test 1 Comments:** | | | | | |
| **Assessor:**<br>**Date:** | **Test 2 Comments:** | | | | | |
| **Assessor:**<br>**Date:** | **Test 3 Comments:** | | | | | |

**TEST ENVIRONMENTS**
**L:** Laboratory/Classroom
**C:** Clinical/Field Testing
**P:** Practicum
**A:** Assessment/Mock Exam

**TEST INFORMATION**
**Test Statistics:** N/A
**Reference(s):**   Houglum (2005)
                    Prentice (2014)

# PROPRIOCEPTIVE NEUROMUSCULAR FACILITATION—STRENGTHENING

| NATA EC 5th | BOC RD6 | SKILL |
|---|---|---|
| TI-11a/b/d | D4-0401 | PNF: Slow Reversal (Upper Extremity D1 Flexion) |

**Supplies Needed:** Table

*This problem allows you the opportunity to demonstrate the PNF technique known as* **slow reversal** *to restore flexibility, strength, and coordination in* **upper extremity D1 flexion.** *You have 2 minutes to complete this task.*

| PNF: Slow Reversal (Upper Extremity D1 Flexion) | Course or Site Assessor Environment | | | | | |
|---|---|---|---|---|---|---|
| | | Test 1 | | Test 2 | | Test 3 |
| **Purpose of treatment** | | Y | N | Y | N | Y | N |
| Increase a muscle's ability to initiate movement and stabilize | | O | O | O | O | O | O |
| **Patient education/safety** | | Y | N | Y | N | Y | N |
| Explains to the patient why the exercise is appropriate | | O | O | O | O | O | O |
| Explains to the patient what the expected treatment goals and outcomes are | | O | O | O | O | O | O |
| Explains to the patient what he/she should or should not feel | | O | O | O | O | O | O |
| Reviews precautions/contraindications with the patient | | O | O | O | O | O | O |
| **Tester places patient in appropriate position** | | Y | N | Y | N | Y | N |
| Places the patient in following: shoulder: extended, internally rotated, abducted; forearm: pronated; wrist: ulnar extended; fingers: extended | | O | O | O | O | O | O |
| **Tester administers the therapeutic exercise according to accepted guidelines** | | Y | N | Y | N | Y | N |
| Places hands on brachium (under arm) and palm (over arm) for resistance | | O | O | O | O | O | O |
| Resists and gives the following verbal cues as the patient completes the movement: "Close your hand, palm up, pull up and across" | | O | O | O | O | O | O |
| Stays in appropriate diagonal throughout test | | O | O | O | O | O | O |
| **Termination of treatment** | | Y | N | Y | N | Y | N |
| Ending position: shoulder: flexed, externally rotated, adducted; forearm: supinated; wrist: radial flexed; fingers: flexed | | O | O | O | O | O | O |
| Provides the patient with feedback | | O | O | O | O | O | O |
| Documents the treatment | | O | O | O | O | O | O |
| **Total** | | __/12 | | __/12 | | __/12 |

*(continued on the next page)*

| Must achieve >8 to pass this examination | Ⓟ | Ⓕ | Ⓟ | Ⓕ | Ⓟ | Ⓕ |
|---|---|---|---|---|---|---|
| **Assessor:**<br>**Date:** | **Test 1 Comments:** | | | | | |
| **Assessor:**<br>**Date:** | **Test 2 Comments:** | | | | | |
| **Assessor:**<br>**Date:** | **Test 3 Comments:** | | | | | |

**TEST ENVIRONMENTS**
**L:** Laboratory/Classroom
**C:** Clinical/Field Testing
**P:** Practicum
**A:** Assessment/Mock Exam

**TEST INFORMATION**
**Test Statistics:** N/A
**Reference(s):** Houglum (2005)
Prentice (2014)

# PROPRIOCEPTIVE NEUROMUSCULAR FACILITATION—STRENGTHENING

| NATA EC 5th | BOC RD6 | SKILL |
|---|---|---|
| TI-11a/b/d | D4-0401 | PNF: Slow Reversal<br>(Upper Extremity D1 Extension) |

**Supplies Needed:** Table

*This problem allows you the opportunity to demonstrate the PNF technique known as* **slow reversal** *to restore flexibility, strength, and coordination in* **upper extremity D1 extension**. *You have 2 minutes to complete this task.*

| PNF: Slow Reversal<br>(Upper Extremity D1 Extension) | Course or Site<br>Assessor<br>Environment | | | | | |
|---|---|---|---|---|---|---|
| | | Test 1 | | Test 2 | | Test 3 |
| **Purpose of treatment** | | **Y** | **N** | **Y** | **N** | **Y** | **N** |
| Increase a muscle's ability to initiate movement and stabilize | | O | O | O | O | O | O |
| **Patient education/safety** | | **Y** | **N** | **Y** | **N** | **Y** | **N** |
| Explains to the patient why the exercise is appropriate | | O | O | O | O | O | O |
| Explains to the patient what the expected treatment goals and outcomes are | | O | O | O | O | O | O |
| Explains to the patient what he/she should or should not feel | | O | O | O | O | O | O |
| Reviews precautions/contraindications with the patient | | O | O | O | O | O | O |
| **Tester places patient in appropriate position** | | **Y** | **N** | **Y** | **N** | **Y** | **N** |
| Places the patient in following: shoulder: flexed, externally rotated, adducted; forearm: supinated; wrist: radial flexed; fingers: flexed | | O | O | O | O | O | O |
| **Tester administers the therapeutic exercise according to accepted guidelines** | | **Y** | **N** | **Y** | **N** | **Y** | **N** |
| Places hands on posterior humerus and hypothenar eminence | | O | O | O | O | O | O |
| Resists and gives the following verbal cues as the patient completes the movement: "Open your hand, palm down, push down and out" | | O | O | O | O | O | O |
| Stays in appropriate diagonal throughout test | | O | O | O | O | O | O |
| **Termination of treatment** | | **Y** | **N** | **Y** | **N** | **Y** | **N** |
| Ending position: shoulder: extended, internally rotated, abducted; forearm: pronated; wrist: ulnar extended; fingers: extended | | O | O | O | O | O | O |
| Provides the patient with feedback | | O | O | O | O | O | O |
| Documents the treatment | | O | O | O | O | O | O |
| **Total** | | ____/12 | | ____/12 | | ____/12 |

*(continued on the next page)*

| Must achieve >8 to pass this examination | Ⓟ | Ⓕ | Ⓟ | Ⓕ | Ⓟ | Ⓕ |
|---|---|---|---|---|---|---|
| **Assessor:**<br>**Date:** | **Test 1 Comments:** | | | | | |
| **Assessor:**<br>**Date:** | **Test 2 Comments:** | | | | | |
| **Assessor:**<br>**Date:** | **Test 3 Comments:** | | | | | |

**TEST ENVIRONMENTS**
**L:** Laboratory/Classroom
**C:** Clinical/Field Testing
**P:** Practicum
**A:** Assessment/Mock Exam

**TEST INFORMATION**
**Test Statistics:** N/A
**Reference(s):** Houglum (2005)
Prentice (2014)

## THERAPEUTIC INTERVENTIONS
# PROPRIOCEPTIVE NEUROMUSCULAR FACILITATION—STRENGTHENING

| NATA EC 5th | BOC RD6 | SKILL |
|---|---|---|
| TI-11a/b/d | D4-0401 | PNF: Slow Reversal (Upper Extremity D2 Flexion) |

**Supplies Needed:** Table

*This problem allows you the opportunity to demonstrate the PNF technique known as **slow reversal** to restore flexibility, strength, and coordination in **upper extremity D2 flexion**. You have 2 minutes to complete this task.*

| PNF: Slow Reversal (Upper Extremity D2 Flexion) | Course or Site Assessor Environment | | Test 1 | | Test 2 | | Test 3 |
|---|---|---|---|---|---|---|---|
| | | Y | N | Y | N | Y | N |
| **Purpose of treatment** | | | | | | | |
| Increase a muscle's ability to initiate movement and stabilize | | ○ | ○ | ○ | ○ | ○ | ○ |
| **Patient education/safety** | | Y | N | Y | N | Y | N |
| Explains to the patient why the exercise is appropriate | | ○ | ○ | ○ | ○ | ○ | ○ |
| Explains to the patient what the expected treatment goals and outcomes are | | ○ | ○ | ○ | ○ | ○ | ○ |
| Explains to the patient what he/she should or should not feel | | ○ | ○ | ○ | ○ | ○ | ○ |
| Reviews precautions/contraindications with the patient | | ○ | ○ | ○ | ○ | ○ | ○ |
| **Tester places patient in appropriate position** | | Y | N | Y | N | Y | N |
| Places the patient in following: shoulder: extended, internally rotated, adducted; forearm: pronated; wrist: ulnar deviated; fingers: flexed | | ○ | ○ | ○ | ○ | ○ | ○ |
| **Tester administers the therapeutic exercise according to accepted guidelines** | | Y | N | Y | N | Y | N |
| Places hands on posterior humerus and dorsal aspect of hand | | ○ | ○ | ○ | ○ | ○ | ○ |
| Resists and gives the following verbal cues as the patient completes the movement: "Open your hand, palm up, push up and out" | | ○ | ○ | ○ | ○ | ○ | ○ |
| Stays in appropriate diagonal throughout test | | ○ | ○ | ○ | ○ | ○ | ○ |
| **Termination of treatment** | | Y | N | Y | N | Y | N |
| Ending position: shoulder: flexed, externally rotated, abducted; forearm: supinated; wrist: radial extended; fingers: extended | | ○ | ○ | ○ | ○ | ○ | ○ |
| Provides the patient with feedback | | ○ | ○ | ○ | ○ | ○ | ○ |
| Documents the treatment | | ○ | ○ | ○ | ○ | ○ | ○ |
| **Total** | | ___/12 | | ___/12 | | ___/12 | |

*(continued on the next page)*

| Must achieve >8 to pass this examination | Ⓟ | Ⓕ | Ⓟ | Ⓕ | Ⓟ | Ⓕ |
|---|---|---|---|---|---|---|
| **Assessor:** **Date:** | **Test 1 Comments:** | | | | | |
| **Assessor:** **Date:** | **Test 2 Comments:** | | | | | |
| **Assessor:** **Date:** | **Test 3 Comments:** | | | | | |

## TEST ENVIRONMENTS
**L:** Laboratory/Classroom
**C:** Clinical/Field Testing
**P:** Practicum
**A:** Assessment/Mock Exam

## TEST INFORMATION
**Test Statistics:** N/A
**Reference(s):** Houglum (2005)
Prentice (2014)

© SLACK Incorporated, 2016. Hauth, J. M., Gloyeske, B. M., & Amato, H. K. (2016). *Clinical Skills Documentation Guide for Athletic Training, Third Edition.* Thorofare, NJ: SLACK Incorporated.

# PROPRIOCEPTIVE NEUROMUSCULAR FACILITATION—STRENGTHENING

| NATA EC 5th | BOC RD6 | SKILL |
|---|---|---|
| TI-11a/b/d | D4-0401 | PNF: Slow Reversal (Upper Extremity D2 Extension) |

**Supplies Needed:** Table

*This problem allows you the opportunity to demonstrate the PNF technique known as* **slow reversal** *to restore flexibility, strength, and coordination in* **upper extremity D2 extension**. *You have 2 minutes to complete this task.*

| PNF: Slow Reversal (Upper Extremity D2 Extension) | Course or Site Assessor Environment | Test 1 | | Test 2 | | Test 3 | |
|---|---|---|---|---|---|---|---|
| **Purpose of treatment** | | **Y** | **N** | **Y** | **N** | **Y** | **N** |
| Increase a muscle's ability to initiate movement and stabilize | | ○ | ○ | ○ | ○ | ○ | ○ |
| **Patient education/safety** | | **Y** | **N** | **Y** | **N** | **Y** | **N** |
| Explains to the patient why the exercise is appropriate | | ○ | ○ | ○ | ○ | ○ | ○ |
| Explains to the patient what the expected treatment goals and outcomes are | | ○ | ○ | ○ | ○ | ○ | ○ |
| Explains to the patient what he/she should or should not feel | | ○ | ○ | ○ | ○ | ○ | ○ |
| Reviews precautions/contraindications with the patient | | ○ | ○ | ○ | ○ | ○ | ○ |
| **Tester places patient in appropriate position** | | **Y** | **N** | **Y** | **N** | **Y** | **N** |
| Places the patient in following: shoulder: flexed, externally rotated, abducted; forearm: supinated; wrist: radial extended; fingers: extended | | ○ | ○ | ○ | ○ | ○ | ○ |
| **Tester administers the therapeutic exercise according to accepted guidelines** | | **Y** | **N** | **Y** | **N** | **Y** | **N** |
| Places hands on brachium (under arm) and palm (over arm) for resistance | | ○ | ○ | ○ | ○ | ○ | ○ |
| Resists and gives the following verbal cues as the patient completes the movement: "Close your hand, turn palm down, pull down and across" | | ○ | ○ | ○ | ○ | ○ | ○ |
| Stays in appropriate diagonal throughout test | | ○ | ○ | ○ | ○ | ○ | ○ |
| **Termination of treatment** | | **Y** | **N** | **Y** | **N** | **Y** | **N** |
| Ending position: shoulder: extended, internally rotated, adducted; forearm: pronated; wrist: ulnar flexed; fingers: flexed | | ○ | ○ | ○ | ○ | ○ | ○ |
| Provides the patient with feedback | | ○ | ○ | ○ | ○ | ○ | ○ |
| Documents the treatment | | ○ | ○ | ○ | ○ | ○ | ○ |
| | Total | ___/12 | | ___/12 | | ___/12 | |

*(continued on the next page)*

| Must achieve >8 to pass this examination | Ⓟ | Ⓕ | Ⓟ | Ⓕ | Ⓟ | Ⓕ |
|---|---|---|---|---|---|---|
| **Assessor:** **Date:** | **Test 1 Comments:** | | | | | |
| **Assessor:** **Date:** | **Test 2 Comments:** | | | | | |
| **Assessor:** **Date:** | **Test 3 Comments:** | | | | | |

## TEST ENVIRONMENTS
**L:** Laboratory/Classroom
**C:** Clinical/Field Testing
**P:** Practicum
**A:** Assessment/Mock Exam

## TEST INFORMATION
**Test Statistics:** N/A
**Reference(s):** Houglum (2005)
Prentice (2014)

# JOINT MOBILIZATIONS—OSCILLATORY

| NATA EC 5th | BOC RD6 | SKILL |
|---|---|---|
| TI-15 | D4-0401 | Joint Mobs: Grade 1 Oscillatory (Tibiofemoral Extension) |

**Supplies Needed:** Table, towel

*This problem allows you the opportunity to demonstrate the therapeutic technique known as* **grade 1 oscillatory joint mobilization** *for the* **tibiofemoral joint (extension)** *to* **reduce pain***. You have 2 minutes to complete this task.*

| Joint Mobs: Grade 1 Oscillatory (Tibiofemoral Extension) | Course or Site Assessor Environment | | Test 1 | | Test 2 | | Test 3 | |
|---|---|---|---|---|---|---|---|---|
| | | Y | N | Y | N | Y | N |
| **Purpose of treatment** | | Y | N | Y | N | Y | N |
| Decrease pain and spasm | | ○ | ○ | ○ | ○ | ○ | ○ |
| **Patient education/safety** | | Y | N | Y | N | Y | N |
| Explains to the patient why the exercise is appropriate | | ○ | ○ | ○ | ○ | ○ | ○ |
| Explains to the patient what the expected treatment goals and outcomes are | | ○ | ○ | ○ | ○ | ○ | ○ |
| Explains to the patient what he/she should or should not feel | | ○ | ○ | ○ | ○ | ○ | ○ |
| Reviews precautions/contraindications with the patient | | ○ | ○ | ○ | ○ | ○ | ○ |
| **Tester places patient in appropriate position** | | Y | N | Y | N | Y | N |
| Prone, beginning with knee in resting position; progress to the end of available range | | ○ | ○ | ○ | ○ | ○ | ○ |
| Places towel under the patient's knee | | ○ | ○ | ○ | ○ | ○ | ○ |
| **Tester administers the therapeutic exercise according to accepted guidelines** | | Y | N | Y | N | Y | N |
| Grasps the distal tibia with the hand that is closer to it and places the palm of the proximal hand on the posterior aspect of the proximal tibia | | ○ | ○ | ○ | ○ | ○ | ○ |
| Applies a small amplitude rhythmic oscillation force at the beginning of the range with the hand on the proximal tibia in an anterior direction | | ○ | ○ | ○ | ○ | ○ | ○ |
| **Termination of treatment** | | Y | N | Y | N | Y | N |
| Applies rapid oscillations for 7 to 10 seconds with a few seconds of rest between cycles | | ○ | ○ | ○ | ○ | ○ | ○ |
| Notes the response and either repeats or discontinues | | ○ | ○ | ○ | ○ | ○ | ○ |
| Documents the treatment | | ○ | ○ | ○ | ○ | ○ | ○ |
| **Total** | | ___/12 | | ___/12 | | ___/12 | |

*(continued on the next page)*

| Must achieve >8 to pass this examination | Ⓟ | Ⓕ | Ⓟ | Ⓕ | Ⓟ | Ⓕ |
|---|---|---|---|---|---|---|
| **Assessor:** **Date:** | **Test 1 Comments:** | | | | | |
| **Assessor:** **Date:** | **Test 2 Comments:** | | | | | |
| **Assessor:** **Date:** | **Test 3 Comments:** | | | | | |

**TEST ENVIRONMENTS**
**L:** Laboratory/Classroom
**C:** Clinical/Field Testing
**P:** Practicum
**A:** Assessment/Mock Exam

**TEST INFORMATION**
**Test Statistics:** N/A
**Reference(s):** Kisner & Colby (2012)
Prentice (2014)

**THERAPEUTIC INTERVENTIONS**
# JOINT MOBILIZATIONS—OSCILLATORY

| NATA EC 5th | BOC RD6 | SKILL |
|---|---|---|
| TI-15 | D4-0401 | Joint Mobs: Grade 2 Oscillatory (Tibiofemoral Extension) |

**Supplies Needed:** Table, towel

*This problem allows you the opportunity to demonstrate the therapeutic technique known as* **grade 2 oscillatory joint mobilization** *for the* **tibiofemoral joint (extension)** *to* **reduce pain**. *You have 2 minutes to complete this task.*

| Joint Mobs: Grade 2 Oscillatory (Tibiofemoral Extension) | Course or Site Assessor Environment | | Test 1 | | Test 2 | | Test 3 | |
|---|---|---|---|---|---|---|---|---|
| **Purpose of treatment** | | Y | N | Y | N | Y | N | |
| Decrease pain and spasm | | O | O | O | O | O | O | |
| **Patient education/safety** | | Y | N | Y | N | Y | N | |
| Explains to the patient why the exercise is appropriate | | O | O | O | O | O | O | |
| Explains to the patient what the expected treatment goals and outcomes are | | O | O | O | O | O | O | |
| Explains to the patient what he/she should or should not feel | | O | O | O | O | O | O | |
| Reviews precautions/contraindications with the patient | | O | O | O | O | O | O | |
| **Tester places patient in appropriate position** | | Y | N | Y | N | Y | N | |
| Prone, beginning with knee in resting position; progress to the end of available range | | O | O | O | O | O | O | |
| Places towel under the patient's knee | | O | O | O | O | O | O | |
| **Tester administers the therapeutic exercise according to accepted guidelines** | | Y | N | Y | N | Y | N | |
| Grasps the distal tibia with the hand that is closer to it and places the palm of the proximal hand on the posterior aspect of the proximal tibia | | O | O | O | O | O | O | |
| Applies a large amplitude rhythmic oscillation force within the range (not reaching the limit) with the hand on the proximal tibia in an anterior direction | | O | O | O | O | O | O | |
| **Termination of treatment** | | Y | N | Y | N | Y | N | |
| Applies rapid oscillation, 2 per second for 1 to 2 minutes | | O | O | O | O | O | O | |
| Notes the response and either repeats or discontinues | | O | O | O | O | O | O | |
| Documents the treatment | | O | O | O | O | O | O | |
| Total | | | /12 | | /12 | | /12 | |

*(continued on the next page)*

| Must achieve >8 to pass this examination | Ⓟ | Ⓕ | Ⓟ | Ⓕ | Ⓟ | Ⓕ |
|---|---|---|---|---|---|---|
| **Assessor:**<br>**Date:** | **Test 1 Comments:** | | | | | |
| **Assessor:**<br>**Date:** | **Test 2 Comments:** | | | | | |
| **Assessor:**<br>**Date:** | **Test 3 Comments:** | | | | | |

**TEST ENVIRONMENTS**
**L:** Laboratory/Classroom
**C:** Clinical/Field Testing
**P:** Practicum
**A:** Assessment/Mock Exam

**TEST INFORMATION**
**Test Statistics:** N/A
**Reference(s):**  Kisner & Colby (2012)
                   Prentice (2014)

## THERAPEUTIC INTERVENTIONS
# JOINT MOBILIZATIONS—OSCILLATORY

| NATA EC 5th | BOC RD6 | SKILL |
|---|---|---|
| TI-15 | D4-0401 | Joint Mobs: Grade 3 Oscillatory (Tibiofemoral Extension) |

**Supplies Needed:** Table, towel

*This problem allows you the opportunity to demonstrate the therapeutic technique known as* **grade 3 oscillatory joint mobilization** *for the* **tibiofemoral joint (extension)** *to* **reduce pain**. *You have 2 minutes to complete this task.*

| Joint Mobs: Grade 3 Oscillatory (Tibiofemoral Extension) | Course or Site Assessor Environment | Test 1 | | Test 2 | | Test 3 | |
|---|---|---|---|---|---|---|---|
| **Purpose of treatment** | | Y | N | Y | N | Y | N |
| Decrease pain and spasm and to increase limited movement toward the end range of motion | | O | O | O | O | O | O |
| **Patient education/safety** | | Y | N | Y | N | Y | N |
| Explains to the patient why the exercise is appropriate | | O | O | O | O | O | O |
| Explains to the patient what the expected treatment goals and outcomes are | | O | O | O | O | O | O |
| Explains to the patient what he/she should or should not feel | | O | O | O | O | O | O |
| Reviews precautions/contraindications with the patient | | O | O | O | O | O | O |
| **Tester places patient in appropriate position** | | Y | N | Y | N | Y | N |
| Prone, beginning with knee in resting position; progress to the end of available range | | O | O | O | O | O | O |
| Places towel under the patient's knee | | O | O | O | O | O | O |
| **Tester administers the therapeutic exercise according to accepted guidelines** | | Y | N | Y | N | Y | N |
| Grasps the distal tibia with the hand that is closer to it and places the palm of the proximal hand on the posterior aspect of the proximal tibia | | O | O | O | O | O | O |
| Applies a large amplitude rhythmic oscillation force up to the limit of range of motion with the hand on the proximal tibia in an anterior direction | | O | O | O | O | O | O |
| **Termination of treatment** | | Y | N | Y | N | Y | N |
| Applies rapid oscillation, 2 per second, for 1 to 2 minutes | | O | O | O | O | O | O |
| Notes the response and either repeats or discontinues | | O | O | O | O | O | O |
| Documents the treatment | | O | O | O | O | O | O |
| **Total** | | __/12 | | __/12 | | __/12 | |

*(continued on the next page)*

| Must achieve >8 to pass this examination | (P) | (F) | (P) | (F) | (P) | (F) |
|---|---|---|---|---|---|---|
| **Assessor:** **Date:** Test 1 Comments: | | | | | | |
| **Assessor:** **Date:** Test 2 Comments: | | | | | | |
| **Assessor:** **Date:** Test 3 Comments: | | | | | | |

**TEST ENVIRONMENTS**
**L:** Laboratory/Classroom
**C:** Clinical/Field Testing
**P:** Practicum
**A:** Assessment/Mock Exam

**TEST INFORMATION**
**Test Statistics:** N/A
**Reference(s):** Kisner & Colby (2012)
Prentice (2014)

# JOINT MOBILIZATIONS—OSCILLATORY

| NATA EC 5th | BOC RD6 | SKILL |
|---|---|---|
| TI-15 | D4-0401 | Joint Mobs: Grade 4 Oscillatory (Tibiofemoral Extension) |

**Supplies Needed:** Table, towel

*This problem allows you the opportunity to demonstrate the therapeutic technique known as* **grade 4 oscillatory joint mobilization** *for the* **tibiofemoral joint (extension)** *to* **increase range of motion**. *You have 2 minutes to complete this task.*

| Joint Mobs: Grade 4 Oscillatory (Tibiofemoral Extension) | Course or Site Assessor Environment | | Test 1 | | Test 2 | | Test 3 | |
|---|---|---|---|---|---|---|---|---|
| **Purpose of treatment** | | Y | N | Y | N | Y | N |
| Increase limited movement toward the end range of motion | | O | O | O | O | O | O |
| **Patient education/safety** | | Y | N | Y | N | Y | N |
| Explains to the patient why the exercise is appropriate | | O | O | O | O | O | O |
| Explains to the patient what the expected treatment goals and outcomes are | | O | O | O | O | O | O |
| Explains to the patient what he/she should or should not feel | | O | O | O | O | O | O |
| Reviews precautions/contraindications with the patient | | O | O | O | O | O | O |
| **Tester places patient in appropriate position** | | Y | N | Y | N | Y | N |
| Prone, beginning with knee in resting position; progress to the end of available range | | O | O | O | O | O | O |
| Places towel under the patient's knee | | O | O | O | O | O | O |
| **Tester administers the therapeutic exercise according to accepted guidelines** | | Y | N | Y | N | Y | N |
| Grasps the distal tibia with the hand that is closer to it and places the palm of the proximal hand on the posterior aspect of the proximal tibia | | O | O | O | O | O | O |
| Applies a small amplitude rhythmic oscillation force at the limit of range of motion and stressed into the tissue resistance with the hand on the proximal tibia in an anterior direction | | O | O | O | O | O | O |
| **Termination of treatment** | | Y | N | Y | N | Y | N |
| Applies rapid oscillation, like manual vibrations | | O | O | O | O | O | O |
| Notes the response and either repeats or discontinues | | O | O | O | O | O | O |
| Documents the treatment | | O | O | O | O | O | O |
| **Total** | | ___/12 | | ___/12 | | ___/12 | |

*(continued on the next page)*

| Must achieve >8 to pass this examination | (P) | (F) | (P) | (F) | (P) | (F) |
|---|---|---|---|---|---|---|
| **Assessor:**<br>**Date:** | **Test 1 Comments:** | | | | | |
| **Assessor:**<br>**Date:** | **Test 2 Comments:** | | | | | |
| **Assessor:**<br>**Date:** | **Test 3 Comments:** | | | | | |

**TEST ENVIRONMENTS**
**L:** Laboratory/Classroom
**C:** Clinical/Field Testing
**P:** Practicum
**A:** Assessment/Mock Exam

**TEST INFORMATION**
**Test Statistics:** N/A
**Reference(s):**  Kisner & Colby (2012)
                   Prentice (2014)

THERAPEUTIC INTERVENTIONS
# JOINT MOBILIZATIONS—OSCILLATORY

| NATA EC 5th | BOC RD6 | SKILL |
|---|---|---|
| TI-15 | D4-0401 | Joint Mobs: Grade 1 Oscillatory (Glenohumeral Abduction) |

**Supplies Needed:** Table, belt

*This problem allows you the opportunity to demonstrate the therapeutic technique known as* **grade 1 oscillatory joint mobilization** *for the* **glenohumeral joint (abduction)** *to* **reduce pain**. *You have 2 minutes to complete this task.*

| Joint Mobs: Grade 1 Oscillatory (Glenohumeral Abduction) | Course or Site Assessor Environment | | | | | |
|---|---|---|---|---|---|---|
| | | Test 1 | | Test 2 | | Test 3 |
| **Purpose of treatment** | | Y | N | Y | N | Y | N |
| Decrease pain and spasm | | O | O | O | O | O | O |
| **Patient education/safety** | | Y | N | Y | N | Y | N |
| Explains to the patient why the exercise is appropriate | | O | O | O | O | O | O |
| Explains to the patient what the expected treatment goals and outcomes are | | O | O | O | O | O | O |
| Explains to the patient what he/she should or should not feel | | O | O | O | O | O | O |
| Reviews precautions/contraindications with the patient | | O | O | O | O | O | O |
| **Tester places patient in appropriate position** | | Y | N | Y | N | Y | N |
| Supine, with belt stabilizing the patient's torso | | O | O | O | O | O | O |
| Arm placed in resting position, support the forearm between trunk and elbow | | O | O | O | O | O | O |
| **Tester administers the therapeutic exercise according to accepted guidelines** | | Y | N | Y | N | Y | N |
| Places one hand in the patient's axilla to provide distraction and the web space of the other hand is placed just distal to the acromion process | | O | O | O | O | O | O |
| Applies small amplitude rhythmic oscillation force inferiorly at the beginning of the range with the hand on the humerus | | O | O | O | O | O | O |
| **Termination of treatment** | | Y | N | Y | N | Y | N |
| Applies rapid oscillations for 7 to 10 seconds with a few seconds of rest between cycles | | O | O | O | O | O | O |
| Notes the response and either repeats or discontinues | | O | O | O | O | O | O |
| Documents the treatment | | O | O | O | O | O | O |
| **Total** | | ___/12 | | ___/12 | | ___/12 |

*(continued on the next page)*

| Must achieve >8 to pass this examination | Ⓟ | Ⓕ | Ⓟ | Ⓕ | Ⓟ | Ⓕ |
|---|---|---|---|---|---|---|
| **Assessor:**<br>**Date:** | **Test 1 Comments:** | | | | | |
| **Assessor:**<br>**Date:** | **Test 2 Comments:** | | | | | |
| **Assessor:**<br>**Date:** | **Test 3 Comments:** | | | | | |

**TEST ENVIRONMENTS**
**L:** Laboratory/Classroom
**C:** Clinical/Field Testing
**P:** Practicum
**A:** Assessment/Mock Exam

**TEST INFORMATION**
**Test Statistics:** N/A
**Reference(s):** Kisner & Colby (2012)
Prentice (2014)

## THERAPEUTIC INTERVENTIONS
# JOINT MOBILIZATIONS—OSCILLATORY

| NATA EC 5th | BOC RD6 | SKILL |
|---|---|---|
| TI-15 | D4-0401 | Joint Mobs: Grade 2 Oscillatory (Glenohumeral Abduction) |

**Supplies Needed:** Table, belt

*This problem allows you the opportunity to demonstrate the therapeutic technique known as* **grade 2 oscillatory joint mobilization** *for the* **glenohumeral joint (abduction)** *to* **reduce pain.** *You have 2 minutes to complete this task.*

| Joint Mobs: Grade 2 Oscillatory (Glenohumeral Abduction) | Course or Site Assessor Environment | Test 1 | | Test 2 | | Test 3 | |
|---|---|---|---|---|---|---|---|
| **Purpose of treatment** | | Y | N | Y | N | Y | N |
| Decrease pain and spasm | | O | O | O | O | O | O |
| **Patient education/safety** | | Y | N | Y | N | Y | N |
| Explains to the patient why the exercise is appropriate | | O | O | O | O | O | O |
| Explains to the patient what the expected treatment goals and outcomes are | | O | O | O | O | O | O |
| Explains to the patient what he/she should or should not feel | | O | O | O | O | O | O |
| Reviews precautions/contraindications with the patient | | O | O | O | O | O | O |
| **Tester places patient in appropriate position** | | Y | N | Y | N | Y | N |
| Supine, with belt stabilizing the patient's torso | | O | O | O | O | O | O |
| Arm placed in resting position, support the forearm between trunk and elbow | | O | O | O | O | O | O |
| **Tester administers the therapeutic exercise according to accepted guidelines** | | Y | N | Y | N | Y | N |
| Places one hand in the patient's axilla to provide distraction and the web space of the other hand is placed just distal to the acromion process | | O | O | O | O | O | O |
| Applies a large amplitude rhythmic oscillation force within the range (not reaching the limit) with the hand on the humerus | | O | O | O | O | O | O |
| **Termination of treatment** | | Y | N | Y | N | Y | N |
| Applies rapid oscillation, 2 per second, for 1 to 2 minutes | | O | O | O | O | O | O |
| Notes the response and either repeats or discontinues | | O | O | O | O | O | O |
| Documents the treatment | | O | O | O | O | O | O |
| **Total** | | ___/12 | | ___/12 | | ___/12 | |

*(continued on the next page)*

| Must achieve >8 to pass this examination | P | F | P | F | P | F |
|---|---|---|---|---|---|---|
| **Assessor:**<br>**Date:** | **Test 1 Comments:** | | | | | |
| **Assessor:**<br>**Date:** | **Test 2 Comments:** | | | | | |
| **Assessor:**<br>**Date:** | **Test 3 Comments:** | | | | | |

## TEST ENVIRONMENTS
**L:** Laboratory/Classroom
**C:** Clinical/Field Testing
**P:** Practicum
**A:** Assessment/Mock Exam

## TEST INFORMATION
**Test Statistics:** N/A
**Reference(s):**  Kisner & Colby (2012)
Prentice (2014)

THERAPEUTIC INTERVENTIONS
# JOINT MOBILIZATIONS—OSCILLATORY

| NATA EC 5th | BOC RD6 | SKILL |
|---|---|---|
| TI-15 | D4-0401 | Joint Mobs: Grade 3 Oscillatory (Glenohumeral Abduction) |

**Supplies Needed:** Table, belt

*This problem allows you the opportunity to demonstrate the therapeutic technique known as* **grade 3 oscillatory joint mobilization** *for the* **glenohumeral joint (abduction)** *to* **reduce pain**. *You have 2 minutes to complete this task.*

| Joint Mobs: Grade 3 Oscillatory (Glenohumeral Abduction) | Course or Site Assessor Environment | Test 1 | | Test 2 | | Test 3 | |
|---|---|---|---|---|---|---|---|
| **Purpose of treatment** | | **Y** | **N** | **Y** | **N** | **Y** | **N** |
| Decrease pain and spasm and to increase limited movement toward the end range of motion | | O | O | O | O | O | O |
| **Patient education/safety** | | **Y** | **N** | **Y** | **N** | **Y** | **N** |
| Explains to the patient why the exercise is appropriate | | O | O | O | O | O | O |
| Explains to the patient what the expected treatment goals and outcomes are | | O | O | O | O | O | O |
| Explains to the patient what he/she should or should not feel | | O | O | O | O | O | O |
| Reviews precautions/contraindications with the patient | | O | O | O | O | O | O |
| **Tester places patient in appropriate position** | | **Y** | **N** | **Y** | **N** | **Y** | **N** |
| Supine, with belt stabilizing the patient's torso | | O | O | O | O | O | O |
| Arm placed in abduction, within range, support the forearm between trunk and elbow | | O | O | O | O | O | O |
| **Tester administers the therapeutic exercise according to accepted guidelines** | | **Y** | **N** | **Y** | **N** | **Y** | **N** |
| Places one hand along distal humerus and provides long axis traction and the web space of the other hand is placed just distal to the acromion process | | O | O | O | O | O | O |
| Applies a large amplitude rhythmic oscillation force up to the limit of range of motion with the hand on the proximal humerus | | O | O | O | O | O | O |
| **Termination of treatment** | | **Y** | **N** | **Y** | **N** | **Y** | **N** |
| Applies rapid oscillation, 2 per second, for 1 to 2 minutes | | O | O | O | O | O | O |
| Notes the response and either repeats or discontinues | | O | O | O | O | O | O |
| Documents the treatment | | O | O | O | O | O | O |
| **Total** | | __/12 | | __/12 | | __/12 | |

*(continued on the next page)*

| Must achieve >8 to pass this examination | Ⓟ | Ⓕ | Ⓟ | Ⓕ | Ⓟ | Ⓕ |
|---|---|---|---|---|---|---|
| **Assessor:** **Date:** | **Test 1 Comments:** | | | | | |
| **Assessor:** **Date:** | **Test 2 Comments:** | | | | | |
| **Assessor:** **Date:** | **Test 3 Comments:** | | | | | |

## TEST ENVIRONMENTS
**L:** Laboratory/Classroom
**C:** Clinical/Field Testing
**P:** Practicum
**A:** Assessment/Mock Exam

## TEST INFORMATION
**Test Statistics:** N/A
**Reference(s):** Kisner & Colby (2012)
Prentice (2014)

## THERAPEUTIC INTERVENTIONS
# JOINT MOBILIZATIONS—OSCILLATORY

| NATA EC 5th | BOC RD6 | SKILL |
|---|---|---|
| TI-15 | D4-0401 | Joint Mobs: Grade 4 Oscillatory (Glenohumeral Abduction) |

**Supplies Needed:** Table, belt

*This problem allows you the opportunity to demonstrate the therapeutic technique known as* **grade 4 oscillatory joint mobilization** *for the* **glenohumeral joint (abduction)** *to* **increase range of motion.** *You have 2 minutes to complete this task.*

| Joint Mobs: Grade 4 Oscillatory (Glenohumeral Abduction) | Course or Site / Assessor / Environment | Test 1 | | Test 2 | | Test 3 | |
|---|---|---|---|---|---|---|---|
| | | Y | N | Y | N | Y | N |
| **Purpose of treatment** | | Y | N | Y | N | Y | N |
| Increase limited movement toward the end range of motion | | O | O | O | O | O | O |
| **Patient education/safety** | | Y | N | Y | N | Y | N |
| Explains to the patient why the exercise is appropriate | | O | O | O | O | O | O |
| Explains to the patient what the expected treatment goals and outcomes are | | O | O | O | O | O | O |
| Explains to the patient what he/she should or should not feel | | O | O | O | O | O | O |
| Reviews precautions/contraindications with the patient | | O | O | O | O | O | O |
| **Tester places patient in appropriate position** | | Y | N | Y | N | Y | N |
| Supine, with belt stabilizing the patient's torso | | O | O | O | O | O | O |
| Arm placed in abduction, within range, support the forearm between trunk and elbow | | O | O | O | O | O | O |
| **Tester administers the therapeutic exercise according to accepted guidelines** | | Y | N | Y | N | Y | N |
| Places one hand along distal humerus and provides long axis traction and the web space of the other hand is placed just distal to the acromion process | | O | O | O | O | O | O |
| Applies small amplitude rhythmic oscillation force at the limit of range of motion and stressed into the tissue resistance with the hand on the proximal humerus | | O | O | O | O | O | O |
| **Termination of treatment** | | Y | N | Y | N | Y | N |
| Applies rapid oscillation, like manual vibrations | | O | O | O | O | O | O |
| Notes the response and either repeats or discontinues | | O | O | O | O | O | O |
| Documents the treatment | | O | O | O | O | O | O |
| Total | | ___/12 | | ___/12 | | ___/12 | |

*(continued on the next page)*

| Must achieve >8 to pass this examination | Ⓟ | Ⓕ | Ⓟ | Ⓕ | Ⓟ | Ⓕ |
|---|---|---|---|---|---|---|
| **Assessor:**<br>**Date:** | **Test 1 Comments:** | | | | | |
| **Assessor:**<br>**Date:** | **Test 2 Comments:** | | | | | |
| **Assessor:**<br>**Date:** | **Test 3 Comments:** | | | | | |

## TEST ENVIRONMENTS
**L:**  Laboratory/Classroom
**C:**  Clinical/Field Testing
**P:**  Practicum
**A:**  Assessment/Mock Exam

## TEST INFORMATION
**Test Statistics:** N/A
**Reference(s):**  Kisner & Colby (2012)
                   Prentice (2014)

## THERAPEUTIC INTERVENTIONS
# JOINT MOBILIZATIONS—SUSTAINED

| NATA EC 5th | BOC RD6 | SKILL |
|---|---|---|
| TI-15 | D4-0401 | Joint Mobs: Grade 1 Sustained (Tibiofemoral Flexion) |

**Supplies Needed:** Table

*This problem allows you the opportunity to demonstrate the therapeutic technique known as* **grade 1 sustained joint mobilization** *for the* **tibiofemoral joint (flexion)** *to* **reduce pain.** *You have 2 minutes to complete this task.*

| Joint Mobs: Grade 1 Sustained (Tibiofemoral Flexion) | Course or Site Assessor Environment | Test 1 | | Test 2 | | Test 3 | |
|---|---|---|---|---|---|---|---|
| | | Y | N | Y | N | Y | N |
| **Purpose of treatment** | | Y | N | Y | N | Y | N |
| Decrease pain and spasm | | O | O | O | O | O | O |
| **Patient education/safety** | | Y | N | Y | N | Y | N |
| Explains to the patient why the exercise is appropriate | | O | O | O | O | O | O |
| Explains to the patient what the expected treatment goals and outcomes are | | O | O | O | O | O | O |
| Explains to the patient what he/she should or should not feel | | O | O | O | O | O | O |
| Reviews precautions/contraindications with the patient | | O | O | O | O | O | O |
| **Tester places patient in appropriate position** | | Y | N | Y | N | Y | N |
| Supine, beginning with feet flat on the table; progress | | O | O | O | O | O | O |
| **Tester administers the therapeutic exercise according to accepted guidelines** | | Y | N | Y | N | Y | N |
| Places wrists together, thumbs on tibial tuberosity and fingers wrapped around proximal tibia | | O | O | O | O | O | O |
| Applies small amplitude distraction in a posterior direction | | O | O | O | O | O | O |
| **Termination of treatment** | | Y | N | Y | N | Y | N |
| Sustained traction for 10 seconds | | O | O | O | O | O | O |
| Notes response | | O | O | O | O | O | O |
| Repeats or discontinues treatment | | O | O | O | O | O | O |
| Provides the patient with feedback | | O | O | O | O | O | O |
| Documents the treatment | | O | O | O | O | O | O |
| **Total** | | ___/13 | | ___/13 | | ___/13 | |

*(continued on the next page)*

| Must achieve >9 to pass this examination | (P) | (F) | (P) | (F) | (P) | (F) |
|---|---|---|---|---|---|---|
| **Assessor:** <br> **Date:** | **Test 1 Comments:** | | | | | |
| **Assessor:** <br> **Date:** | **Test 2 Comments:** | | | | | |
| **Assessor:** <br> **Date:** | **Test 3 Comments:** | | | | | |

## TEST ENVIRONMENTS
**L:** Laboratory/Classroom
**C:** Clinical/Field Testing
**P:** Practicum
**A:** Assessment/Mock Exam

## TEST INFORMATION
**Test Statistics:** N/A
**Reference(s):** Kisner & Colby (2012)

THERAPEUTIC INTERVENTIONS
# JOINT MOBILIZATIONS—SUSTAINED

| NATA EC 5th | BOC RD6 | SKILL |
|---|---|---|
| TI-15 | D4-0401 | Joint Mobs: Grade 2 Sustained (Tibiofemoral Flexion) |

**Supplies Needed:** Table

*This problem allows you the opportunity to demonstrate the therapeutic technique known as* **grade 2 sustained joint mobilization** *for the* **tibiofemoral joint (flexion)** *to* **reduce pain.** *You have 2 minutes to complete this task.*

| Joint Mobs: Grade 2 Sustained (Tibiofemoral Flexion) | Course or Site Assessor Environment | | Test 1 | | Test 2 | | Test 3 |
|---|---|---|---|---|---|---|---|
| | | Y | N | Y | N | Y | N |
| **Purpose of treatment** | | Y | N | Y | N | Y | N |
| Decrease pain and spasm | | O | O | O | O | O | O |
| **Patient education/safety** | | Y | N | Y | N | Y | N |
| Explains to the patient why the exercise is appropriate | | O | O | O | O | O | O |
| Explains to the patient what the expected treatment goals and outcomes are | | O | O | O | O | O | O |
| Explains to the patient what he/she should or should not feel | | O | O | O | O | O | O |
| Reviews precautions/contraindications with the patient | | O | O | O | O | O | O |
| **Tester places patient in appropriate position** | | Y | N | Y | N | Y | N |
| Supine, beginning with feet flat on the table; progress | | O | O | O | O | O | O |
| **Tester administers the therapeutic exercise according to accepted guidelines** | | Y | N | Y | N | Y | N |
| Places wrists together, thumbs on tibial tuberosity and fingers wrapped around proximal tibia | | O | O | O | O | O | O |
| Applies distraction to "take up the slack" in the joint in a posterior direction | | O | O | O | O | O | O |
| **Termination of treatment** | | Y | N | Y | N | Y | N |
| Sustained traction for 10 seconds | | O | O | O | O | O | O |
| Notes response | | O | O | O | O | O | O |
| Repeats or discontinues treatment | | O | O | O | O | O | O |
| Provides the patient with feedback | | O | O | O | O | O | O |
| Documents the treatment | | O | O | O | O | O | O |
| Total | | ___/13 | | ___/13 | | ___/13 | |

*(continued on the next page)*

| Must achieve >9 to pass this examination | Ⓟ | Ⓕ | Ⓟ | Ⓕ | Ⓟ | Ⓕ |
|---|---|---|---|---|---|---|
| **Assessor:** **Date:** | **Test 1 Comments:** | | | | | |
| **Assessor:** **Date:** | **Test 2 Comments:** | | | | | |
| **Assessor:** **Date:** | **Test 3 Comments:** | | | | | |

## TEST ENVIRONMENTS
**L:** Laboratory/Classroom
**C:** Clinical/Field Testing
**P:** Practicum
**A:** Assessment/Mock Exam

## TEST INFORMATION
**Test Statistics:** N/A
**Reference(s):** Kisner & Colby (2012)

THERAPEUTIC INTERVENTIONS
# JOINT MOBILIZATIONS—SUSTAINED

| NATA EC 5th | BOC RD6 | SKILL |
|---|---|---|
| TI-15 | D4-0401 | Joint Mobs: Grade 3 Sustained (Tibiofemoral Flexion) |

**Supplies Needed:** Table

*This problem allows you the opportunity to demonstrate the therapeutic technique known as* **grade 3 sustained joint mobilization** *for the* **tibiofemoral joint (flexion)** *to* **reduce pain.** *You have 2 minutes to complete this task.*

| Joint Mobs: Grade 3 Sustained (Tibiofemoral Flexion) | Course or Site Assessor Environment _____ | | | | | |
|---|---|---|---|---|---|---|
| | | Test 1 | | Test 2 | | Test 3 |
| **Purpose of treatment** | | **Y** | **N** | **Y** | **N** | **Y** | **N** |
| Decrease pain and spasm, increase limited movement toward the end range of movement | | ○ | ○ | ○ | ○ | ○ | ○ |
| **Patient education/safety** | | **Y** | **N** | **Y** | **N** | **Y** | **N** |
| Explains to the patient why the exercise is appropriate | | ○ | ○ | ○ | ○ | ○ | ○ |
| Explains to the patient what the expected treatment goals and outcomes are | | ○ | ○ | ○ | ○ | ○ | ○ |
| Explains to the patient what he/she should or should not feel | | ○ | ○ | ○ | ○ | ○ | ○ |
| Reviews precautions/contraindications with the patient | | ○ | ○ | ○ | ○ | ○ | ○ |
| **Tester places patient in appropriate position** | | **Y** | **N** | **Y** | **N** | **Y** | **N** |
| Supine, beginning with feet flat on the table; progress | | ○ | ○ | ○ | ○ | ○ | ○ |
| **Tester administers the therapeutic exercise according to accepted guidelines** | | **Y** | **N** | **Y** | **N** | **Y** | **N** |
| Places wrists together, thumbs on tibial tuberosity and fingers wrapped around proximal tibia | | ○ | ○ | ○ | ○ | ○ | ○ |
| Applies distraction to stress the joint capsule and surrounding tissue in a posterior direction | | ○ | ○ | ○ | ○ | ○ | ○ |
| **Termination of treatment** | | **Y** | **N** | **Y** | **N** | **Y** | **N** |
| Sustained traction for 10 seconds | | ○ | ○ | ○ | ○ | ○ | ○ |
| Notes response | | ○ | ○ | ○ | ○ | ○ | ○ |
| Repeats or discontinues treatment | | ○ | ○ | ○ | ○ | ○ | ○ |
| Provides the patient with feedback | | ○ | ○ | ○ | ○ | ○ | ○ |
| Documents the treatment | | ○ | ○ | ○ | ○ | ○ | ○ |
| **Total** | | ___/13 | | ___/13 | | ___/13 |

*(continued on the next page)*

| Must achieve >9 to pass this examination | Ⓟ | Ⓕ | Ⓟ | Ⓕ | Ⓟ | Ⓕ |
|---|---|---|---|---|---|---|
| **Assessor:** **Date:** **Test 1 Comments:** | | | | | | |
| **Assessor:** **Date:** **Test 2 Comments:** | | | | | | |
| **Assessor:** **Date:** **Test 3 Comments:** | | | | | | |

**TEST ENVIRONMENTS**
**L:** Laboratory/Classroom
**C:** Clinical/Field Testing
**P:** Practicum
**A:** Assessment/Mock Exam

**TEST INFORMATION**
**Test Statistics:** N/A
**Reference(s):** Kisner & Colby (2012)

## THERAPEUTIC INTERVENTIONS
# JOINT MOBILIZATIONS—SUSTAINED

| NATA EC 5th | BOC RD6 | SKILL |
|---|---|---|
| TI-15 | D4-0401 | Joint Mobs: Grade 1 Sustained (Glenohumeral Joint) |

**Supplies Needed:** Table

*This problem allows you the opportunity to demonstrate the therapeutic technique known as* **grade 1 sustained joint mobilization** *for the* **glenohumeral joint (flexion)** *to* **reduce pain**. *You have 2 minutes to complete this task.*

| Joint Mobs: Grade 1 Sustained (Glenohumeral Joint) | Course or Site Assessor Environment | Test 1 | | Test 2 | | Test 3 | |
|---|---|---|---|---|---|---|---|
| **Purpose of treatment** | | Y | N | Y | N | Y | N |
| Decrease pain and spasm | | O | O | O | O | O | O |
| **Patient education/safety** | | Y | N | Y | N | Y | N |
| Explains to the patient why the exercise is appropriate | | O | O | O | O | O | O |
| Explains to the patient what the expected treatment goals and outcomes are | | O | O | O | O | O | O |
| Explains to the patient what he/she should or should not feel | | O | O | O | O | O | O |
| Reviews precautions/contraindications with the patient | | O | O | O | O | O | O |
| **Tester places patient in appropriate position** | | Y | N | Y | N | Y | N |
| Supine, beginning with shoulder and elbow flexed to 90 degrees; progress | | O | O | O | O | O | O |
| **Tester administers the therapeutic exercise according to accepted guidelines** | | Y | N | Y | N | Y | N |
| Places palm of dominant hand on elbow and nondominant hand on anterior chest for stabilization | | O | O | O | O | O | O |
| Applies small amplitude distraction in a posterior direction | | O | O | O | O | O | O |
| **Termination of treatment** | | Y | N | Y | N | Y | N |
| Sustained traction for 10 seconds | | O | O | O | O | O | O |
| Notes response | | O | O | O | O | O | O |
| Repeats or discontinues treatment | | O | O | O | O | O | O |
| Provides the patient with feedback | | O | O | O | O | O | O |
| Documents the treatment | | O | O | O | O | O | O |
| Total | | ___/13 | | ___/13 | | ___/13 | |

*(continued on the next page)*

| Must achieve >9 to pass this examination | Ⓟ | Ⓕ | Ⓟ | Ⓕ | Ⓟ | Ⓕ |
|---|---|---|---|---|---|---|
| **Assessor:**<br>**Date:** | **Test 1 Comments:** | | | | | |
| **Assessor:**<br>**Date:** | **Test 2 Comments:** | | | | | |
| **Assessor:**<br>**Date:** | **Test 3 Comments:** | | | | | |

**TEST ENVIRONMENTS**
**L:** Laboratory/Classroom
**C:** Clinical/Field Testing
**P:** Practicum
**A:** Assessment/Mock Exam

**TEST INFORMATION**
**Test Statistics:** N/A
**Reference(s):** Kisner & Colby (2012)

## THERAPEUTIC INTERVENTIONS
# JOINT MOBILIZATIONS—SUSTAINED

| NATA EC 5th | BOC RD6 | SKILL |
| --- | --- | --- |
| TI-15 | D4-0401 | Joint Mobs: Grade 2 Sustained (Glenohumeral Joint) |

**Supplies Needed:** Table

*This problem allows you the opportunity to demonstrate the therapeutic technique known as* **grade 2 sustained joint mobilization** *for the* **glenohumeral joint (flexion)** *to* **reduce pain**. *You have 2 minutes to complete this task.*

| Joint Mobs: Grade 2 Sustained (Glenohumeral Joint) | Course or Site Assessor Environment | | | | | |
| --- | --- | --- | --- | --- | --- | --- |
| | | Test 1 | | Test 2 | | Test 3 |
| **Purpose of treatment** | | Y | N | Y | N | Y | N |
| Decrease pain and spasm | | O | O | O | O | O | O |
| **Patient education/safety** | | Y | N | Y | N | Y | N |
| Explains to the patient why the exercise is appropriate | | O | O | O | O | O | O |
| Explains to the patient what the expected treatment goals and outcomes are | | O | O | O | O | O | O |
| Explains to the patient what he/she should or should not feel | | O | O | O | O | O | O |
| Reviews precautions/contraindications with the patient | | O | O | O | O | O | O |
| **Tester places patient in appropriate position** | | Y | N | Y | N | Y | N |
| Supine, beginning with shoulder and elbow flexed to 90 degrees; progress | | O | O | O | O | O | O |
| **Tester administers the therapeutic exercise according to accepted guidelines** | | Y | N | Y | N | Y | N |
| Places palm of dominant hand on elbow and nondominant hand on anterior chest for stabilization | | O | O | O | O | O | O |
| Applies distraction to "take up the slack" in the joint in a posterior direction | | O | O | O | O | O | O |
| **Termination of treatment** | | Y | N | Y | N | Y | N |
| Sustained traction for 10 seconds | | O | O | O | O | O | O |
| Notes response | | O | O | O | O | O | O |
| Repeats or discontinues treatment | | O | O | O | O | O | O |
| Provides the patient with feedback | | O | O | O | O | O | O |
| Documents the treatment | | O | O | O | O | O | O |
| Total | | ___/13 | | ___/13 | | ___/13 |

*(continued on the next page)*

| Must achieve >9 to pass this examination | Ⓟ | Ⓕ | Ⓟ | Ⓕ | Ⓟ | Ⓕ |
|---|---|---|---|---|---|---|
| **Assessor:**<br>**Date:** | **Test 1 Comments:** | | | | | |
| **Assessor:**<br>**Date:** | **Test 2 Comments:** | | | | | |
| **Assessor:**<br>**Date:** | **Test 3 Comments:** | | | | | |

### TEST ENVIRONMENTS
**L:** Laboratory/Classroom
**C:** Clinical/Field Testing
**P:** Practicum
**A:** Assessment/Mock Exam

### TEST INFORMATION
**Test Statistics:** N/A
**Reference(s):** Kisner & Colby (2012)

THERAPEUTIC INTERVENTIONS
# JOINT MOBILIZATIONS—SUSTAINED

| NATA EC 5th | BOC RD6 | SKILL |
|---|---|---|
| TI-15 | D4-0401 | Joint Mobs: Grade 3 Sustained (Glenohumeral Joint) |

**Supplies Needed:** Table

*This problem allows you the opportunity to demonstrate the therapeutic technique known as* **grade 3 sustained joint mobilization** *for the* **glenohumeral joint (flexion)** *to* **reduce pain**. *You have 2 minutes to complete this task.*

| Joint Mobs: Grade 3 Sustained (Glenohumeral Joint) | Course or Site Assessor Environment | Test 1 | | Test 2 | | Test 3 | |
|---|---|---|---|---|---|---|---|
| | | Y | N | Y | N | Y | N |
| **Purpose of treatment** | | Y | N | Y | N | Y | N |
| Decrease pain and spasm, increase limited movement toward the end range of movement | | O | O | O | O | O | O |
| **Patient education/safety** | | Y | N | Y | N | Y | N |
| Explains to the patient why the exercise is appropriate | | O | O | O | O | O | O |
| Explains to the patient what the expected treatment goals and outcomes are | | O | O | O | O | O | O |
| Explains to the patient what he/she should or should not feel | | O | O | O | O | O | O |
| Reviews precautions/contraindications with the patient | | O | O | O | O | O | O |
| **Tester places patient in appropriate position** | | Y | N | Y | N | Y | N |
| Supine, beginning with shoulder and elbow flexed to 90 degrees; progress | | O | O | O | O | O | O |
| **Tester administers the therapeutic exercise according to accepted guidelines** | | Y | N | Y | N | Y | N |
| Places palm of dominant hand on elbow and nondominant hand on anterior chest for stabilization | | O | O | O | O | O | O |
| Applies distraction to stress the joint capsule and surrounding periarticular tissue in a posterior direction | | O | O | O | O | O | O |
| **Termination of treatment** | | Y | N | Y | N | Y | N |
| Sustained traction for 10 seconds | | O | O | O | O | O | O |
| Notes response | | O | O | O | O | O | O |
| Repeats or discontinues treatment | | O | O | O | O | O | O |
| Provides the patient with feedback | | O | O | O | O | O | O |
| Documents the treatment | | O | O | O | O | O | O |
| | Total | ___/13 | | ___/13 | | ___/13 | |

(continued on the next page)

| Must achieve >9 to pass this examination | P | F | P | F | P | F |
|---|---|---|---|---|---|---|
| **Assessor:** <br> **Date:** | **Test 1 Comments:** | | | | | |
| **Assessor:** <br> **Date:** | **Test 2 Comments:** | | | | | |
| **Assessor:** <br> **Date:** | **Test 3 Comments:** | | | | | |

## TEST ENVIRONMENTS
**L:** Laboratory/Classroom
**C:** Clinical/Field Testing
**P:** Practicum
**A:** Assessment/Mock Exam

## TEST INFORMATION
**Test Statistics:** N/A
**Reference(s):** Kisner & Colby (2012)

# APPENDIX

Hauth, J. M., Gloyeske, B. M., & Amato, H. K.
*Clinical Skills Documentation Guide for Athletic Training, Third Edition* (pp. 635-642).
© 2016 SLACK Incorporated.

# ACES
## Amato-Cole Educational Services

### Self-Reporting Assessment of Athletic Training Competencies

NAME: _____     DATE: _____

A = **Extremely confident with skill**
B = **Confident with skill**
C = **Confident, but needs practice with skill**
D = **Not totally confident with skill**
E = **Very little confidence with skill**

*For every "D" or "E" answer provided, please explain what aspect of the skill you are uncomfortable with and how you plan to increase proficiency with that skill.

### I.    Evidence-Based Practice (EBP)
*explain D/E answers below

1.  Define Evidence-Based Practice
2.  Quantitative vs. Qualitative Research
3.  Research Components
4.  Levels of Research Evidence
5.  Five Step Approach
6.  PICO Question (Patients, Intervention....)
7.  Search Techniques/Engines
8.  Types of Articles (Narrative Reviews......)
9.  Standard Criteria & Developed Scales
10. Determine Efficacy & Effectiveness

### II.    Prevention and Health Promotions (PHP)
*explain D/E answers below

11. Injury/Illness Surveillance
12. Monitoring Injury Prevention
13. Risk Factors for Injury/Illness
14. Effectiveness of a Prevention Strategy

*Precautions for Common Health Conditions*

       15. Sickle Cell

       16. Mitral Valve Prolapse

       17. Anemia

18. Universal Precautions (OSHA)

19. Pre-participation Physical Exam

20. Thermoregulatory Mech. Heat Gain/Loss

21. Environmental Factors

*Environmental Assessment*

       22. Sling Psychrometer

       23. WBGT

       24. Heat Index Guidelines

*Participation Guidelines for:*

       25. Weight Loss/Hydration Status

       26. Blood Glucose Levels (glycometer)

       27. Asthma Symptoms (peak flow)

*Etiology/Prevention for Sudden Death*

       28. Cardiac Arrhythmia or Arrest

       29. Asthma

       30. Traumatic Brain Injury

       31. Exertional Heat Stroke

       32. Hyponatremia

       33. Exertional Sickling

       34. Anaphylactic Shock

       35. Cervical Spine Injury

       36. Lightning Strike

37. Ergodynamics

38. Standard Protective Equipment

39. Orthotics/Splints

*Preventative Taping/Wrapping/Padding*

       40. Foot       (Selection/Fabrication/Fit)

       41. Ankle       (Selection/Fabrication/Fit)

       42. Knee       (Selection/Fabrication/Fit)

       43. Hip/Thigh    (Selection/Fabrication/Fit)

       44. Thorax      (Selection/Fabrication/Fit)

       45. Shoulder    (Selection/Fabrication/Fit)

       46. Elbow      (Selection/Fabrication/Fit)

       47. Hand/Wrist/Thumb (Selection/Fabrication/Fit)

48. Components of Physical Fitness

49. Fitness/Wellness Testing

50. Designing a Fitness Program

51. Proper Use Weight Lifting Equipment

52. Nutritional Intake Recommendations     _____   _____
53. Basic Dietary Analysis                  _____   _____
54. Micro- and Macronutrients               _____   _____
55. Components of Food Labels                _____   _____
56. Proper Nutrition                         _____   _____
57. Pre/Post Activity Meals & Hydration      _____   _____
58. Assessing Body Composition               _____   _____
59. Weight Management Strategies             _____   _____
60. Disordered Eating/Eating Disorders       _____   _____

*Bans and Physiological Effects of:*
    61. Performance Enhancing Drugs       _____   _____
    62. Dietary Supplements               _____   _____
    63. Recreational Drugs                _____   _____

## III.   Clinical Examination and Diagnosis (CE)

**\*explain D/E answers below**

64. Basic Anatomy (All Regions)              _____   _____
65. Basic Physiology (All Regions)           _____   _____
66. Gender Specific Risk Factors             _____   _____
67. Normal Osteokinematics                   _____   _____
68. Normal Arthrokinematics                  _____   _____
69. Diagnostic Imaging                       _____   _____
70. Functional Outcome Measurements          _____   _____
71. Clin. Predication Rules (Ottawa Ankle Rules)  _____   _____
72. Identify Differential Diagnosis          _____   _____
73. Return to Play Criteria                  _____   _____
74. Neck/Spine Injuries                      _____   _____
75. Head Injuries/Concussions                _____   _____
76. Facial Injuries                          _____   _____
77. Shoulder Injuries                        _____   _____
78. Elbow Injuries                           _____   _____
79. Hand/Wrist Injuries                      _____   _____
80. Back/Thorax Injuries                     _____   _____
81. Abdominal Injuries                       _____   _____
82. Hip/Pelvis Injuries                      _____   _____
83. Knee Injuries                            _____   _____
84. Foot/Ankle Injuries                      _____   _____
85. HOPS (history/observation/palpation)     _____   _____
86. Manual Muscle Testing                    _____   _____
87. ROM/Goniometry                           _____   _____
88. Special Test (selective tissue examination)  _____   _____
89. Neurological Assessment                  _____   _____
90. Respiratory Assessment                   _____   _____

91. Circulatory Assessment _____ _____
92. Abdominal Assessment _____ _____
93. ENT Assessment (otoscopic evaluation) _____ _____
94. Ocular Assessment (vision, ophthalmoscope) _____ _____
95. Dermatology Assessment _____ _____
96. Posture/Gait Analysis _____ _____
97. Capsular/Ligamentous Stress Testing _____ _____

## IV. Acute Care of Injuries and Illnesses (AC)

**\*explain D/E answers below**

98. Scope of Practice _____ _____
99. Emergency Action Plan _____ _____
100. CPR/AED for the Professional Rescuer _____ _____
101. Vital Signs _____ _____
102. Equipment Removal _____ _____
103. Establishing an Airway _____ _____
104. Airway Adjuncts _____ _____
105. Supplemental Oxygen _____ _____
106. First Aid/Wound Care _____ _____
107. Spine Boarding/Cervical Stabilization _____ _____
108. Splinting _____ _____
109. Ambulatory Aid _____ _____

*Signs/Symptoms/Care/Return-to-Play for:*

110. Heat Illnesses _____ _____
111. Asthma (metered-dose inhaler) _____ _____
112. Allergic Anaphylaxis _____ _____
113. Concussion _____ _____
114. Spine Trauma _____ _____
115. Sickle Cell Trait _____ _____
116. Rhabdomyolysis _____ _____
117. Internal Hemorrhage _____ _____
118. Diabetes _____ _____
119. Seizures (epileptic/non-epileptic) _____ _____
120. Shock _____ _____
121. Cold Illnesses _____ _____
122. Drug Overdose _____ _____

## V.    Therapeutic Interventions (TI)

*explain D/E answers below

123. Pain Management
124. Pain Theories/Modulation
125. Tissue Healing
126. Edema Control
127. Joint Mobilizations
128. Rehabilitation Principles
129. Stretching/PNF
130. Neuromuscular Control/Balance
131. Exercise for Strength/End/Speed/Power
132. Exercise for Gait/Posture/Body Mechanics
133. Cardiovascular Fitness
134. Functional Exercise/Progression
135. Home Exercise Programs
136. Aquatic Therapy
137. Return to Play Guidelines
138. Ankle/Foot Rehab
139. Knee Rehab
140. Hip/Low Back Rehab
141. Shoulder Rehab
142. Elbow Rehab
143. Hand/Wrist Rehab
144. Tape/Wrap/Splint/Brace for RTP
145. Common Surgical Techniques

*Therapeutic Modalities*
146. Superficial Thermal Agents
147. Electrical Stimulation
148. Therapeutic Ultrasound
149. Diathermy
150. Laser
151. Biofeedback

*Mechanical Modalities*
152. Traction
153. Intermittent Compression
154. CPM
155. Massage
156. Myofascial Techniques
157. Muscle Energy Techniques

*Therapeutic Medications*

158. Proper Storage/Disposal/Dispensing    _____     _____
159. Indication/Contraindications    _____     _____
160. Pharmacokinetics    _____     _____
161. Pharmacodynamic Principles    _____     _____
162. Patient Education    _____     _____

*Common Medication Principles for:*

163. Asthma
164. Diabetes
165. Hypertension
166. Infections
167. Depression
168. GERD
169. Allergies
170. Pain
171. Inflammation
172. Common Cold

## VI. Psychosocial Strategies and Referral (PS)

**\*explain D/E answers below**

173. Cognitive Appraisal Model
174. Stress Response Model
175. Motivation Techniques
176. Psychological Interventions/Referral
177. Psychosocial Factors & Persistent Pain
178. Sociocultural Issues
179. Types of Mental Healthcare Workers
180. Mental Health Disorders
181. Eating Disorders
182. Substance Abuse
183. Crisis Intervention
184. Counseling Techniques

## VII. Healthcare Administration (HA)

**\*explain D/E answers below**

185. Developing a Business Plan
186. Budgeting Process
187. Facility Design
188. Medical Record Keeping
189. State/Federal Statutes
190. Personnel Management

191.  OSHA
192.  Key Regulatory Agencies
193.  Legal Issues
194.  Risk Management Plan
195.  Emergency Action Plan
196.  Health Care Insurance
197.  Documentation Codes
198.  Administrative Policies & Procedures

## VIII.  Professional Development & Responsibility (PD)

**\*explain D/E answers below**

199.  NATA History/Development

*Organizations*
  200.  NATA
  201.  BOC
  202.  CAATE
  203.  State Regulatory Boards
  204.  State Practice Acts

*Essential Documents*
  205.  NATA Education Competencies
  206.  BOC Standards Professional Practice
  207.  NATA Code of Ethics
  208.  BOC Role Delineation
  209.  NATA Position Statements

210.  Credentialing
211.  Education Strategies
212.  Professional Development Plan
213.  Identify Healthcare Provider's Role
214.  Referral Strategies

**NATA: Athletic Training Education Competencies 5ᵗʰ Edition (Released 2011)**

# BIBLIOGRAPHY

Amato, H., Hawkins, C. D., & Cole, S. L. (2006). *Clinical skills documentation guide for athletic training* (2nd ed.). Thorofare, NJ: SLACK Incorporated.

Armstrong, L. E., & Pandolf, K. B. (1988). Physical training, cardiorespiratory physical fitness and exercise-heat tolerance. In K. B. Pandolf, M. N. Sawka, & R. R. Gonzalez (Eds.), *Human performance physiology and environmental medicine at terrestrial extremes* (pp. 199-226). Indianapolis, IN: Benchmark Press.

Bacharach. (2010). *Instruction manual*. New Kingston, PA: Author.

Baechle, T. R., & Earle, R. W. (Eds.). (2008). *Essentials of strength training and conditioning* (3rd ed.). Champaign, IL: Human Kinetics.

Beam, J. W. (2012). *Orthopedic taping, wrapping, bracing, & padding*. Philadelphia, PA: F. A. Davis Co.

Board of Certification. (2010). *The 2009 athletic trainer role delineation study*. Omaha, NE: Stephen B. Johnson.

Board of Certification. (2011). *BOC role delineation study/ practice analysis* (6th ed.). Omaha, NE: Author.

Casa, D. J. (2012). *Preventing sudden death in sport and physical activity*. Sudbury, MA: Jones and Bartlett.

Casa, D. J., Armstrong, L. E., Hillman, S. K., Montain, S. J., Reiff, R. V., Rich, B. S. E., ... Stone, J. A. (2000). National Athletic Trainers' Association position statement: Fluid replacement for athletes. *Journal of Athletic Training, 35*(2), 212-224.

Cook, C. E., & Hegedus, E. J. (2013). *Orthopedic physical examination tests: An evidence-based approach* (2nd ed.). Upper Saddle River, NJ: Pearson Prentice Hall.

Cuppett, M., & Walsh, K. M. (2012). *General medical conditions in the athlete* (2nd ed.). St. Louis, MO: Elsevier Mosby.

Gorman, P. P., Butler, R. J., Plisky, P. J., & Kiesel, K. B. (2012). Upper Quarter Y Balance Test: Reliability and performance comparison between genders in active adults. *Journal of Strength and Conditioning Research, 26*(11), 3043-3048.

Gorse, K. M., Blanc, R., Feld, F., & Radelet, M. (2010). *Emergency care in athletic training*. Philadelphia, PA: F. A. Davis Co.

Gribble, P. A., Hertel, J., & Plisky, P. (2012). Using the Star Excursion Balance Test to assess dynamic postural-control deficits and outcomes in lower extremity injury: A literature and systematic review. *Journal of Athletic Training, 47*(3), 339-357.

Gulli, B., Piazza, G. M., & Rahm, S. J. (2012). *Health care provider CPR* (4th ed.). Sudbury, MA: Jones and Bartlett.

Hislop, H. J., & Montgomery, J. (2007). *Daniels and Worthingham's muscle testing: Techniques of manual examination* (8th ed.). St. Louis, MO: Saunders.

Houglum, P. A. (2005). *Therapeutic exercise for musculoskeletal injuries* (2nd ed.). Champaign, IL: Human Kinetics.

Hauth, J. M., Gloyeske, B. M., & Amato, H. K.
*Clinical Skills Documentation Guide for Athletic Training, Third Edition* (pp. 643-645).
© 2016 SLACK Incorporated.

Karachalios, T., Hantes, M., Zibis, A. H., Zachos, V., Karantanas, A. H., & Malizos, K. N. (2005). Diagnostic accuracy of a new clinical test (the Thessaly test) for early detection of meniscal tears. *Journal of Bone and Joint Surgery, 87*(5), 955-962.

Kendall, F. P., McCreary, E. K., Provance, P. G., Rodgers, M. M., & Romani, W. A. (2005). *Muscles: Testing and function with posture and pain* (5th ed.). Baltimore, MD: Lippincott Williams & Wilkins.

Kisner, C., & Colby, L. A. (2012). *Therapeutic exercise: Foundations and techniques* (6th ed.). Philadelphia: F. A. Davis Co.

Konin, J. G., Lebsack, D., Valier Synder, A., & Isear, J. A., Jr. (2016). *Special tests for orthopedic examination* (4th ed.). Thorofare, NJ: SLACK Incorporated.

Lueken, J., Aguilar, A., Kingma, J., & Johnson, S. (2013a). Cardiac assessment. *Building Blocks of Clinical Practice, 6.*

Lueken, J., Aguilar, A., Kingma, J., & Johnson, S. (2013b). Chest percussion and auscultations. *Building Blocks of Clinical Practice, 8.*

Magee, D. J. (2005). *Orthopedic physical assessment* (5th ed.). Philadelphia, PA: Elsevier Saunders.

Makhmalbaf, H., Moradi, A., Ganji, S., & Omidi-Kashani, F. (2013). Accuracy of Lachman and anterior drawer tests for anterior cruciate ligament injuries. *Archives of Bone and Joint Surgery, 1*(2), 94-97.

Malanga, G., Andrus, S., Nadler, S. F., & McLean, J. (2003). Physical examination of the knee: A review of the original test description and scientific validity of common orthopedic tests. *Archives of Physical Medicine and Rehabilitation, 84*(4), 592-603.

Malanga, G. A., Landes, P., & Nadler, S. F. (2003). Provocative tests in cervical spine examination: Historical basis and scientific analyses. *Pain Physician, 6*(2), 199-205.

McChesney, J. A., & McChesney, J. W. (2001). Auscultation of the chest and abdomen by athletic trainers. *Journal of Athletic Training, 36*(2), 190-196.

Meserve, B. B., Cleland, J. A., & Boucher, T. R. (2008). A meta-analysis examining clinical test utilities for assessing meniscal injury. *Clinical Rehabilitation, 22*(2), 143-161.

Michlovitz, S. L., Bellew, J. W., & Nolan, T. P., Jr. (2012). *Modalities for therapeutic intervention* (5th ed.). Philadelphia, PA: F. A. Davis Co.

Mucha, A., Collins, M. W., Elbin, R. J., Furman, J. M, Troutman-Enseki, C., Dewolf, R., ... Kontos, A. P. (2014). A brief vestibular/ocular motor screening (VOMS) assessment to evaluate concussions: Preliminary findings. *American Journal of Sports Medicine, 42,* 2479-2486.

National Athletic Trainers' Association. (2011). *Athletic training education competencies* (5th ed.). Dallas, TX: Author.

National Athletic Trainers' Association Board of Certification. (1995). *Role delineation study* (3rd ed.). Philadelphia, PA: F. A. Davis Co.

Norkin, C. C., & White, D. J. (2009). *Measurement of joint motion: A guide to goniometry* (4th ed.). Philadelphia, PA: F. A. Davis Co.

Occupational Safety and Health Administration. *Bloodborne pathogens* (29 CFR 1919.1030). Retrieved from https://www.osha.gov/pls/oshaweb/owadisp.show_document?p_table=STANDARDS&p_id=10051

Omron. (2001). *Body fat analyzer instruction manual.* Vernon Hills, IL: Author.

Ostrowski, J. (2006). Accuracy of 3 diagnostic tests for anterior cruciate ligament tears. *Journal of Athletic Training, 41*(1), 120-121.

Pieper, S., Fulcher, K., Sundre, D., & Erwin, D. (2008). What do I do with the data now? Analyzing assessment information for accountability and improvement. *Research and Practice in Assessment, 2*(1).

Prentice, W. E. (2014). *Principles of athletic training: A competency-based approach* (15th ed.). New York, NY: McGraw-Hill.

Rehberg, R. S. (2013). *Sports emergency care: A team approach* (2nd ed.). Thorofare, NJ: SLACK Incorporated.

Reider, B. (2004). *The orthopaedic physical examination* (2nd ed.). Philadelphia, PA: Elsevier Saunders.

Reiman, M. P., Goode, A. P., Cook, C. E., Holmich, P., & Thorborg, K. (2015). Diagnostic accuracy of clinical tests for the diagnosis of hip femoroacetabular impingement/labral tear: A systematic review with meta-analysis. *British Journal of Sports Medicine, 49,* 811.

ReliOn. (2008). *Blood glucose monitoring system user instruction manual.* Minneapolis, MN: Author.

Salazar, J. V. (2009). *Oxygen administration.* Sudbury, MA: Jones and Bartlett.

Scheinberg, S. (2005). *SAM splint user's guide and reference card.* Newport, OR: SAM Medical.

Scifers, J. (2008). *Special tests for neurologic examination.* Thorofare, NJ: SLACK Incorporated.

Skyndex. (2013). *Professional skinfold caliper instruction manual.* Albuquerque, NM: Author.

Sman, A. D., Hiller, C. E., & Refshauge, K. M. (2012). Diagnostic accuracy of clinical tests for diagnosis of ankle syndesmosis injury: A systematic review. *British Journal of Sports Medicine, 47,* 620-628.

Starkey, C. (2013). *Therapeutic modalities* (4th ed.). Philadelphia, PA: F. A. Davis Co.

Starkey, C., & Brown, S. D. (2015). *Examination of orthopedic and athletic injuries* (4th ed.). Philadelphia, PA: F. A. Davis Co.

Stevens, S. (2007). Test distance vision using a Snellen chart. *Community Eye Health, 20*(63), 52.

Thygerson, A. L., Thygerson, S. M., Gulli, B., & Piazza, G. (2012). *First aid* (6th ed.). Sudbury, MA: Jones and Bartlett.

Wainner, R. S., Fritz, J. M., Irrgang, J. J., Boninger, M. L., Delitto, A., & Allison, S. (2003). Reliabilty and diagnositic accuracy of the clinical examination and patient self-report measures for cervical radiculopathy. *Spine (Phila Pa 1976), 28*(1), 52-62.

# *Websites*

ACES Written Exams: http://www.nata.org/nata-study-guide-faqs (must be NATA member to log into this site and to register for the exams)

Assessment Progress Template: http://www.jmu.edu/assessment/visitor/assessmentresources.shtml#APT

Athletic Training Education Competencies (5th Edition/Released 2011): http://caate.net/wp-content/uploads/2014/06/5th-Edition-Competencies.pdf

BOC Exam Crosswalk Analysis: http://www.bocatc.org/images/stories/educators/boc_rdpa6_and_nata_ec5_crosswalk_analysis_1212af.pdf

BOC Self-Assessment: Integrated Test Mode: http://www.bocatc.org/index.php?option=com_content&task=view&id=136&Itemid=149

Guidelines of the New Leadership Alliance: Committing to Quality Guidelines for Assessment and Accountability in Higher Education: http://www.chea.org/alliance_publications/default.asp

Mapping Program Objectives: https://www.jmu.edu/assessment/Visitor/AssessmentResources.shtml

National Athletic Trainers' Association Study Guides: http://www.nata.org/nata-study-guide-boc-exam/

NATA Online Exams Breakdowns: http://www.nata.org/sites/default/files/sample-cert-for-website-combined.pdf (must be NATA member to log into this site and to register for the exams)

Selecting Assessment Tools: https://www.jmu.edu/assessment/Visitor/AssessmentResources.shtml

Six-Step Assessment: https://www.jmu.edu/assessment/Visitor/AssessmentResources.shtml

What Is Program Assessment? http://www.jmu.edu/assessment/Visitor/AssessmentResources.shtml

Writing Program Objectives: http://www.jmu.edu/assessment/Visitor/AssessmentResources.shtml